Neurological
Rehabilitation

For Elsevier

Commissioning Editor: *Rita Demetriou-Swanwick*
Development Editor: *Louisa Welch*
Project Manager: *Elouise Ball*
Designer: *Kirsteen Wright*
Illustration Manager: *Merlyn Harvey*
Illustrator: *Robert Britton*

2nd
Edition

Neurological Rehabilitation
Optimizing Motor Performance

Janet H. Carr MA, EdD (Columbia), FACP

Honorary Associate Professor, Physiotherapy, Faculty of Health Sciences, The University of Sydney, Australia

Roberta B. Shepherd MA, EdD (Columbia), FACP

Honorary Professor, Physiotherapy, Faculty of Health Sciences, The University of Sydney, Australia

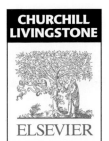

CHURCHILL
LIVINGSTONE

ELSEVIER

Edinburgh   London   New York   Oxford   Philadelphia   St Louis   Sydney   Toronto   2010

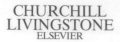

CHURCHILL
LIVINGSTONE
ELSEVIER

First edition 1998
Second edition 2011

ISBN: 978-0-7020-4468-7
Formerly: 978-0-7020-4051-1

British Library Cataloguing in Publication Data
A catalogue record for this book is available from the British Library

Library of Congress Cataloging in Publication Data
A catalog record for this book is available from the Library of Congress

Notices
Knowledge and best practice in this field are constantly changing. As new research and experience broaden our understanding, changes in research methods, professional practices, or medical treatment may become necessary.

Practitioners and researchers must always rely on their own experience and knowledge in evaluating and using any information, methods, compounds, or experiments described herein. In using such information or methods they should be mindful of their own safety and the safety of others, including parties for whom they have a professional responsibility.

With respect to any drug or pharmaceutical products identified, readers are advised to check the most current information provided (i) on procedures featured or (ii) by the manufacturer of each product to be administered, to verify the recommended dose or formula, the method and duration of administration, and contraindications. It is the responsibility of practitioners, relying on their own experience and knowledge of their patients, to make diagnoses, to determine dosages and the best treatment for each individual patient, and to take all appropriate safety precautions.

To the fullest extent of the law, neither the Publisher nor the authors, contributors, or editors assume any liability for any injury and/or damage to persons or property as a matter of products liability, negligence or otherwise, or from any use or operation of any methods, products, instructions, or ideas contained in the material herein.

The Publisher

ELSEVIER your source for books,
journals and multimedia
in the health sciences

www.elsevierhealth.com

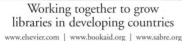

Working together to grow
libraries in developing countries

www.elsevier.com | www.bookaid.org | www.sabre.org

ELSEVIER   BOOK AID International   Sabre Foundation

The publisher's
policy is to use
paper manufactured
from sustainable forests

Printed in China

Contents

Contributors

Julie Bernhardt BSc, PhD
Director, Very Early Rehabilitation Research Program,
Senior Research Fellow, National Stroke Research Institute
(Florey Neuroscience Institute),
Melbourne,
Australia

Colleen Canning BPhty (Qld), MA (Columbia), PhD
(Syd)
Senior Lecturer,
Faculty of Health Sciences,
The University of Sydney,
Australia

Leanne Hassett BAppSc (Physio), MHlthSc(NeuroPhty),
PhD
Senior Physiotherapist,
Brain Injury Rehabilitation Unit,
Liverpool Health Service,
Australia

Phu D Hoang PhD (Syd)
NHMRC Post-doctoral Training Fellow,
Research Officer, Prince of Wales Medical Research Institute,
University of NSW, Australia
Physiotherapist, Multiple Sclerosis Society,
Australia

Anne Moseley BAppSc (Physio), Grad Dip (ExSpSc),
PhD
Senior Research Fellow,
The George Institute for International Health,
The University of Sydney,
Australia

Preface
to the first edition

This book represents an attempt to set down a philosophy and model of rehabilitation for individuals with movement dysfunction which is an alternative to models most commonly in use throughout the world, the eponymous facilitation–inhibition models. The view taken here is that research in the areas of neuromuscular control, biomechanical aspects of performance, the link between cognition and action, together with recent developments related to pathology and adaptation can inform rehabilitation methods.

In this book, we argue that consideration of movement science research implies that movement rehabilitation should focus on motor performance, on exercises and training to ensure appropriate muscle strength, on endurance and physical fitness to enable the desired physical activities to be carried out and on increased cognitive engagement with the environment. The clinician is then coach to the individual with the disability, one who is skilled in methods of training action, and of organizing independent practice. Too often therapists underestimate the capacity of individuals, including small children and the elderly, to work hard, pay attention and actively engage with a training regime over which they have some control. One-to-one therapy remains the preferred style in many rehabilitation settings, yet the available evidence points to the need for disabled individuals to be actively involved in their rehabilitation for several hours a day. This requires that there be a plan for group practice, and work stations for independent practice; that therapists work with engineers, computer scientists, orthotists and the makers of gymnasium equipment to design training devices which will enable independent practice and promote the wanted actions. The clinician as problem-solving scientist is both a user of research and an adaptor of technology.

The chapters are clustered into three groups. Chapters 1 to 3 focus on three major issues critical to neurorehabilitation: the nature of the adaptive system, the optimization of functional motor performance and methods of measurement. It is increasingly being shown that the brain, neural system, muscles and other soft tissues reorganize and adapt according to patterns of use and experience. We argue that what happens to an individual and what that person does will affect positively or negatively the reorganization and adaptation which are naturally occurring phenomena. Focus in the second chapter is therefore on skill learning, physical training and exercise in neurorehabilitation, stressing the importance of cognitive engagement and practice. The third chapter sets out a selection of, for the most part, reliable and valid measures which are appropriate for use in neurorehabilitation. Tests are grouped according to the level of measurement – whether global tests of function or specific biomechanical measures of motor performance, tests of muscle strength or perception; whether tests of impairment or of anxiety or self-efficacy. Emphasis throughout the book is on the need to measure the effects of the interventions that make up rehabilitation.

Chapters 4 to 7 focus on actions critical to an independent and effective lifestyle: standing up and sitting down, walking, reaching and manipulation, and balancing, in which biomechanical models of the action are presented as a framework upon which training and exercise to improve performance are based.

Chapters 8 to 10 focus on pathological and adaptive aspects of lesions of the motor system (upper motor neuron, cerebellum) and of the sensory-perceptual system.

Chapters 11 to 14 contain descriptions of the particular pathological impairments, adaptations and disabilities associated with stroke, traumatic brain injury, Parkinson's disease and multiple sclerosis, with specific points about rehabilitation which are of significance for these conditions.

Throughout the book, we have provided references in order to illustrate the process of utilizing theoretical and data-based information in clinical practice. Where these are available, we have included reference to outcome studies because it is such evidence-based material which is a powerful determinator of theory and direction, enabling the development and testing of protocols (or strictly observed guidelines) as a means of establishing best practice. Our aim in writing this book was to assist clinicians to become more informed and effective practitioners and to raise questions intended to stimulate clinical and laboratory research which will in turn lead to dynamic and effective methodologies. Finally, we hope the book will give the reader an appreciation for what are currently unexplored possibilities of movement rehabilitation.

J.H.C.
R.B.S.

Preface
to the second edition

In the first edition of this book we set out to illustrate how to develop science-based rehabilitation methods designed to optimize functional motor performance of individuals with acute and chronic lesions of the brain. Ten years later the evidence from clinical trials and systematic reviews makes it clear that methods used in neurorehabilitation should provide a sufficient stimulus to learning and to the acquisition of skill. It is also clear that sufficient time must be spent practising everyday actions, and exercising vigorously to increase muscle strength, endurance and aerobic fitness to the level required for general wellbeing and participation in daily life.

In this new edition, we have been joined by colleagues whose research and clinical practice skills reflect their education in the brain, movement and medical sciences. Education in these fields is critical for rehabilitation professionals as a solid knowledge base upon which to build practical clinical skills. Together we have brought fresh insights to the content of the new volume.

The new edition continues with themes developed in the first edition. There is now an increased understanding of the nature of impairments of central origin, secondary changes that occur in soft tissues, in intersegmental biomechanics and in cardiorespiratory function that are associated with physical inactivity and disuse. In addition, new insights into motor learning and cognitive science, developments in exercise science, and in technology are providing the rehabilitation team with increased opportunities to develop and test potentially more effective rehabilitation methods. The development of rehabilitation practice also takes place with the growing recognition of the factors that have a positive influence on brain plasticity and recovery. Optimal progress seems to be dependent on the opportunities available to an individual. It is now acknowledged that what people do, what opportunities are available for intensive, meaningful and challenging practice, the process of rehabilitation itself, can really make a difference. The rehabilitation team is making changes not only to the methods used in acute care and rehabilitation but also to the mode of delivery and to influencing what occurs after discharge. Opportunities for supervised group practice and exercise, increased use of exercise machines, and interactive practice are increasing the time spent in task-relevant physical and mental activity.

Physiotherapists are making a major change away from methodologies developed in an earlier time for with there is no evidenciary support, and increasingly using methods that are congruent with current knowledge and for which there is encouraging evidence. The results of suitably rigorous clinical trials eventually contribute to evidence-based practice. The current interest in rehabilitation research and the quality of that research are grounds for optimism.

J.H.C.
R.B.S.

He who has not endured the stress of study will not taste the joy of knowledge …
Abd al-Latif
Medical scholar of Baghdad
1162/3-1231

Acknowledgements

We wish to express our thanks to the contributors to this book, Julie Bernhardt, Colleen Canning, Leanne Hassett, Phu Hoang and Anne Moseley, who worked with us to update the second edition; it was a pleasure and a privilege to work with them.

We wish to thank the people who so kindly agreed to be photographed for this book and the physiotherapists from Sydney hospitals who have given us generous support, in particular Karl Schurr, Simone Dorsch and their colleagues at Bankstown-Lidcombe Hospital, Fiona Mackey at Illawarra Health Service, Jill Hall and colleagues at War Memorial Hospital, Waverley, and Anne Løge and colleagues, Trondheim, Norway. We also wish to thank Jeanette Blennerhassett for reading and commenting on the Appendix to Chapter 11.

The authors and publishers of this book express their appreciation for being granted permission to reproduce figures and photographs as indicated throughout.

J.H.C.
R.B.S.

Part | 1 |

Introduction: adaptation, training and measurement

Chapter | 1 |

The adaptive system: plasticity and recovery

All living organisms have an inherent capacity to self-organize throughout life, and organizational processes affecting all systems are reflective of the organism's history, i.e., learning, experience and use. Specific molecular, biochemical, electrophysical and structural changes take place throughout life in central nervous system (CNS) neurons and neuronal networks in response to activity and behaviour (Weiller 1998; Johansson 2000; Nudo et al 2001). Learning how both the normal and lesioned brain functions provides insights into how these processes can be manipulated to drive optimal recovery. Developments over the last two decades in brain imaging during functional activity provide the means to explore the reorganizational processes related to normal behaviour and learning. It is becoming increasingly clear that the brain retains a plastic potential to reorganize in adult humans, even in old and/or lesioned brains and that neural plasticity can be influenced by drugs, training, rehabilitation and the environment (Weiller & Rijntjes 2005).

Functional improvement after a brain lesion results from changes in spared sections of the brain. The mechanisms may vary with the type and location of lesion, and can involve improved connectivity with individual neurons, modification of cortical representations, cortical maps and non-synaptic transmission (Johansson 2005).

Hemiparesis after stroke provides a good model for studying cerebral reorganization. An important question is to what extent post-ischaemic events can influence lesion-induced plasticity and improve functional restoration. Half a century ago, Hebb (1947) hypothesized that neural cortical connections had the capacity to remodel throughout life by strengthening synapses thus enabling improved function.

A brain lesion, such as a stroke, affects both the anatomy and the physiology of the nervous system. It interferes with (or destroys) nerve cell bodies, dendrites and axons and indirectly affects the 'programming' or networking of nerve impulses throughout intact brain tissue. This chapter addresses issues related to neural plasticity after stroke as a means of stressing the potential for rehabilitation to affect such processes. Concurrent with brain changes, muscles and other soft tissues also adapt and reorganize according to patterns of use, and this issue is discussed throughout the book. We have hypothesized (Carr & Shepherd 1987, 1996, 2000, 2003) that training following a stroke involves people learning again how to perform actions and mental processes that were performed with ease pre-lesion. Training appears to be a critical stimulus to making new or more effective functional connections within remaining brain tissue.

What seems certain is that for rehabilitation (including physiotherapy) to be effective in the restoration of optimal function, there needs to be more emphasis on providing an activity-stimulating environment, and repetitive and intensive task-related exercise and training of the partly compromised limbs. There is mounting evidence that neural reorganization reflects patterns of use. It also seems likely that sensory feedback provided by the use of the affected limbs may play a major role in reshaping remaining circuits.

©2010 Elsevier Ltd
DOI: 10.1016/B978-0-7020-4051-1.00008-4

Following a stroke, those individuals who survive begin to demonstrate behavioural recovery, and the underlying biological manifestations of recovery reflect the inherent reorganizational ability of the system. The notion of the brain (indeed the entire human system) as adaptable is filtering through to the clinical community together with an understanding that events occurring post-lesion, the rehabilitation environment and the actual methods of training affect recovery; that some methods may facilitate and others actually inhibit recovery. It is necessary to accept that there is a link between brain plasticity (i.e., anatomical, physiological and functional reorganization) and the methods used in rehabilitation and recovery. Major clinical research emphasis should now be on studying the effects of rehabilitation methods upon brain morphology and function.

PLASTICITY OF THE INTACT BRAIN

The term 'plasticity' refers, in general, to the capacity of the CNS to adapt to functional demands and therefore to the system's capacity to reorganize. Following from experimental studies of both animals and humans, brain processes are now acknowledged to be remodelled by our experiences, particularly by the use to which we put the system. Plasticity includes the process of learning. Substantial evidence has emerged that the human brain is dynamic, flexible and problem solving throughout life (Weiller 1998). This view is in contrast to an earlier view of the brain as functionally static (for discussion, see Merzenich et al 1991).

Mechanisms of brain plasticity include the capacity for neurochemical, neuroreceptive and neuronal structural changes. Furthermore, the parallel and distributed nature of brain organization appears to play an important role in its capacity for flexibility and adaptation. Extensive intracortical axonal collaterals provide input to many different movement representations of a given body part, and their pattern of recruitment may determine the execution of complex movements. There is a wide overlap in cortical neuronal networks targeting different body parts, and these networks, in part, share common neuronal elements (Schieber 1992). Cellular populations within the brain are dynamically organized, with the possibility for variability in structure and function according to behavioural needs (Edelman 1987). Even the simplest task requires coordination of several distinct brain areas. Individual cells and neuronal systems have the ability to subserve more than one function. Regulation of both transient and long-term effectiveness of synapses occurs daily throughout life and is also determined by experience. Receptors themselves demonstrate plasticity, synaptic transmission becoming stronger or weaker according to use. Specific mechanisms underlying brain plasticity are described in detail elsewhere (Kolb 1995; Kandel 2000).

Remodelling of cortical neuron responses occurs between columnarly arrayed and cooperative groups of neurons of which there are hundreds of millions. Merzenich and colleagues (1991) describe a continual competition between neural groups for the domination of neurons on their mutual borders. This competition for cortical territory appears to be use-dependent. Cortical maps differ in ways that reflect their use (Merzenich et al 1983), appearing to be subject to modification on the basis of activity of peripheral sensory pathways. For example, a monkey was trained for 1 hour a day to perform a task that required repeated use of two, three and occasionally four fingers to obtain food. After a period of repeated stimulation, with several thousand repetitions, the area of cortex representing the tips of the stimulated fingers was substantially greater than in an untrained monkey (Jenkins et al 1990) (Fig. 1.1). A human subject trained to do a rapid sequence of finger movements improved in accuracy and speed after 3 weeks of daily (10–20 min) training. Magnetic resonance imaging (MRI) scans showed that the region activated in the primary motor cortex of the trained subject was larger than the region activated by the control subject who performed random finger movements of the same hand. The change in cortical representation was retained for several months. In these examples, repetitive practice may have acted on pre-existing patterns of connections to strengthen their effectiveness (Kandel 2000).

Studies of humans following surgery to transpose muscle or with congenital blindness have also shown the capacity of the brain to reorganize. For example, reorganization of cortical outputs has been reported in individuals with amputation of a limb or segment of a limb. Following amputation, neighbouring networks expand into the area previously devoted to activity of the amputated segment (Hall et al 1990; Fuhr et al 1992). In congenital upper limb amputees and early following amputation of part of a limb, the remaining muscles in the limb received more descending connections than those muscles of the uninvolved limb (Hall et al 1990). Changes reported include increased size of cortical motor representation area and recruitment of a larger percentage of the alpha motor neuron pool of muscles ipsilateral and immediately proximal to the side of the amputation.

It seems clear, therefore, that neuronal elements are inherently flexible, responding according to use and experience and the capacity for functional gain for that individual. In contrast, a significant shrinkage in cortical representation of inactive muscles in healthy subjects was found after only 4–6 weeks of unilateral ankle immobilization and this was more pronounced when duration of immobilization was longer (Liepert et al 1995).

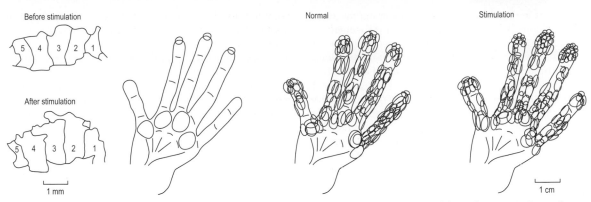

Before stimulation

After stimulation

1 mm

Normal

Stimulation

1 cm

Figure 1.1 Repetitive use of fingers 2, 3, 4 caused expansion of the cortical representation of these fingers. Outlines of regions in cortical area 3b represent surfaces of fingers before and after training. Maps of glabrous fields are identified for recording sites within area 3b before and after training. *(From Jenkins et al 1990, with permission).*

Motor learning, training and plasticity

Evidence of the effects of different environments, of learning and of training on brain reorganization, including functional changes in cortical motor and sensory neurons, comes from numerous studies (e.g., Merzenich et al 1990; Sanes et al 1992). For example, rats housed in enriched environments after brain infarction performed significantly better on motor tasks such as narrow-beam walking, ladder-rung walking and skilled forearm reaching than rats housed alone or in standard cages (Held et al 1985; Ohlsson & Johansson 1995). Aspects of an enriched environment found to result in the best performance were the opportunity for physical activity combined with social interaction (Johansson & Ohlsson 1996; Biernaskie & Corbett 2001; Risedal et al 2002). Training rats on specific tasks such as reaching increases selectively the dendritic arborization in the forelimb representation of the motor and sensory cortex (Greenough et al 1985). Such changes are found for both unimanual and bimanual reaching either on one side of the motor cortex or on both sides (Kolb 1995).

Skill learning in humans is associated with similar nervous system changes as seen in animals (see Merzenich 1986 for review). Humans with an intact brain have shown functional changes in the brain associated with training and use, specifically with increased use of a body part or enhanced sensory feedback from it. This is particularly so where the increase in use is accompanied by functional gain for the subject. Increased use of a body part or enhanced sensory feedback from it may lead to a shift in the balance of intracortical networks towards that body part (Gracies 1996). For example, skilled Braille reading is associated with a relative enlargement of the cortical

sensorimotor representation of the reading finger (Pascual-Leone & Torres 1993), with brain changes mapped by focal transcranial magnetic stimulation (TMS). Flexible modulation of corticomotor outputs may represent a first stage in learning, with further practice of a task eventually leading to structural changes in intracortical and subcortical networks (Pascual-Leone et al 1995). In addition, the size of the representation fluctuates with the amount of reading activity (Pascual-Leone et al 1995).

Learning is reflected in alterations in the pattern of interconnections in those sensory and motor systems involved in learning a specific task, in particular changes in the effectiveness of neural connections (Kandel 2000). Specific motor training can increase the size of different components of motor maps. For example, brain maps in humans have demonstrated that cortical representations of muscles of the fingers of the left but not the right hand were expanded in right-handed skilled violin players who regularly perform (Elbert et al 1995).

There is now substantial evidence from biomechanical studies of healthy subjects that neuromuscular as well as brain adaptations occur in response to physical activity, strength training and immobilization (Enoka 1995). The gain in strength occurring in the first few weeks of a strength-training programme is accompanied by a comparable increase in electrical activity in muscle which precedes a significant change in muscle size (Moritani & deVries 1979; Narici et al 1989). This time course implicates a role for neural adaptation. Qualitative and quantitative changes in neural drive occurring in association with exercise appear to be task specific.

There is increasing evidence that altered physical activity is likely to involve functional and structural adaptations in the motor pathway (e.g., Cracraft & Petajan 1961; Sale et al 1982; Hakkinen & Komi 1983). It has been shown that strength training can result in a greater improvement in performance than in either muscle bulk or muscle strength (Rutherford & Jones 1986). Descending drive on to spinal motor neurons appears to increase following strength training and decrease after a period of inactivity (McComas 1993).

In acquiring a motor skill, the learner must combine movements of individual segments into the pattern or synergy, in both spatial and temporal domains, that ensures successful performance of the action. Practice enables the movements to become smoother, more coordinated and usually more rapid. Such biomechanical changes are reflective of changes at the neural level.

It is not only physical practice that can promote modulation of neural circuits but also mental practice (Ch. 2). In the early stage of learning a complicated finger exercise, changes to cortical motor output maps show that mental practice alone can lead to the same plastic changes in the motor system as those occurring with repetitive physical practice (Pascual-Leone et al 1995).

Do comparable brain changes occur in ageing brains? Histologically there is a loss of neurons as we age. However, there is evidence that one mechanism that enables the adaptation associated with learning a new skill at any age is an increase in the number of synapses per neuron (Buell & Coleman 1981). It appears that the effectiveness of existing connections is increased by practice and learning at any age.

PLASTICITY FOLLOWING A BRAIN LESION

The logical question arising from studies of brain plasticity is whether an enriched environment, use, training and experience would have similar effects on the damaged brain and whether these effects would enhance functional recovery (Kolb 1995). Conversely, do environmental impoverishment and non-use inhibit recovery? Technological advances that enable brain processes to be more closely examined demonstrate that recovery of function following a brain lesion occurs as a result of structural and functional reorganization.

As might be expected, recovery mechanisms are widespread throughout the brain. Ipsilateral motor pathways may play a role in recovery of motor function (Chollet et al 1991; Fisher 1992; Weiller et al 1992; Silvestri et al 1993). Extensions of cortical motor fields into undamaged areas have also been demonstrated (Asanuma 1991; Weiller et al 1993). Differences in levels of motor unit synchronization have been found during recovery following stroke, paralleling improvements in fine motor control (Farmer et al 1993). Environmental factors and learning bring out specific capabilities by altering the effectiveness (and anatomical connections) of pre-existing pathways

(Kandel 1991) and these two factors probably play key roles in determining the extent of functional recovery.

The mechanisms underlying recovery from brain damage in humans are known to be complex and multi-factorial, including functional and anatomical reorganization, altered neurotransmission and metabolism. Only recently have direct studies of brain function in humans become possible with the introduction of imaging techniques, such as positron emission tomography (PET), functional magnetic resonance imaging (fMRI) and transcranial magnetic stimulation (TMS). The results have demonstrated functional reorganization in intact cortical tissue both adjacent to the injury and in more remote cortical areas after recovery of lost motor function (e.g., Johansson 2000; Liepert et al 2001; Nelles et al 2001; Nudo et al 2001; Kolb 2003; Nudo 2003; Nelles 2004). Several studies have correlated changes in activation patterns with physiotherapy/training-induced improvement in function (Nelles et al 1999, 2001; Liepert et al 2000) (Fig. 1.2). Reorganization may take a number of forms: perilesional extensions of representations, shifts from primary to secondary parallel processing systems, and recruitment of homologous areas of the unaffected hemisphere (Weiller & Rijntjes 2005). It appears that the greater the involvement of the ipsilesional network, the better the recovery.

The actual mechanisms underlying reorganization and therefore recovery are still not entirely understood but are currently being explored using new technologies. In a current hypothesis, functional loss is seen as a disconnection phenomenon and recovery may mean, as Weiller & Rijntjes (2005) suggest, reconnection or better recoordination of a whole set of areas. The challenging aspect for each stroke patient is the question to what degree will he or she recover.

Of critical importance for the patient's rehabilitation is that experience, with the opportunity to work with the physiotherapist to acquire motor skill by training active use of the paretic limbs, modulates the adaptive reorganization that inevitably occurs. However, post-injury plastic changes occurring over time can have beneficial or negative effects driven in part by the individual's physical and mental activity levels following the stroke. Immobility and lack of use induces negative effects. For example, muscle structure, like any physical structure, is dependent upon and reflects patterns of use, and inactivity imposed by a stroke can result in adaptation in the musculoskeletal system. Sustained physical inactivity also involves a reduction in aerobic capacity, limiting the performance of everyday activities and increasing the risk of falls and dependence on others.

The use of animal models permits tight control of factors that may confound the outcomes of human studies, given the complexities inherent in working with people who are active participants in the recovery process. It is in the patient's best interest for those working in

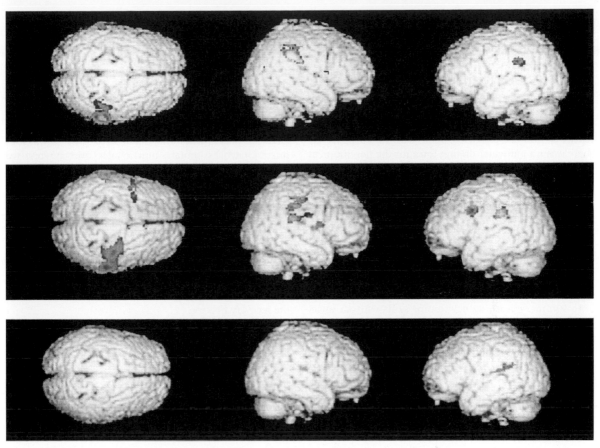

Figure 1.2 Functional reorganization in bilateral motor and sensory systems illustrated by increases in regional blood flow when the subject's paretic arms are moved passively. Area of activation: (top) before training, (middle) after task-oriented training of the experimental group, (lower) in the control group. *(Reproduced from Nelles et al 2001, with permission).*

rehabilitation to remain current with advances in this area. In order to examine lesion-induced plasticity in the primary motor cortex of primates, Nudo and colleagues used intracortical microstimulation techniques (ICMS) to map the hand representation in adult squirrel monkeys before and after focal ischaemic lesions. Unilateral damage to the forelimb area of the sensorimotor cortex resulted in preferential use of the unimpaired limb. It was found that hand movement representations that were adjacent to the infarct but were spared from direct injury underwent a loss of cortical tissue (Nudo & Milliken 1996).

Since the animals in this study did not have any specific training post-injury, the losses in the representational area of the paretic hand may have been the direct result of diminished use (Nudo & Milliken 1996). Therefore, in a subsequent study, lesioned monkeys were trained on a small-object retrieval task. To obtain a small food pellet, they were trained to insert one or two fingers into a small-diameter container to pick out the pellet, a task that required fine control of their digits and hand. The unimpaired limb was restrained. For the first few days after the infarct, movements were slow and monkeys had difficulty placing their digits into the small holes. However, skill improved over time and the number of misses decreased rapidly. Comparison of ICMS maps before and after the infarct showed that the spared hand representation area adjacent to the infarct had expanded (Nudo et al 1996).

These results suggest that specific training to induce motor learning can shape subsequent reorganization in the undamaged motor cortex and that this may play an important part in functional recovery (Nudo et al 1996). Interestingly, restraint of the unimpaired limb without additional training of the paretic limb resulted in a decrease of total hand representation. Specifically, the size of finger, wrist and forearm representations of the paretic limb decreased. That is to say, it was the enforced practice of a desirable task with the paretic limb, not the constraint alone, that brought about improved performance of that limb (Friel & Nudo 1998).

In a further study using identical neurophysiological techniques but with an easy task, monkeys were trained on the reach and retrieval task, this time with a large-diameter container. The lesioned monkeys were able to perform the retrieval task efficiently early in training and performance remained stereotypic and unchanged over time. In addition, comparison of pre- and post-injury ICMS revealed no task-related representational changes. These results suggest that simple use of the limb was insufficient to produce plasticity in cortical maps. Apparently there was no particular driving force for the development of motor skill or new strategies – the task was too easy (Plautz et al 2000). Since motor skill learning can only be inferred when there is a stable and measurable change in motor performance over time, the results show that the task was too easy and, as a result, further practice had no benefit and indeed had a negative effect (Plautz et al 2000). This has particular significance for physiotherapy practice, pointing out the importance of patients practising actions that are difficult and challenging rather than those that are too easy and are already achievable.

In summary, learning new motor skills with an intact CNS and regaining skill after a lesion of the CNS are similar in many respects. At the motor performance level, the biomechanical changes in the regaining of skill after stroke are similar to those that occur when non-lesioned individuals are learning a new skill. Nudo (2003) summarizes the empirical evidence underpinning current understanding of the neuroplasticity that can modulate functional recovery:

- Injury to the motor cortex, as in stroke, induces functional changes in the cortical tissue spared by the injury.
- Acquisition of skilled movement induces predictable functional changes within the motor cortex. The two events interact so that, following cortical injury, acquisition of motor skill influences the type and growth of functional plasticity that occurs in the undamaged cortex.
- Neural organization and motor skill learning are optimized when the focus is on tasks that are engaging, challenging and meaningful.
- Many repetitions are required for an individual to become skilled in a complex motor task.
- Repetition of movements that are too easy or of a non-meaningful task is insufficient to produce long-term neural reorganization.

These neurobiological guidelines should be incorporated into clinical practice.

Recovery of function

Recovery of function can be categorized as:

- *spontaneous recovery* (restitution) due to reparative processes occurring immediately following the lesion that restore the functionality of neural tissue, and

- *reorganization of neural mechanisms* influenced by use and experience.

This distinction has not typically been made, physicians assuming that all recovery is 'spontaneous' and that no relationship exists between what the person does (including physiotherapy) and recovery. The implicit assumption was that rehabilitation enables the person to take advantage of a 'natural' recovery process unaffected in itself by what the person does and experiences. This past lack of interest in what stimulates functional recovery has resulted in little research and a reluctance to test the effects of different rehabilitation methods on brain plasticity and behaviour (Bach-y-Rita 1990, 1996). Physiotherapy intervention was typically regarded as enabling the individual to make the most of what is left after the lesion, inferring a static system, rather than as affecting or driving the recovery (reorganization) process itself. There is, however, increasing support in the neurosciences for the argument that what the person does and experiences in rehabilitation, and the rehabilitation environment itself, must affect the recovery process.

Early after a lesion, accumulation of intracellular fluid (oedema) can produce local functional depression in areas immediately surrounding the primary area of injury and remote functional depression of distant structures (diaschisis). Local factors such as resolution of oedema, absorption of necrotic tissue debris and opening of collateral channels for circulation to the lesioned area enable a return to function of undamaged parts of the brain. Tissue recovery seems to be a relatively fast process whereas recovery through representational plasticity has a far longer time course, and time since stroke is not a limiting factor (Calautti & Baron 2003). There is mounting evidence that intensive and repetitive training can positively affect motor recovery and that the voluntary contribution by the patient is critical.

Too broad an interpretation of spontaneous recovery reflects a lack of understanding of how all recovery beyond the immediate reparative stage must be affected by what the person experiences, by what the person actually does and what is learned. It is certain that the brain will reorganize (adapt) after a lesion whatever happens to the individual. However, given the evidence from investigations of the differential and context-dependent effects on reorganization from animal and human studies, it is reasonable to hypothesize that the nature of that reorganization depends largely on the inputs received and the outputs demanded post-lesion.

It is now possible to monitor a person's recovery after the immediate reparative period in terms of that person's experiences, their immobility or activity, opportunities for training and practice (i.e., the specific intervention available) and the physical features of the environment and its demands. Such data can be matched against changes occurring within the nervous system itself, via such techniques as PET, fMRI and TMS. The results may enable us to determine the critical components of best practice in rehabilitation and to identify those factors that have the potential for a negative effect. It is, however, most important that the details of methods used, and time spent in practice and training (i.e., dosage) are provided.

In the absence of appropriate experience and training, new connections may be *maladaptive*. Furthermore, maladaptive changes occur in the musculoskeletal system, with a negative impact on the capacity of the effector apparatus, the muscles, to generate and time appropriate force for the intended action. These mechanisms may underlie the development over time of stiff 'spastic' muscles (see Ch. 8). Muscle and soft tissue adaptations occur rather quickly, and are discussed in Chapter 2.

Muscle structure, like any physical structure, is dependent upon and reflects patterns of use. Following an acute brain lesion, the potential exists for muscles and soft tissues to adapt as a result of muscle inactivity imposed by the brain lesion itself and secondarily as a result of subsequent disuse.

Compensatory or adaptive behaviour illustrates the individual's attempt to respond, after the lesion, on the basis of the systems available. The way in which a person attempts to achieve a goal illustrates the 'best' that can be done given the state of both the neural and musculoskeletal systems (Shepherd & Carr 1991). The action is performed in the most advantageous manner given the effects of the lesion, the dynamic possibilities inherent in the musculoskeletal linkage and the environment in which the action is performed (Carr & Shepherd 1996). The person uses whatever muscles can generate sufficient force to move the body segments in an attempt to achieve a goal. The biomechanical flexibility inherent in the musculoskeletal system may result in a rough approximation of the action and is a reflection of the imbalance caused by greater activity of some muscles of a synergy compared to others (see Fig. 2.11). Muscle imbalance is the direct result of reduced corticomotor neuronal connectivity with absent or reduced and slowed intensity of muscle activation, as well as changes in disused muscle such as increased stiffness (see Ch. 8).

Setting up conditions that might preserve muscle extensibility and contractility, forcing the required movements and enabling intensive practice must surely become a major part of rehabilitation. The opportunity to do this may only be available if an enriched and challenging environment is built within the rehabilitation setting for humans as has been done for animal experimentation, and if staff attitudes can shift to provide a more stimulating 'coaching' role and a more challenging environment.

In the absence of appropriate experience and specific training of a paretic limb, an individual may learn *not* to use the limb. As in animal studies, focusing on tasks that are engaging, challenging and meaningful to the individual seems to be effective in optimizing the neural plasticity

that parallels functional recovery. Evidence of brain changes related to task-specific training post-stroke suggest that it is possible to entrain or 'lead' the brain toward a more efficient activation pattern (Calautti & Baron 2003).

Effect of the environment on behaviour and recovery

After a stroke people have to contend not only with impairments resulting from the lesion itself but also with emotional effects, depression and lack of motivation which may be associated with their own sense of loss. The patient's own attitude and approach to activity and social interaction influence functional outcome and quality of life (Johansson 2005). Expectations play a significant role in all treatments. Experimental evidence suggests that the post-ischaemic lesion environment can significantly improve functional outcome, influence gene expression (Johansson 2005) and interact with skill training. Contrast this with the debilitating effects of a non-stimulating environment in which an individual may feel he/she has no personal control. What happens to an individual after a stroke can not only inhibit brain reorganization but also inhibit synaptic connections not directly affected by the lesion and which, potentially, could adapt and mediate some functional improvement.

It is apparent from studies of animals that the nature of the environment (physical structure, possibilities for social interaction, physical activity and exercise) affects brain reorganization after a lesion. Anatomical, physiological, biochemical and behavioural differences are known to occur in lesioned and non-lesioned animals kept in an enriched environment compared to those in an impoverished environment (e.g., Rosenzweig et al 1973; Finger 1978; Rosenzweig 1980; Walsh 1981; Held et al 1985; Camel et al 1986; Isseroff & Isseroff 1987). Furthermore, the beneficial effects of enrichment are lost if the animal is subsequently moved to an impoverished milieu. Housing animals in an enriched environment can result in such brain changes as greater cortical depth and weight, increased glial proliferation, an increase in number of synapses in the cortex and in the number of dendritic spines, and increased capillary density (see Kolb 1995 for review).

Motor control research and clinical observations also make it clear that the environment (i.e., objects, their position and orientation) drives the motor pattern in an action. For example, reaching to grasp an object depends on the characteristics (position and orientation) of the object and where it is in the environment. The environment is increasingly being seen as a potent facilitator or inhibitor of behaviour.

It is important, therefore, to consider what effects the typical post-lesion or rehabilitation environment has on human brain reorganization. A person's environment includes the physical structure and the people within it. In human research, behavioural and ecological studies illustrate the close relationship between the environment and behaviour, including the extent and type of physical activity in which the individual engages.

There are no experiments we know of which have investigated the effect of environmental modification on brain reorganization in humans. However, several ecological studies give us information about the behaviour of people under different conditions. From these findings it is possible to infer that human brain reorganization may occur, as it does in animals, according to the richness or poverty of the environment in which people may find themselves post-lesion. The field of human ecology offers many insights into the effects of the environment on human behaviour by observing people in their particular settings. Such observations of a hospital or rehabilitation unit can provide insight into a person's behaviour. For example, a person's poor recovery may be partially explained by the impoverishment of a non-challenging environment. The rehabilitation environment may also affect people in different ways – compare, for example, how a young person after a traumatic brain injury and an elderly person would view their new environment in a hospital or rehabilitation centre.

What is the nature of a rehabilitation environment? Studies of environments in several rehabilitation settings provide some insights. A group of individuals with spinal cord injury were found to be more 'independent' in corridors and the cafeteria than in the therapy rooms (Willems 1972). Another group spent 16% of their time in face-to-face contact with therapists, and 40% in 'isolated disengagement' or inactive. Only 6% of time was spent in interactions with other patients.

The evidence from environmental studies over many years is that stroke rehabilitation tends not to be intensive enough for many groups of patients even when it is planned to be so. It appears that more time is spent in passive pursuits, 'watching others or looking out of the window', than in meaningful and task-related activity and exercise, with little evidence of self-directed exercise (Lincoln et al 1989; Tinson 1989; Mackay et al 1996).

A recent observational study of physical activity within the first 14 days of acute stroke found that although most patients, 84.5%, were free to move out of bed, only 13% were engaged in activities that might have the potential to improve mobility and prevent secondary complications (Bernhardt et al 2004). More than 50% of the patients' time was actually spent resting in bed. The recent multi-centre longitudinal project comparing inpatient care and recovery patterns between four European rehabilitation centres (CERISE) reported that patients in a UK centre spent a long time doing nothing by their beds while therapists spent time doing legally required administration (de Wit et al 2005, 2007). Clearly, there is a need for patients to be active during their rehabilitation period. However,

it is not only the time spent with the physiotherapist but also whether what the individual is doing in that time is sufficiently vigorous to induce a training effect.

The results of a longitudinal observational study of patients in physiotherapy and occupational therapy between 2 and 14 weeks after stroke indicated that, on average, in a physiotherapy session, 42% of the time was spent inactive in lying, 11% active in lying, 16% active in sitting and 31% active in standing (Mackay-Lyons & Makrides 2002). Much of the inactive time involved physiotherapists performing passive interventions, particularly passive ranging. When present, aerobic capacity of a typical session took less than three minutes. During occupational therapy a considerable percentage of inactive time was spent in sitting discussing issues related to discharge, equipment needs and home management.

Another study compared physical activity levels of rehabilitation patients in the acute phase after stroke in Melbourne, Australia and Trondheim, Norway. Patients had similar baseline characteristics. Melbourne patients spent 21% more time in bed and only 12% undertook moderate to high activity compared with 23% in Trondheim. These results are only meaningful if it can be shown that early physical activity improves patient outcome. There is some indirect evidence that early mobilization has a positive effect on outcome (Indredavik et al 1999). There is also some evidence that greater intensity and frequency of therapy improves outcome (Kwakkel et al 1997).

Decline in intellectual activity seen in some individuals after stroke may be explained by the extent of the lesion and/or by the person's age. However, such decline can also be explained by other factors. The rehabilitation environment is complex, unfamiliar and unpredictable to those who suddenly find themselves in it and such situations have been suggested to evoke fewer adaptive responses in the older person, particularly when there are also high stress levels and limited processing or response time is available. Difficulty coping with an unfamiliar environment can cause an erosion of the feeling of competence. Several decades ago it was suggested that 'learned helplessness' generated by an overly assistive and protective environment may cause symptoms of passivity and poor performance in individuals where they have little control over their role (Seligman 1975).

It has been clearly shown in early ecological studies that the physical setting, for example the structure of a room and the furniture in it, can itself affect behaviour (Sommer 1969), even motor performance itself. Biomechanical studies make it clear that inability to stand up from a chair may be due to a physical barrier to foot placement backward or to the therapist or nurse standing too close in front of the patient when trying to help. A well-designed height-adjustable chair can make a large contribution to a person's wellbeing and independence; standing up from a higher chair, by decreasing the extensor muscle force required through the lower limbs, is easier than from a low chair, particularly if it has a backward-sloping seat. If patients sit for most of the day in a wheelchair, for example, muscle length adapts and lower limb flexor muscles may become stiffer and shorter, particularly the soleus muscle. If an individual propels a one-arm wheelchair, it is the non-paretic arm and leg that are exercised. Kolb (1995) points out the probable effects of using one limb to substitute for another paretic limb – learning to depend on one arm to substitute for an impaired limb, for example, reduces the use of the impaired limb. A patient is likely, therefore, to lose any residual capacity in this limb. This phenomenon was called by Taub (1980) 'learned non-use'.

There are, however, some promising new developments in design of rehabilitation units and activities. Physiotherapists are slowly moving away from reliance on one-to-one individual therapy and introducing semi-supervised group and circuit training. Treadmills, electromechanical-assisted gait devices, stair climbing and arm training devices (Hesse et al 2006), exercise bicycles, and computerized systems that enhance motivation, focus attention on critical aspects of a task and provide automated feedback, are becoming more evident in rehabilitation. Entertaining games and interactive machines are reported to lead to improved performance.

Therapists may need to consider that there may be a mismatch between rehabilitation equipment and goals of therapy. Compare, for example, what might be a patient's impression on sighting a treadmill or a wheelchair. A wheelchair signifies an alternative mode of getting about, to be used when walking is difficult or impossible. The treadmill, on the other hand, is a symbol of exercise, activity, a little exciting perhaps, and can suggest that activity and participation are expected and necessary.

It is very likely that the provision of a challenging environment, structured in a way that is relevant to the everyday tasks that people need to learn and stimulating to mental and physical functioning, has direct effects upon reorganization of the brain after a lesion. Meanwhile, neuroscientists are exploring the effects of various drugs (Walker-Batson et al 2004), repetitive transcranial magnetic stimulation (rTMS) (Liepert et al 2007) and transcranial direct cortical stimulation (tDCS) (Hummel et al 2005) to enhance functional recovery. To keep up with these changes, therapists need to incorporate neurobehaviourally- and neurobiologically-informed rehabilitation into their clinical practice. The development of more effective rehabilitation requires joint effort and collaboration between neuroscientists and therapists working in the clinic.

In the first edition of this book we argued that task-oriented training along with preservation of musculoskeletal integrity provides the opportunity to drive neural reorganization and optimize functional recovery for individuals with brain lesions, using post-stroke as an example. The assumption was that if training is effective, it will be associated with cellular change. Some 10 years later, there are promising signs that intensive task-oriented training *can* induce brain reorganization, for example a change in activation patterns in favour of the lesioned hemisphere, in parallel with improved motor function. Understanding motor recovery in humans is far from complete; most of our knowledge about recovery after stroke is observational (Calautti & Baron 2003). However, the study of neuroplasticity has rapidly expanded in past decades. In testing the efficacy of neurological rehabilitation, including physiotherapy, consideration needs to be given not only to motor performance measures but should also include tests of the individual's personal wellbeing and quality of life, their ability to carry out activities that give them independence, opportunities for social integration and participation. Visualization of neural activity after a brain lesion (PET and fMRI) can now be used to investigate the effects of physiotherapy training on brain reorganization. We agree with Nelles (2004) that the recent explosion in neurorehabilitation research is grounds for optimism and promises an exciting scientific future.

REFERENCES

Asanuma C 1991 Mapping movements within a moving motor map. Trends Neurosci 14:217–218.

Bach-y-Rita P 1990 Receptor plasticity and volume transmission in the brain: emerging concepts with relevance to neurologic rehabilitation. J Neurol Rehabil 4:121–128.

Bach-y-Rita P 1996 Conservation of space and energy in the brain. Restor Neurol Neurosci 10:1–3.

Bernhardt J, Dewey H, Thrift A et al 2004 Inactive and alone – physical activity within the first 14 days of acute stroke unit care. Stroke 35:1005–1009.

Biernaskie J, Corbett D 2001 Enriched rehabilitative training promotes improved forelimb motor function and enhanced dendritic growth following focal ischemic injury. J Neurosci 21:5272–5280.

Buell SJ, Coleman DP 1981 Dendritic growth in aged human brain and failure of growth in senile dementia. Science 206:854–856.

Calautti C, Baron J-C 2003 Functional neuroimaging studies of motor recovery after stroke in adults: a review. Stroke 34:1553–1566.

Camel JE, Withers GS, Greenough WT 1986 Persistence of visual cortex dendritic alterations induced by post-weaning exposure to a 'superenriched' environment in rats. Behav Neurosci 100:810–813.

Carr JH, Shepherd RB 1987 A motor relearning programme for stroke. Butterworth Heinemann, Oxford.

Carr JH, Shepherd RB 1996 'Normal' is not the issue: it is 'effective' goal attainment that counts. Behav Brain Sci 19:72–73.

Carr JH, Shepherd RB 2000 A motor learning model for rehabilitation. In: Carr JH, Shepherd RB (eds) Movement science. Foundations for physical therapy in rehabilitation, 2nd edn. PRO Ed, Gaithersburg, MD:33–110.

Carr JH, Shepherd RB 2003 Stroke rehabilitation guidelines for exercise and training to optimize motor skill. Butterworth Heinemann, Oxford.

Chollet F, DiPiero V, Wise RJS et al 1991 The functional anatomy of motor recovery after stroke in humans: a study with positron emission tomography. Ann Neurol 29:63–71.

Cracraft JD, Petajan JH 1961 Effect of muscle training on the pattern of firing of single motor units. Am J Phys Med 56:183–194.

de Wit L, Putman K, Dejaeger E et al 2005 Use of time by stroke patients. A comparison of 4 European rehabilitation centres. Stroke 36:1977–1983.

de Wit L, Putman K, Schuback B 2007 Motor and functional recovery after stroke. A comparison of 4 European rehabilitation centres. Stroke 38:2101–2107.

Edelman GM 1987 Neuronal Darwinism: the theory of neuronal group selection. Basic Books, New York.

Elbert T, Pantev C, Wienbruch C et al 1995 Increased cortical representation of the fingers of the left hand in string players. Science 270:305–307.

Enoka RM 1995 Neural adaptations with chronic physical activity. Proceedings of XVth Congress of ISB. Jyvaskyla, Finland:20–21.

Farmer SF, Swash M, Ingram DA et al 1993 Changes in motor unit synchronisation following central nervous lesions in man. J Physiol 463:83–105.

Finger S 1978 Environmental attenuation of brainlesion symptoms. In: Finger S (ed.) Recovery from brain damage. Plenum Press, London:297–329.

Fisher CM 1992 Concerning the mechanism of recovery in stroke hemiplegia. Can J Neurol Sci 19:57–63.

Friel KM, Nudo RJ 1998 Restraint of the unimpaired hand is not sufficient to retain spared hand representation after focal cortical injury. Soc Neurosci Abst 24:405.

Fuhr P, Cohen LG, Dang N et al 1992 Physiological analysis of motor reorganisation following lower limb amputation. Electroencephalogr Clin Neurophysiol 85:53–60.

Gracies JM 1996 Personal communication.

Greenough WT, Larson JR, Withers GS 1985 Effects of unilateral and bilateral training in a reaching task on dendritic branching of neurons in the rat motor–sensory forelimb cortex. Behav Neural Biol 44:301–314.

Hakkinen K, Komi PV 1983 Electromyographic changes during strength training and detraining. Med Sci Sports Exerc 15:455–460.

Hall EJ, Flament D, Fraser C et al 1990 Non-invasive brain stimulation reveals reorganised cortical outputs in amputees. Neurosci Lett 116:379–386.

Hebb DO 1947 The effect of early experience on problem-solving at maturity. Am Psych 2:737–745.

Held JM, Gordon J, Gentile AM 1985 Environmental influences on locomotor recovery following cortical lesions in rats. Behav Neurosci 99:678–690.

Hesse S, Schmidt H, Werner C 2006 Machines to support motor rehabilitation after stroke: 10 years of experience in Berlin. J Rehabil Res Dev 43:671–678.

Hummel F, Celnik P, Giraux AF et al 2005 Effects of non-invasive cortical stimulation on skilled motor function in chronic stroke. Brain 128:490–499.

Indredavik B, Bakke RPT, Slordahl SA et al 1999 Treatment in a combined acute and rehabilitation stroke unit. Which aspects are most important? Stroke 30:917–923.

Isseroff A, Isseroff R 1987 Experience aids recovery of spontaneous alternation following hippocampal damage. Physiol Behav 21:469–472.

Jenkins WM, Merzenich MM, Ochs MT et al 1990 Functional reorganisation of primary somatosensory cortex in adult owl monkeys after behaviorally controlled tactile stimulation. J Neurophysiol 63:82–104.

Johansson BB 2000 Brain plasticity and stroke rehabilitation: the Willis lecture. Stroke 31:223–230.

Johansson BB 2005 Regenerative ability in the central nervous system. In: Barnes M, Dobkin B, Bogousslavsky J (eds) Recovery after stroke. Cambridge University Press, Cambridge:67–87.

Johansson BB, Ohlsson A-L 1996 Environment, social interaction, and physical activity as determinants of the functional outcome after cerebral infarction in the rat. Exp Neurol 139:322–327.

Kandel E 1991 Cellular mechanisms of learning and the biological basis of individuality. In: Kandel ER, Schwartz JH, Jessell TM (eds) Principles of neural science, 3rd edn. McGraw-Hill, New York:1009–1031.

Kandel E 2000 Cellular mechanisms of learning and the biological basis of individuality. In: Kandel ER, Schwartz JH, Jessell TM (eds) Principles of Neural Science, 4th edn. McGraw-Hill, New York:1247–1279.

Kwakkel G, Wagenaar R, Partridge C 1997 Effects of intensity of stroke rehabilitation: a research synthesis. Stroke 28:1550–1556.

Kolb B 1995 Brain, plasticity and behavior. Lawrence Erlbaum Associates, Mahwah, NJ.

Kolb B 2003 Overview of cortical plasticity and recovery from brain injury. Phys Med Rehabil Clin N Am 14:S7–S25.

Liepert J, Teggenthoff M, Malin JP 1995 Changes in cortical motor area size during immobilization. Electroencephalogr Clin Neurophysiol 97:383–386.

Leipert J, Bauder H, Miltner W et al 2000 Treatment-induced cortical reorganization after stroke in humans. Stroke 31:1210–1216.

Liepert J, Uhde I, Graf S et al 2001 Motor cortex plasticity during forced-use therapy in stroke patients: a preliminary study. J Neurol 248:315–321.

Liepert J, Zittel S, Weiller C 2007 Improvement of dexterity by single session low-frequency repetitive transcranial magnetic stimulation over the contralesional motor cortex in acute stroke: a double-blind placebo-controlled crossover trial. Restor Neurol Neurosci 25:461–465.

Lincoln NB, Gamlen R, Thomason H 1989 Behavioural mapping of patients on a stroke unit. Int Dis Stud 11:149–154.

McComas AJ 1993 Human neuromuscular adaptations that accompany changes in activity. Med Sci Sports Exerc 26:1498–1509.

Mackay F, Ada L, Heard R et al 1996 Stroke rehabilitation: are highly structured units more conducive to physical activity than less structured units? Arch Phys Med Rehabil 77:1066–1070.

MacKay-Lyons MJ, Makrides L 2002 Cardiovascular stress during a contemporary stroke rehabilitation program: is the intensity adequate to induce a training effect? Arch Phys Med Rehabil 83:1378–1383.

Merzenich MM 1986 Sources of intraspecies and interspecies cortical map variability in mammals: conclusions and hypotheses. In: Cohen MJ, Strumwasser F (eds) Comparative neurobiology: modes of communication in the nervous system. John Wiley and Sons, New York.

Merzenich MM, Kaas JH, Wall JT et al 1983 Topographic reorganization of somatosensory cortical areas 3b and 2 in adult monkeys following restricted deafferentation. Neurosci 10:33–55.

Merzenich MM, Recanzone GH, Jenkins WM et al 1990 Adaptive mechanisms in cortical networks underlying cortical contributions to learning and nondeclarative memory. Cold Spring Harbor Symposium of Quantitative Biology 55:873–887.

Merzenich MM, Allard TT, Jenkins WM 1991 Neural ontogeny of higher brain function: implications of some recent neurophysiological findings. In: Franzen O, Westman J (eds) Information processing in the somatosensory system. Macmillan, London.

Moritani T, deVries HA 1979 Neural factors versus hypertrophy in the time course of muscle strength gain. Am J Phys Med 58:115–130.

Narici MV, Roi GS, Landoni L et al 1989 Changes in force, cross-sectional area and neural activation during strength training and detraining of the human quadriceps. Eur J Appl Physiol 59:310–319.

Nelles G 2004 Cortical reorganization – effects of intensive therapy. Restor Neurol Neurosci 22:239–244.

Nelles G, Spiekmann G, Markus J et al 1999 Reorganization of sensory and motor systems in hemiplegia stroke patients: a positron emission tomography study. Stroke 30:1510–1516.

Nelles G, Jentzen W, Jueptner M et al 2001 Arm training induced brain plasticity in stroke studied with serial positron emission tomography. Neuroimage 13:1146–1154.

Nudo RJ, 2003 Functional and structural plasticity in motor cortex: implications for stroke recovery. Phys Med Rehabil Clin N Am 14:S57–S76.

Nudo RJ, Milliken GW 1996 Reorganization of movement representation in primary motor cortex following focal ischaemic infarcts in adult squirrel monkeys. J Neurophysiol 75:2144–2149.

Nudo RJ, Wise BM, SiFuentes F et al 1996 Neural substrates for the effects of rehabilitation on motor recovery after ischaemic infarct. Science 272:1791–1794.

Nudo RJ, Plautz EJ, Frost SB 2001 Role of adaptive plasticity in recovery of function after damage to motor cortex. Muscle Nerve 8:1000–1019.

Ohlsson A-L, Johansson BB 1995 Environment influences functional outcome of cerebral infarction in rats. Stroke 26:644–649.

Pascual-Leone A, Torres F 1993 Plasticity of the sensorimotor cortex representation of the reading finger in Braille readers. Brain 116:39–52.

Pascual-Leone A, Dang N, Chen LG et al 1995 Modulation of muscle responses evoked by transcranial magnetic stimulation during the acquisition of new fine motor skills. J Neurophysiol 74:1037–1045.

Plautz EJ, Milliken GW, Nudo RJ 2000 Effects of repetitive motor training on movement representation in adult squirrel monkeys: role of use versus learning. Neurobiol Learn Mem 74:27–55.

Risedal A, Mattsson B, Dahlqvist P et al 2002 Environmental influences on functional outcome after a cortical infarct in the rat. Brain Res Bull 58:315–321.

Rosenzweig M 1980 Animal models for effects of brain lesions and for rehabilitation. In: Bach-y-Rita P (ed.) Recovery of function: theoretical considerations for brain injury rehabilitation. University Park Press, Baltimore, MD:172.

Rosenzweig MR, Bennet EL, Diamond M 1973 Effects of differential experience on dendritic spine counts in rat cerebral cortex. J Comp Physiol Psychol 82:175–181.

Rutherford OM, Jones DA 1986 The role of learning and coordination in strength training. Eur J Appl Physiol 55:100–105.

Sale DG, McComas AJ, MacDougall JD et al 1982 Neuromuscular adaptations in human thenar muscles following strength training and immobilization. J Appl Physiol 53:419–424.

Sanes JN, Wang J, Donoghue JP 1992 Immediate and delayed changes of rat motor cortical output representation with new forelimb configurations. Cereb Cortex 2:141–152.

Schieber MH 1992 Widely distributed neuron activity in primary motor cortex area during individuated finger movements. Abstr Soc Neurosci 18:504.

Seligman M 1975 Helplessness. On depression, development and death. WH Freeman, San Francisco.

Shepherd RB, Carr JH 1991 An emergent or dynamical systems view of movement dysfunction. Aust J Physiother 37:5–17.

Silvestri M, Caltagirone C, Cupini LM et al 1993 Activation of healthy hemisphere in post-stroke recovery. Stroke 24:1673–1677.

Sommer R 1969 Personal space: the behavioural basis of design. Saxon House, Englewood Cliffs, NJ.

Taub E 1980 Somatosensory deafferentation in research with monkeys: implications for rehabilitation medicine. In: Ince LP (ed.) Behavioural psychology and rehabilitation medicine. Willimas & Wilkins, Baltimore, MD:371–401.

Tinson DJ 1989 How stroke patients spend their days. Int Dis Stud 11:45–49.

Walker-Batson D, Smith P, Curtis S et al 2004 Neuromodulation paired with learning dependent practice to enhance post stroke recovery. Restor Neurol Neurosci 22:387–392.

Walsh R 1981 Sensory environments, brain damage, and drugs: a review of interactions and mediating mechanisms. Int J Neurosci 14:129–137.

Weiller C 1998 Imaging recovery from stroke. Exp Brain Res 123:13–17.

Weiller C, Rijntjes M 2005 Some personal lessons from imaging brain in recovery after stroke. In: Barnes M, Dobkin B, Bogousslavsky J (eds)

Recovery after stroke. Cambridge University Press, Cambridge:124–134.

Weiller C, Chollet F, Friston KJ et al 1992 Functional reorganisation of the brain in recovery from striatocapsular infarction in man. Ann Neurol 31:463–472.

Weiller C, Ramsay SC, Wise RJS et al 1993 Individual patterns of functional reorganisation in the human cerebral cortex after capsular infarction. Ann Neurol 33:181–189.

Willems EP 1972 The interface of the hospital environment and patient behaviour. Arch Phys Med Rehabil March:115–122.

Chapter | 2 |

Training motor control, increasing strength and fitness and promoting skill acquisition

INTRODUCTION TO TRAINING MOTOR CONTROL

The aim of physiotherapy in neurorehabilitation is to enable individuals with acute and chronic brain lesions to function as effectively as possible in everyday life. The individual with motor impairments must attempt, therefore, to regain optimal motor performance (i.e., as effective as possible) in those everyday actions that are critical to independence. Essential to the regaining of effective performance is the provision of an expert coach or trainer (the therapist) and the opportunity for intensive practice and exercise in a stimulating environment.

A major purpose of this chapter (in conjunction with Chapters 4–7) is to show how everyday actions can be trained in adults with motor disabilities that result from an acute or chronic disruption of the motor control system. Methods used are developed out of the neurosciences, biomechanics and motor learning.

Effective performance of standing up and sitting down, walking, reaching out for a variety of objects and manipulating them to achieve desired goals in real-life environments is critical to independent living. Given the importance of the upright posture to most of our goal-directed motor behaviour, the individual needs the opportunity to concentrate on gaining control over body segments in the two upright postures (sitting and standing) most critical for independence. Early emphasis on being upright is particularly important following acute brain lesions. It enables individuals to start working to regain the necessary orienting behaviours and postural control/stability mechanisms that enable them to explore and attend to their environment, to communicate with others and to regain the ability to formulate and carry out their goals.

An understanding of the biomechanics of everyday actions, of biological characteristics of muscle and nerve and how these change according to patterns of use, plus knowledge of how skill is acquired is essential in physiotherapy practice. So also is an understanding that

©2010 Elsevier Ltd
DOI: 10.1016/B978-0-7020-4051-1.00009-6

the environment and the opportunity to be challenged physically and mentally are essential in driving the brain organization that is critical to improving motor and mental performance.

The training of motor control in individuals with impairments in control involves:

- optimizing soft tissue flexibility, muscle contractility, timing and control of force generation (strength), muscle endurance and physical fitness specific to the particular actions, and
- directing rehabilitation training methods toward the regaining of improved neuromuscular control of body segments and skill in everyday activities, through task-oriented exercise and practice.

The ability to maintain balance in a gravitational environment is a major focus of rehabilitation. Movement is impossible without the ability to preserve stability, and falls are common when the motor system is impaired.

The first section of this chapter contains a discussion on specificity in training and the transfer of training effects. The idea that specificity of practice is critical if learning (i.e., the retention of improved performance) is to occur means that to achieve optimal performance of an action in a particular context, practice conditions should match that context (Magill 2001). There are sound biomechanical reasons why an action to be learned should be practised, if possible, in its entirety, since one component of the action is dependent on preceding components. However, it is also useful to consider in rehabilitation that one of the goals in practising an action is developing the ability to transfer performance of the skill from the practice environment to other environments and contexts in which the action is to be carried out. For example, when training walking, the goal is for improved performance in the rehabilitation gymnasium to transfer into more functional walking in different contexts and environments.

The role of strength training in improving motor control of specific actions is emphasized since it is not possible for an individual to regain the ability to perform effectively in the absence of appropriate amplitude and timing of muscle forces. Muscle strength is a neuromuscular phenomenon, and involves the capacity of muscles and groups of muscles to generate and time the forces necessary to carry out purposeful actions. Techniques proposed for strengthening muscles in neurorehabilitation are those used by able-bodied individuals to improve motor performance, and consist of intensive task-oriented exercises and practice of actions to be learned under conditions of progressive difficulty (i.e., by increasing load, or distance moved, or time spent sustaining muscle activity).

In the training process, methods of intervention take into account motor control processes, movement biomechanics, muscle characteristics and environmental context,

as well as the specific effects of primary impairments, secondary adaptations and recovery processes. Age may also be a factor. Elderly people are likely to have reduced musculoskeletal flexibility, decreased muscle function and strength unrelated to their lesion-induced impairments. In particular they may demonstrate a slowed rate of tension development (Hortobagyi et al 2001). Intervention is designed to ensure the optimal length and flexibility of muscles, and to activate muscles, strengthen muscle groups for specific actions, and promote synergic activity between muscles. Training is task specific and the individual practises a particular action, such as standing up, in a variety of relevant environmental contexts. If it is not possible to practise the whole action because of poor motor function, modification of the action may be necessary, such as raising the height of the seat to decrease force required to stand up.

Whether individuals have suffered an acute lesion or a chronic disability, it is necessary to prevent the cycle of weakness–disuse–weakness that eventually can lead to muscle and joint contracture and changes in muscle properties associated with immobility (Gracies 2005). Exercises are added that are designed to increase muscle contractility, improve their ability to generate and time force, and to preserve or increase muscle compliance. Since physical fitness is critical for vigour and for the ability to move about independently, fitness training is a necessary component of all neurological rehabilitation programmes.

Nearly three decades ago we proposed that the methods used in training for individuals with lesions of the CNS should be similar to those shown to be effective in increasing motor skill in non-disabled subjects (Carr & Shepherd 1980, 1987). We proposed that a learning environment is set up that maximizes the time spent in practice, and that this change in methods requires reorganization of delivery methods to include self-monitored, semi-supervised and group practice in addition to individual training sessions. The second section of the chapter contains a brief review of factors that underlie the process of learning or relearning an action.

For the able-bodied and the disabled person, acquiring skill requires the opportunity for monitored practice of a meaningful task that provides motivation and challenge. The learner needs some understanding of what is involved in the action, and knowledge of the results – whether performance was effective at achieving the goal or not. The process of learning probably involves neural reorganization so that the best possible outcome can be achieved by the individual. To enable learning to occur requires attentional focus, a concrete goal and intensive practice of the action. After an acute lesion the person has to relearn the 'rules', the major (biomechanical) characteristics, of the action.

It has become evident in the last decade that, after an acute brain lesion and in the presence of chronic neural dysfunction, the regaining of effective performance in rehabilitation depends on the capacity of the lesioned system to reorganize. From brain research so far, it is likely that successful outcomes might be best achieved if the rehabilitation process is designed to promote motor learning, if it is sufficiently vigorous to provide a challenge, and if it revolves around intensive task-oriented practice. Such a programme may drive brain reorganization so the best possible outcomes are achieved.

TASK-ORIENTED EXERCISE AND TRAINING TO OPTIMIZE FUNCTIONAL PERFORMANCE

It is intuitive that people learn what they want to learn and what they practise. The area of research related to the specificity of exercise training has produced information of particular relevance to the rehabilitation of patients with neural lesions that result in weakness of muscle force production and lack of movement coordination. It is becoming increasingly evident at different levels of analysis (behavioural, biological, biomechanical) that training aimed at improving performance should be specific to what is to be achieved. Even at the muscle level, muscle activation patterns, amplitude and timing and speed of muscle force, type of muscle contraction (eccentric–concentric, isometric–isokinetic), the length of muscle when peak force is produced, all appear to be specific to the action and the context in which it is performed. This is not surprising given the potential for complex interactions both within the multisegmental linkage that makes up the human body and between this linkage and the external environment.

What is required for the coordination of the multijoint movements which make up most human actions is the control of many muscles performing together (synergistically) in combinations that vary, to a small or large degree, from action to action. A muscle may act as a prime mover or a fixator; it may contract to accelerate movement of a segment or to brake (decelerate) movement of a segment. Biarticular muscles may accelerate one segment and stabilize another. Muscles can affect distant segments by their contraction through reactive forces. Overall, the relative timing of contraction of all muscles involved in an action is critical and may be a major factor in fine tuning an action. Muscles are activated by signals from central (supraspinal) neural systems and in response to sensory inputs processed supraspinally or via the spinal cord.

Bernstein (1967) pointed out that in complex movements, groups of muscles are constrained (by motor control processes) to act as one unit. It is recognized that individual body segments become functionally linked (Jeannerod 1990). It is this ability to constrain a mobile limb and to link segments in such a way that an action is carried out smoothly and effectively that is learned as a result of practice.

Specificity and transfer in exercise and training

The principle of specificity says that training effects derived from an exercise programme are specific to the exercise performed and the muscles involved (American College of Sports Medicine (ACSM) 2006a,b). A common finding from laboratory and clinical studies is that the major change accompanying strength training and exercise occurs in the training context itself (e.g., Sale & MacDougall 1981; Rutherford 1988; Morrissey et al 1995; Miller et al 2006; Lee et al 2008). Exercise effects tend to be specific to task and context, with the greatest changes occurring in the training exercise itself, and the transfer effect is typically not great.

One early experiment by Rasch & Morehouse (1957) showed that men who exercised in standing to increase strength in elbow flexor muscles showed an increase in strength when standing but less so when in supine; i.e., there was little transfer of training effect from one position to another. The authors suggested the result reflected the learning component of strength training. We now know from our understanding of interactive forces that the muscles that stabilized the body while a forceful contraction of elbow flexors was produced in standing would differ from those that would be active as stabilizers in supine. For example, postural muscle activation patterns in standing (but not in supine) involve lower limb muscles, timed to contract prior to as well as during the weightlifting exercise in order to control the anticipated perturbation caused by the exercise.

In another study, Rutherford & Jones (1986) demonstrated the *action-specificity* of strength training. Able-bodied subjects, trained to lift a maximum load through range using knee extensors, were able to increase the load lifted by 200% over 12 weeks. However, maximum isometric knee extensor force increased only 11%. Furthermore, when maximum power output generated during isokinetic cycling was measured after the strength training, no change was found either at slow or fast speeds. In other words, weight training for a muscle group that plays a critical part in generating leg extension force in cycling (quadriceps) was not effective in either increasing power output during cycling or in increasing muscle force under isometric conditions. A major reason for lack of transfer from muscle strengthening exercises performed as above with the foot free (open kinetic chain exercise) to actions performed with the foot as the base of support (closed kinetic chain exercise) as in cycling is the different muscle coordination patterns involved in these two actions. In the open-chain exercise, contraction of knee extensors lifts the foot by movement at the knee. In cycling, however, hip extensors and ankle plantarflexors, as well as knee extensors, work together (as synergists) to produce force down through the pedal.

The specificity effect is also seen in *aerobic training*. An early study showed that running training resulted in increased VO_{2max} but with only limited carry over to another action – swimming (McArdle et al 1978). The results of a recent clinical study by Lee and colleagues (2008) also illustrated the specificity effect of different types of exercise. A group of 52 individuals with a history of stroke were assigned to various exercise groups. Those who trained on aerobic cycling improved their cardiorespiratory fitness only. Those trained with progressive resisted exercise (PRE) improved muscle strength, power and endurance, cycling peak power output, stair climbing power and self-efficacy. Those who trained on aerobic cycling and PRE had greater positive effects for mobility scores and muscle strength. Walking did not improve and the authors point out that other exercise prescriptions need to be employed such as task-specific training, balance and coordination training.

There have been many studies in the last few years that have examined the effect of various strength-training protocols, with variable effects on functional performance. The reader should be cautious in interpreting these results, keeping in mind Rutherford & Jones' 1986 study and the general issue of specificity. Several clinical trials have shown negative results for strength training: either no increase in muscle strength or no increase in functional performance. If a clinical population shows no increase in strength of a muscle on isometric testing but does demonstrate an increase in the number of sit-to-stands or speed of walking, it can be assumed that functional strength has increased. Increased timing and control of muscle force as well as magnitude of force production (strength) may be reflected in improved performance of a specific action, for example the power produced by calf muscles at push-off in walking. Increased strength of quadriceps may enable independence in standing up. A measure of strength and power production of hip and knee extensors throughout active isokinetic hip and knee extension may be a more suitable objective test than isometric testing but there are also simple clinical tests available (e.g. the step-up test).

It is becoming clear that isometric strength testing is unable to detect functional changes in muscle strength. For example, while strength training may be carried out through range at one joint in an open-chain exercise or of many joints in a closed-chain weightbearing exercise (Fig. 2.1), isometric tests measure at only one point in the movement's range. Several recent studies have reported the use of 'functional strength' measures such as the step-up test or number of sit-to-stands in a specific standardized time (Sherrington et al 2003, 2004; Olivetti et al

2007). Isokinetic (throughout range) strength tests, using an isokinetic dynamometer, also give more useful context-related information than isometric tests (see Lomaglio & Eng 2005).

Everyday actions typically involve both *concentric* (shortening) and *eccentric* (lengthening) modes of muscle contraction. The two modes of contraction involve different physiological processes and there is evidence from studies of able-bodied subjects that muscle strengthening exercises have specific effects that differ according to which mode is used (Komi & Buskirk 1972; Friden et al 1983; Miller et al 2006). The eccentric mode of isokinetic exercise has a more highly specific strength-training effect than the concentric mode (e.g., Duncan et al 1989; Engardt et al 1993). For example, eccentric exercise can be followed by a greater increase in concentric strength and in ability to stand up from a seat than concentric exercise alone in individuals after stroke (Engardt et al 1993).

When a muscle is actively stretched while generating force, tension in the series elastic component increases, potential energy is stored, and this stored elastic energy is used in the subsequent concentric contraction (Stanish et al 1986; Svantessen et al 1997). That is, lower levels of muscle activation for greater levels of force are a feature of eccentric work compared to concentric work (Westing et al 1990) and eccentric contractions appear to involve lower motor unit discharge rates more than concentric contractions (Tax et al 1990). Eccentric exercise can produce changes in the myofibrillar architecture (Friden 1984), and tension placed on a muscle during lengthening contractions appears to cause a preferential recruitment of type II muscle fibres (Friden et al 1983; McHugh 2003). Eccentric training can produce greater joint forces and faster time to peak force in both eccentric and concentric actions than concentric exercise (Miller et al 2006). Eccentric exercise can increase muscle stiffness. A recent study

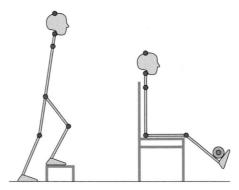

Figure 2.1 Left: Hip, knee and ankle muscles contract in synchrony in kinetic chain (closed-chain) exercises such as step-ups. Right: An exercise for quadriceps femoris that isolates movement to the knee joint, an open-chain exercise.

has demonstrated a short-term increase in stiffness of the gastrocnemius in able-bodied subjects after eccentric strength training. Subjects walked backward downhill on a treadmill for 1 hour. The increase in passive tension occurred principally at the length at which the muscle was exercised (Hoang et al 2007). The authors suggested that eccentric exercises should start at a relatively low load to avoid injury to the muscle. According to the 'repeated bout effect', a single bout of eccentric exercise protects against muscle damage from subsequent eccentric bouts (see McHugh 2003).

A characteristic of eccentric muscle action in functional activities is its effect in stretch-shortening cycles (e.g., Komi 1986). It has been shown in the vertical jump, for example, that when eccentric muscle contraction immediately precedes the generation of concentric force, energy stored by the muscle and released during the subsequent shortening phase augments the amount of force delivered concentrically. This cycle is also illustrated in walking. The viscoelastic properties of the contractile and non-contractile tissues absorb energy when the active soleus muscle is stretched in the stance phase of walking, and this energy increases the concentric force during the subsequent push-off phase. This mechanism may also potentiate quadriceps muscle force for the extensor phase of sit-to-stand (Shepherd & Gentile 1994). Rapid flexion of the upper body causes the knees to flex a few degrees, putting a stretch on the eccentrically contracting quadriceps.

It is generally concluded, therefore, that eccentric contractions can produce more muscle force, have greater mechanical efficiency and involve less metabolic cost than concentric contractions (Komi et al 1987; Chandler & Duncan 1988; Miller et al 2006). Eccentric contractions are a critical producer of muscle forces in activities in which the body mass is lowered (e.g., sitting down, squatting). Therefore, in order to improve motor performance on the many actions that involve lower limb flexion and extension over the feet, a training programme should include practice of body raising and lowering actions (step-ups, squats, standing up and sitting down, stair walking). This programme would be designed to improve coordination of the lower limbs, specifically to control both concentric and eccentric muscle activity, and the ability to switch from one to the other.

The *velocity-specificity of exercise* has been demonstrated in several studies (Kanehisa & Miyashita 1983; Narici et al 1989), but the mechanisms responsible are unknown. As Rutherford (1988) pointed out, exercise might affect the force–velocity characteristics of the muscle itself, or the motor neuron recruitment pattern within the nervous system. One study reported that, despite significant strength improvements in shoulder rotator muscles through both concentric and isokinetic training, tennis serving speed increased only in subjects who received concentric training (Ellenbecker et al 1988). However, findings from a later study (Behm & Sale 1994) suggest that

the *intention* to produce a high rate of force for a fast action appears more important than whether or not the contraction is concentric or eccentric.

Angle-specific training effects have also been reported, showing little transfer from one angle to another in both isometric and isokinetic training (Pavone & Moffat 1985; Kitai & Sale 1989). When muscles are trained isometrically, the greatest increase in strength appears to occur at the angle of training (Sale & MacDougall 1981). There is some electromyographic (EMG) evidence of a greater increase in muscle activity at joint angles trained (Thepaut-Mathieu et al 1985, 1988), suggesting that neural adaptation allows more force to be generated at a particular muscle length (Rutherford 1988; Sale 1988).

It appears, therefore, that strength training is effective primarily for the acquisition of an effective pattern of coordination (skill in performance of the exercise) that is specific to the context in which the action is performed. During training, major changes in strength (load lifted) have been consistently noted to occur early in the training period (Rutherford & Jones 1986) and improvement in strength (force output) is accompanied by increases in neural activation (IEMG) of strengthened muscles (Hakkinen & Komi 1983). It is concluded, therefore, that early changes in strength may be accounted for principally by neural factors (learning), with hypertrophy of the muscles themselves becoming a gradually increasing contribution as training proceeds (Hakkinen & Komi 1983).

Since the context in which muscles must generate force varies from action to action, neural adaptations that become established as a result of, say, lower limb extensor muscle training may not be the adaptations necessary for other actions (Rutherford 1988). Just as training has neural and muscle effects, these effects are reversed by detraining; that is, by relative immobility and disuse.

Hakkinen & Komi (1983) pointed out more than two decades ago that, from a biological viewpoint, variability in training methods is probably advantageous in *increasing the functional capacity of muscle*. The clinical implications from this work are that patients should practise specific actions under as near to natural conditions as possible and at close to natural speed. If individuals with weak lower limb muscles practise exercises involving similar dynamics to those of the everyday actions they must relearn, for example lower limb extension and flexion over fixed feet or reaching actions, there is likely to be a carry over to a variety of actions.

Postural adjustments (muscle activations and segmental movements) that stabilize and balance the body as we move about (reach for a cup of tea in sitting or standing, walk up a hill, stand up from a chair) are also specific to both the action being carried out and the environmental context. This has been shown in biomechanical investigations of *postural adjustments* carried out on able-bodied subjects, particularly in standing, but also in sitting (see

Ch. 7). Muscles that act to balance and stabilize the body mass vary according to such factors as size of base of support, what segments make up the base of support, speed of movement, direction of movement and whether the support surface is stationary or moving (moving walkway or escalators).

Research findings illustrate the ability of the system to utilize whatever muscles are optimally situated to provide support or stability. In standing, when the floor (support) surface is stable, leg muscles ensure a balanced standing position as we pull a lever. By being active prior to the self-initiated voluntary arm movement, they set up the conditions in which the potentially destabilizing pulling movement can be performed effectively. When the floor surface is unstable, we may use a hand for support to ensure that the predicted perturbations will not cause us to lose our balance and fall. Even resting a finger on a stable support surface like a table decreases the work done by lower limbs in balancing.

Specificity in sensory training

In the normal waking state, we are bombarded with sensory inputs from our internal state and from the environment. At any particular point in time, the system selects for attention only those inputs that are relevant. Although the system receives many different sensory inputs from labyrinths, skin, muscle, joint, eyes, ears, it appears to act only on those inputs which provide information relevant to the action we are about to perform or are performing, extinguishing all others. That is, we select what it is we must pay attention to (Wise & Desimone 1988).

Methods of treatment developed several decades ago were based on the belief that therapist-applied sensory inputs, such as fast brushing to specific dermatomes and joint approximation, were likely to initiate muscle activity and improve movement control. There is no evidence that such techniques accomplished what was intended; that is, improved functional performance. Notably, any effect on muscle contractility does not appear to last beyond the administration of the technique (Matyas et al 1986; Bohannon 1987) and carry over into improved function has not been shown.

Arbitrary or non-specific sensory stimulation of a passive recipient is unlikely to affect either the awareness of specific sensations in people with discriminative sensory dysfunction or motor performance. Sensory information appears to be specific to the current state of the system and therefore to the action being performed. An early study showed that when a cat's paw was touched with a rod during the swing phase of walking, there was an increase in flexion of the limb; if it was touched during the stance phase, however, extension of the limb was enhanced (Forssberg et al 1975). That is, the same stimulus had opposite effects depending on the timing of its application and the requirements of the action.

In clinical practice, training of an action such as sit-to-stand, manipulating objects or walking provides the sensory inputs that are normally utilized in the control of these movements. It may help to have the individual pay conscious attention to critical inputs, for example the sense of pressure through the soles of the feet in sit-to-stand, the shape or texture of an object in reaching and grasping. It is likely that extraneous and irrelevant inputs provided by a therapist could either be confusing or redundant and therefore ignored. During practice of a task, the individual may be better able to use the relevant feedback information that is generated internally (from sense receptors) and externally (from vision) that is available from performance itself (Proteau 1992; Abrams & Pratt 1993).

Muscle strengthening and physical conditioning in neurorehabilitation

Muscle strength is relative. A muscle or muscle group has to be strong enough for what it has to do; that is, be capable of generating sufficient force to bring about the intended action. The force generated has to be timed appropriately and synergistic muscle activity coordinated. In addition, muscles have to be capable of generating force over relatively long periods of time. We need endurance in addition to strength in order to walk up a long flight of stairs. We need to be able to build up the necessary force fast enough for the demands of the environment (crossing the street at traffic lights) and the task (using a keyboard or pushing buttons). Ability to produce peak force rapidly (power) is an important function in many actions and may provide a better indication of functional strength than the amplitude of peak force alone.

We also need to be conditioned for the type of activities in which we are involved. Hence, walking up stairs requires the lower limb muscles to generate more force than walking on a level surface; walking up stairs carrying a load of books requires more strength and endurance than walking up without the additional load. Normally our muscles are strong enough and our cardiorespiratory system sufficiently conditioned to enable us to carry out the actions of our daily lives. If, however, we want to do something that requires more muscle strength (or power), endurance or fitness we need to undergo strengthening, endurance or fitness training in addition to specific practice of the task to enable us to perform as well as possible. The link between muscle strength, endurance, fitness and function is therefore intuitively obvious.

In any exercise programme, whether for an able-bodied person or for someone who has just survived a stroke, consideration should be given to the individual's responses to exercise. Physiological and behavioural responses vary between individuals and type of exercise and the intensity, duration and type of exercise will need to be monitored (e.g., heart rate) and adjusted accordingly (ACSM 2006a,b).

The biological and mechanical factors that affect the strength of muscle are:

Structural	Cross-sectional area of muscle, density of fibres
Biomechanical	Efficient mechanical leverage across joints, effects of dynamic intersegmental interactions
Functional	Number, type and frequency of motor units recruited during a contraction, and efficient cooperation between muscles in a synergy.

Strength is therefore a function of the properties of muscle, neural control mechanisms and context. Strength can therefore be increased by increasing muscle size and mechanical efficiency, and by improving neural function (i.e., by learning) (Buchner & de Latour 1991).

It is common for patients with neurological disorders to experience varying degrees of muscle weakness and incoordination, and declining activity is likely to lead to further and more general adaptive decreases in strength. An acute lesion affecting the central motor system commonly results in a disruption to the motor neurons normally activating muscles, causing paralysis or weakness of muscles (Ch. 8). Following a traumatic brain injury, there may be a long period of immobility imposed by skeletal fractures or by a comatose state. Following a stroke, immobility may result from spending a large part of the day, even in rehabilitation, sitting in a wheelchair and inactive. Elderly individuals are likely to have muscle weakness due to neuromuscular changes associated with ageing, and to declining physical activity and a sedentary lifestyle pre-stroke, and may have become deconditioned even before the stroke. Individuals with chronic or progressive neural dysfunction may have experienced decreasing physical activity over the period of their illness. Poor performance on lower limb tasks, including walking and standing up, even in non-disabled people, is said to be predictive of subsequent deterioration in health status including falls and their sequelae (Penninx et al 2000).

A period of immobility is associated with neural and muscular adaptations such as secondary atrophy and weakness of muscles, caused by inactivity (Gracies 2005). Investigations of muscle following disuse have shown decreased muscle volume and cross-sectional area (Ingemann-Hansen & Halkjaer-Kristensen 1980; Young et al 1982). Weakness secondary to movement limitations imposed by a brain lesion may be more debilitating for the individual than the direct effect of the lesion but these secondary changes may be preventable to some extent. A study by Hachisuka and colleagues (1997) proposed that disuse muscle weakness and atrophy are preventable by exercise

that activates high-threshold motor units such as sit-to-stand, stair walking and eccentric knee extension training.

Despite the physiological evidence, old beliefs linger on in physiotherapy, for example that weakness is due to spasticity and that strength training is contraindicated in neurorehabilitation as it may increase spasticity (Bobath 1990). Prejudice against strength training persists despite lack of evidentiary support and increasing evidence not only that strength training can lead to increases in strength, but also improved functional performance. Furthermore, investigators have reported that muscle stiffness, co-contraction and hyperreflexia may actually decrease after strength training. No adverse effects have been reported (e.g., Miller & Light 1997; Sharp & Brouwer 1997; Brown & Kautz 1998; Hsiao & Newham 1999; Teixeira-Salmela et al 1999, 2001; Weiss et al 2000; Kim et al 2001; Sterr & Freivogel 2003; Morris et al 2004). It is likely that task-oriented exercises and training might decrease 'spastic' stiffness both by improving the neural control of muscle and maintaining muscle extensibility. Co-contraction may decrease as a result of improved limb control.

Exercise in able-bodied subjects has a beneficial effect on motor unit activation (Sale 1987) and exercise, including strength training, and should therefore be beneficial where there are decreases in spinal motor neuron activation due to a central lesion and secondary disuse. Recent evidence suggests that repeated high-intensity exercise can overcome the voluntary activation failure present after brain injury (Newham 2005). It is quite clear therefore that exercise (and vigorous activity) has a beneficial effect on both structure and function of muscle.

Strengthening exercises can be carried out as part of task-related practice (with body weight or weight of a limb as resistance), as in repeated standing up and sitting down from seats of progressively lower height, or reaching to pick up an object (of light or heavy weight). Such exercise is likely to have the following results:

- ↑ Muscle strength (increased ability to generate and time muscle forces appropriately for the task).
- ↑ Skill in performance of that task (increased coordination of muscle activations).
- ↑ Extensibility of muscle for the task (decreased resistance to movement).

The first two could involve improved firing and synchronization of motor units and agonist–antagonist and synergic coordination; the third, an increase in muscle length and improved muscle mechanics. Task-related exercises, that is exercises that have similar biomechanical characteristics to the action(s) to be learned, have therefore the potential to increase the control of movement and functional performance of the everyday actions that are the focus of the exercise. Functional strength training is probably critical for regaining control of linked segments.

Strength training in neurological rehabilitation consists of exercises selected according to the individual's needs at a particular time (i.e., according to the threshold of strength for particular actions). The exercises are practised both repetitively and with variations, and at graded levels of difficulty. Examples include (Figs 2.2–2.4):

- Repetitive contractions of a poorly innervated (weak) muscle group. The aim is to regain the capacity to generate and control force concentrically/eccentrically: for example, single or multijoint weightlifting exercise, elastic band exercise, isometric and isokinetic exercise with a dynamometer, electronic cycle trainer, finger flexion/extension, gripping exercises and functional electrical stimulation.
- Functional strength training exercises designed to strengthen muscle force generation, train intersegmenal control of the limb and preserve muscle length, so that force is produced fast enough and at lengths and in modes of contraction related to a particular action. Examples include repetitive closed-chain type step-up, leg press and squatting exercises, sit to stand, treadmill walking.
- Practice of functional actions made ineffective by muscle weakness and reduced control of the limb. For example, stair climbing and descent, ramp walking, overground and treadmill walking are practised with the aim of increasing speed and distance walked; also repetitive standing up and sitting down holding a tray, reaching for, picking up and manipulating objects on the ground and above the head.

The first type of exercise can be effective in helping a person elicit activity in an apparently denervated and paralysed muscle group. Attempts to control the muscles eccentrically may be more successful initially than concentric action. Also, a patient who cannot activate a muscle in a shortened position may be able to do so when that muscle is lengthened, where more torque can typically be generated (Bohannon 1986). A short period using an isokinetic exercise machine to train the quadriceps eccentrically and concentrically, with feedback on torque produced, can enable a person to sustain sufficient contraction to prevent knee collapse in standing. Modified gymnasium equipment provides a means of practising the generation, grading and timing of muscle forces.

The second and third types of exercise are aimed at the person who can contract the relevant muscles but lacks sufficient force, has poor timing of force production such as a slowed rate of force development, poor control of a limb or lack of agility. These exercises are more specific to particular actions and are combined with practice of that action. For example, strengthening of lower limb extensor muscles on an isokinetic machine can be followed by the more task-related step-up exercises and by practice of stair walking. Once muscles can generate sufficient contractile force, progressive increase in resistance is added, in high-intensity training at 80% of maximum voluntary strength (i.e., of 1RM*) (Fiatarone et al 1990; Mazzeo et al 1998). Speed of contraction (i.e., ability to reach peak force fast) is trained in exercises performed faster, or with a moderately explosive quality (e.g., small jumps). It has been shown that both high- and low-intensity (40–50% of 1RM) exercise can be effective in improving muscle strength and the control of muscle contraction in healthy elderly individuals (Hortobagyi et al 2001). Few studies as yet have examined carryover effects from strength training to improved functional motor performance. Cramp and colleagues (2006) reported the results of a feasibility study in which individuals within 6–12 months post-stroke were given a low-intensity progressive strengthening programme for the lower limb, in a group. Participants increased isometric and concentric muscle strength and walking speed and these gains were maintained 4–6 weeks after completion of the programme.

Selecting movements that are critical across similar actions may increase the generalizability or *transferability of exercise*. Controlling a multisegmental linkage to interact with both environmental and task requirements is complex but the motor control system appears to use simplifying strategies to control the segmental linkage. For example, cooperation occurs between muscle forces produced over the three joints of the lower limb, varying according to the task and the conditions under which it is performed. Regaining skill in motor performance requires not only the ability to generate muscle forces but also to time these forces (produced by a large number of muscles) as a means of controlling the complex intersegmental relationships throughout the action required to bring about an effective result. Studies of human movement in neuroscience and biomechanics have led to the development of specifically targeted task-oriented exercises designed to increase muscle strength, preserve soft tissue flexibility and train functional motor control. An exercise programme should contain a variety of experiences and activities to prevent boredom, but also to prevent overuse injury.

For example, with the feet on the floor, the lower limbs become a single functional unit in which hips, knees and ankles flex and extend over the feet as a fixed base of support (Fig. 2.5). This basic action is carried out by the lower limb extensor muscles (monoarticular and biarticular) contracting concentrically and eccentrically to raise and lower the body mass. Many of our taken-for-granted everyday actions involve, to varying degrees, this functional unit, for example standing up and sitting down, squatting to pick up an object, parts of the stance phase of walking including stair walking. The individual has to regain the mechanics of this basic action, characteristics of which can be applied to similar actions with minor modifications. Practice of lower limb weightbearing exercises such as repetitive step-ups and modified squatting does appear to generalize into improvement of other actions

---

*1RM = maximum load that can be lifted once

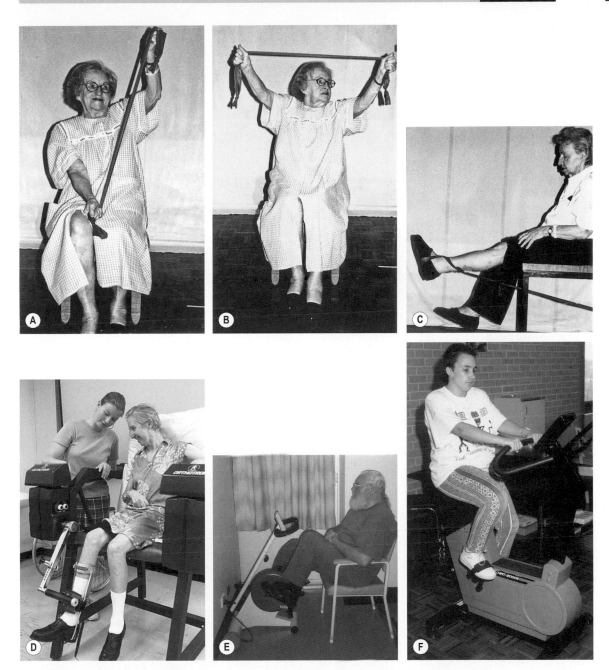

Figure 2.2 (A,B,C) Elastic band exercises focussed on shoulder and shoulder girdle muscles, and on knee extensor muscles in an open-chain exercise. (D) Isokinetic dynamometer training to increase strength of quadriceps muscles concentrically and eccentrically. (E) Reck MOTOmed® provides resistance or assistance in response to the patient's performance. (F) Pedalling a stationary bicycle can improve lower limb muscle strength, control and flexibility, endurance and cardiorespiratory fitness-depending on the mode (dosage) of training.

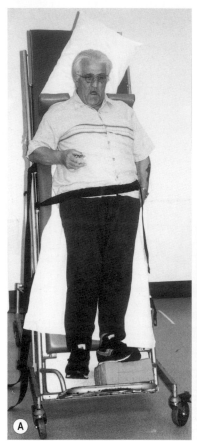

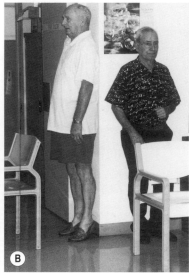

Figure 2.3 (A) Step-ups/downs on a tilt table- a modified closed-chain leg press exercise to train flexion and extension of the affected L leg and increase muscle force generation. (B) Two stations in circuit training. Left: Heels raise and lower with wall as security. Right: Modified squats against the wall. *(Courtesy of F Mackey and colleagues, Illawarra Area Health Service, Australia).*

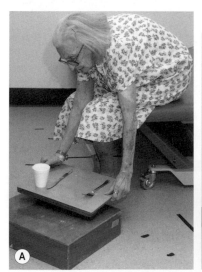

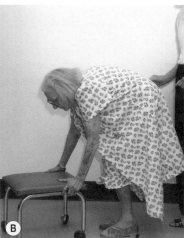

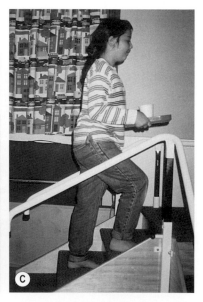

Figure 2.4 (A) Reaching to pick up a tray in sitting- the task was to avoid spilling the water and dislodging the cutlery. (B) Squatting to move a stool on wheels introduces instability. (C) This girl who has ataxia and balance difficulties after a head injury is carrying a tea tray upstairs and downstairs to practise steadiness.

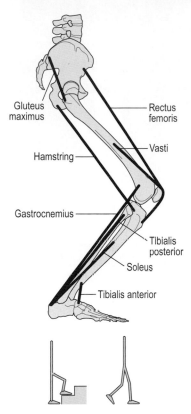

Figure 2.5 Diagram showing lower limb segments and eight functional muscle groups affecting segmental rotation. *(From Kuo and Zajac (1993) by kind permission of Elsevier Science, Amsterdam, The Netherlands).*

that utilize the basic flexion–extension pattern, such as walking (Nugent et al 1994; Dean et al 2000; Sherrington et al 2003, 2004; Salbach et al 2004; Olivetti et al 2007), sit-to-stand (Hsiao & Newham 1999), balance in standing (Sherrington & Lord 1997; Weiss et al 2000; Britton et al 2008) and stair climbing (Bohannon & Walsh 1991).

People who can move about well may, however, lack the agility and speed of reaction time that is necessary to avoid a fall when a trip is imminent. Agility is a function of coordination, strength, power, endurance, reaction time and speed of movement. These variables determine how quickly the body can change direction (ACSM 2006a,b). Practice of quick small steps to the side, forward and backward, stepping on scattered floor markers, small jumps and one-legged hops and ball games may help the development of improved agility.

Weightbearing strength training exercises for the lower limbs

Step up and step down. Hip, knee and ankle extensor muscles are trained to work cooperatively, concentrically

and eccentrically, to raise and lower the body mass. Forces are distributed over the three joints when stepping up and down in a forward direction, and are more concentrated at the knee in lateral step-ups (Agahari et al 1996). Resistance is supplied by the body mass, and effort is increased by raising the step height. The exercise is practised in a safety harness or on a tilt table if necessary (Fig. 2.6).

Heels raise and lower from a step. Ankle plantarflexors are critical muscles, providing power for propulsion in the stance phase of walking and enabling walking up a slope. They contribute to ankle stability and the control of forward postural sway. This exercise actively stretches the calf muscles and is therefore important for preserving the muscle length that is critical for push-off in gait and for the performance of many weightbearing actions (Fig. 2.7).

Squatting. Semi-squatting is practised by reaching down to pick up (or touch) a target object. The depth of squat can be modified, with the target object placed on a stool or on the floor. Repetitive small squats can also be practised (Fig. 2.8).

Sit-to-stand. Major force generation comes from the quadriceps muscles together with other lower limb extensors. If muscles are weak, seat height is increased so less muscle force is required. As muscles become stronger, seat height is lowered and the number of repetitions is increased to improve endurance. The paretic limb is forced to bear weight by placing the paretic foot behind the non-paretic before movement starts. The action is performed at close to normal speed, that is not slowly (Fig. 2.9).

The above exercises are practised repetitively, with maximum repetitions (up to 10 with no rests) in sets of three, with a short break between sets. A counter is a useful aid for the patient to keep track of repetitions. Resisted lower limb flexion/extension exercises can also be practised on an isokinetic dynamometer or exercise trainer (see Fig. 2.2D–F).

Non-weightbearing strength training exercises for the lower limbs

In these exercises, resistance is provided by free weights, weight machines (e.g., dynamometer) and elastic bands. With the goal of increasing the ability of a muscle or group of muscles to generate and control force, these exercises can be practised independently and as part of group exercise and circuit training. Although concurrent task practice is necessary for neural adaptation and learning to occur, in very weak patients small changes in lower limb strength gained by non-weightbearing exercises may produce relatively large changes in motor performance (Buchner et al 1996).

Svantessen and colleagues (2000) suggest that training activities in rehabilitation that emphasise eccentric–concentric exercise may result in more normal function

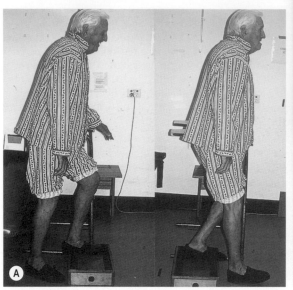
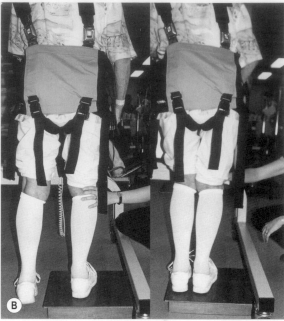

Figure 2.6 (A) Left: Repetitive practice of step-up exercise to train concentric control of the lower limbs & strengthen limb extensor muscles of L leg. He could do 10 reps without a pause. The table is there to give him confidence – he touches it only when he must. Right: Repetitive practice of step-downs to train eccentric control & strengthen limb extensor muscles of L leg. He could do 6 reps without a pause. *(Reproduced from Carr JH, Shepherd RB in Mehrholz J (2008), Frühphase Schlaganfall, with permission from Thieme, Stuttgart).* (B) Training of step-ups and downs in harness. Left: Her R leg extensor muscles are very weak and the therapist guides her knee movement preventing an uncontrolled movement into hyperextension. Right: On this occasion she can do only a few reps with a short pause when she places her foot on the step. She will progress on to more reps with no pauses, with the right foot at the edge of the stool.

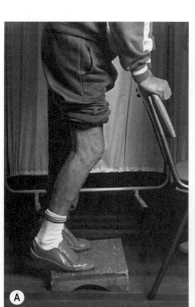
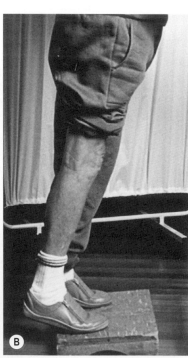
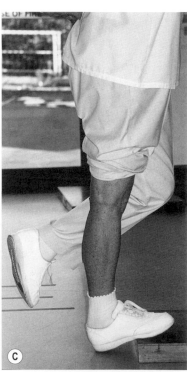

Figure 2.7 Heels raise & lower is an exercise to practise controlling the 3 joints of the lower limb, strengthen and actively stretch the calf muscles. (A) It is difficult to control the right hip and knee while lowering the heels to the floor and raising them. *(Reproduced from Carr JH, Shepherd RB in Mehrholz J (2008), Frühphase Schlaganfall, with permission from Thieme, Stuttgart).* (B) He is getting the idea and although he can lower the heels (an eccentric action) it is difficult to lift them higher (a concentric action) as the calf muscles are weak. (C) This woman has progressed and can do the whole movement on one leg. She is actively stretching and strengthening calf muscles.

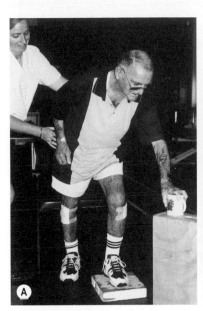
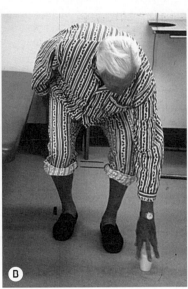
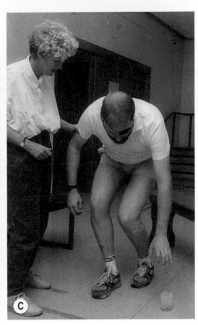

Figure 2.8 Squatting exercise is modified according to the person's ability- the method of practice is progressively challenging as the person improves. (A) He does repetitive small squats with the weak left leg taking most of the load. He alternates legs as his right leg is also weak. (B) This man has progressed and can now squat down to pick up the cup from the floor. He has a rather wide base. (C) A more difficult squat, with a narrow tandem stance.

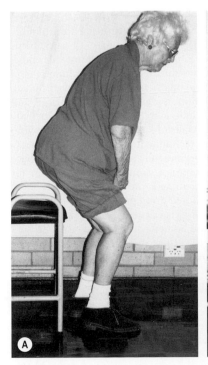
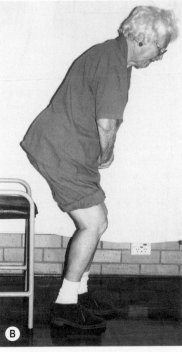

Figure 2.9 Repetitive standing up & sitting down exercise. At this stage she practises from a higher seat which requires less extensor muscle force at hips, knees, ankles. As she gets stronger with more control over the movement the seat will be progressively lowered. (A) The foot of her stronger leg is automatically placed back as this enables the left leg to bear the body weight load. Done this way the exercise will not increase the strength of the weaker right leg. (B) The therapist reminds her to corrects her foot placement so that the weaker right leg is placed back. Now she practises a maximum number of reps with the right leg bearing more of the load. This will increase extensor muscle strength.

and enhance recovery. The weightbearing exercises above meet that criterion but non-weightbearing, open-chain exercises can also be performed in concentric/eccentric combination on an isokinetic machine for example leg press exercises.

As a general rule, in order to increase strength, individuals perform the number of continuous repetitions, without rests, that takes them to the point of mild *muscle fatigue*. They take a short rest, then repeat the exercise with the same number of repetitions for three sets of maximum repetitions. In a study of able-bodied adults training to increase strength of elbow flexors, subjects showed a greater short-term increase in strength when they exercised without rests than when rests were allowed (Rooney et al 1994). They performed 6 (progressing to 10) lifts of a 6RM load (the greatest load that could be lifted 6 times) at each session. Those in the rest group rested for 30 seconds between lifts. These results are interesting since in the clinic patients may perform too few repetitions to enable an increase in muscle strength (or to stimulate learning) for fear that they will tire. The dilemma is, of course, that the less people do the more fatiguable their muscles become. Provided the person's medical condition is satisfactory, repetition as well as progressive effort are critical to a successful training programme and patients need to understand that a degree of muscle fatigue and even some mild muscle soreness is normal after exercise.

Some part of exercise and training of actions involves having the patient move as fast as possible (or at least to increase speed). Difficulty generating and timing peak force in order to move fast is known to be a major problem following acute brain lesion, and *decreased rate of peak force development* (power) affects many functional actions, including manipulation tasks, walking and the ability to balance. Loss of strength and power has significant functional effects for elderly people and those with chronic neural lesions, resulting, for example, in adverse effects on sudden stops and starts, and recovery from a trip (Cao et al 1998; Hortobagyi et al 2001).

Modification of practice is frequently necessary to enable practice to go ahead. For example, everyday actions that require substantial muscle force may need to be modified early in training in order to provide graded practice. For example, sit-to-stand requires a strong burst of muscle activity in the knee extensor muscles in particular, but also in coordination with the hip and ankle extensor muscles, around the time the thighs lift off the seat (see Fig. 4.5). Practice of sit-to-stand without sufficient strength in the muscles of one leg results in adaptive performance in which the other leg is favoured and the hands are used to aid vertical propulsion and balance. When an action is modified by raising the seat height, less muscle force has to be produced to raise the body at thighs-off as the body does not have to move so far and the amplitude of joint movement is not so great. The patient can practise this modified version with the foot of the weaker leg placed

further back than the other, in this way 'forcing' the weaker leg to exercise. As the muscles become stronger, the seat can be incrementally lowered, in this way providing progressive resistance exercise (body mass providing resistance for longer and over a progressively greater joint range) in a task-related manner. This type of exercise is likely to transfer to improved performance of similar actions in which the body mass pivots over the feet as the base of support.

In any comprehensive exercise programme, consideration should be given to details such as *intensity* (how difficult), *duration* (how long), *frequency* (how often) and the *type of activities* to be done. This will depend on clinicians' evaluation of what actions need to be relearned and what impairments create obstacles. A hospital or rehabilitation centre-based programme for a person who has had an acute brain lesion should take place in sessions throughout the day. This may seem idealistic given the present circumstances in many centres, however it is probably unrealistic to continue with therapy sessions that are not active, that do not focus on the patient as a learner or foster an environment that encourages participation and activity. A scientifically-based model is already provided for us by the sports and fitness programmes that are becoming increasingly available not only for elite athletes but also for unfit older members of the community and those who have cardiac dysfunction. The ACSM puts out frequently updated guidelines for mode of exercise, intensity, duration and frequency of exercise, including guidelines for individuals with many clinical conditions, and for the elderly and children.

For each individual, *the programme is designed by the team to address the person's specific needs*. Particular areas of function may take priority at different times; all participants will probably need to increase their flexibility, their functional or task-specific muscle strength, endurance and aerobic fitness. Recreational activities can also be included. A training prescription for an individual (dosage and content) should include exercises specific to the activity being learned and details of specific exercises designed to enhance motor unit recruitment patterns. Repetitive practice engages the neuromuscular system and can enhance subsequent performance. A summary of guidelines for functional strength training is provided in Box 2.1.

Heart rate is monitored throughout exercise if required. An estimate of % HR_{max} is calculated as 220-age (see Box 3.7). For other more accurate measures consult ACSM's guidelines (2006a:144–145). A few minutes of warm-up activities may be helpful before the start of an intensive session. It increases blood flow, increases heart rate gradually and decreases muscle stiffness.

Active muscle stretching. Due to weakness and subsequent inactivity, the natural tendency is for soft tissues to become stiffer and shorter. Increased stiffness in the paretic plantarflexors has been reported to occur as early

- Exercises should be task-oriented – step-ups, squats, push-ups – and specific to tasks being learned plus standing up/sitting down, walking, stair climbing/descent, reaching to targets
- Encourage patient to exercise as intensively as possible, to the point of mild muscle fatigue*
- Grade the amount of resistance and number of repetitions to the individual's ability
- Utilize resistance from body weight, free weights, elastic bands, isokinetic dynamometry, exercise machines, inclined treadmill, depending on specific effects required and the existing muscle control and strength
- Vary body weight resistance by changing step height, chair height, weight of object being lifted
- As a general rule, a maximum number of repetitions should be performed (<10) without a rest and repeated in three sets, with a short break between sets
- In progressive resistance weight training, the person attempts between 3 and 20 repetitions of 50% of the maximum possible load that can be lifted in one attempt. The same principle for repetitions is followed for task-specific exercises, but using body weight for load
- For endurance, a higher number of repetitions is practised at low levels of load and exercises include stationary cycling, arm cycling and treadmill walking
- For very weak muscles, use methods which facilitate muscle activation and force generation, and include simple exercises, biofeedback, mental practice, functional electrical stimulation.
- A normal breathing pattern should be maintained throughout exercise

*Individuals at risk from high levels of blood pressure should avoid high-intensity resistance training.
Refer to American College of Sports Medicine's Guidelines for Exercise Testing and Prescription 2006.

as 2 months after an acute brain lesion (Malouin et al 1997), although it is likely to occur much earlier as shown in both animal and able-bodied human research. Slow-twitch muscles such as the soleus seem particularly vulnerable if they are rarely exposed to active and passive stretch.

Muscle length is variable throughout life as our activities and time spent being active vary. Preservation of functional length of muscles, in particular of the soleus muscle and hip flexors in the lower limbs, normally occurs due to active stretch achieved naturally during our daily activities. For patients who have immobility imposed upon them, practice of functional exercises that make similar length demands to those of functional activities is required. It is particularly important to practise repetitive standing up and sitting down with feet placed behind the knees as early as possible after stroke as a means of preserving the length of the soleus muscle. This muscle shortens rapidly if the person is inactive, and once short, many actions such as standing up may become severely compromised. It is natural for muscle length, stiffness and strength to adapt to an individual's needs, and when our needs change, it is typical for us to stretch and exercise to improve our flexibility when we plan to play an unaccustomed sport. There is evidence that active stretch during repetitive exercise can increase range of motion (Miller & Light 1997, Teixeira-Salmela et al 1999).

Repetitive practice of functional actions is not only necessary for regaining skill but also preserves the necessary muscle length for performance of that action (Fig. 2.10). However, *passive methods of length preservation* in the very early stages may be necessary for some patients. If practice of standing up modified by a raised seat is too difficult standing on a tilt table with the foot on a wedge for 30 minutes will maintain a passive stretch on the soleus muscle (Fig. 2.10A). It is active stretch, however, that is necessary for preserving functional length (Fig. 2.10C–E).

Increased range of motion after stretching involves biomechanical, neurophysiological and molecular mechanisms. Tension in muscle comprises active and passive components. Stretch can affect the active component by altering neural activity (Hummelsheim & Mauritz 1993) and the passive mechanical component by affecting viscous and elastic properties of the muscle. The mechanisms of increasing muscle length and range of motion are not well understood, but may be found eventually in the cellular and adaptive mechanisms of a muscle fibre (De Deyne 2001). One characteristic of viscoelasticity is that tissues respond to stretch and to being held at a constant length with a decrease in tension, called stress relaxation. During stretch, soft tissues also undergo progressive deformation and can be progressively extended with a constant force. This is called creep (Herbert 2005). Studies of passive stretching typically report short-term increase in length which does not persist.

Physiological effects of strength training. So far there have been relatively few investigations of the neurophysiological effects of strength training in individuals with neural lesions. As we have seen earlier in the chapter, strength training exercises can stimulate neuromuscular changes in able-bodied individuals. Changes include increases in muscle excitation, motor unit activation, efficiency of motoneuron recruitment, inhibition of antagonist muscles, improved synchronization of motor unit firing patterns and evidence of enhanced supraspinal influence (Sale et al 1983; McCartney et al 1987). Strength training can stimulate metabolic, mechanical and structural muscle fibre changes, leading to increased mechanical efficiency of muscle and increased strength and muscle

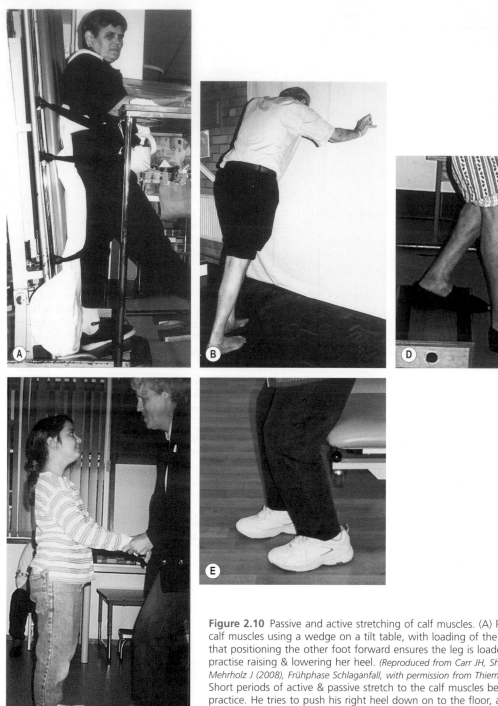

Figure 2.10 Passive and active stretching of calf muscles. (A) Prolonged stretch to calf muscles using a wedge on a tilt table, with loading of the affected leg. Note that positioning the other foot forward ensures the leg is loaded. She can also practise raising & lowering her heel. *(Reproduced from Carr JH, Shepherd RB in Mehrholz J (2008), Frühphase Schlaganfall, with permission from Thieme, Stuttgart).* (B) Short periods of active & passive stretch to the calf muscles between exercise practice. He tries to push his right heel down on to the floor, activating his anterior tibial muscles. (C) As she does repetitive heels raise and lower she actively preserves calf muscle length. (D) Repetitive step-downs actively lengthen calf muscles through full range. (E) Repetitive STS/SIT exercises with the foot of the weaker leg placed well back actively preserves the length of calf muscles.

size. Exercises have the potential to alter passive viscoelastic properties of muscle and tendon. There may also be some advantage gained by an increase in muscle size after stroke (Hakkinen et al 1998), since secondary muscle atrophy can become a factor in disuse weakness. In the elderly, an increase in muscle mass may have functional and metabolic benefits (Harridge et al 1999).

Since the 1980s, increasing numbers of clinical studies are reporting the effects of muscle strengthening in neurorehabilitation. Significant relationships between various measures of muscle strength and measures of motor performance and functional activity have been found in small studies and, more recently, in randomized and controlled trials, in patients with brain lesions and in elderly subjects. Significant increases in muscle strength and/or functional performance have been found in elderly subjects following strength training (Larsson 1982; Frontera et al 1988; Sherrington & Lord 1997; also see ACSM 1998), including high-intensity training (Fiatarone et al 1990, 1994).

Poor functional capacity, muscle weakness and deconditioning are common in older people and can lead to loss of independence. A review in 2002 of the effects of exercise in reducing falls in older people (Gardner et al 2000) concluded that exercise lowered the risk of falls in selected groups. Several clinical studies have reported positive effects in falls prevention after exercise programmes for elderly individuals (e.g., Buchner et al 1997; Lord et al 2003; Li et al 2005; Means et al 2005). Methods used in these programmes included strength training using exercise machines, flexibility and coordination exercises, and Tai Chi practice (see Lord et al 2007 for discussion of this topic).

A review of the literature on weakness after stroke concluded that there was good evidence that strength relates directly to function and that both can be improved by intensive strength training without adverse effects (Ng & Shepherd 2000). Knee muscle (quadriceps) strength in the paretic limb in the first few weeks after stroke and 6 months later was significantly correlated with standing up and walking performance, and also between strength of quadriceps and maximal velocity of movement (Hsiao & Newham 1999). A systematic review of progressive resistance strength training demonstrated increased muscle strength, with some small positive effects of exercise on walking, sit-to-stand and stair climbing (Morris et al 2004). Positive strength–function relationships have been reported by other investigators (Bohannon 1986; Nadeau et al 1999; Teixeira-Salmela et al 1999; Andrews & Bohannon 2001; Chae et al 2002a,b; Ada et al 2006; Olivetti et al 2007; Lee et al 2008).

The results of recent reviews point to the need for investigation of the effects of different types of strength training (van Peppen et al 2004; Ada et al 2006). There is yet to be a substantial body of experimental evidence on the effects of specific strength training methods on functional motor performance, endurance and the ability to function effectively in everyday life in individuals with brain disorders. The evidence from these reviews so far illustrates the paucity of scientific investigation of the effects of strength training on functional performance. There may be many reasons for this, including methods of measuring strength, and the type, quality and intensity of exercise training given to participants. Most studies are carried out on heterogeneous groups, with subjects who have varying degrees of force-generating capacity (strength). Strength training improves muscle strength but we need more evidence related to the carryover from strength training to improvement in functional tasks (Eng 2004), and transfer may only occur between actions with biomechanical and functional similarities. It is likely that strength training will be most effective in neurorehabilitation when it is task oriented, with the objective to improve motor control and functional motor performance. The evidence on specificity of effects is very strong and it is intuitive that motor learning as well as increased efficiency of motor control are major factors in improved performance. For some elderly individuals in particular, a functionally significant result might come from an increase in size of muscle, as well as in strength and motor performance.

The exercise programmes that seem to be the most effective are those that target the specific actions to be regained. A good example comes from a systematic review by Sherrington and colleagues (2008a). Among over 9000 elderly people, the rate of falling was reduced by 17%. The most effective programmes contained a combination of a high total dose (>50 h or a twice-weekly exercise programme for 25 weeks), challenging balancing exercises in standing with the aim of standing with feet close together, or on one leg, minimizing use of the hands to assist while moving the body mass. In other words, where it was necessary to improve balance in standing in order to prevent falls, exercises that challenged balance were provided. It should be noted that an additional criterion for effectiveness/success is that programmes contained no walking exercise, and the authors point out that time spent walking would take away from the time spent regaining effective balance.

Another example is a study by Pang and colleagues (2006) that was designed to improve upper limb function with a group of 63 people more than 1 year after a stroke. The group improved on the Wolf Motor Function and the Fugl-Meyer tests after a circuit-training programme that lasted for 3 hours per week for 19 weeks. The three-station programme included elastic-band-resisted exercises for the shoulder, weightbearing exercises, weight-resisted elbow and wrist exercises, hand muscle strengthening, functional actions and electrical stimulation for those with less than 20° of active wrist extension.

Single joint, open chain exercise against resistance may be most effective in improving a muscle's contractility where a muscle is poorly innervated and very weak, whereas beyond a certain (unknown) threshold strength training should be multijoint and task specific. The major functions of lower limbs are support of body mass and movement of that mass in vertical and horizontal directions in a gravitational environment. It is likely therefore that closed-chain weightbearing strength training exercises performed for many repetitions and at sufficient intensity, using strength training guidelines and against the resistance of body weight and additional weights, are the exercises most likely to improve functional performance of lower limbs. There is increasing evidence that this is so (Ada et al 2006). These exercises take into account motor learning and intersegmental motor control as they are task oriented and allow the possibility of transfer to several actions with similar biomechanics. An interesting study of treadmill exercise over a 3-month period in individuals with stroke showed increases in volitional torque (concentric and eccentric) in hamstrings that correlated with increased mobility and function as measured by timed up-and-go and walking tests (Smith et al 1999).

More research is also needed to establish the optimal methods of strength training for particular groups of individuals. Several theoretical issues about the relationship between strength and function need to be kept in mind; in particular, that the threshold strength for effective function is activity specific (Buchner & de Latour 1991). Related to that is a study by Buchner and colleagues (1996) in which they successfully tested the hypothesis that the relationship between muscle strength and gait speed in an elderly group of subjects would be non-linear. They suggest that a non-linear relationship illustrates a mechanism by which small changes in physiological capacity in frail adults may produce relatively large effects on performance, while large changes in capacity have little or no effect on daily function in healthy adults. This non-linear relationship could help explain the disparate results of recent studies of resistance training. Following Buchner and colleagues on the relativity of strength and strength thresholds (Buchner et al 1996), a very weak muscle(s) may increase in strength to the point where it is sufficient, for example, to enable a person to stand up. Lomaglio & Eng (2005) found a significant relationship between isokinetic strength of ankle dorsiflexors, plantarflexors and knee extensor muscles and sit-to-stand performance (movement time at self-paced and fast speeds, loading symmetry). Similarly, functional strength tests that involve a limb in a multijoint purposeful movement (e.g., number of sit-to-stand-ups in a given period of time from a seat of specific height) may be more valid measures of strength.

In this chapter we emphasize in particular the importance of strength and endurance training of lower limbs. An individual's ability to move about, be active, to balance when moving while in sitting or standing without over-balancing or falling, are all dependent upon the capacity of the lower limbs to support and balance the body mass. Upper limb function is also dependent on muscles producing sufficient force fast enough for us to carry out, with one or both hands, the complex actions so important for daily life. Simple finger exercises performed repetitively and intensively can be effective in improving hand use (Butefisch et al 1995). Strength is relative to the tasks being performed and emphasis in training of upper limbs is on dexterity, with strength training being carried out as part of task practice, using the objects normally involved in those tasks. Bilateral practice is particularly important. Repetition is a critical part of training. Force requirements are increased by increasing the load to be lifted by such means as adding water to the glass, changing from glass to bottle, lifting objects of different sizes and weights down from high shelves, pushing and pulling objects of different weights, and so on. The addition of constraint of the non-paretic limb to the training process after stroke appears to over-ride the natural tendency to use this limb preferentially, thereby forcing use of the paretic limb. Upper limb movement is also dependent on stability; that is, effective balance mechanisms. Training of upper limb function is described in Chapter 6.

In conclusion, there is strong evidence that patients can benefit from exercise programmes in which functional tasks are directly and intensively trained (van Peppen et al 2004). The authors pointed out that additional benefits were gained by the use of treadmill training with and without body weight support and by constraint of the non-paretic arm in appropriate patients after stroke. Patients benefit from circuit training with work stations that target specific tasks (Dean et al 2000; Sherrington et al 2008b), and from strength training programmes that target functional strength and endurance (Duncan et al 2003; Ada et al 2006). There is increasing evidence that improved functional performance is accompanied by brain reorganization (Luft et al 2004; see Chapter 1).

Training for cardiorespiratory fitness

The extent and time course of change in exercise capacity during rehabilitation has not been studied extensively, and the intensity of exercise and of cardiovascular stress induced during rehabilitation have also received little attention (Kilbreath & Davis 2005). It appears from a few studies of stroke, however, that deconditioning after acute brain lesion may to some extent be a consequence of the relatively static nature of typical rehabilitation programmes (Kelley et al 2003; MacKay-Lyons & Howlett 2005). The results suggest that contemporary stroke rehabilitation programmes may not be sufficiently vigorous to prevent physical deconditioning.

Recently MacKay-Lyons and Makrides (2002) investigated the aerobic component of physical and occupational therapy for stroke patients by monitoring heart rate (using heart rate monitors) and therapeutic activities biweekly over a 14-week period without influencing the content. The major finding was that therapy sessions involved low-intensity exercise and activity that did not provide adequate metabolic stress to induce a training effect. A disproportionate amount of time was spent inactive. When present, the aerobic component of a typical physiotherapy session took less than 3 minutes. Although one might expect progressively higher exercise intensities over time as functional status improves, any increase in HR_{mean} and HR_{peak} did not reach statistical significance.

Implementation of a programme to improve cardiorespiratory fitness by increasing the aerobic component of training during the early rehabilitation period may help to prevent the downward degenerative cycle of decreased physical activity and disability that is frequently reported. Low cardiorespiratory fitness in chronic stroke is said to be secondary to a decrease in exercise capacity, decreased mobility and increased energy expenditure. The criterion measure for aerobic capacity†, peak oxygen consumption (VO_2), may be as low as 50–70% of the age- and sex-matched values of sedentary individuals (Eng et al 2004; MacKay-Lyons & Makrides 2004).

It is well documented that stroke patients have low physical endurance when discharged from rehabilitation, limiting their ability to perform household tasks and to walk outside the home. Loss of independent ambulation, especially outdoors, has been identified as one of the most debilitating of stroke sequelae. Among stroke survivors 1 year post-stroke, the most striking area of difficulty was low endurance as measured by a 6-minute walk test (Mayo et al 2005). Subjects able to complete this test were able to walk on average only 250 m, equivalent to 40% of their predicted ability and not far enough for a reasonable and active lifestyle. The detrimental effect of low exercise capacity and muscle endurance on functional mobility and resistance to fatigue can be compounded by the high metabolic demand of adaptive movements. Endurance is likely to decline further after discharge if follow-up exercise programmes are not available. Furthermore, low aerobic fitness is a significant determinant of poor bone health (specifically osteoporosis) in individuals with chronic stroke (Pang et al 2005). Sustained physical inactivity induces a reduction in aerobic capacity,† limiting the performance of activities of daily living, and increasing the risk of falls and dependence on others.

Although it can be difficult to test fitness after acute brain injury, Mackay-Lyons & Makrides (2002) used a treadmill with 15% body weight support in a maximal exercise test given to patients post-stroke. Submaximal tests can also be valid such as the 6-minute walk test. There is some evidence that exercise trainability early after stroke can be both feasible and safe if appropriate screening by

medical practitioners (see ACSM guidelines 2006a,b) and monitoring of heart rate and blood pressure are used (MacKay-Lyons & Howlett 2005). Training is initiated at conservative intensities. Exercise prescription is discussed in Kilbreath & Davis (2005). Table 2.1 gives a guide to exercise prescription with recommended dosages after stroke. ACSM guidelines (2006a,b) provide details for patient groups with other neurological conditions.

Early indications suggest that walking speed, mobility and balance improve with such programmes. Several studies report positive effects of physical conditioning programmes (involving strength, endurance, flexibility, coordination and cardiorespiratory fitness) in older individuals and following stroke (Fiatarone et al 1994; Lord & Castell 1994; Potempa et al 1995; Macko et al 1997, 2005; Teixeira Salmela et al 1999; Lee et al 2008). In people with progressive neurological disease, increases in strength and endurance and a decrease in fatiguability have been found initially after strength training (Milner-Brown et al 1986; Milner-Brown & Miller 1988a,b).

There are several reports of improved aerobic capacity in chronic stroke with appropriate training such as bicycle ergometry (Potempa et al 1995), graded treadmill walking (Macko et al 1997) and a combination of aerobic and strengthening exercises (Teixeira-Salmela et al 1999). As might be expected, the effects tend to be exercise specific. Generalization occurs, however, in the improvements noted in general health and wellbeing that had positive effects on performance of activities they considered meaningful. Teixeira-Salmela and colleagues (1999) assessed the general level of physical activity of their subjects on the Human Activity Profile, a survey of 94 activities that are rated according to their required metabolic equivalents. The results indicated that subjects were able to perform more household chores and recreational activities after strength and aerobic training. These quality of life gains appear to be critical factors for stroke survivors' reintegration into society. A recent systematic review provides good evidence that aerobic exercise, at 50–80% of heart rate reserve, 3–5 days a week for 20–40 minutes, should be an important component of stroke rehabilitation (Pang et al 2005). Kilbreath & Davis (2005) provide an interesting discussion of the reasons why cardiorespiratory training is so important after acute lesions such as stroke.

The implications are clear. The challenge for clinicians and patients is not only of increasing the time spent in physical activity but also of organizing time to provide sufficient intensity to induce a training effect. Time spent in therapy is a crude estimate of actual intensity, and does not allow an estimate of the effort and energy that was expended during training. Intensity and aerobic content of training need to be addressed specifically and early in individuals with neurological impairments in an effort both to increase exercise capacity and to minimize post-lesion deconditioning.

---

†Aerobic capacity is the product of the capacity of the cardiorespiratory system to supply oxygen (i.e., cardiac output) and the capacity of the skeletal muscle to utilize oxygen (Pang et al 2005).

Table 2.1 Recommended dose of aerobic exercise for post-stroke patients

Programme component	Sub-acute stroke		Chronic stroke	
	Threshold[1]	Recommended[2]	Threshold[1]	Recommended[2]
Frequency	2 times weekly	2–3 times weekly	2–3 times weekly	3–4 times weekly
Intensity	>40% VO_{2peak}, 40% HRR[3]	>50% VO_{2peak}, >50% HRR	40–50% VO_{2peak}, 40–50% HRR	>60% VO_{2peak}, >60% HRR, RPE[4] 12–14
Duration	Minimum 15 min	30+ min	Minimum 20 min	30–45 min
Mode	Interval training	Interval training proceeding to continuous exercise	Interval training	Continuous exercise
Type	Isokinetic Cycling, PBWS[5] – treadmill walking	Stationary cycling (semi-recumbent or upright), isokinetic cycling, treadmill or overground walking, elliptical stepping	Treadmill walking (if needed PBWS), isokinetic cycling, stationary cycling (semi-recumbent or upright), overground walking, elliptical stepping	Treadmill walking, overground walking, isokinetic cycling, stationary cycling (semi-recumbent or upright), elliptical stepping, other types for leg muscles based on patient preference
Monitoring	ECG,[6] heart rate, blood pressures (3–5 min), signs and symptoms,[7] RPE	ECG (if appropriate), heart rate, blood pressures, signs and symptoms, RPE	Heart rate, blood pressures (3–5 min), RPE	Heart rate, blood pressures, RPE
Comments				RPE 12–14 ('somewhat hard') may be used with experienced patients to estimate an appropriate exercise intensity

[1]Generally defined as the minimum 'dose' of an exercise programme component to elicit a gain of cardiorespiratory fitness in previously sedentary patients. [2]Generally defined as the 'optimum dose' of an exercise programme component to elicit a gain of cardiorespiratory fitness in patients currently undertaking exercise. [3]Heart rate reserve (HR_{peak}–HR_{rest}). [4]Rating of perceived exertion. [5]Partial body weight supported. [6]Electrocardiogram. [7]For example, clinical symptoms of exertional intolerance, dyspnoea, chest pain, pallor, nausea, headache or other symptoms associated with unstable hypertension.
(Adapted from Kilbreath & Davis 2005).

MOTOR LEARNING AND SKILL ACQUISITION IN THE RESTORATION OF OPTIMAL FUNCTIONAL PERFORMANCE

Skill has been defined in many ways. One definition with explanatory value for the clinic is from Annett (1971):

skill is any human activity that becomes better organized and more effective as the result of practice.

It is also described as the ability to consistently attain a goal with some economy of effort (Gentile 2000). Our everyday motor activities (walking, standing up, picking up a glass of water) are motor skills – they are complex actions made up of body segment movements linked together in an appropriate spatial and temporal sequence to fulfil an intention, to achieve a goal. The development of skill in a novel task takes place in overlapping stages – first the learner gets the idea of the movement (this is the cognitive stage), then he/she must develop the ability to adapt the movement pattern to the demands of different environments (Gentile 2000).

When an adult has a brain lesion affecting the motor control system, skill in action is either lost or severely impaired as a result of disordered voluntary muscle activation and inability to control the pattern of muscle activations. The person can no longer perform actions that were previously easily performed. This process of loss can occur gradually over time in progressive conditions affecting the neural system or suddenly after an acute lesion. After an initial period of recovery from an acute lesion, any change in motor performance probably occurs through a process of learning (adaptation). However, what is it that is learned, what does this involve at the neural level and what are the most effective methods of regaining skill? Is there a difference between these processes and those that occur in non-brain-lesioned individuals when they learn a new skill? There are so far no answers to most of these questions. We do know, however, what methods seem to result in able-bodied individuals increasing their skill and we assume that those methods are likely to be effective with individuals who have neuromuscular dysfunctions. In a distributed system that utilizes multiple connections in order to translate a goal into action, damage to or malfunction of one part requires a process of recovery with reorganization of intact pathways and connections. As a result, the relearning process must resemble in some ways the process that occurs when someone learns a novel action. Increasing attention is being paid to the neural mechanisms underlying brain reorganization using new brain imaging technologies, and some of these findings are presented in Chapter 1.

What do we mean by the term motor learning? We make the assumption that the acquisition of skill, involving practice and exercise, is a manifestation of internal processes making up what is called motor learning. Magill (2001) defines learning as a change in the ability of a person to perform a skill, and points out that learning itself cannot be directly observed but can only be *inferred* from our observations of a relatively consistent improvement in performance of an action, retained over time. We note a relatively stable change in an observable motor behaviour as a result of a set of processes involving exercise and practice (Schmidt 1988; Magill 2001). This is why certain characteristics of motor performance are measured in rehabilitation at the start of training and at various stages throughout and after training. Note, however, that although improved performance is a positive finding, it is not itself evidence of learning. This is obtained by follow-up testing of retention over a period of time.

Another characteristic of learning of relevance to clinical practice is *adaptability*. As Magill (2001) points out, improved performance is adaptable to a variety of different contexts. The context in which we perform a particular action is rarely the same. The clinical implication is, of course, that a training programme must give an individual the opportunity to perform in different contexts. This is illustrated in Chapters 4 to 7.

The process of learning

Two interdependent learning processes, operating in parallel, have been proposed to underlie skill acquisition (Gentile 1998, 2000). Gentile describes these processes and makes implications for training methods that might have the greatest effect on learning within the rehabilitation process.

Explicit learning is directed toward achieving a specific goal, for example standing up from sitting, and, if successful, results in a 'mapping' of the individual's body morphology in relation to environmental conditions. A topographical 'map' of how the body moves through space toward the standing position can be illustrated by the therapist (e.g., see Fig. 2.12). With practice, this relationship is modified to increase the likelihood of success. If small changes are made to the task, for example by holding a tray while standing up (see Fig. 4.24), the system is capable of adapting the movement's topology or shape to suit various environments and tasks of a similar nature.

Implicit learning is about the actual movement dynamics. While the early learning phase takes the learner to the stage where the movement's structure is 'good enough' to meet task demands, with practice, active and passive intersegmental forces become finely tuned, increasing performance efficiency. Since the process of controlling forces is not conscious, learning is referred to as implicit.

In clinical practice, individuals who have movement disabilities of acute onset typically have to learn again how to perform everyday tasks, and understanding the nature of skill learning provides the therapist with a guide to how to organize training. It can be very difficult for a patient to perform even a simple everyday action due to extreme weakness in muscle force generation and loss of coordination. Intensive and repetitive exercises designed to stimulate muscle activity, increase force production and limb coordination, and train balance mechanisms need to be included in the programme of task practice.

The major aim of intervention in neurorehabilitation is ultimately the optimization of motor performance, that is the regaining of effective performance in the motor actions of daily living. Physiotherapists are becoming increasingly aware of patients as active participants and learners rather than as passive recipients of therapy. Patients have to learn again how to perform the functional motor actions in which they were previously skilled, but this time with a lesioned system. They need to know that rehabilitation requires hard work and sustained attentional focus, and that the endeavour has considerable rewards.

Fluency of movement is an important criterion of skilled motor behaviour. Movement becomes more efficient with learning and this is probably due to improvements in timing, tuning and coordination of muscle activations (Rosenbaum 1991). The learning (relearning) process for disabled individuals with muscle paralysis or weakness is closely related to the greater ease of movement arising out of increased efficiency of muscle, that is increased force-generating capacity and timing, increased endurance and physical fitness.

Adaptations. When individuals try to move after an acute lesion, their first attempts reflect the distribution of muscle weakness and the resultant adaptive motor pattern. At initial attempts, adaptive movement emerges spontaneously and appears to reflect the best action possible given the state of the neural and musculoskeletal systems and the dynamic possibilities of a multisegmental system (Fig. 2.11). If walking very slowly, holding the leg stiffly appears reasonably effective initially in achieving the goal of independent mobility; it is repeated and may become habitual. This can be a disadvantage once the person has returned home, since such walking is not so effective outside the sheltered rehabilitation environment.

In attempting to generate sufficient muscle force, output may be relatively uncontrolled. Dyscontrol may be demonstrated by muscle co-contraction to stiffen the limb in order to restrict the degrees of freedom to be controlled, or by excessive force with difficulty reducing it to the level required for the action (see Fig. 6.11). Bernstein (1967) suggested that novices control mobile segmental linkages by cutting down on the joints that are free to move, that is by locking some joints, only freeing them up as they gain more experience. This proposal was confirmed in a study of pistol shooting (Arutyunyan et al 1968). Novices initially held wrists and elbows rigid, then released them as they developed skill. A similar result was reported for dart throwing (McDonald et al 1989). In able-bodied individuals, as skill increases, counterproductive or

unnecessary movements tend to decrease (Sparrow 1983; Sparrow & Irizarry-Lopez 1987).

Reducing unnecessary muscle activity. A skilled performer demonstrates less energy expenditure than one who is unskilled. This is probably due to a number of factors associated with the elimination of unnecessary muscle activity. Training consists therefore of teaching the person to control muscle output, in other words, to match force generation to the needs of the task, to fine tune muscle activation. As skill increases, there should be a minimum expenditure of energy consistent with the goal to be achieved (MacConaill & Basmajian 1969), with greater efficiency of force production and decreased energy expenditure. Decreased EMG output has been noted in several investigations of able-bodied subjects as they increased their skill (e.g., Mulder & Hulstijn 1985; Sale 1987), indicating that, as a result of training, muscles become more effective in producing tension, recruiting fewer motor units or lowering the firing rate of motor units.

Since the environment plays a significant role in modulating motor performance, specific aspects of the environment or of a task can be utilized to channel and drive motor output. Similarly, if an action is too difficult for an individual with movement dysfunction, some feature of the environment can be modified to make the task achievable.

Modifications. The environment can be altered to set up conditions that are likely to elicit muscle activity. Examples include the following:

- Objects are placed so that reaching for them requires increased external rotation of the glenohumeral joint (see Fig. 6.15).
- In training standing up from a seat, pressure down the shank holds the foot on the floor so that contraction of the quadriceps rotates the thigh over the fixed shank rather than extending the knee and lifting the foot from the floor (see Fig. 4.16).
- Walking on a treadmill naturally produces a larger amplitude of hip extension (a longer stride) than overground walking. This stretches the hip flexor and soleus muscles; they contract eccentrically prior to hip flexion and ankle plantarflexion at push-off (see Ch. 5), and facilitate the swing forward of the leg.

The action itself can be modified to provide constraint of unwanted actions. A good example of behaviour modification is the use of physical constraint of the non-paretic upper limb so that use of the paretic limb during task-oriented upper limb training is mandatory (see Ch. 7). Use of the paretic lower limb for bearing weight in standing up is ensured by placing the foot of the paretic limb behind the foot of the stronger leg (see Fig. 2.9). This forces loading of the weaker leg as the stronger is at a mechanical disadvantage. A neck collar enables a person who cannot easily raise the head to sit erect, pay attention

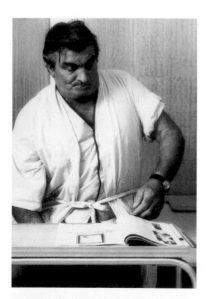

Figure 2.11 After stroke, adaptations to weakness or paralysis of shoulder flexors & external rotators includes for this man activity of muscles that are innervated. The resulting movement is made up of shoulder girdle elevation, lateral flexion of the spine with some spinal rotation. These movements allow him to move his hand forward and place it on the page.

to the surroundings and take in inputs that aid in regaining the sense of horizontality and verticality. Enabling the person to make the most of visual experiences may also increase her level of alertness and participation in surrounding events.

Perceptual and cognitive factors

Action comprises not only motor factors but also cognitive and perceptual factors. The obvious conceptual links between knowing and doing (Newell 1981), that is cognition and action, are increasingly recognized. After acute brain lesion (stroke, traumatic brain injury), poor attentional performance or poor memory can have a negative impact on daily functioning (McDowd et al 2003), since the ability to pay attention and concentrate are critical for motor learning (Schmidt 1988; Magill 2001). There is an increasing body of clinical literature in which the need to recognize and incorporate the action–cognition link in neurorehabilitation is examined (Carr & Shepherd 2000, 2003; Shumway-Cook & Woollacott 2005). In everyday life, most of our actions are linked to an intention. In working toward a goal, we pay attention to the most relevant information available.

In chronic neurological conditions and after acute brain trauma, attentional capacity may be depleted and extra input may be required to help the person pay attention. One of the important functions of the therapist (as coach) is setting up the conditions of practice to facilitate this process. Small details such as engaging eye contact between patient and therapist can encourage attentiveness and increase motivation (Mehrabian 1969). A reminder to look at the object or at particularly relevant aspects of the environment may be necessary when an individual is easily distracted or when attention is inappropriately focused. McDowd and colleagues (2003) have pointed out that minimizing disability after an acute brain lesion requires a better understanding of the link between cognitive abilities and outcome, and the inclusion of attention and memory training in rehabilitation of individuals with cognitive difficulties.

Motivation

We have to want to do what we are learning to do. Motivation can be provided by reward, by positive reinforcement, by an understanding of the goals and their relevance to the individual. With a concrete goal it is clear what is to be done and whether or not the goal was achieved. This may not be so with a more abstract goal. Both success and failure appear to be motivating forces, and in the early stages of learning can increase the person's level of aspiration and preparedness to try hard and take up the challenge. Seeing that an action is possible, even if it is a modified version of the action, seems important to developing the perseverence necessary to develop skill.

Belmont and colleagues (1969) suggested that the possibility of brain-damaged patients requiring 'unique motivating conditions for performance has received little consideration' and this is probably true 40 years later. Some individuals following acute brain lesion may appear unmotivated and relatively passive if left to practise on their own. There may be a number of reasons for this, including poor memory, distractibility, perceptual–cognitive dysfunction, depression and, in non-stimulating surroundings, boredom. Patients can become very isolated from others, even in a busy department, and opportunities for interaction with others may make a difference to the way they view their own difficulties and the rehabilitation process. Group work should begin very early in rehabilitation and people can be encouraged to work together in the supervised environment of the exercise area. Stress, tension and anxiety, although they may not adversely affect motor performance, may depress it under certain conditions (Singer 1980), particularly in terms of complex tasks. Individuals in an institutional environment can develop what has been termed 'learned helplessness', described by Seligman in 1975. Perception of lost effectiveness in events that a person tries repeatedly to control can result in anxiety and this may be followed by depression, characterized by apathy and by giving up that generalizes to other facets of life.

Apparent lack of motivation, however, may also indicate that the tasks to be practised have little meaning or relevance for the patient. Physiotherapy may lack motivating impact if it is not immediately and obviously relevant to the person's needs, or not sufficiently difficult or challenging to require concentration and the person's full attention. The rehabilitation environment may be non-motivating by being undemanding and insufficiently geared to the patient as an active participant and learner. The following sections describe some of the factors that seem critical to learning and the development of effective and efficient motor performance.

Focus of attention: instruction, demonstration and feedback

The ability to focus attention on a task, to shift attention from one task to another or from one environmental feature to another, to sustain concentration and ignore irrelevant inputs, and to do more than one thing at a time (e.g., walk and talk) are critical to everyday functional ability. Magill (2001) has pointed out that we can attend consciously to only so much at one time. We manage in our complex daily lives provided we do not exceed the limits of our information processing system. Attention can be one of the most significant limitations influencing learning and performance. We often have difficulty doing more than one thing at a time, when we need to divide our attention. We have limited resources. In particular, doing two things at once may exceed our limit if both tasks demand a great deal of attention. As an example, driving a car in heavy traffic and having a difficult telephone conversation at the same time may cause us to have an accident or to say something we may regret.

There is some evidence that our capacity to divide our attention declines as we age. Much of the research on the effects of ageing has been carried out using specially-designed and sometimes quite complex laboratory experiments, and other cognitive factors such as memory may not be taken into account. Nevertheless, it does appear that type of task seems to be an important factor. Two more naturalistic studies by Chen and colleagues (1994, 1996) illustrated the effect of overload on the attentional capacities of healthy older compared to younger people. One study compared the performance of subjects presented with an unexpected obstacle that they had to step over while walking. Results showed that differences due to age were present but rather minor (Chen et al 1994). In a later study, subjects were presented with the obstacle but also had to make a vocal response to an unexpected light source. Both younger and older individuals showed significant declines in their walking performance but the decline was much greater in the older group (Chen et al 1996). These and other studies provide information about the potential reasons for falls as people age (see also Lord et al 2007).

Internal and external focus of attention

Paying attention is critical during practice of a task that is difficult for the individual. The early stage of task learning involves identifying what has to be learned, and understanding the ways by which the goal can be accomplished. In motor training, for a goal to be pursued with enthusiasm, it needs to be perceived as worthwhile and meaningful to that individual. As an example, tasks that have goals directed toward controlling one's physical interaction with objects or persons in the immediate environment seem to have more meaning than goals that are directed at movement for its own sake (for review see Wulf 2007). Recent findings with healthy subjects have demonstrated the positive effects on performance and skill development of directing attention toward the effect of the movement, whether or not the goal is achieved (an external focus), rather than to the movement itself (an internal focus) (Wulf et al 1999, 2000, 2002). For example, holding a glass full of water while standing up (two tasks) focuses attention on not spilling the water; when walking among obstacles on the floor, attention is on where they are, how high they are, how wide. Wulf and colleagues suggest that paying attention to the outcome and not the movement helps the system to self-organize (Wulf et al 1998, 2001). Their findings suggest that when learners focus internally on their movements, this may constrain or interfere with automatic control processes that would normally regulate the movement (Wulf et al 2001).

Recent studies of individuals with Parkinson's disease (PD) or stroke have similar findings. Using three everyday tasks involving the upper limb, focusing on the object to be moved (can, apple, coffee mug) produced better movement coordination (shorter movement time, greater peak velocity) in a group of people with PD than focusing on the arm movement (Fasoli et al 2005). Focusing attention on the surface under their feet produced more effective balance control in a group with stroke than focusing on getting equal pressure under each foot (Landers et al 2005). Focusing attention on minimizing movement of the unstable rubber disk (external focus) on which they stood and balanced rather than on reducing movements of their feet (internal focus) resulted in less body sway (Wulf et al 2009).

In the early stages of rehabilitation after an acute brain lesion, however, when the patient is struggling to contract muscles and control movements, the focus may have to be on critical details of the action. However, focus of attention can still be external but directed toward body topology – the shape of the movement described on a diagram ('Swing your shoulders forward and up') or toward taking large steps (in terms of distance covered, not leg movement itself). As muscle function, motor control and skill increase, the patient's focus of attention shifts. In walking, attention may shift from taking a longer step to focusing on the height of the obstacle ahead; the focus in sit-to-stand may change from placing the feet back and increasing the speed of standing up to steadying a glass of water while standing up.

Methods of communication between therapist and patient in neurorehabilitation deserve more consideration than is typical in clinical practice. Commonly used learning methods for conveying information about the goal or the action itself include demonstration (modelling) of the action to be relearned (Fig. 2.12), with verbal instructions about key aspects of the action pattern (e.g., Gentile 1998, 2000). Different instructions can produce different effects on the person's motor performance.

Concrete versus abstract goals. There is evidence that individuals perform better when an action is presented as a concrete rather than an abstract task. These two types of task differ in the degree to which the required action is directed toward controlling one's physical interaction with the environment as opposed to merely moving a limb. van der Weel and colleagues (1991) described an experiment in which the difference between performance on a concrete task (beating a drum) compared to an abstract task which required the same action (pronation and supination of the forearm) was examined. The subjects were nine children with hemiplegic cerebral palsy (CP) aged between 3 and 7 years. The children significantly increased movement range of both pronation and supination during performance of the concrete task, beating two drums by alternately supinating and pronating the forearms,

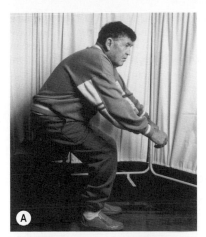

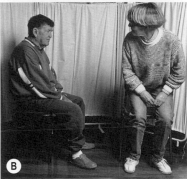

Figure 2.12 (A) He can stand up on most attempts but he produces horizontal momentum to move his body mass forward over his feet by swinging his arms forward. (B) An example of observational learning- he watches as the therapist demonstrates the topology or shape of the movement as she swings the upper body forward (shoulders forward over the knees) and up into standing. She emphasizes to him that the legs must do the work. He could practise repetitive STS-SIT with arms folded over chest.

compared to the abstract task. Supination range increased by more than 20% in the concrete task.

In explanation, the authors point out that movement is not an independent process but an integral part of an act. The extent and quality of movement depend on how much practice the individual has in performing the action, how interested the person is and the quality of the information available. Concrete tasks are associated with more information from the environment than abstract tasks. The drum in this experiment provided visual, auditory and tactile information about the individual's relationship with it and feedback about the attainment of the goal. The abstract task provided no concrete information, just 'reach as far as you can'.

Another study (Leont'ev & Zaporozhets 1960) had patients with restricted range of motion of the elbow or

shoulder as a result of injury raise their arm in four actions that varied from abstract to concrete. The actions were to raise the arm: (1) as far as possible with eyes shut; (2) as far as possible with eyes open; (3) to a specific point on a ruled screen; and (4) to grasp an object. The results indicated that the amplitude of movement increased progressively from task 1 to task 4, as the task became more concrete.

Instructions

Instructions should be short and present a clear goal. Magill (2001) has pointed out that verbal instructions about critical environmental features or critical performance characteristics can have a negative effect. Instructions may cause the learner to pay too much attention to a particular feature and not enough to the task itself. Instructions may actually degrade performance if they are inappropriate or too many, or if they contain too much information. They may make the task so attention demanding that the learner experiences information overload (Wulf & Weigelt 1997).

A patient in the early stages after stroke or brain surgery, who may be confused, depressed and weak, may need frequent instructional cues about where to focus attention. In the early stages of learning, instructions from the therapist should be brief. They should cue the person to one or two critical features of the action. For example: 'Swing your shoulders forward and stand up' conveys key information and a suggestion to speed up. 'Pick up the glass' (on the floor) may be a sufficient cue for a patient; others, however, may respond better to 'Squat down and pick up the glass', as the instruction cues the person into the major feature of the action. A figure drawing of standing up can reinforce key elements (see Fig. 4.1). As the person internalizes these details, they can start to think more of the goal of the action, for example to shake hands, or to walk to another room. At this later stage of learning, instructing the person to focus on details of their performance can be detrimental. Wulf and colleagues (2000) point out that it is clear that the instructions given by the therapist are very important and the therapist needs be observant of the effects.

Verbal instructions and demonstration are used in the early stages of learning to help the patient develop an image of the fit between his/her morphology and the environment. However, these methods may not facilitate implicit learning. Once the person has the idea of the movement and can achieve the movement goal, or an approximation of it, the therapist organizes varied practice. The teaching goal is to provide practice opportunities that challenge force generation and intersegmental control, by varying the task, extending the possible options and encouraging the prolonged practice necessary for learning to occur (Gentile 1998).

Demonstration

The goal of the action and the movements to be executed can be demonstrated either live or on a computer or video. Empirical work on the effectiveness of demonstration has been sporadic and the results equivocal. One of the reasons for this is that the videotaped demonstration is sometimes distant from actual practice in both time and place. Gonella and colleagues (1981), however, demonstrated that self-instruction using an audiovisual medium could be effective in enabling able-bodied subjects to learn the new skill of crutch walking. The hypothesis that subjects could learn the cognitive aspects of the motor task in one viewing of the film was supported and transfer of learning to the physical performance of the task was found to occur.

Modelling of an action, either by videotape or by the 'coach' performing the action, can help the learner develop an understanding, a mental image or 'conceptual representation' of the action (Carroll & Bandura 1982) or template (Keele & Summers 1976) of the action. Demonstration is given by the therapist who models the action (see Fig. 2.12B), and by a videotape of performance.

Cognition plays a significant role in this *observational learning* since the individual must attend selectively to the model and to critical features of the model. Observation is an aid to learning the temporal and spatial aspects of an action, helping the person get the idea of what the movement looks like – the 'shape' or topology of the movement (see Magill 2001). Demonstration may focus on kinematic descriptors, angular displacements or the path of a body part: for example, the shoulders in sit-to-stand move forward in front of the knees and upward (Fig 2.12B). This requires an understanding by the therapist of linked segment dynamics and the biomechanical necessities of the action to be learned.

It appears that the visual system automatically detects invariant information in determining how to produce the observed action. A combination of observation and physical practice seems to permit unique opportunities for learning beyond those available from physical practice alone (Shea et al 1999). The spatial relationship of therapist to patient may be critical to the effectiveness of modelling when the patient is striving to understand the action (see Fig. 4.14A). For example, observational learning may be better if both model and subject maintain the same spatial orientation, that is reaching with the same hand, side by side, providing an 'image of the act' (Whiting & den Brinker 1982). Observation allows the patient to see the amplitude of the movement, appreciate the timing and fluency of the action, and the relationship between body parts. Whiting and colleagues (1987) showed that able-bodied subjects learning a new action who had access to a dynamic model of an expert performer produced more coordinated action than subjects who did not.

A correspondence between observing another person carrying out an action and doing it oneself has been observed using brain imaging (Grezes & Decety 2001). Studies using transcranial magnetic stimulation have reported modulation of motor cortical areas of the brain during observation of another's actions (Fadiga et al 1995; Aziz-Zadeh et al 2002). A recent review paper (Pomeroy et al 2005) hypothesizes that observation of another's motor performance with intent to imitate it may produce activity in the motor execution system (including the paretic muscles) and improve functional activity after stroke.

Augmented feedback

Magill (2001) classifies performance-related feedback as *task-intrinsic*, sensory-perceptual information related to movement that is received through various sense receptors, and *augmented* or *extrinsic*, feedback from other sources, teacher, coach, therapist or feedback device. Augmented feedback is usually categorized as knowledge of results (KR) and knowledge of performance (KP). KR is externally presented information related to achievement of the goal of the action, or outcome (Magill 2003) and is one of the most potent variables in learning. KR comes most readily from a concrete task since the outcome is easily observed. KP provides information about how the movement was performed; that is, it gives information about the performance characteristics that led to the outcome (Magill 2003). This knowledge provides guidance so the individual knows what to do on the next attempt and can be very motivating. Error identification may not be useful in itself; the individual needs to know what to do about it.

There is a considerable body of work on feedback as a tool for motor learning in able-bodied individuals. As long ago as 1927, Thorndike showed that practice with right/wrong feedback could be more effective in bringing about learning than practice alone. His subjects, with vision obstructed, drew 3-, 4-, 5- and 6-inch (5-, 7-, 13-, 15-cm) lines and the experimenter said 'right' if the line was within a tolerance band around the correct length, or 'wrong' if it was not. Subjects who had practised with feedback improved their percentage of 'right' scores from 13% at pre-test to 55% in the final session (after 4200 lines were drawn). When subjects had no feedback, the percentage of correct lines remained similar after 5400 lines were drawn. In another early study, the findings of Trowbridge & Cason (1932) supported Thorndike's work but added another dimension. They showed that quantitative feedback about the *extent* of error produced faster learning than qualitative feedback such as 'right' or 'wrong'.

One function of feedback is to provide an external focus of attention (Wulf et al 1998; Shea & Wulf 1999). During training, paying attention to the task and its outcome enables the person to use feedback naturally for error correction, noting the effects of their movement on whether or not they achieve their goal. Paying attention to the feedback can lead to improvement on the next attempt. Feedback and the need to act on it stimulate concentration and help to focus attention, particularly if the task is challenging.

Feedback may motivate the learner as well as provide information. However, feedback given while the patient is carrying out a task (concurrent feedback) or inappropriate feedback may be ineffective and increase the person's confusion about what is to be done. It is possible that if feedback is given concurrently, any improvement may not be retained because the individual learns to rely on it. Once feedback is withdrawn the individual must rely on other feedback mechanisms. Feedback given constantly can also have detrimental effects on learning (Wulf & Schmidt 1989). The patient may become dependent on the therapist's or a device's feedback as a substitute for their own error-detection abilities (McNevin et al 2000). Developing one's own monitoring capabilities is critical to independent practise.

Feedback probably has a special place in rehabilitation when individuals have problems with motor control and some compromise of feedback mechanisms. KR and KP are provided by the therapist verbally, by demonstration and through the use of electronic devices that give visual or auditory feedback (e.g., videotape, EMG, force plate, computer game). Having a concrete goal, particularly involving an object, provides the most meaningful KR. Although KR and KP are critical to learning, there has been little investigation of the effects of different types of feedback on individuals with neural dysfunction. As pointed out by van Vliet & Wulf recently in their review paper (2006), there has been more interest in investigating the effects of instrumental feedback devices than of the KR and KP given by therapists in rehabilitation. According to a study of clinical practice by Talvitie in 2000, although therapists give a great deal of verbal feedback during therapy sessions, it is particularly for motivational and reinforcing purposes and rarely for providing information. Research into informational feedback from therapists is important, as currently there is a need for feedback to be provided 'in a more focussed and deliberate way' (van Vliet & Wulf 2006).

Verbal feedback as a training technique to provide reinforcement in the attainment of a goal, 'Yes, you did it', might be useful in the early stages of rehabilitation when the task is very challenging for the patient. At another stage, however, it may be more effective to give kinematic or kinetic information related to performance, for example during training of sit-to-stand, 'Try again – this time push down through your left foot'. The feedback instruction (with an internal focus) may need to be rephrased (with an external focus) as '… put your left foot behind the right before you stand up' (when the left is the paretic leg). This information may be more effective at achieving the goals of improving control of the weaker limb, strengthening the extensor muscles and facilitating the relearning of an effective stand up.

Feedback about critical kinematic or kinetic features of an action provides information that is directly relevant to the action the individual is striving to learn. For example, if the therapist has organized a system to monitor a patient's performance objectively, such as chart or video, this information can be fed back to the patient as in 'Today you walked 10 m further than yesterday' (KR). 'Take longer strides this time' or 'walk a little faster' provide KP.

When a patient is experiencing perceptual or cognitive difficulty, verbal feedback may need to be brief, or replaced by demonstration. For individuals with an auditory perception impairment (as in receptive dysphasia), feedback may need to be modified according to the person's capacity to understand the spoken word, and a smile or a nod can also indicate whether an action should be repeated as before. Since accurate feedback is important, repetitive positive exclamations such as 'Good', should be avoided. Reinforcement feedback encourages the individual to keep trying. There should not be a mismatch between the consequence of an action and the feedback.

A major advantage of electronic feedback devices is that they may enable a person to practise relatively independently, with some supervision from the therapist, and to gain pleasure and a sense of achievement from their own intended actions. A potential value of these devices is their use in training at work stations, set up by the therapist, where patients can practise tasks semi-independently, with monitoring but without the one-to-one presence of the therapist. Several feedback devices are described in the literature.

Auditory feedback is provided by pressure-sensitive devices (force plate, foot pad) that detect forces under the feet in walking, standing and in sit-to-stand (e.g., Engardt et al 1993; Fowler & Carr 1996). Engardt & colleagues (1993) reported in their study of standing up and sitting down, using auditory feedback from force plates, that patients who did not receive feedback about loading the paretic limb during training did not improve limb loading when sitting down.

Surface EMG can provide information, visually or by sound, about the presence of muscle activity and its amplitude (Wolf et al 1979, 1980). EMG feedback from paretic muscles can be a guide for both patient and therapist to whether or not muscles can be activated in the early stage after an acute lesion.

Although some studies have shown functional improvements with a device at the end of a period of training, these results were not always retained over time (e.g., Engardt 1994). Overall, the clinical results are ambiguous. Failure to demonstrate efficacy in terms of a long-term effect may result from an inappropriate application of feedback (i.e., not directed at an appropriate goal) or from failure to incorporate the use of the feedback device into the practice of real-life actions (i.e., lack of specificity).

One neglected issue in the debate on augmented visual or auditory feedback is in relation to the onsets and timing of muscle activity (force production). Force produced over a joint or through a limb can be monitored and fed back to the patient instantaneously during strength training on an isokinetic dynamometer. Devices that require the patient to focus on timing during the performance of an action may prove to be more effective than those commonly described in which the focus is more on the mere presence of the signal or the amplitude. Timing of the action can be confused by the signal and the carryover from such a device is reported to be poor. A feedback device may be more effective when combined with specific task practice with a gradual reduction in the feedback as the person progresses. The effectiveness of feedback in rehabilitation practice needs further examination. However, the therapist should consider carefully how best to use feedback and instruction to individuals according to their changing needs as learning and their attempts at more effective functional performance progress. For this, it is necessary to observe the person's response to feedback and instruction, changing it if it does not appear to help.

Practice and intensity of training

Practice is the single most important factor responsible for permanent improvement in the ability to perform a motor skill, that is for learning to occur (Magill 2001). Skill in performance increases as a direct result of practice. The specificity of training principle was referred to in the first section and this same principle underlies motor learning

Specificity of learning

As a general rule the action to be acquired should be practised in its entirety since one component of the action depends on preceding components. The necessary neuromotor and biomechanical mechanisms, including, in particular, the timing mechanisms, can only be activated by performance of the action itself. For example, contraction of plantarflexors at the end of stance phase produces power generation for push-off that is critical to the upcoming swing phase. This power generation affects walking speed and ensures energy exchange (Olney et al 1986). The necessary mechanisms that underpin and bring about the action of walking can only be optimized through the practice of walking. However, exercises that are oriented to a major action component (e.g., ankle plantarflexion) may also need to be practised if the muscles are very weak or too weak to perform the action itself.

Several studies of sit-to-stand (Schenkman et al 1990; Pai & Rogers 1991; Shepherd & Gentile 1994) have reported the significance of upper body flexion at the hips in setting up conditions for raising the body into standing. The implication from these studies is that vertical movement of the body mass is potentiated by the angular momentum generated by the upper body 'swinging' forward over the thighs, and that the two movements of the body mass – forward and upward – overlap. The mechanics of the action and 'learning' of this phenomenon can only be optimized by practice.

Performing the action in its entirety seems important for giving the individual the idea of the action to be achieved. However, when the patient has difficulty activating muscles and generating and timing forces, specifically prescribed exercises may improve motor unit activation and train the muscles to produce and sustain a higher level of force. The patient can practise a modified version of the action with, for example, the seat height raised. As strength and control increase, the seat is progressively lowered, adding variety and increasing difficulty, and working toward re-establishing the functional linkage of the lower limbs.

Practice specificity and transfer lie at the heart of motor learning (Magill 2001). One of the goals of practising a task such as walking is to be able to transfer what is learned into different contexts. In order to function in the community, the patient first practises walking in the rehabilitation gymnasium, but must also transfer this new skill into different, more meaningful, contexts – walk to a shop, walk up a hill, cross the road at traffic lights, carry a bag. After an acute lesion, this capacity to transfer skill may also require practice of exercises that strengthen and improve endurance of leg muscles and improve fitness. In the first section of the chapter we saw that strength training exercises should be planned to approximate the action pattern in specific functional tasks so that the improved muscle strength and limb control gained from strength training will transfer into improved functional performance. Training methods to improve the performance of actions such as walking, standing up and reaching to take an object should also be planned so that what has been learned can transfer to a variety of different contexts and under different constraints.

Reaching for an object in sitting requires the ability to move the body mass and balance over the base of support (the thighs and feet). Practice of reaching for objects on the floor and reaching in different directions enables the person to test the limits of balance stability and to expand these limits to increase reaching distance. By varying the tasks or the placement of objects, the therapist can challenge the person to explore the possibilities and move more confidently. When reaching to one side, the lower limb on that side is used actively as the base of support, the extent of active use of that leg varying according to conditions such as direction, speed and distance to be moved. Such exercise not only improves balance and reaching ability in sitting but also gives practice of weight-bearing through both feet or one foot.

Transfer of training can take place between functionally similar actions. For example, since reaching forward vigorously beyond arm's length in sitting is similar biomechanically to the momentum-producing pre-extension phase of sit-to-stand, it is not surprising that sit-to-stand performance of a group of people post-stroke also improved at the conclusion of a training study directed at improving balance in sitting. The findings from this study provide some evidence of generalizability or transferability from the reaching and balancing exercises (Dean & Shepherd 1997).

The practice sessions in the above study illustrate the way in which task practice and the practice environment can be organized to improve functional performance of, in this case, a balancing task, by organizing variable practice conditions. There has been much interest in the motor learning literature on the relative benefits to the learner of *consistent (blocked) versus variable (random) practice* (e.g., Gentile 2000; Magill 2001). Consistent practice involves repetitive practice of the same action in the same environment; in variable practice the conditions are changed so that the individual performs the action in different locations and for different goals. Blocked practice might be particularly useful when exercises to improve strength and control are necessary as well as in the early stages of learning. Random or variable practice on a range of related tasks or the same task under varying environmental conditions seems to lead to better performance and learning than consistent practice of the one task (Gentile 2000) in the later fine-tuning stage. This leads us to the issue of repetition in practice.

Repetitions. Many repetitions of an action are required to increase muscle strength and limb control, and for the patient to develop an optimal way of performing the action (Bernstein in Latash & Latash 1994). Thousands of repetitions may be necessary to improve strength and control, and to embed the organization of the action in the system. Acquiring skill does not only mean to repeat and consolidate, but also to invent and progress (Whiting 1980), so-called 'repetition without repetition' (Bernstein 1967). Repetition of an action under varying conditions develops the ability to solve motor problems posed by the environment.

Physiotherapy practice may be guilty of neglecting the repetitive element of skill acquisition that forms an essential prerequisite in motor rehabilitation (see Rooney et al 1994; Butefisch et al 1995). A single performance of an exercise or task, or a series of single performances with rests between each attempt, are unlikely to affect learning or limb control. In the initial stage of rehabilitation, if muscle weakness interferes with the performance of an action making it either impossible or ineffective, repetitive exercise in a stable environment may be critical. The objective is to get the muscles contracting and generating force well enough to perform the action. Fine tuning for the skill required for functional performance, however, requires variable practice under a variety of conditions. Therefore, once a basic approximation of an action has been achieved,

patients need the opportunity to practise that action in a variety of different task and environmental conditions in order to develop flexibility.

How difficult a functional task is for a person depends on how challenging the task is relative to the skill level of the individual (Guadagnoli & Lee 2004). This is a useful concept for clinical practice as even very simple tasks may be nearly impossible for an individual with severe impairment. If this is the case, the task and/or the environment in which it is being carried out may need to be modified to enable practice to take place. A task can be modified so less force is required. For example, training reaching forward and upward can start with the arm resting on a table (see Fig. 6.13). A simple modification may increase the effectiveness of prime mover muscles and avoid unnecessary adaptive behaviour. A task can be made less difficult by decreasing the number of segments to be moved. The distance to be moved can be decreased so that the person has more control over the movement. Challenges to balance can be decreased to enable the person to gain some control over balance mechanisms while performing the task; wearing a harness, for example, gives the person confidence and allows practise of different tasks in standing without fear of falling (see Fig. 2.6B).

As the person improves, the task itself can be made more difficult and the action can be practised under different and more difficult environmental conditions, for example walking around and over obstacles, performing more repetitions, increasing range of movement, resistance or load. Progressing training may involve increasing distance walked, or carrying out two tasks at once such as holding a glass full of water while standing up (see Ch. 4).

With practice, the dynamics of force generation become organized according to principles of optimization. The dynamics evolve toward minimization of cost, in terms of energy, time or need for information. When first attempting a new task the learner uses what they already 'know' implicitly about movement dynamics. During practice, refinement of force dynamics occurs due to the self-organizing process of implicit learning. Alexander and colleagues (1992) have pointed out that reinforcement can be viewed as 'increasing the connection strength between neural elements within a richly connected network'.

Variability of performance during practice repetitions need not be considered as error (Manoel & Connolly 1995) but as a necessary step in the gradual optimization of patterns of force production. The individual developing skill is learning to exploit external forces, minimize the generation of muscle forces (including decreasing co-contraction) and smooth out the flow of movement (Bernstein 1967). It appears from studies of children and adults who are learning new skills that achieving a movement goal occurs much earlier than an efficient, smoothly performed movement. Gentile (1998) suggests that it might be beneficial to follow the same course with individuals who are learning to perform functional every-day actions that have become difficult or impossible as a result of brain damage. That is to say, focus should be on goal attainment (success in achieving the goal) in the early stages of task practise. Further practice under variable and more challenging environmental conditions will then enable fine tuning of the action.

Modification of task or context provides a useful concept for physiotherapists who may not allow practice of an action in the early stages after acute brain lesion unless performance is 'correct'. This is a significant issue. We can only improve motor performance by a process of trial-and-error. Simplifying a task enables practice without gross errors. As an example, walking with partial weight support on a treadmill is an effective way of simplifying the action of walking by modifying the task and the environmental context.

One of the advantages of task-specific training is that it enables the individual to see the future benefits of practice to improve performance. Ability to stand up independently and to walk, for example, means independence; practice of overground or treadmill walking in the early stages of rehabilitation suggests an expectation that the person will improve their walking ability.

In general, it can be said that a combination of repetitive and variable practice is required:

- to enable a movement pattern to be learned, i.e., to refine neuromotor processes
- to strengthen muscles and train synergistic activity specifically and with a flow-on to similar actions
- to enable a stable pattern to be modified as necessary according to environmental and other demands, i.e., to develop flexibility of performance, to learn the 'rules' of movement that carry over to different contexts.

Mental practice

Practice is a continuum from overt physical practice to covert or mental practice. Mental practice involves the cognitive rehearsal of a task without overt physical movement (Magill 2001). It has been shown to be a useful aid to learning in able-bodied subjects. It shows great potential for enhancing performance and learning in individuals with disability, particularly when they are unable to physically practise a task or if they are having difficulty putting the action together. Rehearsing a simple physical action in the mind may assist in focusing attention on the action to be performed (Page et al 2001). Mental imagery may be particularly important for the person who is unable to practise a task physically as it improves ability to sustain attention and plan task performance.

Mental practice combined with physical practice has been effectively used for many decades to promote the learning of motor skills in athletes, and to preserve skill when physical practice is not possible (Driskell et al 1994;

Deiber et al 1998). Several early studies found electrical activity in muscles when individuals were asked to imagine performing an action. In one study, subjects visualized bending an arm to lift a weight and EMG activity was noted in the biceps brachii (Jacobson 1932). These results suggest that appropriate motor connections may be activated during mental practice, helping to establish and reinforce an appropriate coordination pattern (Magill 2001). Research findings also support the assumption that the initial stage of learning a task involves a high degree of cognitive activity (Kosslyn et al 2001).

Thinking of the topology or shape of a movement, for example standing up from sitting, can enable a patient to practise by bringing to mind a visuospatial image of the action. The action image is reinforced by the introduction of variability into the environments in which the task is 'performed'. The aim is for an internal model to be established showing the fit between the individual's morphology and the environment, and this internal model or mental image can be the mechanism for mental practice (Gentile 1998).

It appears from recent reviews that mental practice can be effective in improving motor performance in people with neural lesions (Crosbie et al 2004; Liu et al 2004; Malouin et al 2004; Page 2005). Malouin and colleagues (2004) examined the effects of mental practice on performance of sit-to-stand in individuals after stroke. They tested 12 people after stroke and 14 able-bodied subjects, before and after a single session of mental practice using motor imagery. They were asked to reduce the loading through the unaffected leg and increase the load on the affected leg in standing. Subjects were shown a vertical force signal, indicating magnitude and timing of force, from under the feet. The results showed that loading the affected leg improved, and working memory scores (recall in visuospatial, verbal, kinesthetic domains) at follow-up correlated significantly with the level of improvement. Two recent systematic reviews (Braun et al 2006; Zimmermann-Schlatter et al 2008) found evidence that mental practice as an adjunct to therapy has positive effects on outcome after stroke. Mental practice is likely to be most effective when the individual has developed a basic understanding of the action itself, and when combined with physical practice.

NEW APPROACHES TO THE DELIVERY OF PHYSIOTHERAPY: PROVIDING OPPORTUNITIES FOR PRACTICE

Anyone who wants to become skilled at a sporting activity, or playing a musical instrument or at chess will spend many hours a day in practice. Similarly, someone with neural impairment who wants to regain or improve motor skill in everyday actions needs to practise intensively, not only during training sessions with the therapist giving individual advice and assistance.

For meaningful and intensive practice to take place outside individual training sessions requires:

- an environment organized to enable safe, independent, relatively unsupervised practice to take place
- a change in the ways of delivering therapy so that time is allocated to instructing the patient about what to practise, providing workbooks and organizing a physical environment that is challenging and provides frequent and interesting opportunities for practice
- an understanding by rehabilitation staff and patients that an optimally effective rehabilitation process involves active participation and mental and physical practice.

The issue of *how much time is spent in practice* is a critical one for motor training in rehabilitation. Changes in physiotherapy practice are required to make better use of the time allotted, not only in methods used but also in delivery. It is clear from several studies of clinical practice that only a small part of an inpatient's day is made available for practice and learning. This is particularly so for patients who have had an acute lesion. Yet we now have clear evidence that recovery of reasonable functional efficacy after stroke demands a great deal of practice and that rehabilitation methods in large part involve specific training.

Therapists are gradually moving away from reliance on hands-on, one-to-one therapy to a model in which the person practises, not only in individualized training sessions with the therapist, but also at *work stations* set up to encourage practice of specific actions, where they can be semi-supervised by therapist and aides. The work space can also include a suspended harness for balancing tasks, feedback and computer-aided devices, and exercise machines such as treadmill and isokinetic dynamometers.

Supervised practice with patients working together in *groups* and helping each other is another way of increasing the time spent in practice, exercise and activity. Individual assistance and training are given as necessary (Fig. 2.13). One or two therapists with the assistance of aides can supervise several individuals in a group, with relatives helping if they are willing and able (see Fig. 5.15). Patients can move from one work station to another in a circuit training class where they practise specific motor activities with both simple and technological aids to promote strength and skill, photographs or videotapes of the action to be learned, and printed or electronic exercise guidelines. In group work the availability of others with similar disabilities may motivate and encourage individuals to do better and increase their sense of wellbeing and their communication skills by engaging with others. The introduction of group classes can increase the level of social interaction and participation during the day. In one study, patients who attended classes spent 25% more time with their peers (de Weerdt et al 2001). Barreca and colleagues found that participants assigned to a group developed a camaraderie, encouraging each other and celebrating successes (Barreca et al 2004).

Practising with another person in an interactive way increases the learners' motivation by adding competitive and cooperative components to the practice milieu (McNevin et al 2000). Research on 'dyad' training, where two people work together, alternating between physical practice and observation, appears, in able-bodied subjects, to be more effective than individual practice. Shea and colleagues (1999) described the effects of interactive practice between two people. Their results suggest that physical practice, observation and dialogue (suggestions, motivating comments) between learners in an interactive way can produce an effective learning protocol/environment.

The positive results seem to be the result of observation of another performer, that is the demonstration by another learner, with opportunity to observe the action to be learned and any errors in performance (Herbert & Landin 1994; Granados & Wulf 2007). Working with another person provides rest intervals when training is physically challenging, yet the individual has to remain focused in order to assist his/her partner. The interaction between practice partners may be a major factor in enhanced learning effectiveness (Shea et al 1999). It has been shown that observational practice can improve error recognition (Black & Wright 2000). The clinical implications of this research are discussed by McNevin et al (2000).

Computer-aided, virtual reality, robotic and electromechanical training

The potential of devices in motor training has not yet been realized. New technological aids currently being developed and investigated can increase time spent in physical and mental activity by enabling patients to practise more repetitions of an action and practise independently (Mehrholz et al 2008). They can provide feedback, drive physical participation, increase intensity of practice and increase motivation. As Hesse and colleagues (2006) point out, machines open new dimensions in motor rehabilitation. New technologies include:

- robot-aided training (Fasoli et al 2004; Hidler et al 2005; Hesse et al 2006; Hornby et al 2008)
- electromechanical training aids (Hesse et al 2006; Barker et al 2008)
- virtual reality systems (Sisto et al 2002; Fung et al 2006)
- interactive computer games controlled by manipulanda of different types (Hermsdorfer et al 2004).

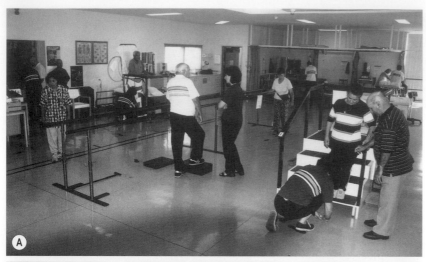

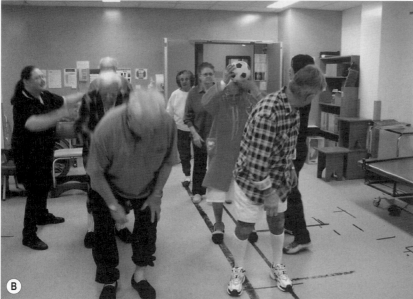

Figure 2.13 (A) An overview of a lower limb circuit class. *(With permission F Mackey, Port Kembla Hospital, Australia).* (B) Part of a balance and upper limb class. *(Courtesy of K Schurr & S Dorsch, Physiotherapy Department, Bankstown-Lidcombe Hospital, Sydney, Australia).*

Robotic systems. Several studies report successful outcomes in terms of isolated arm movements but results of carryover into long-term improved function are equivocal (Volpe et al 2000; Hidler et al 2005; Krebs et al 2002; Lum et al 2002; Hesse et al 2003; Gallichio & Kluding 2004; Lam et al 2006). Functional improvements in individuals with severe upper limb paresis after stroke have been noted after training bilaterally (forearm pronation–supination and wrist flexion–extension) on a robot trainer (Bi-Manu-Track) (Hesse et al 2003). A study of robot-assisted treadmill gait training (Lokomat®) has shown no extra benefit

gained by patients who were independent walkers after a stroke, when compared to treadmill training with a therapist assisting the person to move the paretic limb through swing phase (Hornby et al 2008). Mayr and colleagues (2007) compared the effects of walking training on a treadmill using Lokomat and Bobath therapy with patients who were unable to walk independently. The treadmill-trained group showed significantly greater improvements in functional measures (including Rivermead Motor Assessment, 10-min timed walk test) and in Medical Research Council strength tests compared to the control group whose physiotherapy included rolling, kneeling and facilitation of the paretic limb in sitting and standing.

Electromechanical systems. Barker and colleagues (2008) have reported on the testing of a newly developed non-robotic device (Sensorimotor Active Rehabilitation Training (SMART) Arm) that can be used with or without EMG-triggered triceps brachii (see Fig. 6.21). This device enables individuals with severe upper limb paresis to practise constrained but natural reaching tasks in which the arm extends forward along a normal hand path. Individuals who had a stroke more than 6 months prior to the experiment were divided into three groups. Practice with the SMART trainer, with or without EMG stimulation, significantly increased function at the impairment (triceps strength and resistance to passive movement) and activity (Motor Assessment Scale) level. Changes were maintained for at least 2 months after training ceased. No changes were seen in the control group.

Hesse and colleagues (2006) describe several devices designed for training arm and hand movements and walking. A Cochrane systematic review (Mehrholz et al 2008) provides evidence that suggests that stroke patients who have electromechanical assistance with gait training together with physiotherapy are more likely to achieve independent walking than those who have gait training without these devices.

Virtual reality (VR) systems present simulated or artificially generated sensory information that allows the individual to experience and interact with three-dimensional environments (Holden & Dyar 2002; Sisto et al 2002; Deutsche et al 2004; Holden 2005; Lam et al 2006). The system can involve the patient in variable training, with environmental challenges such as crossing the road, stepping over obstacles (Jaffe et al 2004) and stepping up a kerb (Fung et al 2006), thereby aiding the process of returning to real life environments. Improvements in motor activity and functional performance have been reported, for example a decrease in hemispatial neglect after a training programme using a virtual hand (Castiello et al 2004). Enhanced cortical reorganization has been reported (You et al 2005). A recent review of VR in stroke rehabilitation (Crosbie et al 2007) illustrates the limited evidence base (weak to moderate) so far, while suggesting that VR is an exciting new development in rehabilitation. VR offers stimulating, varied environments and can increase time spent in practice (Malouin & Richards 2005).

It is too early for substantial outcome evidence, but there are early indications that these training aids can result in improvements in limb movement, strength and sometimes functional motor performance (Hesse et al 2006; Barker et al 2008) and promote motor recovery (Hesse et al 2006).

Whether or not functional task performance improves probably depends on what actions are trained using these devices. For example, there was no evidence of improved upper limb function after robot-assisted training of reaching in the horizontal plane although movements at individual joints improved. A systematic review of electromechanical and robot-assisted arm training (Mehrholz et al 2008) showed evidence of positive effects on arm function and strength but not on performance of daily actions. It must be noted that the preferred measures of activities of daily living in this review were Functional Independence Measure and Barthel, both rather general measures of disability and not really of functional performance on everyday actions. It may also be important to select appropriate patients. As Hornby and colleagues (2008) suggested, robot-assisted training may be more appropriate for the most affected individuals. Once people can perform a particular action, learning is likely to proceed more quickly without guidance or assisted movement. Future design of systems and investigations should keep in mind (1) the specificity effects of training and exercise and (2) the need for relevance and validity in the methods of measuring functional performance.

Part of planning for independent practice involves organizing methods of prompting the patient's attention to the actions to be practised. Canning & Adams (1985) reported the results of planned covert monitoring of a woman recovering from a stroke during her independent practice of walking. Although she could walk quite well in the physiotherapy area, elsewhere she reverted to a short-stepped and wide-based gait. She agreed to be monitored by a group of unknown observers, who would score her on stride width and step length. Observations were tallied daily. After 11 days her walking had improved.

The delivery of physiotherapy in circuit and exercise classes has been shown to be effective and feasible, with participants improving strength, fitness and functional performance (Teixeira-Salmela et al 1999, 2001; Dean et al 2000; Eng et al 2003; Salbach et al 2004; Sherrington et al 2008b). Semi-supervised practice can help bridge the gap between individualized training and unsupervised practice in rehabilitation and at home. If patients feel they have some control over practice conditions and are encouraged to see the therapist as a resource person, their problem-solving abilities can improve. These skills become essential when they are at home. Many therapists already acknowledge that it is unrealistic to expect that any patient will reach their potential if they spend only a short period each day in physical activity (Bernhardt et al 2004; Smith et al 2008). It is possible that many hours of each patient's day spent in specialized stroke units and rehabilitation facilities are hours wasted. Challenges to customary delivery of therapy can be difficult for clinicians and may require a change in culture within a rehabilitation unit or health department.

In conclusion, the primary purpose of this chapter is to stress the importance of motor learning and physical

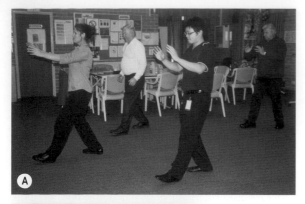

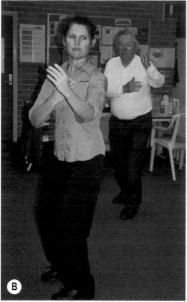

Figure 2.14 Tai Chi class in rehabilitation centre. *(Courtesy of Physiotherapy Department, War Memorial Hospital, Sydney).*

training in neurorehabilitation and of setting up physical conditions and procedures to enable effective and reasonably intensive practice. Changes may need to be made within physiotherapy education so that clinicians are up to date in their knowledge of biomechanics, motor learning, neural and exercise science; in the development of science-based exercise programmes; and have the opportunity to gain skill in the application of training methods. What seems certain is that the process of rehabilitation must become more active and more intensive for patients recovering from acute brain lesions than it currently seems to be, and more specific to the person's impairments when they are struggling to manage with chronic illness. Rehabilitation departments and physiotherapy clinics need to offer facilities for exercise classes as part of the rehabilitation experience. Community facilities, including physiotherapy practices, and other exercise opportunities need to be developed so that they are available when patients return to their community. Recovery after acute brain lesion continues for as long as an individual continues with an active life. For those with chronic neurological conditions, the maintenance of a mentally and physically active life is paramount. As part of their duty of care, therapists encourage individuals to seek out activity programmes offered by local communities. These might include gym classes, exercise classes in water and swimming, walking groups, and Tai Chi classes (Fig. 2.14). Evaluation and knowledge of mechanisms and effects of impairments can clarify the particular emphasis for individuals. However, it is probable that all could benefit from being stronger, mentally and physically more active and more physically fit.

Programmes of exercise and training for optimizing performance of specific tasks are described later in this book. They are designed to promote the relearning of skilled performance specifically in standing up and sitting down, walking, reaching and manipulation, and balancing throughout movement.

REFERENCES

Abrams RA, Pratt J 1993 Rapid aimed limb movements: differential effects of practice on component sub-movements. J Mot Behav 25:288–298.

Ada L, Dorsch S, Canning C 2006 Strengthening interventions increase strength and improve activity after stroke: a systematic review. Aust J Physiother 52:241–248.

Agahari I, Shepherd RB, Westwood PA 1996 A comparative evaluation of lower limb forces in two variations of the step exercise in able-bodied

subjects. In: Lee M, Gilleard W, Sinclair P et al (eds) Proceedings of 1st Australasian Biomechanics Conference, Sydney, Australia:94–95.

Alexander GE, DeLong MR, Crutcher MD 1992 Do cortical and basal ganglionic motor areas use 'motor programs' to control movement? Behav Brain Sci 16:656–665.

American College of Sports Medicine 1998 Position stand: exercise and physical activity for older adults. Med Sci Sports Exerc 30:992–1008.

American College of Sports Medicine 2006a ACSM's guidelines for exercise testing and prescription, 7th edn. Lippincott Williams & Wilkins, Baltimore, MD.

American College of Sports Medicine 2006b ACSM's resource manual for guidelines for exercise testing and prescription, 5th edn. Lippincott Williams & Wilkins, Baltimore, MD.

Andrews AW, Bohannon RW 2001 Discharge function and length of stay for patients with stroke are predicted by lower extremity muscle force on admission to rehabilitation. Neurorehabil Neural Repair 15:93–97.

Annett J 1971 Acquisition of skill. Br Med Bull 27:266–271.

Arutyunyan GH, Gurfinkel VS, Mirskii ML 1968 Investigation of aiming at a target. Biophysics 13:536–538.

Aziz-Zadeh A, Maeda F, Zaidel A et al 2002 Lateralization in motor facilitation during action observation: a TMS study. Exp Brain Res 144:127–131.

Barker RN, Brauer SG, Carson RG 2008 Training of reaching in stroke survivors with severe and chronic upper limb paresis using a novel nonrobotic device. Stroke 39:1800–1807.

Barreca S, Sigouin CS, Lambert C et al 2004 Effects of extra training on the ability of stroke survivors to perform an independent sit-to-stand: a randomized controlled trial. J Ger Phys Ther 27:59–64.

Behm DG, Sale DG 1994 Intended rather than actual movement velocity determines velocity-specific training response. J Appl Physiol 74:359–368.

Belmont I, Benjamin H, Ambrose J et al 1969 Effect of cerebral damage on motivation in rehabilitation. Arch Phys Med Rehabil 50:507.

Bernhardt J, Dewey HM, Thrift AG et al 2004 Inactive and alone: physical activity in the first 14 days of acute stroke unit care. Stroke 35:1005–1009.

Bernstein N 1967 The coordination and regulation of movements. Pergamon Press, London.

Black CB, Wright DL 2000 Can observational practice facilitate error recognition and movement production? Res Q Exerc Sport 71:331–339.

Bobath B 1990 Adult hemiplegia: evaluation and treatment, 3rd edn. Butterworth Heinemann, Oxford.

Bohannon RW 1986 Strength of lower limb muscle related to gait velocity and cadence in stroke patients. Physiother Can 38:204–206.

Bohannon RW 1987 Relative decreases in knee extension torque with increased knee extension velocities in stroke patients with hemiparesis. Phys Ther 67:1218–1220.

Bohannon RW, Walsh S 1991 Association of paretic lower extremity strength and balance with stair climbing ability in patients with stroke. J Stroke Cerebrovasc Dis 1:129–133.

Braun SMBAJ, Borm PJ, Schack T et al 2006 The effects of mental practice in stroke rehabilitation: a systematic review. Arch Phys Med Rehabil 87:842–852.

Britton E, Harris N, Turton A 2008 An exploratory randomized controlled trial of assisted practice for improving sit-to-stand in stroke patients in the hospital setting. Clin Rehabil 22:458–468.

Brown DA, Kautz SA 1998 Increased workload enhances force output during pedalling exercise in persons with post-stroke hemiplegia. Phys Sportsmed 26:598–606.

Buchner DM, de Latour BJ 1991 The importance of skeletal muscle strength to physical function in older adults. Ann Behav Med 13:91–98.

Buchner DM, Larson EB, Wagner EH et al 1996 Evidence for a non-linear relationship between leg strength and gait speed. Age Ageing 25:386–391.

Buchner DM, Cress ME, de Latour BJ 1997 The effects of strength and endurance training on gait, balance, fall risk, and health services use in community-living older adults. J Gerontol A Biol Sci Med Sci 52:M218–224.

Butefisch C, Hummelsheim H, Denzler P et al 1995 Repetitive training of isolated movements improves the outcome of motor rehabilitation of the centrally paretic hand. J Neurol Sci 130:59–68.

Canning C, Adams R 1985 Covert monitoring to promote consistency of walking performance: a case study. Aust J Physiother 31:152.

Cao C, Schultz AB, Ashton-Miller JA et al 1998 Sudden turns and stops while walking: kinematic sources of age and gender differences. Gait Posture 7:45–52.

Carr JH, Shepherd RB 1980 Physiotherapy in disorders of the brain. Heinemann, London.

Carr JH, Shepherd RS 1987 A motor relearning programme for stroke, 2nd edn. Butterworth Heinemann, Oxford.

Carr JH, Shepherd RB 2000 A motor relearning model for rehabilitation. In: Carr JH, Shepherd RB (eds) Movement science. Foundations for physical therapy in rehabilitation, 2nd edn. Aspen, Rockville, MD:31–92.

Carr JH, Shepherd RB 2003 Stroke rehabilitation. Guidelines for training and exercise to optimise motor skill. Butterworth Heinemann, Oxford.

Carr JH, Shepherd RB 2008 Optimierung der Wiederherstellung der Funktion nach Schlaganfall. In: Mehrholz J (ed.) Fruhphase Schlaganfall Physiotherapie und Medizinische Versorgung, Thieme, Stuttgart 63–156.

Carroll WR, Bandura A 1982 The role of visual monitoring in observational learning of action patterns: making the unobservable observable. J Mot Behav 14:153–167.

Castiello U, Lusher D, Burton C et al 2004 Improving left hemispatial neglect using virtual reality. Neurol 62:1958–1962.

Chae J, Yang G, Park BK et al 2002a Delay in initiation and termination of muscle contraction, motor impairment, and physical disability in upper limb paresis. Muscle Nerve 25:568–575.

Chae J, Yang G, Park BK et al 2002b Muscle weakness and cocontraction in upper limb hemiparesis: relationship to motor impairment and physical disability. Neurorehabil Neural Repair 16:241–248.

Chandler JM, Duncan PW 1988 Eccentric vs concentric force velocity relationships of the quadriceps femoris muscle. Phys Ther 68:800.

Chen H-C, Ashton-Miller JA, Alexander NB et al 1994 Effects of age and available response time on ability to step over an obstacle. J Gerontol Med Sci 49:M227–233.

Chen H-C, Schultz AB, Ashton-Miller JA et al 1996 Stepping over obstacles: dividing attention impairs performance of old more than young adults. J Gerontol 51A:M116–122.

Cramp MC, Greenwood RJ, Gill M et al 2006 Low intensity strength training for ambulatory stroke patients. Disabil Rehabil 28:883–889.

Crosbie JH, McDonough SM, Gilmore DH et al 2004 The adjunctive role of mental practice in the rehabilitation of the upper limb after hemiplegic stroke: a pilot study. Clin Rehabil 18:60–68.

Crosbie JH, Lennon S, Basford JR et al 2007 Virtual reality in stroke rehabilitation: still more virtual than real. Disabil Rehabil 29:1139–1146.

Dean CM, Shepherd RB 1997 Task-related training improves performance of seated reaching tasks following stroke: a randomized controlled trial. Stroke 28:722–728.

Dean CM, Richards CL, Malouin F 2000 Task-related circuit training improves performance of locomotor tasks in chronic stroke: a randomized, controlled pilot trial. Arch Phys Med Rehabil 81:409–417.

De Deyne PG 2001 Application of passive stretch and its implications for muscle fibres. Phys Ther 81:819–827.

Deiber MP, Ibanez V, Honda M et al 1998 Cerebral processes related to visuomotor imagery and generation of finger movements studied with positron emission tomography. Neuroimage 7:73–85.

Deutsche JE, Merians AS, Adamovich S et al 2004 Development and application of virtual reality technology to improve hand use and gait of individuals post-stroke. Restor Neurol Neurosci 22:371–386.

de Weerdt W, Nuyens G, Hilde F et al 2001 Group physiotherapy improves time-use by patients with stroke in rehabilitation. Aust J Physiother 47:53–61.

Driskell JE, Copper C, Moran A 1994 Does mental practice enhance performance? J Appl Psychol 79:481–492.

Duncan PW, Chandler JM, Cavanaugh DK et al 1989 Mode and speed specificity of eccentric and concentric exercise training. J Sports Phys Ther 11:70–75.

Duncan P, Studenski S, Richards L et al 2003 Randomized clinical trial of therapeutic exercise in subacute stroke. Stroke 34:2173–2180.

Ellenbecker TS, Davies GJ, Rowinski MJ 1988 Concentric and eccentric isokinetic strengthening of the rotator cuff. Am J Sports Med 16:65–69.

Eng JJ 2004 Strength training in individuals with stroke. Physiother Can 56:189–201.

Eng JJ, Chu KS, Kim CM et al 2003 A community-based group exercise program for persons with chronic stroke. Med Sci Sports Exerc 35:1271–1278.

Eng JJ, Dawson AS, Chu KS 2004 Submaximal exercise in persons with stroke: test-retest reliability and concurrent validity with maximal oxygen consumption. Arch Phys Med Rehabil 85:113–118.

Engardt M 1994 Long term effects of auditory feedback training on relearned symmetrical body weight distribution in stroke. A follow-up study. Scand J Rehabil Med 26:65–69.

Engardt M, Ribbe T, Olsson E 1993 Vertical ground reaction force feedback to enhance stroke patients' symmetrical body-weight distribution while rising/sitting down. Scand J Rehabil Med 25:41–48.

Fadiga L, Fogassi L, Pavesi G et al 1995 Motor facilitation during action observation: a magnetic stimulation study. J Neurophysiol 73:2608–2611.

Fasoli SE, Krebs HI, Stein J et al 2004 Robotic therapy for chronic motor impairments after stroke: follow-up results. Arch Phys Med Rehabil 85:1106–1111.

Fasoli SE, Krebs HI, Stein J et al 2005 Effects of robotic therapy on motor impairment and recovery in chronic stroke. Arch Phys Med Rehabil 84:477–482.

Fiatarone MA, Marks EC, Ryan ND et al 1990 High-intensity strength training in nonagenarians. J Am Med Assoc 263:3029–3034.

Fiatarone MA, O'Neill EF, Ryan ND et al 1994 Exercise training and nutritional supplementation for physical frailty in very elderly people. N Engl J Med 330:1769–1775.

Forssberg H, Grillner S, Rossignol S 1975 Phase dependent reflex reversal during walking in chronic spinal cats. Brain Res 55:247–304.

Fowler V, Carr J 1996 Auditory feedback: effects on vertical force production during standing up following stroke. Int J Rehabil Res 19:265–269.

Friden J 1984 Changes in human skeletal muscle induced by long-term eccentric exercise. Cell Tissue Res 236:365–372.

Friden J, Seger J, Sjostrom M et al 1983 Adaptive responses in human skeletal muscle subjected to prolonged eccentric training. Int J Sports Med 4:177–183.

Frontera WR, Meredith CN, O'Reilly KP et al 1988 Strength conditioning in older men: skeletal muscle hypertrophy and improved function. J Appl Physiol 64:1038–1044.

Fung J, Richards CL, Malouin F et al 2006 A treadmill and motion-coupled virtual reality system for gait training post-stroke. Cyberpsychol Behav 9:157–162.

Gallichio J, Kluding P 2004 Virtual reality in stroke rehabilitation: review of the emerging research. Phys Ther Rev 9:207–212.

Gardner MM, Robertson MC, Campbell AJ 2000 Exercise in preventing falls and fall related injuries in older people: a review of randomized controlled trials. Br J Sports Med 34:7–17.

Gentile AM 1998 Implicit and explicit processes during acquisition of functional skills. Scand J Occup Ther 5:7–16.

Gentile AM 2000 Skill acquisition: action, movement, and neuromotor processes. In: Carr JH, Shepherd RB (eds) Movement science. Foundations for rehabilitation, 2nd edn. Aspen, Rockville, MD:93–154.

Gonella C, Hale G, Ionta M et al 1981 Self-instruction in a perceptual motor skill. Phys Ther 61:177–184.

Gracies JM 2005 Pathophysiology of spastic paresis. 1. Paresis and soft tissue changes. Muscle Nerve 31:535–551.

Granados C, Wulf G 2007 Enhancing motor learning through dyad practice: contributions of observation and dialogue. Res Q Exerc Sport 78:197–203.

Grezes J, Decety J 2001 Functional anatomy of execution, mental stimulation, observation and verb generation of actions: a meta-analysis. Hum Brain Mapp 12:1–19.

Guadagnoli MA, Lee TD 2004 Challenge point: a framework for conceptualizing the effects of various practice conditions in motor learning. J Motor Behav 2:212–224.

Hachisuka K, Umezu Y, Ogata B 1997 Disuse muscle atrophy of lower limbs in hemiplegic patients. Arch Phys Med Rehabil 78:13–18.

Hakkinen K, Komi PV 1983 Electromyographic changes during strength training and detraining. Med Sci Sports Exerc 15:455–460.

Hakkinen K, Newton RU, Gordon SE et al 1998 Changes in muscle morphology, electromyographic activity, and force production characteristics during progressive strength training in young and older men. J Gerontol Biol Sci 53A:B415–B423.

Harridge SDR, Krygen A, Stensgaard A 1999 Knee extensor strength, activation, and size in very elderly people following strength training. Muscle Nerve 22:831–839.

Herbert R 2005 How muscles respond to stretch. In: Refshauge K, Ada L, Ellis E (eds) Science-based rehabilitation. Butterworth Heinemann, Oxford.

Herbert EP, Landin D 1994 Effects of a learning model and augmented feedback on tennis skill acquisition. Res Q Exerc Sport 65:250–257.

Hermsdorfer J, Marquardt C, Heiss J 2004 Evaluation of a feedback-based training of cerebral hand function deficits using kinematic analysis. Physik Med Rehabil 14:187–194.

Hesse S, Schulte-Tigges G, Konrad M et al 2003 Robot-assisted arm trainer for the passive and active practice of bilateral forearm and wrist movements in hemiparetic subjects. Arch Phys Med Rehabil 84:915–920.

Hesse S, Schmidt H, Werner C 2006 Machines to support motor rehabilitation after stroke: 10 years of experience in Berlin. J Rehabil Res Dev 43:671–678.

Hidler J, Nichols D, Pelliccio M et al 2005 Advances in the understanding and treatment of stroke impairment using robotic devices. Top Stroke Rehabil 12:22–35.

Hoang PD, Herbert RD, Gandevia SC 2007 Effects of eccentric exercise on passive mechanical properties of human gastrocnemius in vivo. Med Sci Sports Exerc 39:849–857.

Holden MK 2005 Virtual environments for motor rehabilitation: a review. Cyberpsychol Behav 8:187–211.

Holden M, Dyar T 2002 Virtual environment training: a new tool for neurorehabilitation. Neurol Report 26:62–71.

Hornby TG, Campbell DD, Kahn JH et al 2008 Enhanced gait-related improvements after therapist- versus robotic-assisted locomotor training in subjects with chronic stroke. Stroke 39:1786–1792.

Hortobagyi T, Tunnel D, Moody J et al 2001 Low- or high-intensity strength training partially restores impaired quadriceps force accuracy and steadiness in aged adults. J Gerontol A Biol Sci Med Sci 56:B38–47.

Hsiao S-F, Newham DJ 1999 The non-paretic side of stroke patients:

extent of deficit in mechanical output. Clin Rehabil 13:80–81.

Hummelsheim A, Mauritz K-H 1993 Chronic transformation of muscle in spasticity: a peripheral contribution to increased tone. J Neurol Neurosurg Psychiatry 48:676–685.

Ingemann-Hansen T, Halkjaer-Kristensen J 1980 Computerised tomography determination of human thigh components. Scand J Rehabil Med 12:27–31.

Jacobson E 1932 Muscular phenomenon during imagining. Am J Psychol 49:677–694.

Jaffe DL, Brown DA, Pierson-Carey CD et al 2004 Stepping over obstacles to improve walking in individuals with post-stroke hemiplegia. J Rehabil Res Develop 41:283–292.

Jeannerod M 1990 The neural and behavioral organization of goal-directed movement. Clarendon Press, Oxford.

Kanehisa H, Miyashita M 1983 Specificity of velocity in strength training. Eur J Appl Physiol Occup Physiol 52:104–106.

Keele SW, Summers JJ 1976 The structure of motor programs. In: Stelmark GE (ed.) Motor control: issues and trends. Academic Press, New York.

Kelley JO, Kilbreath SL, Davis GM et al 2003 Cardiorespiratory fitness and walking ability in subacute stroke patients. Arch Phys Med Rehabil 84:1780–1785.

Kilbreath SL, Davis GM 2005 Cardiorespiratory fitness after stroke. In: Refshauge K, Ada L, Ellis E (eds) Science-based rehabilitation: theories into practice. Elsevier, Oxford:131–158.

Kim CM, Eng JJ, MacIntyre DL et al 2001 Effects of isokinetic strength training on walking in persons with stroke: a double-blind controlled pilot study. J Stroke Cerebrovasc Dis 10:265–273.

Kitai TA, Sale DG 1989 Specificity of joint angle in isometric training. Eur J Appl Physiol 58:744–748.

Komi PV 1986 The stretch-shortening cycle and human power output. In: Jones NL, McCartney N, McComas AJ (eds) Human muscle power. Human Kinetics, Champaign, IL:27–39.

Komi PV, Buskirk ER 1972 Effects of eccentric and concentric muscle conditioning on tension and

electrical activity of human muscle. Ergonomics 15:417–434.

Komi PV, Kaneko M, Aura O 1987 EMG activity of the leg extensor muscles with special reference to mechanical efficiency in concentric and eccentric exercise. Intern J Sports Med Suppl 8:22–29.

Kosslyn SM, Ganis G, Thompson WL 2001 Neural foundations of imagery. Nat Rev Neurosci 2:635–642.

Krebs HI, Volpe BT, Ferraro M et al 2002 Robot-aided neuro-rehabilitation: from evidence-based to science-based rehabilitation. Top Stroke Rehabil 8:54–70.

Kuo AD, Zajac FE 1993 A biomechanical analysis of muscle strength as a limiting factor in standing posture. J Biomech 26:137–150.

Lam YS, Man DWK, Tam SF et al 2006 Virtual reality training for stroke rehabilitation. Neurorehabil 21:245–253.

Landers M, Wulf G, Wallmann H et al 2005 An external focus of attention attenuates balance impairment in Parkinson's disease. Physiotherapy 91:152–185.

Larsson L 1982 Physical training effects on muscle morphology in sedentary males at different ages. Med Sci Sports Exerc 14:203–206.

Latash LP, Latash ML 1994 A new book by NA Bernstein: 'On Dexterity and its Development'. J Mot Behav 26:56–62.

Lee M-J, Kilbreath SL, Fiatarone-Singh M et al 2008 Comparison of effect of aerobic cycle training and progressive resistance training on walking ability after stroke: a randomized sham exercise-controlled study. J Am Geriatr Soc 56:976–985.

Leont'ev AN, Zaporozhets AV 1960 Rehabilitation of hand function. Pergamon Press, London.

Li F, Harmer P, Fisher KJ et al 2005 Tai Chi and fall reductions in older adults: a randomized and controlled trial. J Gerontol A Biol Sci Med Sci 60:187–194.

Liu KP, Chan CC, Lee TM et al 2004 Mental imagery for promoting relearning for people after stroke: a randomised controlled trial. Arch Phys Med Rehabil 18:1403–1408.

Lomaglio MJ, Eng JJ 2005 Muscle strength and weight-bearing symmetry relate to sit-to-stand performance in individuals with stroke. Gait Posture 22:126–131.

Lord SR, Castell S 1994 Physical activity program for older persons: effect on balance, strength, neuromuscular control, and reaction time. Arch Phys Med Rehabil 75:648–652.

Lord SR, Castell S, Corcoran J et al 2003 The effect of group exercise on physical functioning and falls in frail older people living in retirement villages: a randomized controlled trial. J Am Geriatr Soc 51:1685–1692.

Lord S, Sherrington C, Menz H et al 2007 Falls in older people, 2nd edn. Cambridge University Press, Cambridge.

Luft AR, McCombe-Waller S, Whitall J et al 2004 Repetitive bilateral arm training and motor cortex activation in chronic stroke. A randomized controlled trial. JAMA 292:1853–1861.

Lum PS, Burger CG, Shor PC et al 2002 Robot-assisted movement training compared with conventional therapy techniques for the rehabilitation of upper-limb motor function after stroke. Arch Phys Med Rehabil 83:952–959.

McArdle WD, Margel JR, Delio DJ et al 1978 Specificity of run training on VO_2 max and heart rate changes during running and swimming. Med Sci Sports 10:16–20.

McCartney N, Moroz D, Garner SH et al 1987 The effects of strength training in patients with selected neuromuscular disorders. Med Sci Sports Exerc 20:362–368.

MacConaill MA, Basmajian JV 1969 Muscle and movements. Basis for human kinesiology. Williams and Wilkins, Baltimore, MD.

McDonald PV, van Emmerick REA, Newell KM 1989 The effects of practice on limb kinematics in a throwing task. J Mot Behav 21:245–264.

McDowd JM, Filion DL, Pohl PS et al 2003 Attentional abilities and functional outcomes following stroke. J Gerontol B Psychol Sci Soc Sci 58:P45–53.

McHugh M 2003 Repeated advances in the repeated bout effect: the protective effect against muscle damage from a single bout of eccentric exercise. Scand J Med Sci Sports 13:88–97.

MacKay-Lyons MJ, Howlett J 2005 Exercise capacity and cardiovascular adaptations to aerobic training early after stroke. Top Stroke Rehabil 12:31–44.

MacKay-Lyons MJ, Makrides L 2002 Cardiovascular stress during a contemporary stroke rehabilitation program: is the intensity adequate to induce a training effect? Arch Phys Med Rehabil 83:1378–1383.

MacKay-Lyons MJ, Makrides L 2004 Longitudinal changes in exercise capacity after stroke. Arch Phys Med Rehabil 85:1608–1612.

Macko RF, DeSpuza CA, Tretter LD et al 1997 Treadmill aerobic exercise training reduces the energy expenditure and cardiovascular demands of hemiparetic gait in chronic stroke patients: a preliminary report. Stroke 28:326–330.

Macko RF, Ivey FM, Forrester LW 2005 Task-oriented aerobic exercise in chronic hemiparetic stroke: training protocols and treatment effects. Top Stroke Rehabil 12:45–57.

McNevin NH, Wulf G, Carlson C 2000 Effects of attentional focus, self control, and dyad training on motor learning: implications for physical rehabilitation. Phys Ther 80:373–385.

Magill RA 2001 Motor learning concepts and applications, 6th edn. McGraw-Hill, New York.

Magill RA 2003 Motor learning concepts and applications, 7th edn. McGraw-Hill, New York.

Malouin F, Richards CL 2005 Assessment and training of locomotion after stroke: evolving concepts. In: Refshauge K, Ada L, Ellis E (eds) Science-based rehabilitation. Theories into practice. Butterworth Heinemann, Oxford:185–222.

Malouin F, Bolleville C, Richard C et al 1997 Non-reflex mediated changes in plantarflexor muscles early after stroke. Scand J Rehabil Med 29:147–153.

Malouin F, Belleville S, Richards CL et al 2004 Working memory and mental practice outcomes after stroke. Arch Phys Med Rehabil 85:177–183.

Manoel E de J, Connolly KJ 1995 Variability and the development of skilled actions. Int J Psychophysiol 19:129–147.

Matyas TA, Galea MP, Spicer SD 1986 Facilitation of maximum voluntary contraction in hemiplegia by concomitant cutaneous stimulation. Am J Phys Med 65:125–134.

Mayo NE, Wood-Dauphinee S, Ahmed S et al 2005 Disablement following stroke. Disabil Rehabil 27:258–268.

Mayr A, Kofler M, Quirbach E et al 2007 Prospective, blinded, randomized crossover study of gait rehabilitation in stroke patients using the Lokomat gait orthosis. Neurorehabil Neural Repair 21:307–314.

Mazzeo RS, Cavanagh P, Evans WJ et al 1998 ACSM position stand: exercise and physical activity for older adults. Med Sci Sports Exerc 30:992–1008

Means KM, Rodell DE, O'Sullivan PS 2005 Balance, mobility, and falls among community-dwelling elderly persons: effects of a rehabilitation exercise program. Am J Phys Med Rehabil 84:238–250

Mehrabian A 1969 Significance of posture and position in the communication of attitude and status relationships. Psych Bull 71:359–372.

Mehrholz J, Werner C, Kugler J et al 2008 Electromechanical-assisted gait training with physiotherapy may improve walking after stroke. Stroke 39:1929–1930.

Miller GJT, Light KE 1997 Strength training in spastic hemiparesis: should it be avoided? Neurorehabil 9:17–28.

Miller LE, Pierson LM, Nickols-Richardson SM et al 2006 Knee extensor and flexor torque development with concentric and eccentric isokinetic training. Res Q Exerc Sport 77:58–63.

Milner-Brown HS, Miller RG 1988a Muscle strengthening through high-resistance weight training in patients with neuromuscular disorders. Arch Phys Med Rehabil 69:14.

Milner-Brown, HS, Miller RG 1988b Muscle strengthening through electric stimulation combined with low-resistance weights in patients with neuromuscular disorders. Arch Phys Med Rehabil 69:20.

Milner-Brown HS, Mellenthin M, Miller RG 1986 Quantifying human muscle strength, endurance and fatigue. Arch Phys Med Rehabil 67:530.

Morris SL, Dodd KJ, Morris M 2004 Outcomes of progressive resistance strength training following stroke: a systematic review. Clin Rehabil 18:27–39.

Morrissey MC, Harman EA, Johnson MJ 1995 Resistance training modes: specificity and effectiveness. Med Sci Sports Exerc 27:648–660.

Mulder T, Hulstijn W 1985 Sensory feedback in the learning of a novel task. J Mot Behav 17:110–128.

Nadeau S, Arsenault B, Gravel D et al 1999 Analysis of the clinical factors determining natural and maximal gait speeds in adults with stroke. Am J Phys Med Rehabil 78:123–130.

Narici MV, Roi GS, Landoni L et al 1989 Changes in force, cross-sectional area and neural activation during strength training and detraining of the human quadriceps. Eur J Appl Physiol Occup Physiol 59:310–319.

Newell KM 1981 Skill learning. In: Holding DH (ed.) Human skills. John Wiley & Sons, New York:203–226.

Newham DJ 2005 Muscle performance after stroke. In: Refshauge K, Ada L, Ellis E (eds) Science-based rehabilitation. Elsevier, Oxford.

Ng S, Shepherd RB 2000 Weakness in patients with stroke: implications for strength training in neurorehabilitation. Phys Ther Rev 5:227–238.

Nugent JA, Schurr KA, Adams RD 1994 A dose–response relationship between amount of weight-bearing exercise and walking outcome following cerebrovascular accident. Arch Phys Med Rehabil 75:399–402.

Olivetti L, Sherrington C, Wallbank G et al 2007 A novel weight-bearing strengthening program during rehabilitation of older people is feasible and improves standing up more than a non-weight-bearing strengthening program: a randomised trial. Aust J Physiother 53:147–153.

Olney SJ, Monga TN, Costigan PA 1986 Mechanical energy of walking of stroke patients. Arch Phys Med Rehabil 67:92–98.

Page J 2005 Effects of mental practice on affected limb use and function in chronic stroke. Arch Phys Med Rehabil 86:399–402.

Page SJ, Levine P, Sisto SA et al 2001 Mental practice combined with physical practice for upper-limb motor deficit in subacute stroke. Phys Ther 81:1455–1462.

Pai Y-C, Rogers MW 1991 Segmental contributions to total body momentum in sit-to-stand. Med Sci Sports Exerc 29:225–230.

Pang MY, Eng JJ, Dawson AS et al 2005 A community-based fitness and mobility exercise program for older adults with chronic stroke: a randomized, controlled trial. J Am Geriatr Soc 53:1667–1674.

Pang MY, Harris JE, Eng JJ 2006 A community-based upper-extremity group exercise program improves motor function and performance of functional activities in chronic stroke: a randomized controlled trial. Arch Phys Med Rehabil 87:1–9.

Pavone E, Moffat M 1985 Isometric torque of the quadriceps femoris after concentric, eccentric and isometric training. Arch Phys Med Rehabil 66:168–170.

Penninx BWJH, Ferrucci L, Leveille SG et al 2000 Lower extremity performance in nondisabled older persons as a predictor of subsequent hospitalisation. J Gerontol Med Sci 55A:M691–697.

Pomeroy VM, Clark CA, Miller SG et al 2005 The potential for utilizing the 'mirror neurone system' to enhance recovery of the severely affected upper limb early after stroke: a review and hypothesis. Neurorehabil Neural Repair 19:4–13.

Potempa K, Lopez M, Braun LT et al 1995 Physiological outcomes of aerobic exercise training in hemiparetic stroke patients. Stroke 26:101–105.

Proteau L 1992 On the specificity of learning and the role of visual information for movement control. In: Proteau L, Elliott D (eds) Vision and motor control. Elsevier Science, New York:67–103.

Rasch PT, Morehouse LE 1957 Effect of static and dynamic exercise on muscular strength and hypertrophy. J Appl Physiol 11:29–34.

Rooney KJ, Herbert RD, Balnave RJ 1994 Fatigue contributes to the strength training stimulus. Med Sci Sports Exerc 26:1160–1164.

Rosenbaum DA 1991 Human motor control. Academic Press, New York.

Rutherford OM 1988 Muscular coordination and strength training. Implications for injury rehabilitation. Sports Med 5:196–202.

Rutherford OM, Jones DA 1986 The role of learning and coordination in strength training. Eur J Appl Physiol Occup Physiol 55:100–105.

Salbach NM, Mayo NE, Wood-Dauphinee S et al 2004 A task-orientated intervention enhances walking distance and speed in the first year post stroke: a randomised controlled trial. Clinic Rehabil 18:509–519.

Sale DG 1987 Influence of exercise and training on motor unit activation. Exerc Sports Sci Rev 15:95–151.

Sale DG 1988 Neural adaptation to resistance training. Med Sci Sports Exerc 20:S135–S145.

Sale DG, MacDougall D 1981 Specificity in strength training: a review for the coach and athlete. Can J Appl Sport Sci 6:87–92.

Sale DG, MacDougall JD, Upton ARM et al 1983 Effect of strength training upon motoneuron excitability in man. Med Sci Sports Exerc 15:57–62.

Schenkman M, Berger RA, O'Riley P et al 1990 Whole-body movements during rising to standing from sitting. Phys Ther 70:638–651.

Schmidt RA 1988 Motor control and learning, 2nd edn. Human Kinetics, Champaign, IL.

Seligman M 1975 In: Helplessness: On depression, development and death. WH Freeman, San Francisco:21–41.

Sharp SA, Brouwer BJ 1997 Isokinetic strength training of the hemiparetic knee: effects on function and spasticity. Arch Phys Med Rehabil 78:1231–1236.

Shea CH, Wulf G 1999 Enhancing motor learning through external-focus instructions and feedback. Hum Mov Sci 18:553–571.

Shea CH, Wulf G, Whitacre C 1999 Enhancing training efficiency and effectiveness through the use of dyad training. J Mot Behav 31:119–125.

Shepherd RB, Gentile AM 1994 Sit-to-stand: functional relationship between upper body and lower limb segments. Hum Mov Sci 13:817–840.

Sherrington C, Lord SR 1997 Home exercise to improve strength and walking velocity after hip fracture: a randomized controlled trial. Arch Phys Med Rehabil 78:208–212.

Sherrington C, Lord S, Herbert R 2003 A randomised trial of weight-bearing versus non-weight-bearing exercise for improving physical ability in inpatients after hip fracture. Aust J Physiother 49:15–22.

Sherrington C, Lord SR, Herbert RD 2004 A randomized controlled trial of weight-bearing versus non-weight-bearing exercise for improving physical ability after usual care for hip fractures. Arch Phys Med Rehabil 85:710–716.

Sherrington C, Whitney JG, Lord SR et al 2008a Effective exercise for the prevention of falls: a systematic review and meta-analysis. J Am Geriatr Soc 56:2234–2243.

Sherrington C, Pamphlett PI, Jacka JA et al 2008b Group exercise can improve participants' mobility in an outpatient rehabilitation setting: a randomised controlled trial. Clin Rehabil 22:493–502.

Shumway-Cook A, Woollacott M 2005 Motor control. Translating research into clinical practice 3rd edn. Lippincott, Philadelphia.

Singer RN 1980 Motor learning and human performance. Macmillan, New York.

Sisto SA, Forrest GF, Gendinning D et al 2002 Virtual reality applications for motor rehabilitation after stroke. Top Stroke Rehabil 8:11–23.

Smith GV, Silver KHC, Goldberg AP et al 1999 'Task-oriented' exercise improves hamstring strength and spastic reflexes in chronic stroke patients. Stroke 30:2112–2118.

Smith P, Galea M, Woodward M et al 2008 Physical activity by elderly patients undergoing inpatient rehabilitation is low: an observational study. Aust J Physiother 54:209–213.

Sparrow WA 1983 The efficiency of skilled performance. J Mot Behav 15:237–261.

Sparrow WA, Irizarry-Lopez VM 1987 Mechanical efficiency and metabolic cost as measures of learning a novel gross motor task. J Mot Behav 19:240–264.

Stanish WD, Rubinovich RM, Aurwin S 1986 Eccentric exercise in chronic tendinitis. Clin Orthop 208:65–68.

Sterr A, Freivogel S 2003 Motor improvement following intensive training in low-functioning chronic hemiparesis. Neurology 61:842–844.

Svantessen U, Sunnerhagen KS 1997 Stretch-shortening cycle in patients with upper motor neuron lesion due to stroke. Eur J Appl Physiol 75:312–318.

Svantessen U, Takahashi H, Carlsson U et al 2000 Muscle and tendon stiffness in patients with upper motor neuron lesion following a

stroke. Eur J Appl Physiol 82:275–279.

Talvitie U 2000 Socio-affective characteristics and properties of extrinsic feedback in physiotherapy. Physiother Res Int 5:173–188.

Tax AA, Denier van der Gon JJ, Erkelens CJ 1990 Differences in coordination of elbow flexor muscles in force tasks and in movement. Exper Brain Res 81:567–572.

Teixeira-Salmela LF, Olney SJ, Nadeau S et al 1999 Muscle strengthening and physical conditioning to reduce impairment and disability in chronic stroke survivors. Arch Phys Med Rehabil 80:1211–1218.

Teixeira-Salmela LF, Nadeau S, McBride I et al 2001 Effects of muscle strengthening and physical conditioning training on temporal, kinematic and kinetic variables during gait in chronic stroke survivors. J Rehabil Med 33:53–60.

Thepaut-Mathieu C, Van Hoecke J, Maton B 1985 Length specificity of strength and myoneural activation improvements following isometric training. In: Johnson B (ed.) Biomechanics 1-A. Human Kinetics, Champaign, IL:513–517.

Thepaut-Mathieu C, Van Hoecke J, Maton B 1988 Myoelectrical and mechanical changes linked to length specificity during isometric training. J Appl Physiol 64:1500–1505.

Thorndike EL 1927 The law of effect. Am J Psychol 39:212–222.

Trowbridge EL, Cason H 1932 An experimental study of Thorndike's theory of learning. J Gen Psychol 7:245–258.

van der Weel FR, van der Meer AL, Lee DN 1991 Effect of task on movement control in cerebral palsy: implications for assessment and therapy. Develop Med Child Neurol 33:419–426.

van Peppen RPS, Kwakkel G, Wood-Dauphinee S et al 2004 The impact of physical therapy on functional outcomes after stroke: what's the evidence? Clin Rehabil 18:833–862.

van Vliet PM, Wulf G 2006 Extrinsic feedback for motor learning after stroke: what is the evidence? Disabil Rehabil 28:831–840.

Volpe BT, Krebs HI, Hogan N et al 2000 A novel approach to stroke rehabilitation: robot-aided sensorimotor stimulation. Neurology 54:1938–1944.

Weiss A, Suzuki T, Bean J et al 2000 High intensity strength training improves strength and functional performance after stroke. Am J Phys Med Rehabil 79:369–376.

Westing SH, Seger JY, Thorstensson A 1990 Effects of electrical stimulation on eccentric and concentric torque-velocity relationships during knee extension in man. Acta Physiol Scand 140:17–22.

Whiting HTA 1980 Dimensions of control in motor learning. In: Stelmark GE, Requin J (eds) Tutorials in motor behavior. North Holland, New York:537–550.

Whiting HTA, den Brinker BPLM 1982 Image of the act. In: Das JP, Mulcahy RF, Wall AE (eds) Theory and research in learning disabilities. Plenum Press, New York.

Whiting HTA, Bijlard MJ, den Brinker BPLM 1987 The effect of the availability of a dynamic model on the acquisition of a complex cyclical action. Q J Exp Psychol 39A:43–59.

Wise SP, Desimone R 1988 Behavioral neurophysiology: insights into seeing and grasping. Science 242:736–741.

Wolf SL, Baker MP, Kelly JL 1979 EMG biofeedback in stroke: effect of patient characteristics. Arch Phys Med Rehabil 60:96–103.

Wolf SL, Baker MP, Kelly JL 1980 EMG biofeedback in stroke: a one-year follow-up of the effect on patient characteristics. Arch Phys Med Rehabil 61:351–355.

Wulf G 2007 Attention and motor skill learning. Human Kinetics, Champaign, IL.

Wulf G, Schmidt RA 1989 The learning of generalized motor programs: reducing the relative frequency of knowledge of results enhances memory. J Exp Psychol Learn Mem Cogn 19:748–757.

Wulf G, Weigelt C 1997 Instructions about physical principles in learning a complex motor skill: to tell or not to tell… Res Q Exerc Sport 68:362–367.

Wulf G, Hof M, Prinz W 1998 Instructions for motor learning: differential effects of internal and external focus of attention. J Mot Behav 30:169–179.

Wulf G, Lauterbach B, Toole T 1999 The learning advantages of an external focus of attention. Res Q Exerc Sport 70:120–129.

Wulf G, McNevin NH, Fuchs T et al 2000 Attentional focus in complex skill learning. Res Q Exerc Sport 71:229–239.

Wulf G, McNevin N, Shea CH 2001 The automaticity of complex motor skill learning as a function of attentional focus. Q J Exp Psychol 54A:1143–1154.

Wulf G, Connel N, Gartner M et al 2002 Feedback and attentional focus: enhancing the learning of sports skills through external-focus feedback. J Mot Behav 34:171–182.

Wulf G, Landers M, Lewthwaite R et al 2009 External focus instructions reduce postural instability in individuals with Parkinson's disease. Phys Ther 89:162–168.

You SH, Jang SH, Kim YH et al 2005 Virtual reality-induced cortical reorganization and associated locomotor recovery in chronic stroke. Stroke 36:1166–1171.

Young A, Hughes I, Round JM et al 1982 The effect of knee injury on the number of muscle fibres in the human quadriceps femoris. Clin Sci 62:227–234.

Zimmermann-Schlatter A, Schuster C, Puhan MA et al 2008 Efficacy of motor imagery in post-stroke rehabilitation: a systematic review. J Neuroeng Rehabil 5:8.

Chapter | 3 |

Measurement

INTRODUCTION

The clinical evaluation of an individual with a neurological diagnosis involves reference to relevant medical history and the results of screening tests, including X-rays, brain scans, electrophysical tests, cognitive-behavioural assessments and current medications. The rehabilitation team works together so as not to overburden the individual by duplicating questions. Where a patient is unconscious or unable to communicate, information from relatives may help the therapist's understanding of the patient's personality and preferences.

The major role of physiotherapy is the analysis and training of everyday motor functions with the aim of enabling the individual to return to or continue with the personal, leisure, household and work-related activities they normally perform. The general purpose of measurement is to detect change over time, whether the individual's performance is better, worse or the same. This requires repeated measurements under the same standardized testing conditions. Data are collected using objective tests in which some measure of functionality is obtained and also by encouraging self-report, from which information about the individual's own perceptions of their health is gathered. Clinical practice therefore involves the collection of relevant, accurate and objective data about the individual's performance in motor tasks most critical to the person's everyday life.

It is important to make a clear distinction between *objective and subjective assessment*. Objective information is critical to the design and ongoing modification of the individual's training programme. Measures used may involve both functional and laboratory tests depending on the questions to be answered and the availability of

©2010 Elsevier Ltd
DOI: 10.1016/B978-0-7020-4051-1.00010-2

equipment and technical expertise. Data are collected on entry to physiotherapy, at regular periods during hospital- or community-based rehabilitation, and on discharge and follow-up. Follow-up data are necessary to provide information about 'real' outcomes such as retention of gains and how the individual is functioning at home. Some clinical research projects also necessitate the collection of baseline data before commencing intervention.

Measurement of motor performance is therefore a critical part of physiotherapy, providing objective information for identifying a problem that may benefit from intervention and for determining the direction and detail of training. Measurement can also provide information about broader issues of, for example, recovery patterns, and effectiveness of intervention that may be used to justify continuing a programme of intervention, or to evaluate the cost-effectiveness of the intervention. The cost–benefit relationship in neurorehabilitation as much as humanitarian concerns has increased the need for the healthcare community to be accountable for the services they provide (Keith 1995). We can expect to see greater reference to the cost–benefits of interventions as researchers begin to examine this issue. Although systematic reviews and meta-analyses are beginning to examine the effects of interventions, there are, in these early stages, some general methodological weaknesses making the findings difficult to interpret. Nevertheless, important clinical findings can usually be inferred. Herbert and colleagues (2005) point out the importance of distinguishing *measures of outcome* (e.g., the presence or absence of shoulder pain tested at discharge) from *measures of specific treatment effects*.

Three major problems in assessing the effectiveness of neurorehabilitation are a lack of consistency in instruments used, the heterogeneity in both patient groups and interventions, and lack of detail about specific exercise and training given, that is, the actual 'dosage'. Two issues requiring further recognition and further research are the clinical significance of an observed effect, and whether the estimate of change in performance is true change or can be attributed to measurement error (Ferreira & Herbert 2008) or natural recovery. Clinically important interventions are those in which effects are large enough to make the costs and the effort involved worthwhile.

Measurement is only part of the assessment process, the quantification of an observation against a standard. Evaluation, however, also involves the analysis and interpretation of the information gathered (Wade 1992a) and provides the knowledge necessary to plan appropriate exercise and training. It is an important means of establishing best practice and making changes to practice as more effective methods of intervention are developed. The usefulness of rehabilitation research depends on the inclusion of details of interventions given and of the intensity of exercise and training in order to make a link between the problems being targeted, methods used and the functional results. A consensus on a few valid and reliable

measurement tools between rehabilitation centres would help in examining the value and effect of neurological rehabilitation.

Some measurement instruments have a *ceiling effect*. This exists when a maximum score is achieved but there is scope for higher levels of functional performance (e.g., walking item on the Motor Assessment Scale (MAS)). Some instruments have *floor effects* and are of limited value for individuals with severe disability who are likely to score 0 (unable to do), preventing identification of any change over time.

Measurement carries with it a number of responsibilities. Terminology makes more sense if it is standardized across professional boundaries. The World Health Organization's (WHO) International Classification of Impairments, Disabilities and Handicaps (ICIDH) has recently been modified and revised to become the International Classification of Function (ICF). The terms impairments, disability and handicap have been replaced by 'body function and structure' for impairments, 'limitations in activities' for disability and 'restriction in participation' for handicap (WHO 2001).

Reliable and valid measures exist for evaluating outcome and testing the effects of interventions, and physiotherapists should use these rather then deciding to spend time and effort in developing their own scale (Hill et al 2005). In a well-organized rehabilitation unit, clinicians will agree on measures to be used, collect essential data routinely and reliably, and act on the results.

Matching the test to the objective. If the objective is to improve performance on a functional task, a method of measuring that task is used, for example sitting to standing item on the MAS, 10-metre walk test, nine-hole peg test for hand function. If calf muscle length is the issue, a different type of measure is used. If reduction in falls is a major concern in an individual with Parkinson's disease, a Falls Efficacy Scale may be appropriate in addition to measuring, for example, gait speed or timed up-and-go.

The rehabilitation team should avoid excessive use of measurement in the clinic. Experience in rehabilitation units where the physiotherapists are enthusiastic about the principle of measurement suggests that, once the idea takes on, it is of such interest that more time can be spent on assessment and measurement than on training.

There are many publications that discuss issues related to measurement or contain details related to the large number of tests available for use in neurological rehabilitation (e.g., Wade 1992a; Finch et al 2002; Hill et al 2005; Lord et al 2007). This chapter outlines some measurements and self-report questionnaires that have been shown to be reliable, valid and clinically relevant. The value of the tests included is that they require little or no equipment and are quick and easy to perform in the clinic. Some training and practice on using a scale helps the therapist develop reliability in administration.

Some tests included are not typically administered by physiotherapists but since they provide critical information about the patient's physical, social and emotional status that can assist in planning appropriate intervention, they are included so therapists have some understanding of what the tests are designed to measure. Biomechanical studies of motor performance that involve equipment such as electromyogram (EMG), load cells, force plates and motion-analysis systems are usually restricted to research laboratories equipped with technical assistance.

In general, we have acknowledged the original developers of the instruments listed and provided additional references where necessary. For a more comprehensive analysis of measurement in neurological physiotherapy and the instruments in current use, we recommend Hill and colleagues' monograph (2005) available from the Australian Physiotherapy Association (www.physiotherapy.asn.au). These authors provide an analysis of the strengths and limitations of instruments, evidence of validity and reliability, include testing procedures and scoring sheets and normative gender- and age-related values where they exist. Many instruments listed have easily accessible Web sites.

GLOBAL MEASURES OF FUNCTION

These tests are more likely to be administered by a physician or nurse than a physiotherapist, who would concentrate on the motor performance measures. The two global measures below tend to be used as measures of dependence.

Barthel Index

The Barthel Index measures performance across a range of commonly performed functional activities. It is said to be the most widely used measurement tool and has been used in many clinical and research settings. Since its introduction there have been several variations developed (e.g., Shah et al 1989). The test has high retest reliability when used with stroke patients and is considered valid. It covers many functions and provides no specific indicators of value to planning intervention other than broad areas of focus. Nevertheless, the Barthel Index does provide a general overview of a person's status. There are 10 categories (Box 3.1).

Reference: Mahoney & Barthel 1965.

Functional Independence Measure (FIM®)

FIM® is a widely used measure of severity of disability, that is of the impact of disease or impairment on performance of daily activities. It was designed to assess the degree of assistance required by a person with a disability to perform

---

Box 3.1 Barthel index

Feeding
Bathing
Grooming
Dressing
Bowels
Bladder
Toilet use
Transfers (bed to chair and back)
Mobility (on level surfaces)
Stairs

Items are scored from 0 (dependent) to 5, 10 or 15 (independent) based on criteria. Scores are usually summed out of 100 although it is an ordinal scale.

---

daily activities (the burden of care). It has been reported to be reliable and valid. Staff who wish to use the FIM® are required to be trained. Information and training are available in Australia through the University of Wollongong, or consult the Web site in Box 3.2. There are six categories and 18 activities (Box 3.2).

References: Granger et al 1986; Keith et al 1987.

MEASURES OF MOTOR PERFORMANCE

Biomechanical measures

The initial step in understanding human motor performance is to measure in some organized fashion how humans move. On one level, observation of an individual's motor behaviour is a form of assessment, however observations usually lack both validity and reliability, making suspect the conclusions drawn (Smith 1990). Understanding the terminology, the tools and techniques of biomechanical research on human motor performance provides the clinician with the knowledge to identify more accurately the nature of motor dysfunction and to base training on a scientific rationale. Understanding the data gathered requires an education that encompasses biomechanics and kinesiology. Physiotherapists working in movement rehabilitation must be familiar with results of biomechanical research and the methods used. The knowledge gained from ongoing research into functional actions in both healthy and disabled subjects should underpin and direct both evaluation and training these actions in clinical practice.

Biomechanical data on functional actions such as standing up, walking and reaching out in both able-bodied and

---

Box 3.2 Functional independence measure®

Personal care
    Feeding
    Grooming
    Bathing
    Dressing (upper body)
    Dressing (lower body)
    Toileting
Sphincter control
    Bladder management
    Bowel management
Mobility
    Transfers (bed/chair/wheelchair)
    Transfers (toilet)
    Transfers (bath/tub/shower)
Locomotion
    Walking or using wheelchair
    Stairs
Communication
    Comprehension
    Expression
Social cognition
    Social interaction
    Problem solving
    Memory

Each category is scored on a 7-point ordinal scale, 1 indicating fully dependent and 7 independent with no aids. The maximum total score is 126. Operational definitions for the 7 levels are provided on the Uniform Data System for Medical Rehabilitation (UDS-MR) home page: http://www.udsmr.org.

Box 3.3 The Motor Assessment Scale for stroke

Supine to side lying on to intact side
Supine to sitting over the side of bed
Balanced sitting
Sitting to standing
Walking
Upper arm function
Hand movements
Advanced hand activities

Each item of the MAS is scored on a 7-point ordinal scale from 0 to 6. Criteria for scoring are provided, together with general rules for administering the scale.

Global clinical tests

Motor Assessment Scale (MAS) for stroke

Two decades ago, in an attempt to provide a reliable and valid method for testing the task-related interventions we were developing, we designed and tested this global motor assessment scale. The updated version consists of eight items (Box 3.3). Reliability of individual physiotherapists is tested, after practice sessions with five patients, by rating individual's scores made against a criterion rating from observations of videotapes of patients. No importance is attached to the 'quality' of movement when testing, as the therapist must concentrate on following the standardized 'rules' of the test.

The scale has test–retest and inter-rater reliability (Carr et al 1985; Loewen & Anderson 1988; Poole & Whitney 1988;) and is a valid instrument (Malouin et al 1994; Lennon & Hastings 1996). The validity of the *sitting to standing* item is supported by several biomechanical studies of the action, showing that improvement on the scale occurs in conjunction with increasing normalization of certain biomechanical parameters (Ada & Westwood 1992; Ada et al 1993).

A study comparing MAS scores with scores on the Fugl-Meyer Assessment (FMA) (Malouin et al 1994) showed good correlation between the two except for the sitting balance item. This may not be surprising, given that the FMA assesses the ability to sit still, whereas the MAS assesses the ability to balance while moving about (reaching in different directions) and may, therefore, be the better indicator of balance.

An advantage of the test is that it takes a short time to administer (10–15 minutes) if the tester is experienced (Carr et al 1985; Malouin et al 1994). It measures each item as a separate entity since items bear no particular relationship to each other but are separate actions. Therefore, individual items, for example *sitting to standing*, can be used depending on what information is needed. Although a summative score has been used in several

disabled populations provide input into the more subjective observational analysis and provide an indication of the accuracy of observations that have formed the basis of training that particular task. Neurological physiotherapy cannot rely on clinical observation alone in clinical practice.

Rehabilitation departments with easy access to motion analysis laboratories and technical assistance have the greatest potential to produce reliable and meaningful biomechanical data for clinical research. Such laboratories also assist the clinician to identify more accurately the nature of the motor performance dysfunction. However, due to cost, space and resources it is not possible for all patients to have a biomechanical analysis, and there are simpler tests suitable for use in the clinic. As with all measurement tools, particular attention is paid to standardization issues when testing.

clinical trials, this is of questionable validity since it is an ordinal scale and the criteria were not hierarchically organized. The MAS is routinely used in many stroke units and in clinical trials. Its major advantage seems to be in providing information related to the performance of actions that acute neurological patients have a great interest in improving; everyday actions such as standing up and sitting down, walking and hand use.

The MAS appears to be a useful measure of functional ability both in clinical data collection and for laboratory research. It has been shown to be predictive of stroke recovery and suggested as a means of prioritizing rehabilitation management (Loewen & Anderson 1990). Muscle tone was included in the original version but has been omitted given that the term 'tone' is vague in meaning and its reliability is questionable since a subjective clinical test like this cannot separate muscle stiffness from reflex hyperexcitability. The MAS has been translated into several languages including Chinese, Norwegian, Danish, Swedish and Portuguese.

Reference: Carr et al 1985.

Rivermead Motor Assessment (RMA)

The scale was designed as a measure of motor function after stroke. Its three sections include both impairments and disabilities: *gross function, leg and trunk, arm*. Each section contains 10–15 items. For example, *gross function* includes walking, sitting to standing, lying to sitting over the side of the bed. Each item is scored 0 or 1 and the total for each section is summed.

The scale has a number of problems that raise the question of validity. Each section is based on a hierarchy of actions, which, since they are unrelated to each other in a biomechanical or a functional sense, cannot be considered to reflect a progression. The RMA assumes without evidentiary support that motor recovery post-stroke occurs in a proximal to distal sequence that is inaccurate (Poole & Whitney 2001). The scale is long and we are not aware that it has been formally tested for reliability (Lincoln & Leadbitter 1979; Collin et al 1990). A prospective study concluded that much of the scale is outdated (Adams et al 1997). Nevertheless, the scale is still sometimes used and may be encountered in journal articles.

Fugl-Meyer Assessment (FMA)

The FMA tool is used in some centres in North America. It is based on Brunnstrom's stages of recovery which assumed, in the 1950s, that motor recovery proceeds in a sequence from mass stereotypical flexor or extensor movement patterns to movements that combine the two, to voluntary isolated movements at each joint (Poole & Whitney 2001). It is divided into five domains: *motor function, sensory function, balance, joint range of motion*, and *joint pain*. It has been criticized for being too lengthy and difficult to understand (Wade 1992a). The test has been

shown to have moderate inter-rater reliability (Sanford et al 1993) but its validity is questionable given that it is based on what appears to be an inaccurate view of the pattern of recovery from stroke (e.g., Malouin et al 1994). The FMA has been reported to discriminate better in the early stage of recovery, probably because it assesses isolated joint movement rather than task-related actions. The MAS has been suggested as a replacement for the FMA (Poole & Whitney 1988).

Reference: Fugl-Meyer et al 1975.

Specific performance tests

Gait

MAS walking item

The *walking* item of the MAS can be used as a measure of gait function. Due to the ceiling effect, individuals who achieve the highest score can be tested on other measures, such as speed and endurance.

6–10-Metre walk test

Speed can be measured by timing the subject while he or she walks a known distance between two marks on the floor. The distance walked is a matter of convenience but somewhere in the region of 6–10 m (20–33 ft) is probably adequate. The 10-m test has been tested for validity and reliability (Wade et al 1987; Maeda et al 2000; Green et al 2002; Flansbjer et al 2005). The subject is asked to walk at their natural pace or can be asked to walk as fast as he/she can safely walk (Moseley et al 2004). The distance to be walked is marked out on the floor with two additional metres either end to allow the individual to get into their stride before measurement starts and to slow down after crossing the finishing line. Time taken from when the patient crosses the starting line to the finishing line is measured with a stopwatch. Note is taken of any aids used. The result can be expressed as time taken (seconds) or speed (metres/second). This test should be reliable if it is standardized and a careful record is kept of details. A graph of the patient's performance can provide feedback over time and be kept by the patient as a record of progress.

Walking speed over a short distance is a commonly used outcome measure in stroke rehabilitation providing information about change in walking. However, it does not provide an indication of a person's ability as a competent walker in the community. The findings of a recent study show that walking speed over a short distance can overestimate locomotor capacity (Dean et al 2001). To assess 'real' walking ability, both speed and endurance (6-minute walk test) need to be measured.

Reference: Wolfson et al 1990.

Measures of specific temporal and spatial variables

Several methods of measuring *cadence* (steps per minute) and *length of stride* (metre) have been reported. The commercially available clinical Stride Analyzer (B & L Engineering, Sante Fe, CA, USA) consists of a pair of foot switches, a start–stop controller and data storage unit. This system enables data to be collected for a subject's gait speed, stride length (distance covered in two steps), cadence and percentage of gait cycle spent in double support.

Reference: Morris et al 2002.

A simple method of quantifying these parameters is to attach two felt-tip marking pens with washable ink to the heels of the subject who walks on a walkway of suitable length on paper taped to the floor. A stopwatch is used to record time taken. Step and stride lengths and width of base can be measure and cadence calculated.

Reference: Cerny 1983.

Balance

There is no single test that can measure every aspect of balance since balance is an integral part of all the actions we perform and postural adjustments have a high degree of specificity. Many tests can measure significant improvements in task performance from which we can infer that balance has improved. One needs to be clear what question is being asked, since different tests measure different aspects of balance and there is little indication as yet about generalizability.

Balance can be classified under three broad classes of action: when we make a volitional movement, when the support surface moves unexpectedly and when we maintain a posture against external interference. In our view the most relevant tests of balance in the clinic test the person's ability to remain balanced during a self-initiated action. Postural adjustments throughout actions, such as walking, standing up, stair climbing and descent, when reaching for an object in sitting and standing, or when turning the head to look around the room, are critical to the performance of these actions. Without appropriate postural muscle activity and segmental rotations, the person would fail to achieve the goal or fall; if the person thinks they will fall, they will be reluctant to move. Whether or not measures that test only the person's response to unexpected support surface movement or to perturbation (pushes) initiated by the examiner are relevant to balance under the dynamic conditions of self-initiated movement is not known, but they might give insight into a person's ability to respond quickly. Testing an individual's ability to respond to a trip or slip to prevent a fall is difficult to assess in the clinic without a safety harness and virtual reality equipment. Below is a selection of valid and reliable tests that measure important aspects of balance during self-initiated actions.

MAS balanced sitting item

The *balanced sitting* item requires the patient to sit unsupported and reach in different directions without losing balance.

Functional reach test

This test measures maximum reach forward in standing. It is reliable and valid in that it measures an action that is common in everyday life and because reach distance scores correlate with biomechanical change (centre of pressure excursion). It is therefore a more dynamic test than tests of ability to stand still. The patient stands next to a wall to which a metre stick (yardstick) is attached. Starting position is with feet a standardized few centimetres apart. The arm is flexed forward to 90° in line with the stick. The patient makes a fist and the position of the third metacarpal relative to the stick is noted. The patient reaches forward as far as possible without taking a step and the position of the third metacarpal is again noted. Distance reached is compared to age- and gender-related norms (Box 3.4). The test has been found to be predictive of falls in the elderly.

Reference: Duncan et al 1990.

Sit-and-reach test

This test measures maximum reach forward in sitting. The subject sits with hips, knees and ankles at 90° flexion, feet flat on the floor. Using the non-paretic upper limb, the subject makes a fist, extends the elbow and flexes the shoulder to 90°. The position of the third metacarpal along a tape measure or metre stick secured to the wall at the level of the acromial process is recorded. The subject is instructed to reach as far forward as possible without rotating the trunk or losing balance. The final position of the third metacarpal is recorded. Distance reached is defined as the difference between the initial and final positions. Subjects have two practice trials before performing three test trials. The test has test–retest reliability.

Reference: Tsang & Mak 2004.

Standing balance test

This is a simple ordinal scale in which patients stand with eyes open (Box 3.5). It is said to be reliable. Its validity,

Box 3.4 **Functional reach test: age- and gender-related norms**		
Age	Male mean cm (in)	Female mean cm (in)
20–40	42 (16.7)	37 (14.6)
41–69	38 (15.0)	35 (13.8)
70–87	33 (13.1)	27 (10.5)

Box 3.5 **Standing balance test: scoring**
0 Unable to stand
1 Able to stand with feet apart, but for less than 30 seconds
2 Stands with feet apart for 30 seconds, but not with feet together
3 Stands with feet together, but for less than 30 seconds
4 Stands with feet together, for 30 seconds or more

including its generalizability to more dynamic situations, is uncertain and the ability to stand still may not be a suitable goal for all patients with brain lesions.

References: Bohannon 1989; Bohannon et al 1993.

Step test

This test measures the ability to support and balance the body mass on one limb while taking a step with the other. The patient stands with feet parallel and 5 cm (2 in) in front of a 7.5-cm (3-in) high block and steps with one foot on then off the block repeatedly as fast as possible. The number of steps made in 15 seconds is counted. The test is reliable and valid.

Reference: Hill et al 1996.

Timed 'up-and-go' (TUG) test

The TUG test measures speed of performance of a functionally significant linked series of tasks which threaten balance and which are known to cause falls in the elderly. The patient is required to stand up from a seat, walk 3 m (10 ft), turn, walk back and sit down while being timed with a stopwatch. Performance can be significantly influenced by the height of the seat which should be standardized. Its validity is supported by its high correlation with functional capacity as recorded on the Barthel Index. Average normative age and gender data for healthy older adults from 60 to 89 years have been recorded (Steffen et al 2002).

Reference: Podsialo & Richardson 1991.

Berg Balance Scale (BBS)

The BBS was specifically designed to assess balance of elderly individuals and monitor change over time. It is sometimes used in stroke rehabilitation. The scale measures the ability to balance while performing 14 static and dynamic balance tasks. All items are graded on a 5-point scale, 0–4. The maximum total score is 56. Items include *sitting and standing unsupported, sitting to standing, retrieving an object from the floor in standing, and turning 360° in standing.* A score of 0 is given if the person is unable to do the task and a score of 4 indicates that the person is able to complete the task based on criteria assigned to it. While

some authors have found the BBS to be a useful predictor of falls, others have not. It has been reported to be reliable and appears to have content validity. The BBS takes about 15 minutes to administer.

Reference: Berg et al 1989, 1992.

Choice stepping reaction time test

This test was devised as a simple measure of the complex response we make to avoid a fall. The subject is required to perform quick, correctly targeted steps in response to visual cues. The test appears to have validity as a composite measure of falls risk in older people.

Reference: Lord et al 2007.

Standing postural sway

The reliability and validity of measures of postural sway (e.g., centre of foot pressure) are not known, and there is some criticism of postural sway as a meaningful measure of functional balance (e.g., Goldie et al 1989). Recent useful developments include a portable sway meter which records displacement of the body at the lower trunk which gives an indication of a person's ability to balance in quiet standing and on a foam rubber mat (see Fig. 7.2).

Reference: Lord et al 2007.

Clinical test of sensory interaction in balance (CTSIB)

This test measures the number of seconds (30 s max) a person can stand in six different sensory conditions that involve reduced or conflicting visual and support surface conditions: *eyes open – firm support surface; eyes closed – firm support surface; visual conflict – firm support surface; eyes open – standing on foam; eyes closed – standing on foam; visual conflict – standing on foam.* It is said to be useful in identifying utilization of various sensory modalities, in particular identifying vestibular dysfunction.

References: Shumway-Cook & Horak 1986; Horak 1987.

Falls-related measures

Definitions of falling usually fail to distinguish between fear of falling and falls efficacy – the perceived ability to undertake activities of daily living confidently without falling (Lord et al 2007). Much work has been done recently to determine how these parameters affect the lives of elderly and disabled people.

Falls Efficacy Scale (FES)

The FES is a self-report questionnaire to assess an individual's confidence in his or her ability to avoid falling while undertaking 10 activities that include house cleaning and dressing. Since the original FES is most relevant for housebound individuals, the *Modified Falls Efficacy Scale* (MFES), that includes four additional items during activities outside the house, has been developed (Hill et al 1996).

Reference: Tinetti et al 1990.

The Activities-Specific Balance Confidence (ABC) Scale

A questionnaire asks a person to rate his or her confidence in the ability to perform 16 items without falling. The scale includes activities outside the house and is suitable for older individuals with higher levels of performance. The administration of the scale does require the individual to have reasonably intact cognition. The individual needs to understand that what is being assessed is confidence in doing the activity, not the ease with which the activity can be performed (Hill 2005).

Reference: Powell & Myers 1995.

Upper limb function

MAS upper limb items

These three items include upper arm function, hand movements and advanced hand activities.

Nine-hole peg test (NHPT)

This is a useful test for patients who have a relatively high level of performance since it measures dexterity and speed in a task that requires movement of the arm and hand. It is a suitable test to administer to people who have achieved top scores in the upper arm function and hand movements items of the MAS.

The apparatus consists of nine wooden pegs and a wood base with nine holes. The time taken by the patient to place all the dowels in the holes is measured with a stopwatch or, alternatively, how many pegs can be placed in a given time is recorded, for example 50 seconds. The test is reliable and valid. Able-bodied individuals take approximately 18 seconds to complete the task. There is also a 10-hole peg test (Turton & Fraser 1986).

References: Mathiowetz et al 1985; Sunderland et al 1989.

Frenchay arm test (FAT)

This short test consists of five tasks to be performed with the affected hand: *stabilize a ruler; grasp a cylinder; drink from a glass; place a spring clothes peg on a dowel; comb the hair*. Criteria for each task are provided and standardization is critical. The test is valid and reliable. It is simple and quick to carry out. The test is performed sitting with the hands in the lap, and each task starts from this position. A score of 1 is given for successful performance, 0 for failure, yielding an overall score of 5. The FAT has limited validity (Poole & Whitney 2001).

References: DeSouza et al 1980; Heller et al 1987; Sunderland et al 1992.

Action research arm test (ARAT)

The ARAT is a shortened version of Carroll's upper extremity function test (Carroll 1965). The test is divided into four subsections with items arranged in hierarchical order of difficulty: *grasp, grip, pinch* and *gross movement*. Each item is scored on a 4-point ordinal scale ranging from 0 (no movement possible) to 3 (movement performed normally). It is a responsive, reliable and valid test to assess recovery in upper limb function following cortical damage (van der Lee et al 2001). A standardized approach to performing the test has recently been published (Yozbatiran et al 2008).

Reference: Lyle 1981.

The spiral test

This test was developed as a measure of coordination and tested on two patients, one with cerebellar ataxia, the other with Parkinson's disease (Fig. 3.1). Two spirals are printed on a sheet of paper, with 1 cm between the lines. The subject must draw a line from a starting position (the arrow) to the central point as quickly as possible and without touching the lines. The subject is scored on time taken to perform the test in seconds. Each time a line is touched, 3 seconds are added to the time taken, and 5 seconds every time a line is crossed. The test appears to be reliable and is a valid measure of accuracy and speed. It is also a useful way of providing qualitative feedback to a patient.

Reference: Verkerk et al 1990.

MEASURES OF BODY STRUCTURE AND FUNCTION (IMPAIRMENTS)

Measures of specific factors related to movement such as muscle strength, spasticity and joint range are included below.

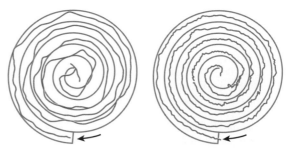

Figure 3.1 Spiral test results of individuals with cerebellar ataxia (Left) and Parkinson's disease (Right). *(From Verkerk et al (1990) by kind permission of Elsevier, Amsterdam).*

Muscle strength

The Medical Research Council (MRC) grades

These grades are used as an indication of the strength of muscle (Box 3.6). They provide a subjective impression of the ability to contract a muscle under certain conditions. In no sense do they provide an objective measure. They have been found to be reliable when raters are trained (Gregson et al 2000). The validity of the test is doubtful for a number of reasons, one of which is that the ability of a target muscle to contract is diminished if its synergists are inactive. Since grades 4 and 5 require a 'normal' side, this presents difficulties following stroke, where muscles on the non-paretic side may also be affected by the lesion.

Reference: Medical Research Council (MRC) 1976.

Motricity Index

The Motricity Index was devised based on the MRC grades. It appears to be reliable and valid for stroke patients (Collin & Wade 1990). The index sums scores for one limb and for one side of the body.

References: Demeurisse et al 1980; Wade 1992a.

Dynamometry

Maximum isometric force can be measured using a hand-held dynamometer or an isokinetic dynamometer under standardized conditions. The subject performs a maximum muscle contraction against a known force in a standardized position. A grip force dynamometer is used to measure grip or pinch force. Given the possible variability between instruments, it is wise to use the same device for pre- and post-tests. The provision of normative values can increase usefulness (Andrews et al 1996). The isokinetic dynamometer is also used to measure dynamic muscle force. Such devices need to be checked for reliability (see Tripp & Harris 1991).

References: Bohannon & Andrews 1987a,b.

Box 3.6 **The Medical Research Council grades**
0 No contraction
1 Palpable contraction
2 Movement without gravity
3 Movement against gravity
4 Movement against resistance lower than the resistance overcome by the healthy side
5 Movement against resistance equal to the maximum resistance overcome by the healthy side
Strength for each muscle is graded on an ordinal scale from 0 to 5.

Gracies (2005) points out that strength measurement in this population (e.g., MRC scales, dynamometry) may not provide a reliable assessment of voluntary agonist activation as the results can be confounded by resistance from soft tissue contracture or increased intrinsic stiffness. It is unlikely that isometric strength tests that are used in clinical studies can provide any information of value beyond evidence that a specific muscle group can generate more or less peak force. Although positive correlations between these strength tests and function have been reported from some studies, in others no relationship has been found (Bohannon 1995; Boissy et al 1999; Eriksrud 2003). Functional strength tests that involve a limb in a multijoint purposeful movement (e.g., number of sit-to-stands in a given period of time from a seat of a specific height) may be more valid measures of strength.

Functional strength

Two simple methods of measuring lower limb strength and coordination have been developed in an attempt to measure 'functional' strength in a closed kinetic chain action. Normative values for males/females for different age groups have not been investigated.

Lateral step test

The patient starts with the foot of the leg to be tested on a 15-cm (6-in) or a 20-cm (8-in) step placed beside the foot, with feet parallel and shoulder width apart. Weight is shifted to this side, the leg is extended, raising the body mass over the step to a position within 10° of knee extension. Body weight is lowered by flexion at the hip, knee and ankle until the heel of the moving leg touches the floor. For the 15-second test, the number of repetitions in 15 seconds is counted. For the 50-rep test, the patient is timed while performing the repetitions as quickly as possible. Both tests have high test–retest reliability.

Reference: Ross 1997.

The timed-stands test

The subject is timed while standing up from a seat 10 times as quickly as possible. Seat dimensions and height influence performance so must be standardized.

Reference: Csuka & McCarthy 1985.

Joint range of motion (ROM)

It is often important to record *passive* joint range, for example before and after intervention to stretch stiff and contracted calf muscles. The reliability of ROM measures depends on the standardization of procedures. A hand-held dynamometer is used to apply a known force to produce movement and a standard goniometer (or electrogoniometer) measures range (Moseley & Adams 1991). Body weight in standing or walking can also be used as a means of standardization. A test of joint range using a goniometer should always be standardized in terms of factors such as anatomical landmarks and force application (see Fig. 12.4), otherwise the test is unreliable (Gajdosik & Bohannon 1987).

Active joint range is measured during some relevant action, for example during stance or swing phase of walking or during sit-to-stand. In a biomechanics laboratory, the test is done using a computerized motion analysis system. In the clinic, range can be measured at a particular point during an action using a video camera or still photography under standardized conditions.

Muscle stiffness can also be quantified using a dynamometer or torque motor (Moseley & Adams 1991) to gauge the resistance to passive movement. In order to separate the neural component from the mechanical properties of soft tissues, EMG activity in muscles is collected simultaneously. This enables the detection of any neural response to stretch as it is applied at different velocities.

Spasticity

Two commonly used clinical tests, the Modified Ashworth Scale and the Tardieu Scale, are flawed as measures of spasticity. They cannot separate mechanical causes of resistance to movement (increased intrinsic stiffness of muscle) from neural causes (stretch reflex hyperactivity) (Fowler et al 1997; Morris 2002; Alibiglou et al 2008). Patrick & Ada (2006) compared the two scales and a laboratory measure of spasticity with a group of people post-stroke. The percentage exact agreement between the Tardieu and the laboratory measure was 100% in identifying the presence or absence of spasticity but only 63% between Ashworth Scale and laboratory measure. The Ashworth Scale overestimated spasticity in all the subjects who had contracture while the Tardieu could differentiate. The Tardieu Scale may be more valid than the Modified Ashworth Scale but both measure spasticity only during passive movement. Measures of stretch reflex activity during active functional movement are carried out in a biomechanics laboratory (e.g., see Crenna 1999), but there have been few studies published.

The Modified Ashworth Scale (MAS)

The scale is an example of a scale that sets out to test one impairment (spasticity) but really tests another (increased muscle stiffness). Muscle tone is graded subjectively by the examiner according to the amount of resistance felt in response to passive movement. Doubts have been raised about the validity of the MAS as a measure of spasticity by studies that have found no relationship between these scores and the results from laboratory tests of reflex hyperactivity (Vattanasilp & Ada 1999; Pandyan et al 2001; Alibiglou et al 2008).

References: Ashworth 1964; Bohannon & Smith 1987.

The Tardieu Scale

This is an ordinal scale that attempts to quantify the neural component of spasticity by measuring the intensity of the muscle response to joint movement at specified velocities. It is important to assess passive range of motion first so that the muscle being tested has experienced the movement before the velocity is increased. The joint angle at which the muscle response occurs is recorded. The scale appears to be more reliable and probably a more valid measure in patients with traumatic brain injury and stroke than the Modified Ashworth (Mehrholz et al 2005; Patrick & Ada 2006).

Reference: Gracies et al 2000.

Cardiorespiratory fitness/exercise capacity

Exercise capacity refers to an individual's ability to respond to the physiological stresses induced by performing large muscle, moderate-to-high intensity exercise for prolonged periods. Before participation in an exercise test, patients should be screened to determine their suitability for exercise testing and the need for an ECG-monitored test. The American College of Sports Medicine (ACSM) has developed screening protocols for different populations (ACSM 2006). Exercise testing should probably become a standard tool used as part of building up the fitness of neurological patients in rehabilitation, particularly following traumatic brain injury, brain surgery, stroke and in Parkinson's disease.

Fitness is typically tested using gymnasium equipment (e.g., treadmill, cycle ergometer) or field tests (e.g., sit-to-stand, modified 20-m shuttle test, 12-minute walk test). A *submaximal test* or *peak exercise test* is performed. A submaximal test involves calculating training heart rate, which is a percentage of heart rate reserve for that individual.

Peak aerobic testing is performed submaximally or maximally. Peak aerobic testing may be carried out using a modified version of a standardized protocol such as the modified Balke treadmill test (Palmer-McLean et al 2002). Peak testing frequently requires simultaneous ECG monitoring and is carried out by specially trained staff. The choice of fitness test should reflect the characteristics of the individual being tested, the level of information required, the equipment and staff available (and their level of expertise), and the mode of exercise that will be presented in an exercise programme.

Measurement of peak aerobic capacity (VO_{2peak}) enables comparison with normative data and with the estimated aerobic requirements of the individual's pre-injury work and/or leisure activities. VO_{2peak} can be measured directly from a peak exercise test by measuring expired ventilation and expired gas fractions, although this requires specialized equipment not usually available in the clinical setting. Alternatively, VO_{2peak} can be estimated from performance on a peak exercise test or in submaximal tests by using a regression equation of heart rate and oxygen uptake at submaximal work loads, or estimated from protocol-specific regression equations.

References: Ward et al 1995; American College of Sports Medicine 1998, 2006; MacKay-Lyons & Howlett 2005.

Heart rate monitoring

Monitoring heart rate is a simple method of ensuring that exercise is sufficiently vigorous to improve fitness and to test whether or not a patient's cardiovascular system is adapting to exercise. It provides an indication of intensity of exercise and is typically used when it is necessary to monitor the level of exercise. This test may be used to monitor intensity of training in any patient with a brain lesion. To exercise at the appropriate level to improve cardiorespiratory fitness, the training heart rate is determined using a heart rate monitor and calculated using the heart rate reserve method (Box 3.7).

Reference: Karvonen et al 1957.

Borg Rating of Perceived Exertion (RPE) Scale

The RPE is a 15-grade rating scale of perceived exertion (Box 3.8). It has been validated in several different age and gender groups, both healthy and disabled. Individuals are familiarized with the scale and asked to rate an estimate of physical effort (degree of work) as accurately and naively as possible throughout the exercise session. The ACSM (2006) provides standardized instructions for administering the scale that are displayed on a poster or board placed so that it is visible to all areas of the exercise area.

Reference: Borg 1970.

6-Minute walk test (6MWT)

Endurance can be tested specifically for walking by measuring the distance walked in 6 minutes. As walking is a self-paced and familiar activity, the score on this test may reflect activities of daily living that are performed at submaximal levels of exertion. An indoor, flat, straight walkway or corridor, at least 30 m long without obstacles is required. Subjects are able to stop and rest with the timer still running. The distance an individual is able to walk in 6 minutes is recorded. Use of a treadmill is not recommended as it is externally paced. The test has been used extensively in individuals with cardiopulmonary problems and is particularly appropriate for use with patients who have had an acute neurological lesion. The 6MWT is useful since some normative data are available (Enright & Sherill 1998). The test can also be performed for 12 minutes (McGavin et al 1976).

Reference: Guyatt et al 1985.

Human activity profile (HAP)

The HAP samples 94 activities across a broad range of energy requirements. The items are based on estimated metabolic equivalents that allow quick and meaningful measurement of changes in activity levels. Respondents answer each item with one of three responses: 'Still doing activity', 'Have stopped doing this activity', 'Never did this'.

Reference: Fix & Daughton 1988.

Sensation

Tests of sensation performed clinically by physicians and therapists, such as light touch, pinprick, heat and cold, passive movement and position sense, have been shown to be subjective and unreliable (Garraway et al 1976; Tomasello et al 1982; Carey 1995). Standardization of testing procedures is essential.

The Nottingham Sensory Assessment for Stroke Patients

The revised version of this test provides standardized measures with known limits to its reliability. The assessment's validity in terms of relevance to function is not

---

Box 3.7 **Formula to determine training heart rate (HR)**
Training HR range = $[40\%–85\%(HR_{max\text{-}pred} – HR_{rest})] + HR_{rest}$
• Calculate maximum age-predicted HR ($HR_{max\text{-}pred}$) by subtracting the patient's age from 220
i.e. $HR_{max\text{-}pred} = 220 – age$
• Measure resting heart rate (HR_{rest})
For example, for a 50-year-old person with a measured HR of 80 bpm
$HR_{max\text{-}pred} = 220 – 50 = 170$
Therefore, training HR range = [40%–85% of (170 – 80)] + 80 = 116 to 157

Box 3.8 **Borg scale giving RPE values**	
6	14
7 Very, very light	15 Hard
8	16
9 Very light	17 Very hard
10	18
11 Fairly light	19 Very, very hard
12	20
13 Somewhat hard	

clear. Each test is demonstrated to the patient who is then blindfolded. The non-paretic side is tested for light touch and temperature. If these are normal, only the paretic side is tested.

Tactile sensation

The patient is asked to indicate either verbally or by a body movement when they feel the test sensation. The skin is touched with the test object in random order. Distal sections of the body are tested first. Six aspects of tactile sensation can be tested: *light touch, pressure, pinprick, temperature, tactile localization, and bilateral simultaneous touch*. Responses are scored as: 0, Absent; 1, Impaired; 2, Normal; 9 Unable to test.

Kinaesthetic sensation

Appreciation/recognition of movement, direction of movement and joint position sense are tested simultaneously. The paretic limb is moved in various directions by the examiner. The patient is asked to mirror the movement with the other limb or indicate whether or not a movement has occurred. Three practice movements are performed before blindfolding. Responses are scored as: 0, Absent; 1, Appreciation of movement taking place; 2, Direction of movement; 3, Joint position sense; 9, Unable to test.

Stereognosis

The ability to recognize common objects by touch alone (blindfolded) is tested by placing a common object in the patient's hand for a maximum time of 15 seconds. The patient identifies the object by naming it, describing it or by pair-matching with an identical object. Objects used include: *coin, ball-point pen, pencil, comb, cup, glass, sponge and flannel*. Scoring is: 0, Absent; 1, Impaired; 2, Normal; 9, Unable to test.

Two-point discrimination

Using blunt dividers, points are applied simultaneously to the skin for approximately 5 seconds. The patient is asked whether one or both points were felt. Minimum distance (millimetres) where two separate points are detected is recorded. Scoring is: 2, Less than 3 mm on fingertips or 8 mm on the palm; 1, Greater than 3 mm at fingertips or 8 mm on the palm; 0, Unable to detect two points.

Reference: Lincoln et al 1998.

Find-the-thumb test

This simple test can be used to give an indication of a person's ability to locate this body part in space. The patient is blindfolded, the arm is moved passively and the patient is asked to find the thumb.

References: Prescott et al 1982; Smith et al 1983.

Visuospatial function

Unilateral spatial neglect can be identified by observation of a patient's behaviour. The position of the patient's head, eyes and trunk is observed at rest and during activities, or when the person is being spoken to. A simple test is to ask the patient to track a visual target from the space ipsilateral to the lesion into contralateral space and maintain fixation for 5 seconds.

The behavioural inattention test (BIT)

This test has been standardized. It comprises six conventional tests: *line crossing (Albert's test), letter cancellation, star cancellation, figure and shape copying, line bisection, representational drawing*; and nine behavioural tests: *picture scanning, telephone dialling, menu reading, article reading, testing and setting the time (digital clock), coin sorting, address and sentence copying, map navigation, card sorting*. One advantage of these tests is that they suggest tasks that the therapist should pay particular attention to in training. Individual tests can be taken from this battery. For example, the star cancellation test is reported to be the most sensitive at detecting neglect (Halligan et al 1989) and the letter cancellation test has been used in clinical trials (e.g., Dean & Shepherd 1997). Since the BIT was standardized on chronic stroke people, it has been modified and shortened for use with acute stroke patients (Stone et al 1991).

References: Albert 1973; Wilson et al 1987.

Memory

Mini-mental state (MMS) examination

This is a widely used clinical test for detecting cognitive impairment. It is scored out of 30 with a score of 20–26 or less used to identify some cognitive deficit; 10–19 moderate to severe cognitive impairment, and below 10 severe cognitive impairment. The test is reliable and valid. It takes only a few minutes to complete. The test includes simple questions and mental tasks in a number of areas: *the time and place of the test, repeating lists of words, calculation, language use* and *comprehension*, and *basic motor skills such as copying a drawing*.

References: Folstein et al 1975; Beatty & Goodkin 1990.

HEALTH-RELATED QUALITY OF LIFE SCALES

The need for a valid and sensitive instrument to measure the patient's subjective health is increasingly being recognized. It is helpful to the rehabilitation process to elicit input from the patient about such issues as their own perceptions of health and wellbeing, of limitations in activities and restrictions to participation at home, work and leisure. Quality of life scales may be a better predictor of need for utilization of health services than 'hard' data such as morbidity and mortality statistics (WHO 1971). As Lembcke (1952) wrote, the best measure of quality is not how well, or how frequently, a medical service is given, but how closely the result approaches the fundamental objectives of prolonging life, relieving distress, restoring function and preventing disability.

The medical outcome survey Short Form-36 (SF-36®) health state questionnaire

The SF-36® measures physical, psychological and social aspects that may, from the patient's perspective, be affected by health status. The SF-36® is a self-administered questionnaire that takes about 5 minutes to complete. It measures health on multi-item dimensions covering functional status, wellbeing and overall evaluation of health. Areas tested include physical and social functioning, role limitations (physical and emotional), mental health, vitality, pain and general health perception. For each dimension, item scores are coded, summed and recorded on a scale from 0 (most healthy) to 100 (least healthy). The questionnaire is easy to use, acceptable to patients and has strong reliability and validity.

References: Brazier et al 1992; McDowell & Newell 1996.

The Nottingham Health Profile

This is another standardized measure of subjective health status in the physical, social and emotional domain

Reference: Hunt et al 1981.

Self-efficacy scales

Self-efficacy scales provide the patient's input regarding the rehabilitative process and help to guide the process. Gathering such information should not be done without consultation with other relevant staff, lest an individual be swamped with questionnaires.

Patient Health Questionnaire-9 (PHQ-9)

Self-rating mood scales such as PHQ-9 may be useful in giving an indication of how people feel. These scales may be indicators of misery and distress rather than clinical depression (Wade 1992b). They are not necessarily reliable for use with neurological patients. However, since they give an indication of how people feel, they enable clinicians to set about instituting changes in the rehabilitation environment and staff and family attitudes. Some form of depression commonly occurs in the first year after stroke. However, there are many complexities in the recognition, assessment and diagnosis of abnormal mood in those with stroke-related disabilities (Hackett et al 2005).

Reference: Kroenke et al 2001.

DIAGNOSIS-SPECIFIC MEASURES

Traumatic brain injury (TBI) or post-surgery coma

Glasgow Coma Scale (GCS)

This is a method of testing state of arousal, and is in common use after traumatic brain injury. It is valid, reliable and sensitive. It has three sections: *eye opening, motor response and verbal response* (Box 3.9). The overall state of arousal can be expressed by summing the three component scores. The summed score on admission to hospital is used to classify injury severity as severe (GCS ≤8), moderate (GCS 9–12) or mild (GCS 13–15). In general, a score of <8 is taken to separate a comatose state from non-coma (Wade 1992a).

References: Jennett & Bond 1975; Jennett & Teasdale 1981.

Box 3.9 **Glasgow Coma Scale**		
Eye opening		
Spontaneous	Opens eyes spontaneously	E4
To speech	Opens eyes on verbal approach	3
To pain	Pain from stimulus to limbs	2
Nil		1
Motor response		
Obeys	Follows simple commands	M6
Localizes	Arm attempts to remove supraorbital/chest pain	5
Withdraws	Arm withdraws from pain, shoulder abducts	4
Abnormal flexion	Shoulder flexes, adducts	3
Extensor response	Shoulder adducted/ internally rotated, forearm pronated	2
Nil		1
Verbal response		
Oriented	Aware of time, place, person	V5
Confused conversation	Responds with conversation, but confused	4
Inappropriate words	Intelligible, exclamatory or random	3
Incomprehensible sounds	Moans, groans, no words	2
Nil		1
Coma score (E + M + V) = 3 to 15		

Modified Oxford and Westmead Post-Traumatic Amnesia (PTA) Scale

This scale is used to measure the length of PTA: a period of impaired consciousness that extends from the initial injury until continuous memory for ongoing events is restored (Levin et al 1982). The scales incorporate both memory and orientation items. The length of time that a patient is in PTA is an indicator of the severity of the injury. Patients are assessed to be out of PTA if they score 12/12 once (if PTA >28 days) or if they score 12/12 for 3 consecutive days (if PTA <28 days) (Tate et al 2006). The validity of this scale was tested by a comparison of scores on the scale with results on standardized neurobehavioral tests. It should be noted that, although some patients may no longer be in a state of PTA as defined, they may still suffer from amnesia to some extent.

References: Shores et al 1986; Levin et al 1982; Tate et al 2006.

Glasgow Outcome Scale (GOS)

The GOS is the most widely used scale to measure outcome from head injury. It is considered useful as a global measure of outcome for these patients and its value lies in the general vision it gives of their status. This 5-point scale has been shown to be reliable. It comprises five states (Box 3.10). There is also an 8-point extended version.

References: Jennett & Bond 1975; Maas et al 1983.

Box 3.10 Glasgow Outcome Scale

Death
Vegetative state
Severe disability; conscious but dependent
Moderate disability; independent but disabled
Good recovery

The Galverston Orientation Amnesia Test (GOAT)

The GOAT is a 10-item rating scale that measures disorientation and amnesia serially during the process of recovery after traumatic brain injury. The scale measures orientation to person, place and time, and memory for events preceding and following the injury. It obviates the need for relying on terms such as 'stupor' and 'confused'. Scoring: abnormal range <66; borderline-abnormal 66–75; normal range >75.

Reference: Levin et al 1979.

The High Level Mobility Assessment Tool (HIMAT)

Retraining running following TBI has the potential to enhance quality of life. The HIMAT is a mobility scale

developed to address the ceiling effects of outcome scales in current use.

Reference: Williams et al 2004.

Stroke

The Stroke-Adapted 30-Item Sickness Impact Profile (SA-SIP30)

The SIP is a valid and reliable 136-item quality of life measure. The SA-SIP was developed as a shorter, more feasible version of the SIP to address issues relevant to stroke. The test can be completed by the individual (self-report) or by an interviewer.

Reference: van Straten et al 1997.

Parkinson's disease

The Hoehn and Yahr Scale

This scale is an attempt to classify stages in Parkinson's disease (Box 3.11).

Reference: Hoehn & Yahr 1967.

Box 3.11 Modified Hoehn and Yahr staging

0	No sign of disease
1	Unilateral disease
1.5	Unilateral plus axial involvement
2	Bilateral disease, without impairment of balance
2.5	Mild bilateral disease, with recovery on pull test
3	Mild to moderate bilateral disease; some postural instability; physically dependent
4	Severe disability; still able to walk or stand unassisted
5	Wheelchair bound or bed-ridden unless aided

United Parkinson's Disease Rating Scale

This scale tests impairment and disability across a number of tasks. The information is collected by interview with the patient (see Ch. 13 for Web site).

ENVIRONMENTAL ANALYSIS

Behaviour mapping

A behaviour map demonstrates the distribution of behaviour in a particular setting. This is a time-sampling technique for studying environmental influences on behaviour. Data are collected that enable various predetermined behaviours to be related to the physical spaces in which they are observed. The picture that emerges is an indication of where patients spend their day and the effects on their behaviour of the environmental features. There have been several studies of rehabilitation environments using behaviour mapping that provide information about the otherwise unnoticed events that can influence a patient's progress (e.g., Lincoln et al 1989; Tinson 1989). The results of some are discussed in Chapter 1.

Reference: Keith 1980.

Behaviour stream analysis

A behaviour stream is a detailed sequential record of a segment of a person's behaviour. One study of patients with spinal cord injuries (Willems 1972) set out to seek answers to these questions: how do patients spend their time and in what settings? With whom do they interact? Is the distribution of the patient's time in keeping with the aims of therapy? In this study, a patient was followed for one waking day from 5.00am to 11.00pm while the observer(s) dictated a description of activities into a tape recorder. The information was coded into episodes with categories of time, activity, who was involved and ratings of initiation of behaviour (Keith 1988). The method of collecting information has been used to find out what potentially damaging events occurred, for example to a paretic upper limb.

References: Willems 1972; Keith 1988.

In conclusion, therapists need to be able to cope with the fact that sometimes the results of their measurement may be negative, and face up to the possibility of a less than positive outcome for a patient. Was poor outcome on a walking test due to the effects of the lesion (not all patients will be able to regain optimal function) or was it due to inappropriate and ineffective physiotherapy (methods available can differ considerably) or to insufficient intensity of exercise (30–60 minutes/day)? For a patient who may have deteriorated over time, objective measurement may assist with decisions between therapist, patient and relatives about a significant shift in management. It really is rewarding to sort these issues out.

REFERENCES

Ada L, Westwood P 1992 A kinematic analysis of recovery of the ability to stand up following stroke. Aust J Physiother 38:135–142.

Ada L, O'Dwyer NJ, Neilson PD 1993 Improvement in kinematic characteristics and coordination following stroke quantified by linear systems analysis. Hum Mov Sci 12:137–153.

Adams SA, Pickering RM, Ashburn A et al 1997 The scalability of the Rivermead Motor Assessment in nonacute stroke patients. Clin Rehabil 11:52–59.

Albert ML 1973 A simple test of visual neglect. Neurology 23:658–664.

Alibiglou L, Rymer WZ, Harvey RL et al 2008 The relation between Ashworth scores and neuromechanical measurements of spasticity following stroke. J Neuroeng Rehabil 5:18.

American College of Sports Medicine 1998 Position stand: the recommended quantity and quality of exercise for developing and maintaining cardiorespiratory and muscular fitness, and flexibility in healthy adults. Med Sci Sports Exerc 30:975–991.

American College of Sports Medicine 2006 ACSM's guidelines for exercise testing and prescription. Lippincott Williams & Wilkins, New York.

Andrews AW, Thomas MW, Bohannon RW 1996 Normative values for isometric muscle force measurements obtained with hand-held dynamometers. Phys Ther 76:248–259.

Ashworth B 1964 Preliminary trial of carisoprodol in multiple sclerosis. Practitioner 192:540–542.

Beatty WW, Goodkin DE 1990 Screening for cognitive impairment in multiple sclerosis. An evaluation of the Mini-Mental State Examination. Arch Neurol 47:297–301.

Berg K, Wood-Dauphinee S, Williams JI et al 1989 Measuring balance in the elderly: preliminary development of an instrument. Physiother Can 41:304–311.

Berg KO, Maki BE, Williams J et al 1992 Clinical and laboratory measures of postural balance in an elderly population. Arch Phys Med Rehabil 73:1073–1080.

Bohannon RW 1989 Correlation of lower limb strength and other variables with standing performance in stroke patients. Physiother Can 41:198–202.

Bohannon RW 1995 Internal consistency of dynamometer measurements in healthy subjects and stroke patients. Percept Mot Skills 81:113–114.

Bohannon RW, Andrews AW 1987a Interrater reliability of hand-held dynamometry. Phys Ther 67:931–933.

Bohannon RW, Andrews AW 1987b Relative strength of seven upper extremity muscle groups in hemiparetic stroke patients. J Neurol Rehabil 1:161–165.

Bohannon RW, Smith MB 1987 Interrater reliability of a modified Ashworth scale of muscle spasticity. Phys Ther 67:206–207.

Bohannon RW, Walsh S, Joseph MC 1993 Ordinal and timed balance measurements: reliability and validity in patients with stroke. Clin Rehabil 7:9–13.

Boissy P, Bourbonnais D, Carlotti MM et al 1999 Maximal grip force in chronic stroke subjects and its relationship to global upper extremity function. Clin Rehabil 13:354–362.

Borg G 1970 Perceived exertion as an indicator of somatic stress. Scand J Rehabil Med 2–3:92–98.

Brazier JE, Harper R, Jones NMB et al 1992 Validating the SF-36 health survey questionnaire: new outcome measure for primary care. BMJ 305:158–164.

Carey LM 1995 Somatosensory loss after stroke. Crit Rev Phys Rehabil Med 7:51–91.

Carr JH, Shepherd RB, Nordholm L et al 1985 Investigation of a new motor assessment scale for stroke patients. Phys Ther 65:175–180.

Carroll D 1965 A quantitative test of upper extremity function. J Chronic Diseases 18:479–491.

Cerny K 1983 A clinical method of quantitative gait analysis. Phys Ther 63:1125–1126.

Collin C, Wade D 1990 Assessing motor impairment after stroke: a pilot reliability study. J Neurol Neurosurg Psychiatry 53:576–579.

Collin FM, Wade DT, Bradshaw CM 1990 Mobility after stroke: reliability and measures of impairment and disability. Int Dis Stud 12:6–9.

Crenna P 1999 Pathophysiology of lengthening contractions in human spasticity: a study of the hamstring muscles during locomotion. Pathophysiology 5:283–297.

Csuka M, McCarty DJ 1985 Simple method for measurement of lower extremity muscle strength. Am J Med 78:77–81.

Dean CM, Shepherd RB 1997 Task-related training improves performance of seated reaching tasks following stroke: a randomised controlled trial. Stroke 28:1–7.

Dean CM, Richards CL, Malouin F 2001 Walking speed over 10 metres overestimates locomotor capacity after stroke. Clin Rehabil 15:415–421.

Demeurisse G, Demol O, Robaye E 1980 Motor evaluation in vascular hemiplegia. J Eur Neurol 19:381–389.

DeSouza LH, Langton Hewer R, Miller S 1980 Assessment of recovery of arm control in hemiplegic stroke patients. Arm function test. Int Rehabil Med 2:3–9.

Duncan PW, Weiner DK, Chandler J et al 1990 Functional reach: a new clinical measure of balance. J Gerontol 45:M192–M197.

Enright PL, Sherrill DL 1998 Reference equations for the six-minute walk in healthy adults. Am J Respir Crit Care Med 158:1384–1387.

Eriksrud O, Bohannon RW 2003 Relationship of knee extensor force to independence in sit-to-stand performance in patients receiving acute rehabilitation. Phys Ther 83:544–551.

Ferreira ML, Herbert RD 2008 What does 'clinically important' really mean? Aust J Physiother 54:229–230.

Finch E, Brooks D, Stratford PW et al 2002 Physical rehabilitation outcome measures: a guide to enhanced clinical decision making, 2nd edn. Canadian Physiotherapy Association, Toronto, Ontario.

Fix A, Daughton D 1988 Human activity profile professional manual. Psychological Assessment Resources, Odessa, FL.

Flansbjer UB, Holmback AM, Downham D et al 2005 Reliability of gait performance tests in men and women with hemiparesis after stroke. J Rehabil Med 37:75–82.

Folstein MF, Folstein SE, McHugh PR 1975 'Mini-Mental State': a practical method for grading the cognitive state of patients for the clinician. J Psychiatr Res 12:189–198.

Fowler V, Canning CG, Carr JH et al 1997 The effect of muscle length on the pendulum test. Arch Phys Med Rehabil 79:169–171.

Fugl-Meyer AR, Jaasko L, Leyman I et al 1975 The post-stroke hemiplegic patient. 1. A method of evaluation of physical performance. Scand J Rehabil Med 1:13–31.

Gajdosik RL, Bohannon RW 1987 Clinical measurement of range of motion: review of goniometry emphasizing reliability and validity. Phys Ther 67:1867–1872.

Garraway WM, Akhtar AJ, Gore SM et al 1976 Observer variation in the clinical assessment of stroke. Age Ageing 5:233–239.

Goldie PA, Bach TM, Evans OM 1989 Force platform measures for evaluating postural control: reliability and validity. Arch Phys Med Rehabil 70:510–517.

Gracies JM 2005 Pathophysiology of spastic paresis. 11: Emergence of muscle overactivity. Muscle Nerve 31:552–571.

Gracies JM, Marosszeky JE, Renton R et al 2000 Short-term effects of dynamic lycra splints on upper limb in hemiplegic patients. Arch Phys Med Rehabil 81:1547–1555.

Granger CV, Hamilton BB, Sherwin FS 1986 Guide for the use of the Uniform Data Set for medical rehabilitation. Project Office, Buffalo General Hospital, New York.

Green J, Forster A, Young J 2002 Reliability of gait speed measured by a timed walking test in patients one year after stroke. Clin Rehabil 16:306–314.

Gregson JM, Leathley MJ, Moore AP et al 2000 Reliability of measurements of muscle tone and muscle power in stroke patients. Age Ageing 29:223–228.

Guyatt GH, Sullivan MJ, Thompson PJ et al 1985 The 6-minute walk: a new measure of exercise capacity in patients with chronic heart failure. Can Med J 132:919–923.

Hackett ML, Yapa C, Parag V et al 2005 Frequency of depression after stroke: a systematic review of observational studies. Stroke 36:1330–1340.

Halligan PW, Marshall JC, Wade DT 1989 Visuospatial neglect: underlying factors and test sensitivity. Lancet ii:908–910.

Heller A, Wade DT, Wood VA et al 1987 Arm function after stroke: measurement and recovery over the first three months. J Neurol Neurosurg Psychiatry 50:714–719.

Herbert R, Jamtvedt G, Mead J et al 2005 Outcome measures measure outcomes, not effects of intervention. Aust J Physiother 51:3–4.

Hill K 2005 Commentary: Activities-specific and balance confidence (ABC) scale. Aust J Physiother 51:197.

Hill K, Schwarz J, Kalogeropoulos A et al 1996 Fear of falling revisited. Arch Phys Med Rehabil 77:1025–1029.

Hill K, Denisenko S, Miller K et al 2005 Clinical outcome measurement in adult neurological physiotherapy, 3rd edn. Australian Physiotherapy Association, Camberwell, Vic.

Hoehn MM, Yahr MD 1967 Parkinsonism: onset, progression, and mortality. Neurology 17:427–442.

Horak FB 1987 Clinical measurement of postural control in adults. Phys Ther 67:1881–1885.

Hunt SM, McKenna SP, McEwen J et al 1981 The Nottingham health profile: subjective health status and medical consultations. Soc Sci Med 15A:221–229.

Jennett B, Bond M 1975 Assessment of outcome after severe brain damage. A practical scale. Lancet i:480–484.

Jennett B, Teasdale GM 1981 Management of head injuries. FA Davis, Philadelphia.

Karvonen M, Kentala K, Mustala O 1957 The effects of training heart rate: a longitudinal study. Ann Med Exp Biol Fenn 35:307–315.

Keith RA 1980 Activity patterns in a stroke rehabilitation unit. Soc Sci Med 14A:575–580.

Keith RA 1988 Observations in the rehabilitation hospital: twenty years of research. Arch Phys Med Rehabil 69:625–631.

Keith RA 1995 Conceptual basis of outcome measures. Am J Phys Med Rehabil 74:73–80.

Keith RA, Granger CV, Hamilton BB et al 1987 The Functional Independence Measure: a new tool for rehabilitation. In: Eisenberg MG (ed.) Advances in clinical rehabilitation. Springer-Verlag, New York:6–18.

Kroenke K, Spiltzer RL, Williams JB 2001 The PHQ 9: validity of a brief depression severity measure. J Gen Int Med 16:606–613.

Lembcke PA 1952 Measuring the quality of medical care through vital statistics based on hospital service areas. 1. Comparative study of appendectomy rates. Am J Public Health 42:276.

Lennon S, Hastings M 1996 Key physiotherapy indicators for quality of stroke care. Physiotherapy 82:655–664.

Levin HS, O'Donnell VM, Grossman RG 1979 The Glaverston orientation and amnesia test: a practical guide to assess congnition after head injury. J Nerv Mental Dis 167:675–684.

Levin HS, Benton AL, Grossman RG 1982 Anterograde and retrograde amnesia. In: Neurobehavioural consequences of closed head injury. Oxford University Press, New York:73–98.

Lincoln N, Leadbitter D 1979 Assessment of motor function in stroke patients. Physiother 65:48–51.

Lincoln NB, Gamlen R, Thomason H 1989 Behavioural mapping of patients on a stroke unit. Int Dis Stud 11:149–154.

Lincoln NB, Jackson JM, Adams SA 1998 Reliability and revision of the Nottingham Sensory Assessment for stroke patients. Physiother 84:358–365.

Loewen SC, Anderson BA 1988 Reliability of the Modified Motor Assessment Scale and the Barthel Index. Phys Ther 68:1077–1081.

Loewen SC, Anderson BA 1990 Predictors of stroke outcome using objective measurement scales. Stroke 21:78–81.

Lord S, Sherrington C, Menz H et al 2007 Falls in older people. Risk factors and strategies for prevention, 2nd edn. Cambridge University Press, New York.

Lyle R 1981 A performance test for assessment of upper limb function in physical rehabilitation treatment and research. Int J Rehabil Res 4:483–492.

Maas AIR, Braakman R, Schouten HJA et al 1983 Agreement between physicians on assessment of outcome following severe head injury. J Neurosurg 58:321–325.

McDowell I, Newell C 1996 Measuring health. A guide to rating scales and questionnaires, 2nd edn. Oxford University Press, New York.

McGavin CR, Gupta SP, McHardy GJ 1976 Twelve-minute walking test for assessing disability in chronic bronchitis. BMJ 1:822–823.

MacKay-Lyons MJ, Howlett J 2005 Exercise capacity and cardiovascular adaptations to aerobic training early after stroke. Topics Stroke Rehabil 12:31–44.

Maeda A, Yuasa T, Nakamura K et al 2000 Physical performance tests after stroke: reliability and validity. Am J Phys Med Rehabil 79:519–525.

Mahoney RI, Barthel DW 1965 Functional evaluation: the Barthel Index. Maryland Med J 14:61–65.

Malouin F, Pichard L, Bonneau C et al 1994 Evaluating motor recovery early after stroke: comparison of the Fugl-Meyer Assessment and the Motor Assessment Scale. Arch Phys Med Rehabil 75:1206–1212.

Mathiowetz V, Weber K, Kashman N et al 1985 Adult norms for the nine-hole peg test of finger dexterity. Occup Ther J Res 5:24–37.

Medical Research Council 1976 Aids to the examination of the peripheral nervous system. Her Majesty's Stationery Office, London.

Mehrholz J, Wagner K, Meissner D et al 2005 Reliability of the Modified Tardieu Scale and the Modified Ashworth Scale in adult patients with severe brain injury: a comparison study. Clin Rehabil 19:751–759.

Morris S 2002 Ashworth and Tardieu Scales: their clinical relevance for measuring spasticity in adult and paediatric neurological populations. Phys Ther Rev 7:53–62.

Morris ME, Cantwell C, Vowels L et al 2002 Changes in gait and fatigue from morning to afternoon in people with multiple sclerosis. J Neurol Neurosurg Psychiatry 72:361–365.

Moseley A, Adams R 1991 Measurement of passive ankle dorsiflexion: procedure and reliability. Aust J Physiother 37:175–181.

Moseley A, Lanzarone S, Bosman J et al 2004 Ecological validity of walking speed assessment after traumatic brain injury. J Head Trauma Rehabil 19:341–348.

Palmer-McLean K, Harbst K, Harbst T 2002 Brain injury. In: Myers J, Herbert W, Humpheys R (eds) ACSM's resources for clinical exercise physiology musculoskeletal, neuromuscular, neoplastic, immunologic and hematologic conditions. Lippincott, Williams & Wilkins, Philadelphia:98–108.

Pandyan AD, Price H, Rodgers MP et al 2001 Biomechanical examination of a commonly used measure of spasticity. Clin Biomech 16:859–865.

Patrick E, Ada L 2006 The Tardieu Scale differentiates contracture from spasticity whereas the Ashworth Scale is confounded by it. Clin Rehabil 20:173–182.

Podsialo D, Richardson S 1991 The timed 'Up & Go': a test of basic functional mobility for frail elderly persons. J Am Geriatr Soc 39:142–148.

Poole JL, Whitney SL 1988 Motor Assessment Scale for stroke patients: concurrent validity and interrater reliability. Arch Phys Med Rehabil 69:195–197.

Poole JL, Whitney SL 2001 Assessments of motor function post stroke: a review. Phys Occup Ther Geriatr 19:1–22.

Powell L, Myers A 1995 The Activities-Specific Balance Confidence (ABC) scale. J Gerontol 50A:M28–M34.

Prescott RJ, Garraway WM, Akhtar AL 1982 Predicting functional outcome following acute stroke using a standard clinical examination. Stroke 13:641–647.

Ross M 1997 Test–retest reliability of the lateral step-up test in young adult healthy subjects. J Orthop Sports Phys Ther 25:128–132.

Sanford J, Moreland J, Swanson LR et al 1993 Reliability of the Fugl-Meyer assessment for testing motor performance in patients following stroke. Phys Ther 73:447–454.

Shah S, Vanclay F, Cooper B 1989 Improving the sensitivity of the Barthel Index in stroke rehabilitation. J Clin Epidemiol 42:703–709

Shores EA, Marosszeky JE, Sandanam J et al 1986 Preliminary validation of a clinical scale for measuring the duration of post-traumatic amnesia. Med J Aust 144:569–572.

Shumway-Cook A, Horak F 1986 Assessing the influence of sensory interaction on balance. Phys Ther 66:1548–1550.

Smith A 1990 The measurement of human performance. In: Ada L, Canning C (eds) Key issues in neurological physiotherapy. Butterworth Heinemann, Oxford:51–80.

Smith DL, Akhtar AJ, Garraway WM 1983 Proprioception and spatial neglect after stroke. Age Ageing 12:63–69.

Steffen T, Hacker T, Mollinger L 2002 Age- and gender-related test performance in community-dwelling elderly people: six minute walk test, Berg Balance Scale, Timed Up & Go test, and gait speeds. Phys Ther 82:128–137.

Stone SP, Wilson B, Wroot A et al 1991 The assessment of visuo-spatial neglect after acute stroke. J Neurol Neurosurg Psychiatry 54:345–350.

Sunderland A, Tinson D, Bradley L et al 1989 Arm function after stroke. An evaluation of grip strength as a measure of recovery and a prognostic indicator. J Neurol Neurosurg Psychiatry 52:1267–1272.

Sunderland A, Tinson DJ, Bradley EL et al 1992 Enhanced physical therapy improves recovery of arm function after stroke. A randomised controlled trial. J Neurol Neurosurg Psychiatry 55:530–535.

Tate RL, Pfaff A, Baguley IJ et al 2006 A multicentre randomized trial

examining the effect of test procedures measuring emergence from post-traumatic amnesia. J Neurol Neurosurg Psychiatry 77:841–849.

Tinetti M, Richman D, Powell L 1990 Falls efficacy as a measure of fear of falling. J Gerontol 45:239–243.

Tinson DJ 1989 How stroke patients spend their days. Int Dis Stud 11:45–49.

Tomasello F, Mariani F, Fieschi C et al 1982 Assessment of interobserver differences in the Italian multicenter study on reversible cerebral ischaemia. Stroke 13:32–34.

Tripp EJ, Harris SR 1991 Test–retest reliability of isokinetic knee extension and flexion torque measurements in persons with spastic hemiparesis. Phys Ther 71:390–396.

Tsang YL, Mak MK 2004 Sit-and-reach test can predict mobility of patients recovering from acute stroke. Arch Phys Med Rehabil 85:94–98.

Turton AJ, Fraser CM 1986 A test battery to measure the recovery of voluntary movement control following stroke. Int Rehabil Med 8:74–78.

van der Lee JH, de Groot V, Beckerman H et al 2001 The intra- and inter-rater reliability of the action research arm test: a practical test of upper extremity function in patients with stroke. Arch Phys Med Rehabil 82:14–19.

van Straten A, De Haan RJ, Limburg M et al 1997 A stroke-adapted 30-item version of the sickness impact profile to assess quality of life (SA-SIP30). Stroke 28:2155–2161.

Vattanasilp W, Ada L 1999 The relationship between clinical and laboratory measures of spasticity. Aust J Physiother 45:135–139.

Verkerk PH, Schouten JP, Oosterhuis HJGH 1990 Measurement of the

hand coordination. Clin Neurol Neurosurg 92:105–109.

Wade DT 1992a Measurement in neurological rehabilitation. Oxford University Press, Oxford.

Wade DT 1992b Evaluating outcome in stroke rehabilitation. Scand J Rehabil Med Suppl 26:97–104.

Wade DT, Wood VA, Heller A et al 1987 Walking after stroke. Scand J Rehabil Med 19:25–30.

Ward A, Ebbeling CB, Ahlquist LE 1995 Indirect methods for estimation of aerobic power. In: Maud PJ, Foster C (eds) Physiological assessment of human fitness. Human Kinetics, Champaign, IL:37–56.

Willems EP 1972 The interface of the hospital environment and patient behaviour. Arch Phys Med Rehabil March:115–122.

Williams GP, Morris ME, Greenwood KM et al 2004 The high-level mobility assessment for traumatic brain injury: user manual. La Trobe University, Australia.

Wilson B, Cockburn J, Halligan P 1987 Development of a behavioral test of visuospatial neglect. Arch Phys Med Rehabil 68:98–102.

Wolfson L, Whipple R, Amerman P et al 1990 Gait assessment in the elderly: a gait abnormality rating scale and its relation to falls. J Gerontol 45:12–19.

World Health Organization 1971 Statistical indicators for the planning and evaluation of public health program. Technical report series no. 472. WHO, Geneva.

World Health Organization 2001 International classification of functioning, disability and health. WHO, Geneva.

Yozbatiran N, Der-Yeghiaian L, Cramer SC 2008 A standardized approach to performing the Action Research Arm test. Neurorehabil Neural Repair 22:78–90.

Part | 2 |

Task-related exercise and training

Chapter | 4 |

Standing up and sitting down

INTRODUCTION

Standing up from a seat is one of the most commonly performed functional activities. The ability to stand up effectively is essential to independent living and is a critical prerequisite for upright mobility. In standing up, the feet act as a fixed base of support over which the body mass is rotated and raised to reposition the centre of body mass (COM) over the feet in standing (Fig. 4.1). Bending the knees to lower the body mass over the feet, moving the hips back until they reach the seat, also requires fine control of the lower limb muscles working eccentrically.

These tasks are particularly difficult for individuals with neurological and/or lower limb musculoskeletal problems. Standing up is one of the most physically demanding actions we perform regularly, requiring greater lower limb strength and range of motion than walking and stair climbing (Berger et al 1988). Lack of independence in standing up and sitting down is one of the most likely factors associated with risk of institutionalization (Branch & Meyers 1987) and is a common source of falls (Nyberg & Gustafson 1995; Cheng et al 1998).

Standing up requires the ability to translate the body mass forward from a relatively stable sitting position (thighs and feet) to a small base of support, the feet. Generating angular and linear momentum sufficient to perform this smooth translatory movement is potentially destabilizing. Therefore, the ability to balance the body mass by segmental movement and lower limb muscle activity while propelling it away from the seat is an important feature of standing up. The individual with motor impairment has to learn not only how to generate and control considerable muscle forces but also how to harness the interactional effects of segmental rotations so that the action becomes balanced and energy efficient.

Support, propulsion and balance are major attributes of the lower limbs. Standing up (STS) and sitting down (SIT) belong to a group of significant weightbearing actions in which the feet act as a fixed segment over which the lower limbs flex and extend. Other significant weightbearing actions include stance phase of gait, walking up and down stairs, squatting and rising from squats, and the initial weightbearing phase of jumping and hopping. Lack of practice of this flexion/extension synergy in relatively immobile individuals is associated with weakness of lower limb extensor muscles and adaptive stiffening of calf muscles, particularly the soleus, making it mechanically more difficult or impossible to perform the actions. Repetitive practice and training of STS and SIT under different varied task and contextual conditions can strengthen weak muscles using body weight resistance concentrically and eccentrically, also providing an active stretch to the

©2010 Elsevier Ltd
DOI: 10.1016/B978-0-7020-4051-1.00012-6

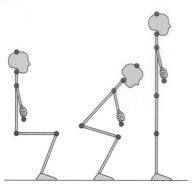

Figure 4.1 This drawing illustrates in a simplified form the essential kinematic features of standing up in the sagittal plane.

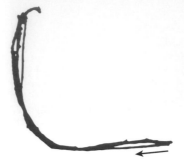

Figure 4.2 Note the smooth continuous curvilinear path of the shoulder marker, recorded as an able-bodied person moved from sitting to standing.

soleus if the feet are placed optimally. Such training improves intersegmental control of the lower limbs and upper body.

BIOMECHANICAL DESCRIPTION

Over the past two decades there has been an increasing interest in examining the dynamics of STS and SIT. The majority of studies have focused on sagittal plane movement using two-dimensional video or optoelectric analysis systems, with the subject standing up with feet on one or two force plates. Laboratory studies of both able-bodied individuals and individuals with motor impairment provide biomechanical data from which we can gain insight into the nature of motor control and develop guidelines for training these actions.

Standing up

STS can be divided into a *pre-extension and an extension phase* (Carr & Gentile 1994; Shepherd & Gentile 1994), the transition occurring at the time the thighs are lifted off the seat, called thighs-off (TO). There are other methods of identifying phases of STS (Kralj et al 1990; Pai & Rogers 1990; Schenkman et al 1990) but this may be the simplest classification for clinical purposes and it has some mechanical validity. In reality, the pre-extension and extension phases form a continuous movement that can be seen from the smooth curved path of the shoulder as the person moves from sitting to standing erect (Fig. 4.2).

In the pre-extension phase, the feet are moved backward to position the ankle joint posterior to the knee joint. The upper body (head, arms, trunk) rotates forward by flexion at the hips and dorsiflexion at the ankles. Reactive forces generated by the angular velocity of the upper body cause

ankle dorsiflexion as the knees move forward (Fig. 4.3). In the extension phase, extensor muscles crossing the hips, knees and ankles accelerate the body mass vertically.

Kinematics and kinetics

Optimal performance of standing up involves a mechanically efficient movement pattern and a basic underlying coordination, regardless of the goal or the environmental context. In the pre-extension phase, STS requires an initial generation of horizontal linear momentum of the body mass to move it forward over the feet, and the translation of horizontal momentum to vertical momentum at the start of the extension phase that propels the body mass vertically into standing. Horizontal momentum is brought about principally by angular rotation of the trunk segment at the hips. Vertical momentum is brought about by extension at the hips, knees and ankles (see Fig. 4.3). It should be noted that the trunk segment (pelvis, spine and head) behaves as one 'virtual' segment, with the spine erect as it rotates forward, almost in one piece in the pre-extension phase and then rotates backward at the hips during the extension phase. Biomechanical analysis indicates that movement at the spinal joints is minimal.

The extent of angular displacement at the hips varies depending on the height and type of seat, presence or not of chair arms, starting position (e.g., presence or not of a back rest), and whether the arms are free to move or used for support and balance. In spite of seat variations, there is a remarkable and repeatable consistency in performance in this relatively simple action brought about essentially by flexion and extension at the hips, knees and ankles.

Flexion and extension at the hips, knees and ankles occur not only by *muscle forces* but also by gravitational, inertial and interactive forces. Major extensor force generation in STS occurs around the time the thighs are lifted off the seat in order to accelerate the body mass vertically. On

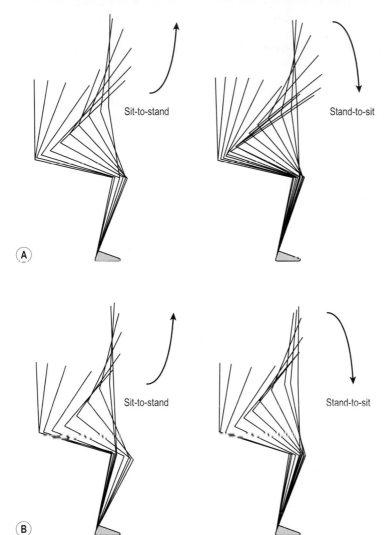

Figure 4.3 Sagittal plane stick figures taken from a biomechanical study of standing up and sitting down. (A) A typical young adult. (B) A typical older adult. Note: 1) movement of the shank segment (ankle dorsiflexion) in both activities. 2) Greater hip flexion in SIT in younger compared to older person. *(Reproduced from Dubost et al 2005, with permission).*

Sit-to-stand

Stand-to-sit

Sit-to-stand

Stand-to-sit

average, peak support moments of force (an algebraic summation of hip, knee and ankle moments of force) range from 4.00 to 5.50 Nm/kg in young able-bodied subjects, that is approximately four to five times body weight, when standing up at their preferred speed (Shepherd & Gentile 1994). When conditions demand it, able-bodied subjects can stand up with weight evenly distributed between the two lower limbs. However, in everyday life, the distribution of weight borne between the lower limbs varies depending on environmental demands and context of the action.

Since the thighs and feet are supported, *ground reaction forces* play an important part in the movement. STS requires coordinated muscle activity to generate forces against both the seat and ground. These ground or supportive reaction forces (GRFs) enable the propulsion of the body mass in the desired direction horizontally and

vertically in standing up and the control of the body mass during descent. Peak vertical GRFs under the feet occur immediately following TO and reach over 100% body weight. These peak forces immediately decrease after TO and eventually stabilize to body weight once the person has settled in standing (Fig. 4.4). Anteroposterior horizontal forces are considerably smaller than vertical forces. Generated in a posterior direction, they propel the body mass forward and are followed by anterior forces of similar magnitude that brake the forward momentum of the body mass.

Muscle activity

Many mono- and bi-articular muscles spanning the hip, knee and ankle joints are involved in STS and SIT. In addition, trunk muscles, rectus abdominus and lumbar paraspinal muscles are active to stabilize the erect trunk segment, turning it into a virtual segment. Extensor muscle strength is a major contributor to successful performance (Cameron et al 2003; Eriksrud & Bohannon 2003; Bohannon 2007).

Muscles investigated using electromyogram (EMG) have included rectus abdominus, lumbar paraspinals, trapezius, gluteus medius, quadriceps, hamstrings, tibialis anterior, gastrocnemius and soleus (Munton et al 1984; Richards 1985; Arborelius et al 1992; Khemlani et al 1998). Tibialis anterior is one of the first muscles to be activated reflecting its role in foot placement backward and in stabilizing the heel on the ground as the trunk swings forward, driving forward movement of the shank (Fig. 4.5). Lumbar paraspinal, hip and knee extensor muscles reach peak activity together at TO to accelerate the body mass vertically once preparatory muscle activity has ensured the centre of gravity (COG) is appropriately placed. Preparatory and ongoing postural adjustments are very important in complex multisegmental actions such as STS in which the individual changes from a position of stability to a much less stable position (Goulart &

Valls-Sole 1999). Variable patterns of EMG activity have been found in gastrocnemius and soleus reflecting their additional role in balancing the body mass during the extensor phase and in standing. A major goal of postural muscle activity is to keep the COG within the base of support.

Iliopsoas, by its action in flexing the pelvis (and trunk) forward at the hip joints, probably initiates this hip flexion (Fig. 4.6), however this relatively deep muscle is difficult to monitor. Simultaneous onsets of bi-articular rectus femoris and biceps femoris contribute to the control of limb movement – rectus femoris contributing to hip flexion and knee extension and biceps femoris exerting a

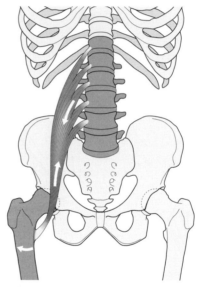

Figure 4.6 Anterior view of the R psoas major – the major muscle contributing to flexion of the trunk and pelvis at the hip in standing up. *(Reprinted from Musculino 2005, with permission).*

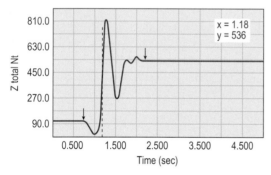

Figure 4.4 Typical vertical (z) ground reaction force profile of an able-bodied subject standing up at a preferred speed of approximately 1.5s. Vertical line indicates thighs-off. Arrows indicate movement onset and movement end.

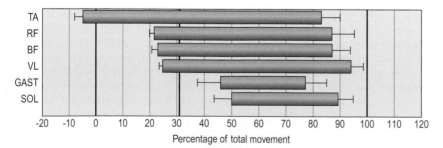

Figure 4.5 Mean and standard error of time-normalized onsets and durations of six lower limb muscles as able-bodied subjects stand up at their preferred speed. TA: tibialis anterior; RF: rectus femoris; BF: biceps femoris; VL: vastus lateralis; GAST: gastrocnemius; SOL: soleus. 0%: movement onset, 31%: thighs-off, 100%: movement end. *(Reproduced from Khemlani et al 1998, with permission).*

braking force in preparation for extension of the hips, knees and ankles to raise the body into standing.

Biomechanical factors influencing performance

STS involves a mechanically efficient movement pattern and a basic underlying musculoskeletal coordination, regardless of the goal or the environment. However, flexibility of performance is critical to meet the demands of daily life and we adapt the action to internal (changing weight in pregnancy) and external (seat height) constraints. Although able-bodied subjects can stand up and sit down with weight evenly distributed between the two limbs, in everyday life the motor strategy employed to rise to standing may vary as it depends on the intention and on the relative loading of the limbs. For example, standing up does not always end in quiet standing. It is often a transitional movement, standing up merging into another action such as walking.

Investigations of standing up to walk have shown that the two tasks merge smoothly in healthy subjects (Magnan et al 1996). One study showed that when subjects were asked to stand up, forward momentum of the body's COM ended in standing. When standing up to walk, however, forward momentum continued into the first step, before the erect standing position was reached (Malouin & Richards 2005). Many stroke patients are unable to merge the two tasks, probably because they have difficulty controlling forward momentum. Instead they stand up first and only then walk off (Dion et al 1999; Malouin & Richards 2005). In measuring functional motor performance, the timed up-and-go test is particularly useful as an indication of functional progress as it tests the ability to adapt the basic STS pattern to the task of standing up and walking.

Mechanical effect of different foot placements. Foot placement specifies the distance the body mass has to be moved forward in order to position the COM over the feet. Foot placement is a major factor in lower limb muscle force production and therefore in the amount of effort required. Standing up from sitting with the feet drawn back, the ankle joint posterior to the knee joint, is easier than with the feet forward. It reduces the distance the body mass has to move in a forward direction and requires less force generation from muscles crossing the hips and knees compared with more anterior foot placements (Shepherd & Koh 1996). Standing up with the ankles dorsiflexed (approximately 75°) puts an active stretch on the soleus (Fig. 4.7), thus preserving length and extensibility – another reason for ensuring the paretic foot is bearing weight.

Standing up with one foot in front of the other increases the loading through the posterior limb and decreases it through the anterior limb. GRFs and magnitude of EMG activity in quadriceps and tibialis anterior increase significantly in the posterior limb with corresponding decreases in the forward limb (Brunt et al 2002). Stroke patients are

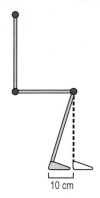

Figure 4.7 Preferred foot placement (approximately 75° ankle dorsiflexion) requires less force generation to stand up.

spontaneously adapting standing up when they can move only the non-paretic foot back. This response sets up the action to be performed principally by the non-paretic limb and must be discouraged in order to prevent the individual from 'favouring' the stronger limb and neglecting the paretic or weaker limb.

Timing and speed of trunk rotation. Trunk angular momentum, produced as the large upper body swings forward at the hip joints, is the major contributor to horizontal momentum of the body mass. It facilitates lower limb extension, requiring less overall muscle force in the lower limbs in order to raise the body mass to the standing position (Schenkman et al 1990; Shepherd & Gentile 1994). Standing up slowly, as many neurological patients do, reduces momentum, with the result that more lower limb muscle force must be produced for a longer period of time (Carr et al 2002). There is a similar effect when a patient moves the upper body forward, pauses, and stands up from a hip flexed position. That is to say, absence of the facilitating effect of horizontal momentum means that greater lower limb muscle forces are produced for a longer time, which is why, in training, the patient is advised to move a little faster.

Seat height influences STS. A higher seat requires lower moments of force at the hip and knee joints, with seat height having a greater influence on the moments of force at the knee than at the hip (Fig. 4.8). Lowering seat height increases the amount of momentum, peak muscle force and muscle strength required to get into standing (see Janssen et al 2002 for review).

Contribution of upper limbs to balance and propulsion. Able-bodied subjects have no difficulty standing up with arm movement restricted. However, variations in the extent of arm movement do have an effect on the dynamics of the action. When the arms are free to move, a lower level of extensor force is produced for a shorter time than when the arms are constrained (Carr & Gentile 1994). Holding the paretic upper limb in front of the body with

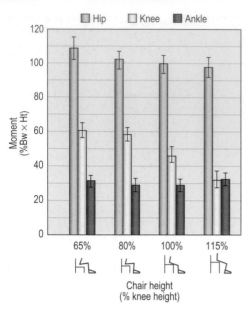

Figure 4.8 As seat height is raised, note that moments of force at the knee decrease. *(Reproduced from Rodosky et al (1989), with permission).*

the non-paretic limb, a common clinical practice, restricts movement of both arms and is not effective as an aid to standing up, and it does not encourage more symmetrical weightbearing (Seelen et al 1995).

Sitting down

Although sitting down appears to be the same as STS only in reverse, there are some important differences. Each is performed under different mechanical constraints. Sitting down is performed by gravity, and movement from the start involves eccentric (lengthening) contractions of extensor muscles that cross the hips, knees and ankles in order to slow descent of the body mass. Just before the seat is reached, forward rotation of the trunk at the hips increases and the knees flex as the body mass moves back at the ankles. This is a particularly destabilizing movement, and the balancing, muscular and mechanical constraints are challenging. As the hips near the seat, tibialis anterior contracts strongly to control the backward path of descent, while quadriceps control the flexing knees, otherwise the individual would 'fall' back onto the seat. Maximum shank angle (dorsiflexion) occurs just before seat-on; maximum trunk flexion angle (at the hips) at seat-on (Dubost et al 2005).

AGE-RELATED CHANGES

Healthy elderly subjects standing up without using arm rests demonstrate motor performance similar to young adults, although they have a tendency toward an increased trunk–thigh angle resulting in a more anterior position of the COM at TO. Movement time may be increased, however the action can be speeded up when required (Vander Linden et al 1994). Older subjects sitting down showed a decreased trunk–thigh angle (i.e., decreased flexion at the hips) compared with young adults (Dubost et al 2005).

Lower limb muscle force generally correlates with balance and is the strongest predictor of success in STS for older individuals with impairments (Schenkman et al 1996). In frail elderly subjects, sitting down is characterized by difficulty in movement initiation followed by rapid descent to the seat that is comparable to a backward fall (Dubost et al 2005). Factors such as joint pain, reduced range of movement, muscle stiffness, muscle weakness and poor vision adversely affect performance. The minimum seat height for successful standing up for community-dwelling and nursing home individuals with standing up difficulties (aged 64–105 years) appears to be about 120% of lower leg length (Weiner et al 1993) – this increased seat height minimizes the effort required.

In a group of older community-dwelling adults (age range 75–90 years), Lord and colleagues (2002) found that a diverse number of physiological and psychological factors were associated with the time taken to stand up. Visual contrast sensitivity, lower limb proprioception, tactile sensitivity, simple reaction time, postural sway, body weight, knee flexor, extensor and ankle dorsiflexor strength, and pain, anxiety and vitality were all significant and independent predictors of standing up performance. However, quadriceps isometric strength was the most reliable predictor and correlated with movement time (Lord et al 2002). This was consistent with Schenkman and colleagues' finding (1996) that isometric strength was relatively more important than balance (functional reach test, static standing postural sway) in predicting movement time in older subjects. Another group of older individuals generated less isokinetic knee extensor strength than young subjects when standing up, using up to 87% of their available knee extensor torque compared with about 49% in the young adults (Alexander et al 1995). Muscle strength is further impaired in individuals who have had a stroke and they may take longer to stand up compared with older subjects without neurological impairments (Adams et al 1990).

MOTOR DYSFUNCTION

Individuals vary in their capacity to stand up and sit down, depending on their impairments and overall level of activity. However, common problems arising from muscle weakness and lack of motor control can be observed as the individual attempts to stand up, and these problems

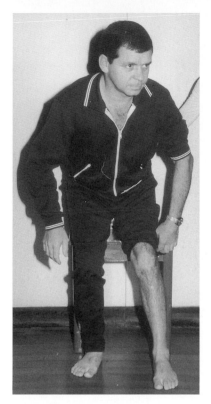

Figure 4.9 Asymmetrical weight-bearing. Failure to move paretic L foot back forces his weight on to the stronger R. leg. Note also the wide base of support.

Standing up

- Weightbearing through a weaker limb is avoided due to limb instability and weakness (Engardt & Olsen 1992; Hesse et al 1994; Cheng et al 1998; Lomaglio & Eng 2005):
  - Foot of stronger limb is spontaneously moved back, weaker limb is not (see Fig. 4.9)
  - If feet are parallel, stronger limb is spontaneously loaded as weight shifts to that side (Fig. 4.10B)
  - Shift to stronger leg may not occur until TO
- Moving the body far enough forward prior to TO is avoided due to inability to stabilize the foot of the weaker leg, fear of falling forward, lack of vigour (Fig. 4.11):
  - Hands are used for support, balance and upward lift (Fig. 4.12)
  - Upper body is moved forward, with a pause, before extension phase begins
  - Feet are placed wide apart for balance
- Movement is performed slowly – stroke patients, for example, take 25–60% longer to stand up than able-bodied adults (Engardt & Olsson 1992; Cheng et al 1998)

Sitting down

- Body mass moves back too soon with reduced shank angle (dorsiflexion), hip flexion and knee flexion (Fig. 4.13):
  - Hands may be used on chair arms

provide the focus for training. Lower limb muscle weakness (particularly of quadriceps and dorsiflexors) and contracture of the soleus muscle are common factors that interfere with performance of standing up and sitting down. So too are hip and knee flexion contractures that may occur during a prolonged period of coma associated with traumatic brain injury.

When individuals have muscle weakness, and difficulty generating, timing and sustaining muscle forces, certain limitations are evident as they try to stand up. The most significant adaptation seen in stroke patients is asymmetrical weightbearing during both standing up and sitting down (Fig. 4.9). These individuals are particularly prone to falling because of muscle weakness and slowness in making postural adjustments that are essential in balancing the body mass throughout these destabilizing movements. It is interesting to note that there is some evidence that increased loading through the paretic limb, that is more symmetrical weightbearing, following postural symmetry and repetitive STS–SIT training is associated with a reduction in falls (Cheng et al 2001). Common limitations and resultant adaptations are listed in Box 4.1

TASK-ORIENTED TRAINING

Standing up is one of the most common daily activities we perform and independence in this action, a critical goal for rehabilitation, is dependent on getting the training right. Training involves repetitive practice of standing up and sitting down, from seats with different characteristics (height, shape) and with a variety of different goals. This provides opportunities for the individual to learn to adapt to task and environmental demands. Varied practice of standing up and sitting down is essential in order to train balance. Functional strength training is included in order to increase concentric and eccentric strength of lower limb extensors and ankle dorsiflexors, and intersegmental control of lower limbs.

Successful standing up and sitting down is critical to the achievement of many different functional goals. Although muscle weakness and lack of vigour may be limiting factors, training and repetitive practice of standing up and sitting down, with other weightbearing exercises to

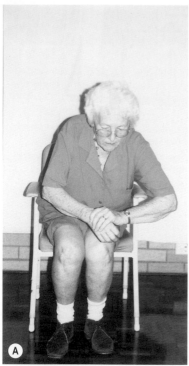

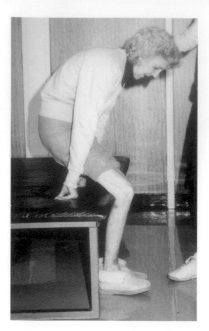

Figure 4.11 Failure to move her body mass far enough forward – she flexes her lumbar spine instead of her hips. Note the use of her arms – using the arms interferes with learning of independent standing up – it prevents the generation of horizontal momentum.

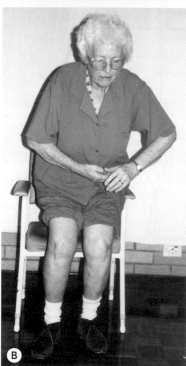

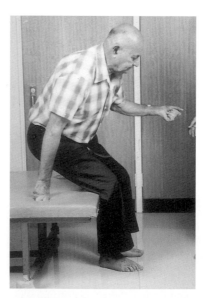

Figure 4.10 Although she can stand up independently, note that she loads the more posterior (stronger) L leg more than R, evident as early as thighs-off.

Figure 4.12 Failure to move his COM far enough forward (↓ hip flexion and ↓ ankle dorsiflexion). Note how he uses his R arm as he attempts to stand up.

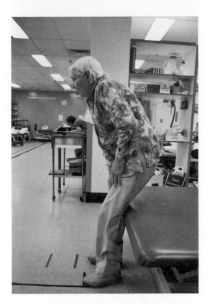

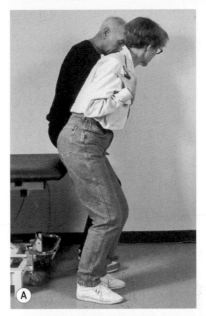

Figure 4.13 Sitting down. Failure to control descent causes her to 'fall' back on to the seat. Her hips, knees and ankles should be flexed. Note tibialis anterior should be working strongly to stabilize the ankle, keeping the knees forward and controlling the backward path of descent.

increase muscle strength and endurance, should enable the majority of people to learn again how to stand up independently and efficiently. Effective standing up and sitting down obviates the necessity for a person to be 'pulled up' into standing by others, with the possibility of damage to soft tissues around the shoulder (Wanklyn et al 1996). Safety procedures in hospitals may result in a weak person after stroke being lifted from bed to chair in a hoist. Once the person is sitting on a suitable seat, training standing up can begin.

Practice of the whole action is necessary in order to develop the necessary sequencing and timing of segmental rotations to both generate and utilize momentum. Use of the hands is discouraged. Those individuals who have difficulty activating and sustaining leg muscle activity may require simple exercises to help them get the idea of activating key muscle groups. Repetition is necessary for three reasons: to strengthen the extensor muscles of the lower limbs, to improve intersegmental control of the lower limbs by training linked segment mechanics, and to optimize learning. The individual is learning again, with an altered nervous system, how to utilize the characteristics of the segmental linkage in order to optimize intersegmental transfer of power and to minimize energy requirements.

Invariant biomechanical characteristics of standing up that are critical to successful performance provide the 'rules' of standing up, from which a standardized set of guidelines can be developed for all members of the therapy and nursing staff, the patient and relatives to follow. The

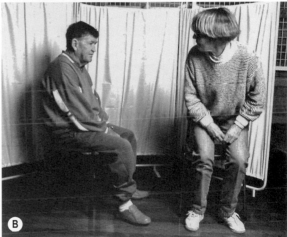

Figure 4.14 The therapist models the action to demonstrate the extent of trunk flexion at the hips (A) beside the patient so he can line his trunk up with hers, (B) providing a sagittal plane view to show him how far forward shoulders are moved.

therapist models the action for the patient to demonstrate the 'shape' or form of the action (Fig. 4.14). Nurses are trained in the STS guidelines so they develop confidence in their ability to give the necessary assistance and advice. Barreca and colleagues (2004) found that a coordinated effort on the part of all staff helped stroke survivors with multiple problems learn to stand up effectively. The practice environment, combined with consistent feedback from all staff, resulted in more stroke patients learning to stand up independently than a control group who had usual care.

Key biomechanical features incorporated into the training guidelines are shown in Box 4.2.

Standing up: foot placement and loading the weaker leg

The patient sits on a flat surface, feet together. To load the weaker leg, the foot of the stronger leg is placed in front of the other. This will force loading of the weaker leg (Fig. 4.15).

> The feet placed approximately 10 cm behind the knee facilitates lower limb extensor muscle force production and requires less effort. The therapist positions the paretic foot back if the patient cannot, to ensure that standing up is practised from an optimal starting position. The foot can be stabilized with the heel on the ground by pushing down along the shank (Fig. 4.16).

Brunt and colleagues (2002) studied standing up with a group of people after stroke in order to investigate the effects of foot placement on loading the paretic limb. There were three conditions: A, normal condition – feet parallel, both knees in 100° flexion; B, foot of non-paretic limb placed in front of paretic foot with non-paretic knee in 75° flexion; and C, foot of non-paretic limb placed on a raised box support, height-adjusted to 25% of seat height. The results showed that patients increased loading of the paretic limb in conditions B and C compared with the normal condition. Peak vertical force under the paretic foot was increased, and EMG amplitude was increased in quadriceps (B, 34%; C, 41%), and tibialis anterior (B, 29%; C, 51%). No instructions were given to the patients to increase the use of the paretic limb – the load increased naturally because the stronger leg was at a biomechanical disadvantage.

A more recent study measured the vertical ground reaction forces under the feet and thighs in stroke patients during standing up and sitting down under four conditions: 1) spontaneous foot placement; 2) symmetrical foot placement; 3) paretic foot placed backward; and 4) non-paretic foot placed backward. Similar to Brunt's findings, when the paretic foot was placed behind the non-paretic foot, asymmetrical loading was reduced, reaching values similar to those reported in able-bodied subjects (Chou et al 2003). The condition in which the non-paretic foot was placed behind the paretic foot resulted in the greatest loading asymmetry. In other words, positioning the paretic foot behind reduced asymmetry whereas positioning the non-paretic foot behind increased asymmetry.

Both studies make it clear that loading asymmetry favouring the non-paratic limb must be avoided if the goal of training is to prevent non-use of the paretic limb. It is interesting to note that asymmetrical loading was evident

---

Box 4.2 **Training guidelines at a glance**

Standing up

- 'Pull your feet back.' Feet placed 10 cm behind the knees. To load the weaker leg, the foot of the stronger leg is placed in front of the other
- Seat height adjusted to match lower limb strength
- Flat seat with no arms or back rest
- Start movement from a trunk vertical position
- 'Swing upper body forward, push down through the feet and stand up' to create horizontal momentum of body mass
- 'Speed up' if too slow
- Focus eyes on an object at sitting eye height
- Do three sets of maximum number of repetitions (e.g., if 5 = max, do three sets of five repetitions) and increase number as soon as possible

Sitting down

- Place feet back near the seat – the foot of the weaker leg back further than the other foot to force limb loading through that leg and eccentric contraction of muscles (particularly quadriceps)
- Flexion at hips, knees flex, ankles dorsiflex to lower the body mass down and back to the seat
- If necessary, assist the final lowering stage by steadying the knees as the person moves the hips back to the seat

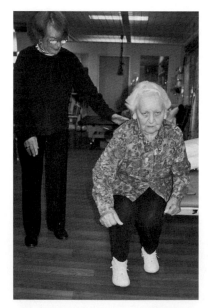

Figure 4.15 She is practicing STS/SIT with the paretic leg placed well back, loading the L leg. Here, she is focusing on swinging her shoulders and trunk forward a little faster in order to develop the momentum to rise to stand.

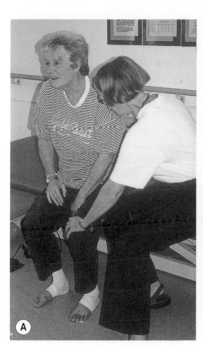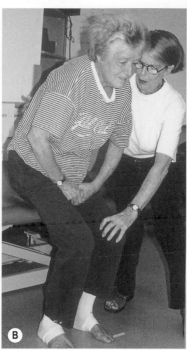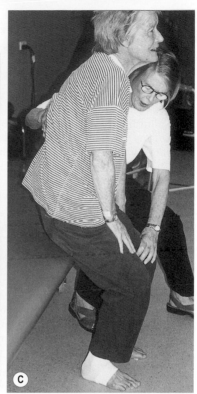

Figure 4.16 Practice of standing up and sitting down. (A) Therapist stabilizes paretic foot on the floor by pushing down along the shank. (B) As she stands up therapist moves the L leg sideways to increase loading of this leg. (C) Lateral view – she has not moved her shoulders far enough forward (i.e. flexed at the hips sufficiently) – she can focus on this during her next set of repetitions.

just before thighs-off in standing up and at thighs-on in sitting down in all foot conditions (spontaneous, symmetrical, paretic foot back, non-paretic foot back) except when the paretic foot was placed back (Roy et al 2006).

Seat height

Seat height is adjusted to match the individual's lower limb's strength – a higher seat makes it possible to stand up when the lower limb muscles are very weak. Seat height is progressively lowered as performance improves.

Adjusting seat height is used to make the action easier or progressively harder in order to strengthen the lower limb extensor muscles concentrically and eccentrically using body weight resistance; that is, by progressively increasing the load (resistance), dynamic strength through range is increased. Adjusting seat height increases or decreases the distance the body weight must be raised to achieve the standing position. It also changes the length at which the quadriceps generates peak force and the joint angle at which inertia is overcome. The lower the seat height, the greater the distance body mass has to be raised and the further it has to move in order to get forward over the feet.

Pivoting the trunk forward

Pivoting the upper body forward at the hips is initiated from a trunk vertical position. Increasing the amplitude of angular rotation in this way optimizes forward and upward momentum. Instructions are given to speed up the action so that forward momentum merges into upward momentum making a smooth translational movement. The instruction can be: 'Swing your shoulders forward, push down through your feet and stand up'.

Directing vision and attention toward a target during STS/SIT provides an external focus for erect body alignment by affecting the path of the head and shoulders forward and up. Attention can be drawn to a target a few metres ahead at sitting eye level. Encourage an increase in speed – a slow performance requires more effort.

Controlling descent in sitting down

Clinical observation suggests that individuals with motor impairment who are not able to stand up may be able to sit down. However, their attempts may be comparable to a backward fall. It is therefore essential to train both standing up and sitting down specifically. Sitting down may appear to be an easier action than standing up. However, although not so much effort is involved, controlling the descent requires good coordination and good balance.

> The feet are placed back near the seat. Flexion at the hips, knees and ankles lower the body down and back to the seat. The paretic foot can be stabilized on the floor (Fig. 4.17).

Specific attention to loading the weaker limb is necessary to ensure an eccentric contraction of quadriceps throughout the action. In a study by Engardt and colleagues (1995), stroke patients who received feedback about loading the paretic limb during sitting down training improved loading more than those who received no feedback.

Repetitions

There is evidence that greater strength gains may be achieved when repetitions are carried out without a rest between each repetition (Rooney et al 1994). The number of repetitions can be prescribed at the beginning of the session. The individual is encouraged to perform three sets of his/her maximum number, taking a rest between sets, not after each stand up. Using a counter enables the physiotherapist and patient to record the number of repetitions during the session (Fig. 4.18), providing feedback and incentive. The number of repetitions during the day can

be monitored using an activity monitor (ActivPal™ single-axis accelerometry).

Several studies have demonstrated positive effects of repetitive STS/SIT practice (Dean et al 2000; Cheng et al 2001; Monger et al 2002; Britten et al 2008). In a recent pilot study, Britten and colleagues (2008) tested a training protocol for patients following stroke in a UK rehabilitation unit. They assessed the effect of a 30-minute programme each day over 2 weeks. STS/SIT practice with training was provided by a physiotherapy assistant. People were included if they could stand up with 'standby' supervision without using their hands for support, but were unable to stand up more than three times in 10 seconds. The control group received an equivalent period of arm therapy. In the STS/SIT training group, training emphasized foot placement at the start of the movement, speed (particularly of forward movement of the trunk), with increased weightbearing through the paretic leg to generate symmetrical GRFs. Visual feedback of GRF was provided to the patients with a balance performance monitor. The assistant gave instructions and verbal feedback to aid learning. Practice was varied by changes in seat height and sitting surfaces. The aim of each session was to increase the number of repetitions and the number of STS each day was recorded using an ActivPal™ single-axis accelerometry activity monitor. Other strengthening exercises were incorporated if a patient fatigued. The assistant kept a log of training times for analysis of frequency of STS/SIT.

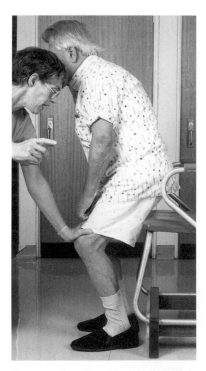

Figure 4.17 Sitting down on to a high seat. The therapist is stabilizing the paretic foot on the floor while keeping his knee forward. This gives him the idea of the amount of flexion necessary. The exercise trains the ability to control descent of the body by eccentric muscle activity of the quadriceps.

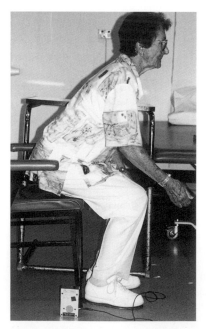

Figure 4.18 Partially supervised repetitive practice of STS and SIT. She is getting feedback about loading the limb from a limb load monitor and is recording the number of repetitions on a hand-held counter.

The results of this interesting study showed that the number of repetitions of STS/SIT increased on average from as few as 18 stands per day to 50 stands. There was a significant mean difference of 10% body weight through the paretic leg after 1 week of training. In contrast, the control group reduced the weight they put through the paretic leg during the period of the clinical trial. The strength of this study comes from the use of a standardized protocol so that the results can provide a clear indication of the effects resulting from what the patients actually did and how much they did (the dosage).

This study demonstrates that 1 week of extra practice can improve performance of patients who can stand up but who are unsteady. After this study, there is absolutely no reason why all neurological patients who can participate do not immediately start on such a programme. The challenge now is to use a training protocol in clinical practice with people with varied impairments who are unable to stand without help and see how many achieve independence in this important action.

Simple exercises to encourage muscle activation and encourage movement

Difficulty *activating the plantarflexors and hamstrings of the paretic leg to move the foot back* behind the knee may require specific training. A slippery surface or roller skate decreases resistance and encourages the patient to slide the foot backward. A line on the floor marking the distance to be moved provides an external focus (Fig. 4.19). The individual is reminded to position the feet to prepare for standing up. This is also important before sitting down, in order to avoid having too great a distance to move the body mass back to the seat.

Early post-stroke, fear of falling forward may be a major barrier to *swinging the body mass forward*. Practice of reaching forward with the hands on a table or reaching forward beyond arm's length enables the patient to get the idea of the extent of movement so it can be incorporated into standing up practice (Fig. 4.20). The table needs to be far enough forward to ensure the shoulders move well forward of the feet.

Loading the paretic leg and training balance

When we reach forward beyond arm's length, ground reaction forces increase under the foot indicating increased loading of one or both legs depending on the direction of the reach (Dean & Shepherd 1997) (Fig. 4.21). Alternate leg lifting gives the idea of loading and unloading (Fig. 4.22).

FUNCTIONAL STRENGTH TRAINING

Effective standing up depends on strength and coordination of muscles that cross the hips, knees and ankles. There is some evidence that knee extensor strength is a major

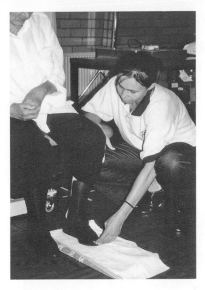

Figure 4.19 A towel reduces the friction between the shoe and floor while she practises activating hamstrings and muscles crossing the ankle to move her foot back. Her goal is to move her toes behind a line on the floor.

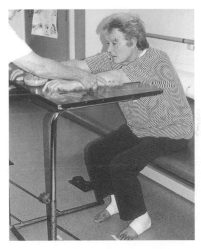

Figure 4.20 This woman was afraid of moving forward over her feet to stand up. With a table to rest her arms on, she is getting the idea of moving the shoulders forward and backward over her feet (flexion and extension at the hips) to improve her confidence.

contributor to successful STS (Cameron et al 2003; Eriksrud & Bohannon 2003; Bohannon 2007). Knee extension strength may only be a predictor of standing up ability when considered in combination with synergic control of other muscles. In addition to knee extensor strength, Lomaglio & Eng (2005) have identified two additional muscle groups, ankle dorsiflexors and plantarflexors, that relate significantly to standing up performance. They point

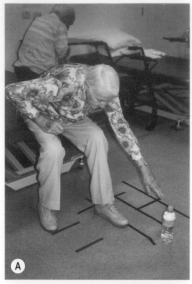

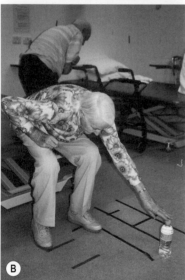

Figure 4.21 Reaching forward beyond arm's length. (A) Initially she does not move her foot back and therefore cannot reach the bottle. (B) She can now extend her reach and is loading her L leg. Note her thighs are leaving the seat. This type of exercise boosts confidence in use of lower limbs.

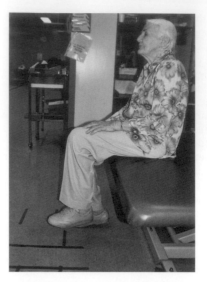

Figure 4.22 Reciprocal leg lifting – as one leg lifts, the other loads. Note she is moving backward. She tries to keep her knee flexed – if it is too difficult the therapist can place a block in front of the foot. She also needs to practice lifting her knees higher.

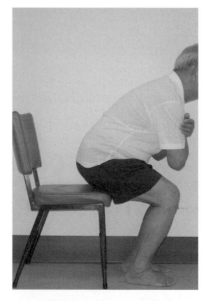

Figure 4.23 Repetitive practice with arms folded increases lower limb extensor force strength. Focus can also be on increasing speed. *(Courtesy of K Schurr and S Dorsch, Physiotherapy Department, Bankstown-Lidcombe Hospital, Sydney).*

out that other muscles, for example gluteus medius, must also be active in standing up to provide lateral stability. At the start of standing up, tibialis anterior actively stabilizes the foot on the ground, explaining its significance and correlation with STS performance. In fast-paced standing up, activation of plantarflexors controls forward momentum of the body mass (Lomaglio & Eng 2005).

Since the lower limb joints and muscles are harnessed together to act as a functional unit, an efficient strength

training method is repetitive performance of the action: standing up and sitting down, positioning the stronger foot in front of the weaker foot, progressively increasing difficulty by lowering the height of the seat, folding the arms (Fig. 4.23), and even adding a weighted belt or vest.

Additional functional weightbearing exercises are discussed in Chapter 2, and include squats, step-ups and step-downs.

Seat selection

Appropriate chair design makes a considerable contribution to an individual's wellbeing and independence, particularly for the less mobile. Britton and colleagues (2008) have observed that when STS is not a specific focus of training, seat height may not be optimal for an individual's height or strength, and patients are often encouraged or allowed to push on the chair arm with their non-paretic hand. This is a common observation. Similarly, teaching a person to 'transfer' is common clinical practice, in our opinion taking valuable therapy time away from a specific focus on training standing up and sitting down.

The most important features in chair design to assist standing up are seat height adjusted to the individual's height and strength, and absence of any structural block to posterior foot placement. A survey in which elderly people were asked to rank in order of importance the five factors they considered important in chair design, 'easy to get out of' was considered to be the most important and was ranked before comfort (Munton et al 1981). Toilet seat raises should also be provided in rehabilitation centres and on discharge if needed.

Mental practice

There may be several factors that limit the amount of physical practice in rehabilitation, including physical frailty, poor balance and lack of endurance, or lack of staff time. The addition of mental practice as a means of increasing practice time has been investigated by Malouin et al (2004). In this study, stroke patients were trained with mental practice to increase loading of the paretic limb while standing up and sitting down, initially using a visual display, then relying on their memory. A single training session of 30 minutes included seven physical repetitions combined with 35 mental rehearsals. This session resulted in improved loading of the paretic limb and improvement was retained 24 hours later, suggesting a learning process. The amount of motor improvement in follow-up was strongly associated with working memory ability, particularly in the visuospatial domain.

Maximizing skill

As the patient improves, gets stronger and more vigorous, and has a clear idea of the movement, emphasis changes from foot placement and speed of trunk rotation to training flexible performance. Practice is varied by incorporating the sort of goals normally encountered in daily life, and provides the opportunity for the individual to perform different tasks and adapt to different environmental contexts. Examples include talking while standing up and sitting down, holding a large object with both hands, steadying a glass of water or a tray (Fig. 4.24), stopping and changing direction without losing balance during

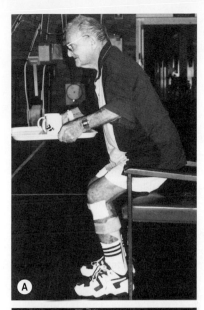

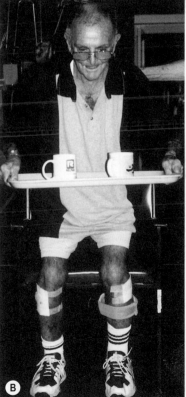

Figure 4.24 Balancing the mugs changes the focus of attention from standing up to steadying the tray. It encourages keeping the body mass forward over the feet at thighs-off.

sitting down practice (Fig. 4.25), and merging standing up into walking off in different directions.

There is no evidence that repetitive practice of STS increases physical fitness. However, for the frail elderly, ability to stand up may be initially limited by poor fitness and endurance. It may be wise to monitor heart rate while increasing the number of repetitions each day.

MEASUREMENT

The following functional tests (see Ch. 3) have been found reliable when performed under standardized conditions:

- Standing up item of Motor Assessment Scale (MAS)
- Timed up-and-go test
- Rise-to-walk test (Malouin et al 2003).

Strength of quadriceps is tested using a hand-held dynamometer or spring scale. Despite the significance of strength in the performance of standing up, no readily available clinical test can measure strength as it is functionally used (Buchner & de Lateur 1991). Number of repetitions can, however, be used as an indicator of functional strength.

The MAS is a valid and reliable indicator of performance. A biomechanical study to test the effectiveness of training standing up after stroke demonstrated that as patients progressed from 2 to 6 on the scale, hip and knee joint velocity profiles became smooth and bell shaped, typical of well-coordinated movement (Ada & Westwood

1992). Further analysis showed that the hip and knee joints had become perfectly coupled at MAS 6 (Fig. 4.26), the highest score, similar to skill acquisition in able-bodied subjects (Ada et al 1993).

In conclusion, lack of independence in standing up limits participation in everyday activities, including socializing and recreation, and it contributes to the overall deterioration of lower limb muscle strength, flexibility and function. Standing up and sitting down are important actions to train in rehabilitation, not only for increasing the individual's independence but also for the role of these actions in increasing muscle strength, motor control of the lower limbs and balance and preventing falls. There is some evidence of increased symmetrical weightbearing during standing up resulting in a reduction in falls (Engardt et al 1995; Cheng et al 2001).

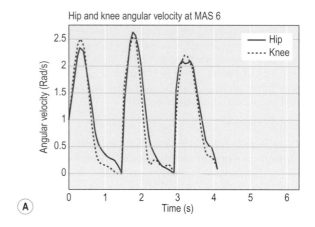

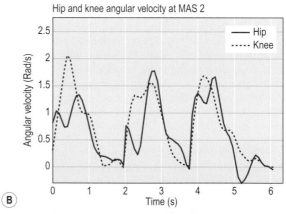

Figure 4.26 Hip (solid line) and knee (dashed line) joint velocities are almost perfectly coupled at MAS 6 (A) whereas there was significant independent activity (lack of coordination) at MAS 2 (B). *(Ada L, O'Dwyer, NJ, Neilson PD (1992) Improvement in kinematic characteristics and coordination following stroke quantified by linear systems analysis. Human Move Sci, **12**, 137–153, by kind permission of Elsevier Science, Amsterdam, The Netherlands).*

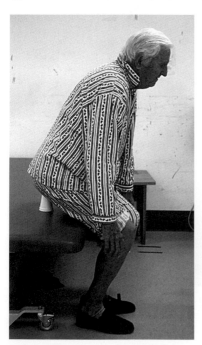

Figure 4.25 An exercise for improving balance that involves stopping and changing direction without losing balance.

REFERENCES

Ada L, Westwood P 1992 A kinematic analysis of recovery of the ability to stand up following stroke. Aust J Physiother 38:135–142.

Ada L, O'Dwyer N, Neilson PD 1993 Improvement in kinematic characteristics and coordination following stroke quantified by linear systems analysis. Hum Mov Sci 12:137–153.

Adams RW, Gandevia SC, Skuse NF 1990 The distribution of muscle weakness in upper motorneuron lesions affecting the lower limb. Brain 113:1459–1476.

Alexander NB, Gu MJ, Branch M et al 1995 Geriatrics: does leg torque influence rising from a chair in older adults. Rehabil R D Prog Rep 32:101–102.

Arborelius UP, Wretenberg P, Lindberg F 1992 The effects of armrests and high seat heights on lower-limb joint load and muscular activity during sitting and rising. Ergonomics 35:1377–1391.

Barreca S, Sigouin CS, Lambert C et al 2004 Effects of extra training on the ability of stroke survivors to perform an independent sit-to-stand: a randomized controlled trial. J Geriatr Phys Ther 27:59–64.

Berger RA, Riley PO, Mann RW et al 1988 Total body dynamics in ascending stairs and rising from a chair following total knee arthroplasty. In: Proceedings of the 34th Annual Meeting of the Orthopedic Research Society, Atlanta, GA.

Bohannon RW 2007 Knee extension strength and body weight determine sit-to-stand independence after stroke. Physiother Theory Pract 23:291–297.

Branch LG, Meyers AR 1987 Assessing physical function in the elderly. Clin Geriatr Med 3:29–51.

Britton E, Harris N, Turton A 2008 An exploratory randomized controlled trial of assisted practice for improving sit-to-stand in stroke patients in the hospital setting. Clin Rehabil 22:458–468.

Brunt D, Greenberg B, Wankadia S et al 2002 The effect of foot placement on sit to stand in healthy young subjects and patients with hemiplegia. Arch Phys Med Rehabil 83:924–929.

Buchner DM, de Lateur BJ 1991 The importance of skeletal muscle strength to physical function in older adults. Ann Behav Med 13:91–98.

Cameron DM, Bohannon RW, Garrett GE et al 2003 Physical impairments related to kinetic energy during sit-to-stand and curb-climbing following stroke. Clin Biomech 18:332–340.

Carr JH, Gentile AM 1994 The effect of arm movement on the biomechanics of standing up. Hum Mov Sci 13:175–193.

Carr JH, Ow JE, Shepherd RB 2002 Some biomechanical characteristics of standing up at three different speeds: implications for functional training. Physiother Theory Pract 18:47–53.

Cheng P-T, Liaw M-Y, Wong M-K et al 1998 The sit-to-stand movement in stroke patients and its correlation with falling. Arch Phys Med Rehabil 79:1043–1046.

Cheng P-T, Wu S-H, Liaw M-Y et al 2001 Symmetrical body-weight distribution training in stroke patients and its effect on fall prevention. Arch Phys Med Rehabil 82:1650–1654.

Chou SW, Wong AMK, Leong CP et al 2003 Postural control during sit-to-stand and gait in stroke patients. Am J Phys Med Rehabil 82:42–47.

Dean CM, Shepherd RB 1997 Task-related training improves performance of a seated reaching task after stroke: a randomized controlled trial. Stroke 28:722–728.

Dean CM, Richards CL, Malouin F 2000 Task-related circuit training improves performance of locomotor tasks in chronic stroke: a randomized, controlled pilot trial. Arch Phys Med Rehabil 81:409–417.

Dion L, Malouin F, McFadyen BJ et al 1999 Assessment of the sit-to-walk capacity after stroke: a validation study. Gait Posture Suppl 1:S24.

Dubost V, Beauchet O, Manckoundia P et al 2005 Decreased trunk angular displacement during sitting down: an early feature of aging. Phys Ther 85:404–412.

Engardt M, Olsson E 1992 Body weight-bearing while rising and sitting down in patients with stroke. Scand J Rehabil Med 24:67–74.

Engardt M, Knutsson E, Johnsson M et al 1995 Dynamic muscle strength training in stroke patients: effects on knee extension torque, electromyographic activity, and motor function. Arch Phys Med Rehabil 76:419–425.

Eriksrud O, Bohannon RW 2003 Relationship of knee extension force to independence in sit-to-stand performance in patients receiving acute rehabilitation. Phys Ther 83:544–551.

Goulart FR, Valls-Sole J 1999 Patterned electromyographic activity in the sit-to-stand movement. Clin Neurophysiol 110:1634–1640.

Hesse S, Schauer M, Malezic M et al 1994 Quantitative analysis of rising from a chair in healthy and hemiparetic subjects. Scand J Rehabil Med 26:161–166.

Janssen WGM, Bussmann HBJ, Stam HJ 2002 Determinants of the sit-to-stand movement: a review. Phys Ther 82:866–879.

Khemlani M, Carr JH, Crosbie WJ et al 1998 Muscles synergies and joint linkages in sit-to-stand under two different initial foot positions. Clin Biomech 14:236–246.

Kralj A, Jaeger RJ, Munih M 1990 Analysis of standing up and sitting down in humans: definitions and normative data presentation. J Biomech 23:1123–1138.

Lomaglio MJ, Eng JJ 2005 Muscle strength and weight-bearing symmetry relate to sit-to-stand performance in individuals with stroke. Gait Posture 22:126–131.

Lord SR, Murray SM, Chapman K et al 2002 Sit-to-stand performance depends on sensation, speed, balance, and psychological status in addition to strength in older people. J Gerontol 57A:M539–M543.

Magnan A, McFadyen BJ, St-Vincent G 1996 Modification of the sit-to-stand task with the addition of gait initiation. Gait Posture 4:232–241.

Malouin F, Richards CL 2005 Assessment and training of locomotion after stroke: evolving concepts. In: Refshauge K, Ada L, Ellis E (eds) Science-based rehabilitation. Butterworth Heinemann, Oxford:185–222.

Malouin F, McFadyen B, Dion L et al 2003 A fluidity scale for evaluating the motor strategy of the rise-to-walk task after stroke. Clin Rehabil 17:674–684.

Malouin F, Belleville S, Richards CL et al 2004 Working memory and mental practice outcomes after stroke. Arch Phys Med Rehabil 85:177–183.

Monger C, Carr JH, Fowler V 2002 Evaluation of a home-based exercise and training program to improve sit-to-stand in patients with chronic stroke. Clin Rehabil 16:361–367.

Munton JS, Ellis MI, Chamberlain MA et al 1981 An investigation into the problems of easy chairs used by the arthritic and the elderly. Rheumatol Rehabil 20:164–173.

Munton JS, Ellis MI, Wright V 1984 Use of electromyography to study leg muscle activity in patients with arthritis and in normal subjects during rising from a chair. Ann Rheumatic Dis 43:63–65.

Muscolino JE 2005 The muscular system manual: the skeletal muscles of the human body, 2nd edn. Elsevier Mosby, St Louis, MO.

Nyberg L, Gustafson Y 1995 Patient falls in stroke rehabilitation. A challenge to rehabilitation strategies. Stroke 26:838–842.

Pai Y, Rogers MW 1990 Control of body mass transfer as a function of speed of ascent in sit-to-stand. Med Sci Sports Exerc 22:378–384.

Richards CL 1985 EMG activity level comparisons in quadriceps and hamstrings in five dynamic activities. In: Winter DA, Norman RW, Wells RP eds International series on biomechanics, IX-A. Human Kinetics, Champaign, IL:313–317.

Rodosky MV, Andriacchi TP, Andersson GBJ 1989 The influence of chair height on lower limb mechanics during rising. J Orthoped Res 7:266–271.

Rooney KJ, Herbert RD, Balnave RJ 1994 Fatigue contributes to the strength training stimulus. Med Sci Sports Exerc 26:1160–1164.

Roy G, Nadeau S, Gravel D et al 2006 The effect of foot position and chair height on the asymmetry of vertical forces during sit-to-stand and stand-to-sit tasks in individuals with hemiparesis. Clin Biomech 21:585–593.

Schenkman M, Berger RA, O'Riley P et al 1990 Whole-body movements during rising to standing from sitting. Phys Ther 70:638–651.

Schenkman M, Hughes MA, Samsa G et al 1996 The relative importance of strength and balance in chair rise by functionally impaired older individuals. J Am Geriatr Soc 44:1441–1446.

Seelen HAM, van Wiggen KL, Halfens JHG et al 1995 Lower limb postural responses during sit-to-stand transfer in stroke patients during neurorehabilitation. In: Hakkinen K, Keskinen KL, Komi PV et al (eds) Book of abstracts of the XVth Congress of the International Society of Biomechanics. University of Jyvaskyla, Jyvaskyla, Finland:826–827.

Shepherd RB, Gentile AM 1994 Sit-to-stand: functional relationships between upper body and lower limb segments. Hum Mov Sci 13:817–840.

Shepherd RB, Koh HP 1996 Some biomechanical consequences of varying foot placement in sit-to-stand in young women. Scand J Rehabil Med 28:79–88.

Vander Linden DW, Brunt D, McCulloch MU 1994 Variant and invariant characteristics of the sit-to-stand task in healthy elderly adults. Arch Phys Med Rehabil 75:653–660.

Wanklyn P, Forster A, Young J 1996 Hemiplegic shoulder pain (HSP): natural history and investigation of associated features. Dis Rehabil 18:497–501.

Weiner DK, Long R, Hughes MA et al 1993 When older adults face the chair-rise challenge. J Am Geriatr Soc 41:6–10.

Chapter | 5 |

Walking

INTRODUCTION

The purpose of walking or running is to transport the body safely, effectively and efficiently across the ground, on the level, uphill and downhill, avoiding obstacles, negotiating uneven terrain, changing speed and direction as needed and responding to slips and trips. The ability to walk independently is a life-enriching activity and the most efficient way of getting from one place to another in the course of our daily lives. Limited walking ability can be a significant handicap restricting the individual's independent mobility about the house and in the community. The principal substitute for walking is propelling a wheelchair and, although this is preferable to not being able to get about at all, individuals who must use this substitution miss out on the considerable versatility of behaviour and experience associated with walking.

There is a large body of literature on biomechanics and control of walking in able-bodied subjects and in different age groups and in people with disability (e.g., Bernstein 1967; Inman et al 1981; Winter 1987, 1989, 1991; Perry 1992; Winter & Eng 1995; Rose & Gamble 2006). Continuing technological developments in measurement based on electronics enable results to be produced in minutes rather than days. Furthermore, mathematical modelling using high-speed computers has the potential to provide greater insights into the mechanics of normal and pathological gait.

Clearly there are idiosyncratic differences in the way we walk and individuals walk differently when exhilarated and when depressed. Each of us learn to integrate the numerous variables with the result that normal walking is an energy-efficient activity and one of the most consistent yet flexible actions we perform. Individuals display the same pattern of movement, presumably geared to optimum efficiency, from one cycle to the next (Murray et al 1964; Bernstein 1967; Inman et al 1981). Individual variations in size of joint angular displacements are relatively small: all we do is accomplish the same pattern in less or more time (Winter 1989). Although the

©2010 Elsevier Ltd
DOI: 10.1016/B978-0-7020-4051-1.00013-8

segmental interactions occurring as we walk are complex, the control system utilizes simplifying strategies, converting that complexity into an action that looks easy and requires little attention. We are freed up from motor control concerns to scan the environment and talk to our companions. This is not the case for individuals with motor disability for whom walking can provide considerable threats.

BIOMECHANICAL DESCRIPTION

Biomechanics now has the tools to perform functional analyses and replace guesswork in the clinic with a scientific framework (Sutherland 2002). Clear and clinically relevant biomechanical descriptions of gait are now readily available. As a result there are now serious attempts being made to transfer information from the research laboratory into clinical practice. The availability of joint movements and power data from gait analysis has advanced significantly the development of guidelines for improving strength and control of critical muscle groups and for training gait.

Biomechanical and behavioural criteria for effective walking

The production of a basic locomotor rhythm, support through the lower limbs, propulsion of the body forward, dynamic balance and the ability to adapt the movement to changing environmental demands and goals are the main functions that must be performed in effective walking (Forssberg 1982). The strength and control of the lower limbs play a significant role in these requirements (Winter 1987).

In the *stance phase*, as the body mass moves forward over the feet, the lower limbs' principal functions are:

- Support: the upper body is supported over one or both feet by the action, in particular, of the lower limb extensor muscles, and mechanical effects that prevent lower limb collapse.
- Balance: maintenance of upright posture over a changing base of support, by postural adjustments in lower limbs and limb–trunk segmental linkage.
- Propulsion (acceleration of the body in space): generation of mechanical energy to drive forward motion of the body.
- Absorption: mechanical energy is harnessed for shock absorption and to decrease the body's forward momentum.

In the *swing phase*, as the foot moves on a smooth path through swing from toe-off to heel contact, the lower limbs are involved in:

- Toe clearance: to clear the foot from the ground.
- Foot trajectory: to prepare the foot for safe landing on the support surface.

The gait cycle

It is necessary to be familiar with the biomechanical terminology used to describe gait. The gait cycle is the time interval between two successive events. It is divided into a stance phase, which commences at heel contact, and a swing phase that lasts from toe-off to the next initial contact. Each leg in turn has a stance phase when the foot is on the support surface and the body moves forward from over one foot to the other, and a swing phase when one foot is in the air as the other, swings forward. There is also a brief double support phase when both feet are in contact with the support surface. Stance and swing times reported for natural cadences are: stance 58–61%; swing 42–39%. Stance percentages increase at slower walking speeds. If symmetry is assumed, two double support periods at 8–11% of the stride occur. The short double support phase is critical in the transfer of weight from one limb to the other, and in the control of balance and posture of the upper body (Winter 1989). As walking speed increases, double support times decrease progressively and double support is replaced with a free flight phase in running. When distinguishing between the two legs, for example in walking over obstacles, the leg in front is known as the 'lead' leg and the one behind is the 'trail' leg.

For the purpose of description, the stance or support phase can be subdivided into weight acceptance/loading response, mid-stance and terminal stance, and pre-swing (push-off), while the swing phase is divided into lift-off (initial swing), mid-swing and reach (terminal/late swing). The terms used to describe foot placements on the ground are shown in Figure 5.1. Natural cadences vary from 101–122 steps/minute with gender differences of 6–11 steps higher in females compared with males. Walking speed (distance/time) is the average speed of forward progression of the body and is typically reported in metres per second (m/s) or centimetres per second (cm/s). Stride length may be correlated with stature and therefore walking speed tends to increase with stature, although there is contemporary debate about this.

The pathway described by the total body centre of gravity as the body moves forward is a smooth, sinusoidal curve (see Fig. 7.4). The centre of gravity is displaced twice in the vertical direction from heel contact of one foot to subsequent heel contact of the same foot. The centre of gravity is also displaced laterally in the horizontal plane in a smooth sinusoidal curve, the summits of which move to the right and to the left in relation to support of the stance leg. By keeping the walking base narrow, lateral movement needed to preserve balance is also reduced (Whittle 2007).

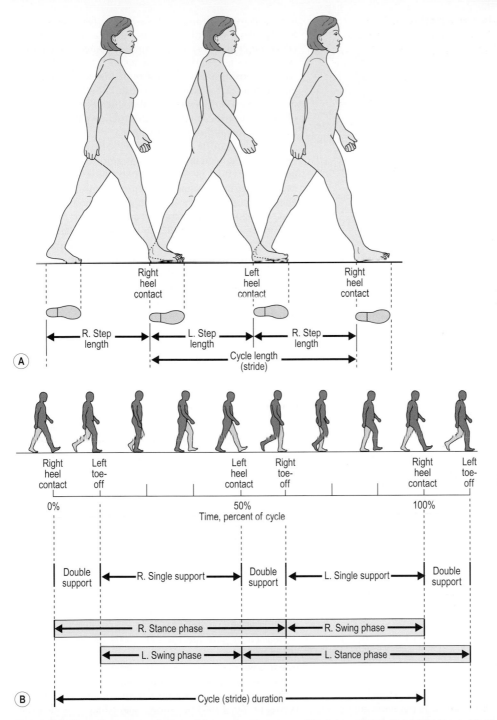

Figure 5.1 Time dimensions of the walking cycle. *(From Inman, V.T., Ralston HJ & Todd F (1981) Human Walking. Baltimore: Williams & Wilkins, by permission).*

Spatiotemporal characteristics

Speed is probably the most important variable in competent walking. We naturally adopt a walking speed that conserves most energy. Slow walking is associated with poor health outcomes (Cress et al 1995), disability (Potter et al 1995) and increased risk of falling (Hausdorff et al 2001; Jorgensen et al 2002). Many individuals with neurological impairments walk slowly. If speed is slow, little intersegmental exchange of energy takes place resulting in a high total energy cost per metre walked (Olney 2005). Several studies in which speed of walking was targeted in training have shown not only significant increases in speed but also similar gains in quality of life issues (Teixeira-Salmela et al 1999; Eng et al 2003). Walking faster also improves efficiency of energy transfer.

Kinematics

Kinematics is the term used to describe joint movement, independent of internal and external forces. Although significant movements occur in three planes, sagittal, frontal and transverse, the major angular changes occur in the sagittal plane. Since the mediolateral base of support is small in walking, little movement in the frontal plane is required. Of particular interest are the angles between segments (joint angles) and their relationship to events in the gait cycle (Fig. 5.2). Joint angle displacements provide helpful information for observational analysis but yield little information about the mechanisms producing the gait pattern.

The stance phase begins at heel contact (ankle dorsiflexed, knee extended). The ankle plantarflexes to bring the forefoot in contact with the ground. The hip extends and the ankle dorsiflexes (shank pivots over the fixed foot) to move the centre of body mass from behind the stance foot to a position in front of the foot. Early in the phase, the knee flexes (the 'yield' of the knee). The knee functions in this way to smooth the path of the centre of gravity. There is some internal rotation at the hip until full weightbearing, when there is a reversal into external rotation as the foot is about to leave the ground.

At mid-stance the angle at the hip is about zero and the knee is extended. Lateral horizontal pelvic shift (4–5 cm) toward the stance leg reaches its maximum and is controlled by hip abductors, particularly gluteus medius.

At termination of stance, the hip is extended (10–15° at the angle between the pelvis and the femur), the knee is flexing (40–50°) and the ankle is plantarflexing ready for push-off and initiation of swing phase. The hip flexes (pull-off) to swing the leg forward, and the knee flexes rapidly to a maximum of 63° for toe clearance. The swing phase is executed with considerable precision, with average toe clearance of about 1 cm (Winter 1987). Flexion at the

knee effectively 'shortens' the swinging leg, enabling the foot to take a forward path without contacting the ground (Eberhart et al 1965). Extension of the knee at the end of swing serves to lengthen the leg again before heel contact so as to position the leg in a more stable configuration and minimize lowering of the trunk. Speed of walking depends to a large extent on the efficiency of the swing phase, since stride length depends on how far the foot can be moved forward during this time.

The pelvis can be regarded as a rigid structure for the purpose of gait analysis. There is some rotation of the pelvis at the hips in the horizontal plane, its maximum excursion at heel contact countered by thoracic rotation. The magnitude of pelvic rotation is typically small. Murray and colleagues (1964) reported an absence of pelvic rotation in some subjects and also pointed out that rotation may vary with stride length and gender. Anterior and posterior pelvic tilting (at the hips and lumbar spine) is also minimal. The fluidity and efficiency of walking depends to some extent on the motions of the trunk and arms while lower limb movements provide the driving and braking forces. Movements of the pelvis and lower trunk appear to occur in response to lower limb movements, and it has further been suggested that thoracic spine movements occur principally in response to arm swing (Crosbie & Vachalathiti 1997).

Kinetics

These variables are calculated from force plate and kinematic data. They included horizontal and vertical ground reaction forces (GRFs), moments of force at the joints, mechanical power transferred between body segments and mechanical energy of segments. The forces that produce movements of the lower limb are muscular, gravitational and interactive, the latter being the result of dynamic interactions between segments.

The ability to propel the body mass forward manifests itself in the generation of appropriate forces on the support surface. These GRFs, *measured by a force plate embedded in the floor*, are the simplest kinetic variables to record (Fig. 5.3). They reflect the vertical and horizontal acceleration and deceleration of the body's centre of mass during weightbearing (Winter 1987).

Moments of force are the net effects of all agonist and antagonist muscles crossing that joint. In actions such as walking, when the body is supported over the feet, muscles that cross the three lower limb joints act cooperatively to support the body mass and prevent collapse of the limb. Winter (1980, 1984) has shown that collapse of the lower limb in stance is prevented by an overall extensor moment of force called a support moment of force (SM). This SM is consistently extensor despite variability that occurs at the hip, knee and ankle. In effect, there is a flexible stride-to-stride trade-off between the muscles crossing the hip

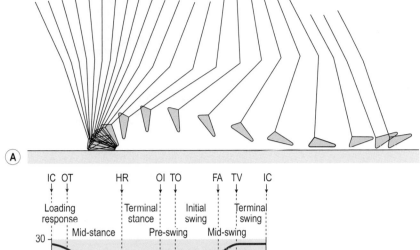

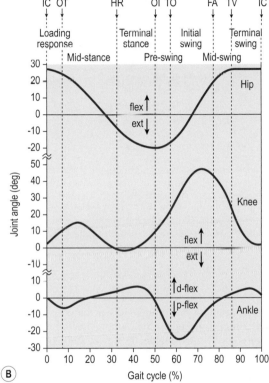

Figure 5.2 (A) Position of the R leg in the sagittal plane at 40ms intervals during a single gait cycle. (B) Sagittal plane joint angles (degrees) during a single gait cycle. IC = initial contact; OT = opposite toe-off; HR = heel rise; OI = opposite initial contact; TO = toe off; FA = feet adjacent; TV = tibia vertical. *(Reproduced from Whittle MW (2007) with permission).*

and knee joints. In this way the limb is controlled as a functional unit or synergy when moments at two or more joints cooperate toward a common goal that is independent of the muscle activity at individual joints.

The major work occurs in the sagittal plane since the goals of walking are to support the body against gravity while generating movement to propel the body forward. However, three-dimensional analysis reveals that a considerable amount of work is done in the frontal plane at the hips to control the pelvis and trunk against gravitational forces (Eng & Winter 1995). More recently, mathematical modelling indicates that gluteus medius is a large

contributor to support and to forward progression, especially during single-limb stance (Liu et al 2006).

An analysis of *mechanical power* (net moment × angular velocity at the joint) provides information about the muscles that are generating energy and those absorbing energy. This analysis is the most valuable of all the gait variables since it describes the magnitude and direction of flow of power into (generation) and out of (absorption) muscles (Winter 1987). Power at a joint (measured in watts) is the product of the net muscle moment at the joint and the angular velocity and is the rate at which energy is generated and absorbed. Negative power results from

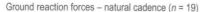

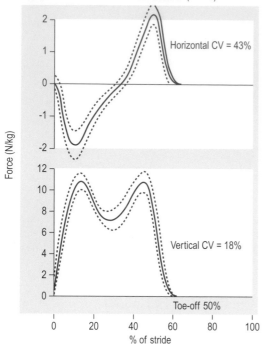

Figure 5.3 Averaged horizontal (top trace) and vertical (bottom trace) ground reaction forces. Horizontal force has a negative phase during the first half of stance, indicating a slowing down of the body, and a positive phase, indicating forward acceleration of the body, during the latter half of stance. Vertical force has the characteristic double hump, the first related to weight-acceptance and the second to push-off. CV: coefficient of variation. *(From Winter, D.A. (1987) The Biomechanics and Motor Control of Human Gait, Waterloo Biomechanics, by permission).*

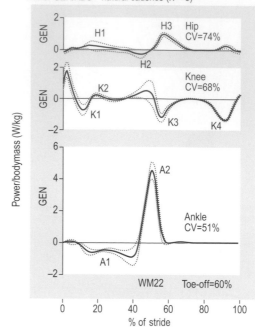

Figure 5.4 Ensemble averages of power patterns of able-bodied subjects walking at their preferred cadence plotted over a single gait cycle indicating the most important power phases for hip (H), knee (K) and ankle (A). 60% indicates the beginning of swing phase. CV: coefficient of variation. *(From Winter, D.A. (1987) The Biomechanics and Motor Control of Human Gait, Waterloo Biomechanics, by permission).*

eccentric contraction and positive power from concentric contraction. Power profiles of the three lower limb joints for healthy subjects are shown in Figure 5.4. These profiles reveal that the major generation of energy (A2, >80%) takes place at push-off by the plantarflexor activity that moves the body mass forward. It is the largest and most important energy burst during the gait cycle. The knee extensors (contracting eccentrically) are primarily absorbing energy during stance. The second most important source of power is provided by hip flexors in late stance and early swing for pull-off (H3). In the third significant energy burst (H1), hip extension is dominant in early stance as the hip extends to position the body in front of the stance foot, pushing from behind. Magnitude of power profiles varies according to speed but tends to remain constant in shape. Power profiles of stroke patients walking slowly are similar to these normative details but the amplitude of power is less or barely perceptible (Olney 2005). Training during walking practice to increase and vary speed may enable the lower limb muscles to build up peak force faster, therefore increasing power and speed.

The three major power bursts provide the propulsive force for forward progression. An understanding of power patterns is used as a guide to training, demonstrating the need to select strengthening exercises that include concentric and eccentric muscle activity and the switch between the two. Another energy conserving mechanism is the energy storage and recovery that take place in the passive elastic tissues in the tendon and muscle when an eccentric contraction precedes a concentric contraction, as in repetitive standing up and sitting down, and in walking, but unlikely in slow walking (Winter & Eng 1995).

Muscle activity

Although the kinematics of walking remain relatively stable, one of the interesting things about walking is that the same movement may be achieved using different combinations of muscles, some of which may be explained by biological differences (Shiavi 1985; Whittle 2007). Even with the improved kinesiological EMG measurement tools available at the present time, technical difficulties make it difficult to identify 'normal' patterns of muscle usage (Sutherland 2001). Physiological walking strategies may also include some variation in muscle timing stride-to-stride (Perry 1992).

Many muscles are active primarily in stance phase or primarily in swing phase. They contract and relax in a precise, orchestrated manner (Boakes & Rab 2006). As the cycle progresses, muscle action becomes primarily isometric and eccentric, both of which are efficient forms of contraction to maintain upright posture against gravity and to transfer energy between segments. Concentric contractions of muscle (positive work) provide brief bursts of power to accelerate the limbs and power forward motion when required. The muscle groups that do most of the propulsive/generative work are the ankle plantarflexors at push-off, the hip extensors at heel strike and the hip flexors at pull-off (Olney 2005). Additional force is required when walking fast or when climbing a slope or stairs. Muscle contraction that is prolonged and out of phase during walking may reflect abnormalities of motor control such as those seen following stroke and in cerebral palsy (Boakes & Rab 2006).

There is some redundancy in the motor system such that if a particular muscle cannot be used, another muscle may take over the function (Winter 1987; Whittle 2007). For example, the knee angle during stance phase is under control of at least three joint moments and many muscles, both mono- and bi-articular (Winter et al 1991). Ankle muscle activity appears the most consistent across trials and individuals. This may reflect the joint's position closest to the base of support while knee and hip muscles have multiple roles, and tend to show more variability. Signals in mono-articular muscles show less variability than bi-articular muscles, reflecting different roles in producing and transferring power.

Stair walking

The biomechanics of walking up and down stairs or steps have been described in many articles and texts (Andriacchi et al 1980; McFadyen & Winter 1988; Nadeau et al 2003). Although it is another action involving the lower limbs in support, balance and propulsion, stair walking is mechanically different from level walking in terms of joint range, muscle activity, magnitude of joint forces (Andriacchi et al 1980) and powers. Stair walking can be very challenging for elderly people and those with disability. The major challenge in ascent is conservation of energy while that of descent is principally that of ensuring safety.

Lower limb function in stair ascent and descent differs from level walking due to the necessity for a greater raising and lowering of the body mass while progressing a short distance. This results in increased demands on both duration and intensity of muscle activity and increased ranges of motion at the lower limb joints (Andriacchi et al 1980). Greater demands are also made on balance, particularly during the period of single stance. Stair descent has been found to have a shorter double support phase than stair ascent, probably reflecting different mechanical demands (Zachazewski et al 1993).

An essential feature of walking up stairs is the ankle dorsiflexion that occurs after the foot has been placed on the stair. Forward translation of the body mass takes place at the ankle, while the body remains in the same relative alignment. The back leg pushes the body forward and upward diagonally over the front foot while this leg lifts the body along a vertical inclination. Failure to move the centre of body mass far enough forward over the foot can result in a fall backward. In contrast, when descending, the body mass is kept back over the supporting leg which flexes at the hip, knee and ankle to lower the body mass and place the foot onto the lower step. Thus a smooth ascent or descent results from coordination of forces produced by both legs. Assessment of stair walking kinematics in able-bodied subjects has revealed increased lower limb joint ranges in the sagittal plane; for example, approximately 12-20° more flexion and extension is required at the knee joint than in level walking (Nadeau et al 2003).

During ascent, concentric contraction of lower limb extensor muscles raises the body mass vertically; in descent, the body mass is lowered by eccentric muscle activity controlling gravitational forces. Extensor muscles in stair walking have to generate much larger forces than in level walking with the largest increase in the sagittal plane occurring at the knee joint (McFadyen & Winter 1988). Stair ascent and descent and level walking all exhibit a support moment of force similar in shape. However, the magnitude of support moment for stair walking is greater. During ascent it is about twice the magnitude produced during level walking depending on the height of the step (Bradford et al 1988). Extensor muscle strength is, therefore, particularly critical to this activity since the body mass must be raised or lowered essentially by one limb. In contrast to level walking, it is the knee extensors that generate most of the energy assisted by ankle plantarflexors and hip extensors.

An interesting finding in a study designed to investigate the adaptation of foot clearance to reduced lighting revealed that whereas young subjects increased their foot clearance, older subjects' foot clearance tended to remain the same. This lack of adaptation to a changing environment may contribute to falls on stairs in the elderly (Hamel et al 2005).

AGE-RELATED CHANGES

The ability to maintain effective walking with increasing age is important for the health and wellbeing of older people. How many of the changes observed in older individuals are due to an ageing process and how many to the reduced activity that may accompany getting older, however, is not clearly understood.

It is a common observation that the walking pattern changes with increasing age. Investigators have described age-related decreases in aerobic capacity, joint flexibility, muscle strength and bone mass. Interestingly, these decrements are similar to those following extended periods of bed rest and even with relative inactivity (Bortz 1982). It is also of note that certain aspects of physical performance are strongly influenced by both the level and type of activity. In a longitudinal study of aerobic capacity in elite athletes aged between 50 and 82 years, those who continued competitive levels of training maintained their aerobic capacity irrespective of their age. Those who decreased training showed significant reductions in aerobic capacity (Pollock et al 1987).

Murray and colleagues (1969) reported that if individuals with pathology were excluded, the walking performance of older men was a 'slowed down' version of the gait of younger men and did not resemble a pathological gait. A subsequent study confirmed this observation on female subjects (Murray et al 1970). More recently Winter and colleagues (1990) studied a group of active and healthy men and women with an age range of 62–78 and compared their performance with younger subjects. The most consistent finding was that older people walked more slowly. This was a function of shortened steps, reduced cadence and an increase in time spent in double-limb support (leading to a reduction in the percentage of the gait cycle in which there was single limb support), and of decreased push-off power with a more flat-footed floor contact. The nature of these adaptations suggests that they may involve a more conservative or less destabilizing gait. However, when older subjects were instructed to walk at specified, fixed speeds, no significant differences were apparent (Jansen et al 1982).

Studies of range of motion suggest that decreased mobility at the ankle joint may be associated with an increasingly sedentary lifestyle, and acute and chronic pathology (Vandervoort et al 1990). Reduced push-off power in subjects aged 62–78 years, compared with younger subjects, has been reported (Winter et al 1990), and significantly smaller peak torque and power values were found in ankle and knee muscles in a group of fallers compared with a group of non-fallers (Whipple et al 1987).

Individuals with limited ankle joint mobility may be particularly at risk of stumbling, tripping and falling. However, the control of stability in walking has not received the same level of attention as standing balance. More recently, biomechanical investigations of walking in the elderly have attempted to investigate variables that more directly reflect instability during walking. Laboratory-based experiments on slips (Strandberg & Lanshammar 1981) and trips (Pavol et al 1999), walking on uneven terrain (Marigold & Patla 2008), and stepping to regain balance (Rogers et al 2003) have advanced the mechanical and physiological understanding of these actions. Although the generalizability to real-life events remains unclear, the fact that older adults find these events challenging provides a scientific basis for training to improve functional mobility and reduce the possibility of falls. A generalized slowing in reaction time is also a consistent factor in ageing and among the strongest predictors of falls (Lord & Fitzpatrick 2001). A number of studies have shown significant improvement following training in initiation of stepping to regain balance (Rogers et al 2003) and in obstacle avoidance (Weerdesteyn et al 2006).

Difficulty maintaining body and head stability may affect the visual system and therefore impact on postural stability by interfering with normal gaze stability (Winter & Eng 1995; Lord et al 2007). Impaired vestibular function is also a factor in falls (Lord et al 2007).

Falls are a frequent hazard for elderly people. Epidemiological studies have implicated many factors: poor initiation of walking, turning, stepping over, and avoiding obstacles, slips and trips, walking on uneven terrain, stairs, and visual problems (Gabell & Nayak 1984; Startzell et al 2000). A number of studies have shown that reduction in temporospatial parameters of gait (speed and step length) are significantly associated with the physiological factors of falls, including lower limb strength, slow reaction time, increased postural sway and impaired peripheral sensation. Research continues to examine the best way of modifying these parameters with training (see Lord et al 2007 for discussion). Fear of falling and the possible consequences of a fall may also influence performance.

MOTOR DYSFUNCTION

Walking in healthy subjects is achieved with relative ease and modest energy consumption, and with an identifiable pattern of biomechanical characteristics. Pathology affecting the locomotor system can lead to gait patterns that are clearly abnormal. Some may be identified through observation but others can only be identified with appropriate instrumentation.

Walking dysfunction is common in individuals with neurological impairments, arising not only from the lesion itself but also from adaptations arising from secondary musculoskeletal and cardiorespiratory consequences of disuse and physical inactivity. Muscle weakness, increases in intrinsic muscle stiffness, disordered motor control and soft tissue contracture are major contributors to walking dysfunction. Functional walking, however, also depends on level of fitness. Since the energy cost of walking is speed dependent, an important aim in gait training is to increase strength and control of lower limb muscles in order to decrease the energy cost of walking. Research has shown that a healthy subject's comfortable walking speed is associated with the minimum metabolic cost. Walking, either more slowly or faster, increases the metabolic cost.

Understanding motor control and the mechanics of walking helps elucidate the performance and control deficits in individuals with neural lesions. In this section we discuss major aspects of movement dysfunction that are associated with acute brain lesions, such as stroke and traumatic brain injury. Impairments affecting walking in cerebellar ataxia, Parkinson's disease and multiple sclerosis are discussed in Chapters 9, 13 and 14. However, the need to train critical biomechanical characteristics of walking, together with strength, motor control and fitness, is similar in all of these conditions.

There are several mechanical problems that commonly interfere with the ability to walk, irrespective of the age of the individual and the underlying pathological mechanisms. Although decreased speed of activation and peak muscle contraction and slowness in reaching peak amplitude of force are probably major contributors to slow walking and lack of dynamic stride length, walking may also be slowed in response to feelings of instability or unsteadiness.

After an upper motor neuron (UMN) lesion (Ch. 8), gait problems arise primarily from impairments of *muscle weakness and disorders of motor control* but also from adaptive musculoskeletal changes that occur over time, some quite quickly, due to immobility (Gracies 2005). Weakness is due to a loss of neuromotor control of voluntary muscle action, that is depression of motor function. There is insufficient motor unit activation, a decline in the rate and amplitude of recruitment resulting in weakness.

Research findings

Since the first edition, a large number of biomechanical examinations of kinematics and kinetics of gait in individuals following stroke in particular enable a clearer picture of what may be the most significant gait deficits limiting activity in many individuals:

- ↓ self-selected and maximum speed
- ↓ magnitude of flexion/extension joint angle range in both lower limbs (Olney et al 1991)

- ↓ hip extension at end of stance (Olney & Richards 1996; Richards et al 1999)
- ↑ double support phase associated with a sense of poor balance (Olney 2005)
- ↓ vertical ground reaction force at push-off implicating weak plantarflexion (Carlsoo et al 1974)
- ↓ power generation at the ankle for push-off and at the hip for pull-off (Olney & Richards 1996; Dean et al 2000).

In clinical practice, the therapist can observe adaptive step and stride lengths and differences in stance and swing ratios. These are the outcomes of the invisible kinetic forces.

For those individuals post-stroke who can walk relatively independently, the most consistent finding is that they walk more slowly than their able-bodied peers (von Schroeder et al 1995; Witte & Carlsson 1997). Slow walking can result from inability of lower limb muscles to generate and control muscle force concentrically and eccentrically, and to time these forces. It can also reflect lack of vigour and a pre-lesion habit in an elderly person. There is very little exchange of energy in slow-speed walking and the individual has much higher total energy costs per metre walked (see Olney 2005). Gait speed has been found to correlate with strength of lower limb muscles (Bohannon & Andrews 1990), magnitude of push-off power (Olney et al 1991) and hip extension angle at the end of stance – the smaller the angle, the slower the speed (Olney & Richards 1996). Speed also correlates with increased time spent in double support phase (Olney & Richards 1996) and reduced hip abduction/adduction power (Kim & Eng 2004).

It is also clear from research that the following are common problems:

- ↓ Endurance – a group of individuals post-stroke were unable to maintain their comfortable walking speed over 6 minutes. They walked only about 50% of the distance predicted for healthy individuals with similar physical characteristics (Dean et al 2001).
- ↓ Adaptability to changing environmental conditions, for example catching the toe or heel while stepping over objects (Said et al 1999).

Evaluation of motor performance

Although instrumented gait analysis techniques are widely used in research, it is not possible or practical for every patient to have a full biomechanical assessment. Instrumentation and technical know-how are not readily available in the clinic because of cost in terms of money, space and time.

However, physiotherapists working in movement rehabilitation must be familiar with results of biomechanical research, and the methods used. The knowledge gained from ongoing research into gait in both healthy and disabled subjects should underpin and direct both evaluation and training of gait in clinical practice.

A videotape or a DVD plus a computer on which to record a patient walking has many advantages. The physiotherapist can review the tape many times; having the taped record reduces the number of times the patient walks for the purpose of observation; patients can see how they are walking and over time it can help to convince them that they are or are not improving. Sagittal plane movement is best observed and filmed from the side, frontal plane movement from the front or back. Videotaping performance does not provide quantitative data but there are some simple methods of measurement without the need for complex and expensive instrumentation (Smith 1990). For example, freeze-frame videotapes and still photography can be used to measure angular displacements or segmental alignment at different points in time throughout the gait cycle (van Vliet 1988) and to confirm (or not) the therapist's observations. A tape measure, stopwatch and marking pens attached to the heels can be used to measure step and stride lengths in order to calculate cadence and speed.

Physiotherapists routinely observe gait in clinical practice to establish the patient's functional status, to identify movement limitations and to make decisions about intervention. Observation depends on the skill of the observer, and an understanding of normative biomechanics and muscle function relative to gait can assist in treatment decisions. Although walking in healthy individuals has a fairly predictable and consistent topology, marked variations can be observed in persons with incoordination due to stroke. The observed gait pattern is the result of an individual's attempts to walk despite muscle weakness, lack of motor control and postural instability. Adaptations to fear of falling and feelings of instability may include a widening of the walking base and dependence on arms for support and balance.

The only observable movement characteristics are the kinematics – how the individual's body segments are coordinated in space and time. Spatiotemporal and kinematic variables can give clues to the underlying dynamics. However, it is clear that without the necessary knowledge, observational analysis of walking can be inaccurate and erroneous conclusions may be drawn (Eastlake et al 1991; Malouin 1995).

The focus of one's observations is important and where we look and how we look depend on our knowledge of gait and the impairments. For example, Olney (2005) points out that without understanding the importance of push-off at the end of stance, physiotherapists have not known what aspects of walking to focus attention on when observing a patient with a flat-footed gait. Figure 5.5 provides some examples of common problems that can be easily observed. The reader can check their observations against the captions.

TRAINING GAIT

Over the past decade or two, with measurement of progress and outcome becoming mandatory in the clinic, it is now possible to base clinical practice on scientific and clinical evidence rather than experience as a form of evidence. We now have a good indication of which methods have long-term/lasting benefits and which do not (Eng & Tang 2007). It is imperative that physiotherapists embrace change and where there is evidence of effectiveness, these methods must be used (Herbert et al 2001) and other ineffective methods discarded. Valid, objective and reliable functional scales and timed walking tests listed in Chapter 3 provide baseline, outcome and retention data.

The major emphasis in training for independent walking is on training support and push-off through the lower limbs, balance of the body mass over the changing base of support, and control of the foot and knee paths through swing. The emphasis is on early activity in standing (Fig. 5.6). The use of the hands for support is discouraged to enable the regaining of dynamic balance and the ability to support the body through the lower limbs.

As soon as the person attempts to walk again in the first few days after stroke, certain gait limitations are evident. They are predictable to some extent given the typical effects of muscle weakness, lack of control of the lower limb, poor balance and, if the period of immobility has been prolonged, increased soft tissue stiffness or contracture. In general, training to optimize walking involves:

- practice of treadmill and overground walking
- exercises to increase strength and control of lower limb muscles, with active stretching of muscles to preserve muscle extensibility
- training to maximize skill, speed, endurance and fitness.

It is usual for physiotherapy to begin within 1 week post-stroke when many patients cannot stand up and walk independently, and some have little ability to activate lower limb muscles. The tendency for the paretic limb to collapse, lack of propulsion for forward progression and poor balance are common problems in the early stages. There are several critical mechanical functions occurring at specific stages in the gait cycle that are a focus in training gait and in the exercise programme:

- $10-15°$ hip extension of the paretic limb in late stance provides some mechanical advantage to hip flexion for power generation for pull-off.
- Plantarflexion at the ankle at the end of stance for push-off. A strong push-off is the most important trigger for knee flexion in early swing.
- Flexion at the hip for pull-off.

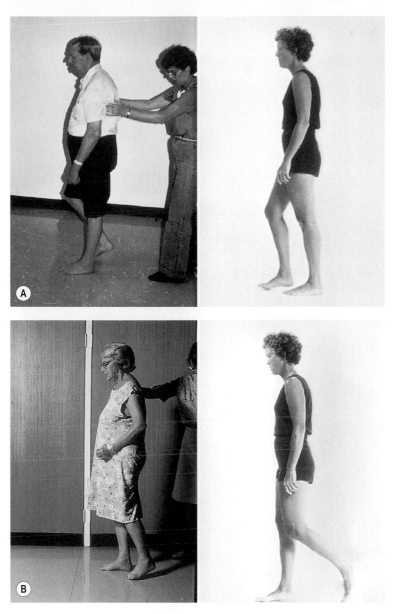

Figure 5.5 (A) L mid-stance – decreased ankle dorsiflexion and hip extension. Normally extension at the hip occurs as the COM moves forward over the stance foot. Compare with figure on the right. (B) Start of L swing – lack of push-off and pull-off. Compare with figure on the right.

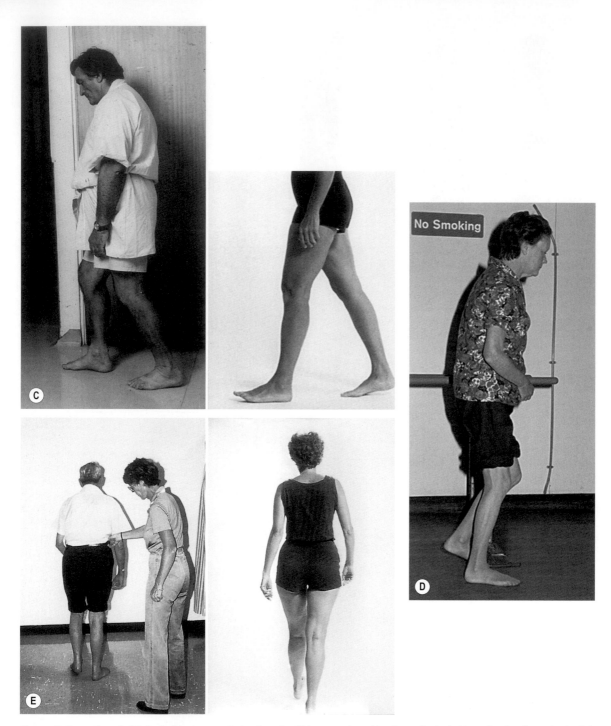

Figure 5.5 *continued* (C) End of L stance – lack of push-off (concentric ankle plantarflexion). Note the flat-footed gait. (D) R mid stance – knee remains flexed showing poor control of the limb. Knee position in stance is normally controlled by the muscles that cross the joint plus soleus that controls movement of the shank over the ankle. (E) Note the wide base compared with the figure on the right.

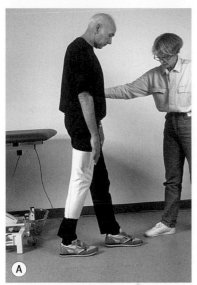

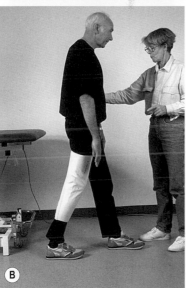

Figure 5.6 The splint is a temporary aid to prevent his knee from collapsing. He practices stepping with the L leg while loading the paretic R leg. (A) He is reluctant to load the R leg and does not move his COM (by extending his hip) over the L foot. (B) When the therapist directs him to step to her foot (a concrete goal) he is more successful.

Loading the paretic limb

The opportunity for weightbearing through the feet seems critical for promoting muscle function in the lower limbs. In an animal experiment in which the hind legs of a rat were suspended, depriving the animal of weightbearing and limb loading, the animal ceased moving the suspended limbs. Examination of gastrocnemius muscle revealed evidence of muscle atrophy within 7 days of suspension even though the muscle was free to contract (Musacchia et al 1980). Inability to bear weight through the lower limbs has also been reported in humans after prolonged bed rest (Haines 1974) and after space travel.

These findings support the critical importance of early practice of weightbearing and loading the paretic limb which should be an urgent and early focus of attention. Functional weightbearing exercises to train muscle force generation and limb control such as repetitive standing up and sitting down and standing balance activities (Fig. 5.7) are trained concurrently with gait training since these activities can force limb loading and improve strength and coordination (see Chs. 2 & 7).

Walking-treadmill and overground

There are many reasons, mechanical, physiological and behavioural, why practice of walking itself is critical to improving performance. Walking requires multiple levels of neural control to support the body against gravity and propel it forward. This necessitates control by the neuromuscular system of many joints and coordination of multiple mono- and bi-articular muscles. At the same time the system must exercise active control to balance the moving body and adapt the walking pattern to environmental and social demands. Although sensory input does not appear to be essential for the generation of a rhythmic walking pattern, speed and coordination are reduced in the absence of peripheral input. It appears that the ease with which we walk can be attributed to intrinsic spinal circuits that take care of the complex coordination of muscle contraction needed to generate rhythmic stepping of the legs (Gordon 1991). Animal research has demonstrated the existence of spinal circuits capable of generating sustained rhythmic outputs without input from either supraspinal structures or sensory receptors (Brown 1914; Grillner & Shik 1973). Spinal cat, for example, can produce stepping movements on a moving treadmill with external support. Although central pattern generators have not been located in the spinal cord in humans, it is considered that human walking may be organized in a similar way. Coordinated networks in the spinal cord would be controlled by descending pathways from higher centres and receive feedback from the periphery (Duysens & van de Crommert 1998). These networks, or a similar mechanism, may be capable of generating a rhythmic pattern thus simplifying the control of walking. It is possible that repetitive gait training could modify these networks, and thus improve walking after stroke (Macko et al 2005). This concept, if several networks can be located, may provide a physiological reason for the reported effectiveness of treadmill walking in individuals with upper motor neuron lesions.

A treadmill, with or without supportive harness, provides an opportunity to practise walking under challenging conditions. The moving belt physically drives and

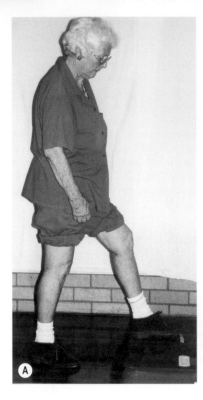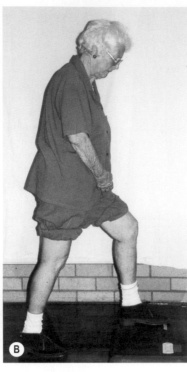

Figure 5.7 This exercise improves control of the limb, particularly hip extension – stepping with the non-paretic leg to load the paretic leg. As she practices she is able to move further forward over the L leg with confidence. She will progress to stepping with alternate legs.

maximizes the extent of hip extension and ankle dorsiflexion, thereby setting up two of the necessary conditions for the swing phase of that leg. In addition, loading the lower limbs while weightbearing in a harness occurs without fear of the leg collapsing and provoking a fall. A harness enables patients to bear some weight and to walk, even in the presence of considerable dysfunction.

Overground walking

There appears to be some confusion in the clinic with regard to walking practice. At one end of the spectrum there are reports of therapists who are reluctant to allow patients to practise walking on their own in case they should practise incorrectly. At the other end, patients are supplied with a quadripod stick (four-point cane), an ankle orthosis and possibly a leg splint, and are 'walked' by the therapist or nurse with little regard for the fact that there is negligible muscle activity in the limb. In between the two extremes is the training of walking by a therapist who understands the biomechanics and muscle activity of walking and can apply exercise and learning strategies. Balance, weightbearing and stepping are trained simultaneously when the individual practises walking. Dependent individuals can train on a treadmill with body weight support.

Gait initiation, the transition from upright stance to steady-state walking, is a challenging activity in which each limb has distinctive responsibility. The individual is encouraged to initiate walking by taking a step forward with the non-paretic limb. In this way, the hip of the paretic limb is extended, and the ankle dorsiflexed that may provoke a stronger push-off, a more effective swing forward and a longer step. Initially it is important that the person regains a sense of the idea of walking, that is of the rhythmical, cyclical nature of gait. The individual can be steadied at the upper arm or with a safety 'grab' belt (see Fig. 7.14) while the individual's attention is on taking big steps with both legs.

Increasing speed may be counter-intuitive to those who consider it important to emphasize slow walking in order to improve the walking pattern. The results of many motor learning studies suggest that focusing attention on the outcome of an action (e.g., walking to a pre-arranged place as quickly as possible) produces more effective performance than focusing attention on the movement itself (see intrinsic vs extrinsic training in Ch. 2). Walking practice at a reasonable speed is also critical to improve exchange between kinetic and potential energy (Olney 2005). Walking sideways and backward involve different patterns of muscle activation and train flexibility and balance. Walking sideways is a useful exercise for training weightbearing and control of mediolateral postural sway while shifting the body mass from one leg to another (Fig. 5.8). Walking backward is an exercise to train the bi-articular hamstrings to control hip extension and knee flexion.

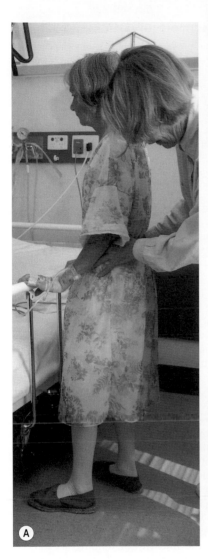
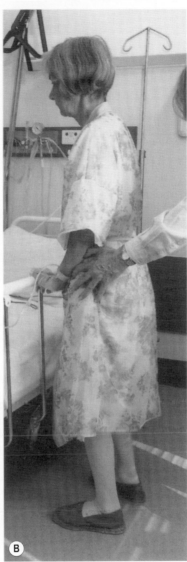

Figure 5.8 Walking sideways early after stroke – one leg loads, other leg lifts. Note she steps forward with her L leg rather than holding her hip extended while abducting it. She is successful on her next attempt. A line on the floor or a small object can provide a concrete goal.

Treadmill training with and without body weight support

Based on findings from investigations of the spinal cat (Barbeau & Rossignol 1967; Rossignol et al 1986), treadmill walking as a dynamic means of providing walking training was proposed several decades ago (Finch & Barbeau 1985; Carr & Shepherd 1987). It was suggested that the patient should walk on a treadmill with a percentage of body weight supported by an overhead harness (body weight support; BWS) in order to reduce the amount of active support through the weak limb(s) (Finch & Barbeau 1985). The adaptations to BWS were few and BWS did not produce an abnormal gait (Finch et al 1991).

Walking on a treadmill with some BWS via a harness connected to an overhead support system is increasingly being shown to be an effective means of promoting rhythmical vigorous walking and increasing endurance, and an effective method of task-related training (Fig. 5.9). The results of a Cochrane systematic review (Moseley et al 2005) suggest that treadmill training is a valuable part of gait training particularly in weak patients (Barbeau & Visintin 2003), and as a means of increasing gait speed and endurance (Ada et al 2003). Treadmill training with BWS is well-tolerated and effective in the early phase of recovery and may be the only means of practising gait for more severely affected, dependent walkers (Barbeau & Visintin 2003). For dependent walkers, BWS

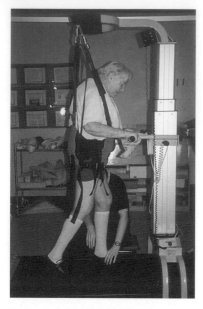

Figure 5.9 Treadmill walking with body weight support. The therapist may need to assist the path of the foot (toe clearance) and step length during swing phase of the paretic L leg.

Box 5.1 **Treadmill training – effects**

- The moving belt stimulates a rhythmic gait pattern. It induces a shift toward more consistent temporal phasing and a symmetrical gait pattern that are associated with changes in the timing of muscle activations (Hesse et al 1999; Harris-Love et al 2004)
- The belt provides a mechanical stimulus to the hip flexors, optimizing pull-off (Harris-Love et al 2004)
- The harness removes some of the biomechanical and balance constraints of full weightbearing
- Treadmill training has the potential to increase the time spent in practice of walking
- Walking uphill on a treadmill can increase strength, endurance and aerobic fitness

---

is essential. For independent walkers, BWS is usually not required.

Although some physiotherapists have expressed concern that treadmill walking is different from overground walking, the mechanical differences in gait pattern are insignificant. The only real differences are in the visual information received by the individual and the impact of the facilitatory action of the belt on the paretic limb.

In summary, the positive effects of a treadmill in walking training may result from the factors shown in Box 5.1 and Box 5.2.

Box 5.2 **Treadmill training – details**

Body weight support (BWS)

- Use the minimum BWS necessary to maintain active hip and knee extension (<30% of BWS; Hesse et al 1997)
- ↓ BWS as patient improves
- Encourage patient to reduce hand support

Speed

- Adjust speed to achieve an optimal step length – if speed is too slow there is little benefit
- Adjust both speed and inclination of the treadmill to challenge the individual
- ↑ speed

Note: Guidance by the therapist may be necessary initially to assist the paretic limb to swing through and to guide foot trajectory.

Several factors, for example speed, amount of BWS support, assistance by the therapist and dosage, are likely to impact on efficacy of treadmill training with or without BWS. All of these can be adjusted in order to provide a sufficient training intensity. Increasing the treadmill slope and using a portable heart rate monitor during training may optimize the training currently provided (Moseley et al 2005). A Lite-Gait® or similar device may help the individual make the transition from treadmill walking to overground walking without fear of falling.

Several studies of treadmill training with and without BWS have demonstrated effective results, showing significantly better results than those obtained by Bobath therapy/neurodevelopmental treatment (NDT) (Richards et al 1993; Hesse et al 1995a) or combined proprioceptive neuromuscular facilitation (PNF) and Bobath therapy (Pohl et al 2002). The large increase in walking speed in the experimental group in Pohl and colleagues' study probably reflected the intensity of training, as subjects were rapidly progressed to increased speeds compared with limited speed increases in the control group.

Programmes of treadmill training combined with other task-oriented exercises are effective at enhancing walking ability (Dean et al 2000; Ada et al 2003; Salbach et al 2004). A key factor may be the varied and intensive practice of weightbearing activities that include functional strength training for both lower limbs, with exercises that provide similar functional stresses to walking, in addition to treadmill walking. The experimental group in Dean and colleagues' study (2000) demonstrated significantly increased walking speed and endurance, increased vertical force production through the paretic foot during standing up, and an increased number of repetitions in the step test, and these results were retained at 2 months' follow-up. Treatment effect is highly dependent on the intensity of the training protocol. A combination of treadmill, task-specific training and practice appears therefore to be optimal (Eng & Tang 2007).

A recent randomized and controlled study has provided evidence of increased activation of cortico–subcortical networks produced by repetitive treadmill training in a group of chronic stroke-affected individuals (Luft et al 2009). Similar changes were not found in the control group that had equal time and exposure in a programme that provided neither aerobic stress nor required many active repetitions.

Electromechanical-assisted gait training

The development of these devices has the potential to enhance walking rehabilitation. Hesse and colleagues (2006) working in Berlin describe the Gait Trainer 1™ (GT1), that removes the need for physiotherapists to assist movement of the paretic leg and provides the opportunity for increasing the time spent practising, and the Haptic Walker, on which patients can train for stair climbing. A recent systematic review provides evidence that the use of an electromechanical-assisted gait training device in combination with physiotherapy increases the likelihood of regaining independent walking. Mehrholz and colleagues (2007) recommend that further research should include outcome measures of activities of daily living and effects on the quality of life. The review indicates that walking speed did not change. However, practice at increased speeds may help.

Functional strength training

Although the individual needs the opportunity to walk early after a brain lesion, it is also necessary to have an additional programme of specific exercises designed to increase strength and control of the lower limbs. Timing relationships between segmental rotations are critical to effective and efficient gait and can only be learned through practice of walking itself or of actions that require a similar biomechanical pattern.

Muscle weakness can be severe on the paretic side in stroke compared with healthy older individuals, but some muscle groups are more important in walking, in particular for regulating speed (Winter 1991) and should be the focus in strength training. Ankle plantarflexors at push-off, hip flexors at pull-off and hip extensors in early stance perform most of the work in walking (see Olney 2005 for discussion). The strength of hip flexors and ankle plantarflexors is significantly related to gait speed with the plantarflexor burst of power explaining about 72% of the variance in gait speed on level surfaces (Bohannon 1986; Kim & Eng 2003).

An investigation of strength, voluntary activation and antagonist co-contraction over the first 6 months following stroke demonstrated that stroke patients have a potential for increasing voluntary strength that should be, but is currently not being, addressed during rehabilitation (Newham & Hsiao 2001). Muscle activation failure is probably the major factor underlying functional disability in gait together with adaptive changes to muscle (increased intrinsic stiffness and decreased length). Results of several recent studies have reported significant increases in motor performance and health outcomes when strength training has been included in the exercise programme (Teixeira-Salmela et al 1999, 2001; Dean et al 2000). For example, at the completion of a physical conditioning programme, subjects were able to generate higher levels of power and increases in positive work by plantarflexors, hip flexors and extensors, and there was a significant increase in walking speed (Teixeira-Salmela et al 1999, 2001). It is possible that many stroke patients maintain significant gait disability because rehabilitation has not targeted strength and endurance due to the dogma related to spasticity. With our present understanding this is a serious clinical error. An examination of the relationship between muscle torque generated by muscles of both lower limbs in level walking and stair climbing shows that weakness in muscles of the non-paretic limb also contributes to slow walking speed and gait disability and should be addressed in training (Kim & Eng 2003). It is important for rehabilitation staff to understand that slow walking speeds can be a major reason for absence of community walking post-discharge and are a major contributor to falls.

Emphasis in training is on the hip, knee and ankle extensor muscles since the force generating capacity in these muscle groups provides the basic support, balance and propulsive functions. An efficient and functionally relevant way to increase muscle strength and control is practice of weightbearing actions (step-ups, standing up and sitting down, heels raise and lower and semi-squats) against body weight resistance (see Ch. 2). Functional weightbearing exercises can be progressed by increasing the number of repetitions (up to 10 with no break between repetitions, in sets of three, with a short break between sets), by decreasing support, increasing the height of the step or decreasing the height of the chair, and increasing speed. There was no evidence of an increase in spasticity due to strengthening exercise in a systematic review of progressive resistance exercises (Morris et al 2004) or in a meta-analysis of methods of intervention in stroke that involve effortful muscle contraction (Ada et al 2006).

Step up and down exercises. Hip, knee and ankle extensors are trained to work cooperatively, concentrically and eccentrically, to raise and lower the body mass (Fig. 5.10). Forces are distributed evenly over the three joints when stepping in a forward direction, and are more concentrated at the knee in lateral step-ups (Agahari et al 1996). Stepping sideways also requires adductor and abductor muscle force and control. Resistance is supplied

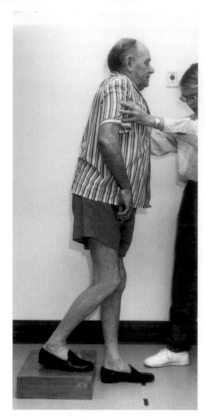

Figure 5.10 Stepping down requires eccentric activity of hip, knee and ankle extensors to lower the body mass. Shoulder elevation shows how difficult this action is.. He needs to practise many repetitions of stepping down and back up repetitively in this range (eccentric changing to a concentric contraction).

by the body weight and effort can be increased by raising step height. The exercises are practised in a safety harness if necessary (see Fig. 2.6B).

Heels raise and lower. Ankle plantarflexors are critical muscles, providing power for propulsion for walking, stair walking, walking up a slope and balancing. Their dominant role in push-off and in energy generation (Winter 1989), as well as their contribution to walking speed (Olney et al 1986) are well documented. They also contribute to ankle stability and the control of forward postural sway. A heels raise and lower exercise actively stretches the calf muscles during the eccentric phase and can therefore preserve the muscle length that is critical to push-off in gait and to performance of other weightbearing actions. It is interesting to note that Marks, as long ago as 1953, following a biomechanical analysis of walking in individuals following stroke, recommended the inclusion of gastrocnemius training for a forceful push-off.

Every attempt should be made to elicit concentric plantarflexor activity during push-off when the angular

position of the foot, shank and thigh are in an ideal alignment to push the body forward (Fig. 5.11). This exercise ensures optimal muscle length as well as training the muscles to generate force in the range from 8–10° dorsiflexion to 16–19° plantarflexion necessary for push-off (Winter 1983). The exercise should be practised routinely by anyone in whom shortened muscle fibres and intrinsic muscle stiffness due to immobility and disuse can be predicted. At the very least, prevention of these peripheral mechanical components of hypertonus is possible, and it is also likely that optimal muscle length and elasticity enable the individual to improve performance.

Non-weightbearing exercises. In these exercises, resistance is provided by free weights, weight machines (e.g., isokinetic dynamometer) and elastic bands (see Ch. 2). With the goal of increasing the ability of a muscle or groups of muscles to generate and control force, these exercises can be practised independently and as part of circuit training. Although task practice is necessary for neural adaptation (Rutherford 1988; Scarborough et al 1999) and learning to occur, in weak elderly individuals small changes in lower limb strength gained by non-weightbearing exercises may produce relatively large changes in motor performance and walking speed (Buchner et al 1996).

Following stroke, graded muscle strengthening can improve the ability to generate force but does not always translate into improved function (Eng & Tang 2007). Significant increases in muscle strength after concentric training of knee extensors have been reported (Engardt et al 1995; Sharp & Brouwer 1997). However, only Sharp & Brouwer (1997) were able to relate the increased strength to a small but significant increase in walking speed. A possible explanation for the lack of marked effects of increased quadriceps strength on walking speed may be the relatively small contribution of quadriceps to propulsive force during gait (Olney et al 1991; Winter 1991).

Until recently, investigations of strengthening effects have provided insufficient quantification of intensity, dosage and type of exercises, and outcome measures have focused on the effects of strengthening on impairments rather than on activities and participation. Exercises provided tend to be arbitrary, with progression and intensity (dosage) rarely administered as recommended by the American College of Sports Medicine (2002), the current authority on strength training in the able bodied and disabled.

The findings of several systematic reviews on the role of strengthening after stroke are inconclusive (Morris et al 2004; van Peppen et al 2004; Ada et al 2006; Eng & Tang 2007). This lack of evidence raises many questions. Reduction in functional capacity in skeletal muscle after stroke together with the likelihood of reduced levels of daily physical exercise highlight the need to examine the functional, neural and morphological effects of strength

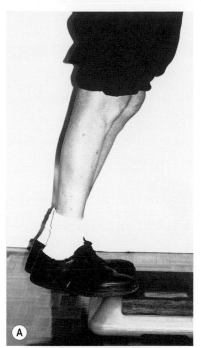

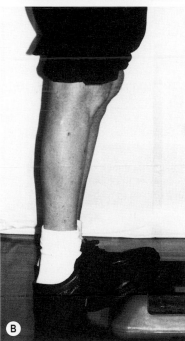

Figure 5.11 Heels raise and lower is controlled by concentric and eccentric action of the calf muscle. This exercise preserves optimal muscle length of plantarflexors as well as training the muscles to generate force (8–10° dorsiflexion to 16–19° plantarflexion) in the relevant range for push-off at the end of stance. *(From Winter 1983).*

training. We know that strength training does not increase spasticity and is not harmful.

Activating weak or paretic muscles

Patients who are unable to generate and sustain sufficient muscle force to support the body in standing and take a step require exercises to elicit contraction of a single muscle or group. Exercises and electrical stimulation may stimulate weak or inactive muscles to twitch and sustain force generation in a simplified context. It may be possible for the individual to elicit an eccentric contraction before a concentric contraction can be achieved. Emerging muscle activity is then utilized in simplified task practice. Interventions may include:

- simple exercises (Fig. 5.12)
- functional electrical stimulation (FES), EMG feedback
- isokinetic dynamometry (Fig. 5.13)
- taping to assist activating a muscle, e.g., gluteal taping.

Early after stroke, if the person is relatively inactive, FES can be used as an adjunct to exercise to maintain the contractibility and functional integrity of muscle. It is given to those muscles likely to adapt negatively to physical inactivity.

Hesse and colleagues (1995b) combined FES to ankle dorsiflexors, hamstrings, quadriceps, gluteus medius and minimus, and treadmill training with BWS for a group of severely affected non-ambulatory chronic stroke patients, with an average time since stroke of 25 weeks (range 11 weeks to 6 years). An A–B–A design was used: A, 15 treadmill/FES sessions; B, 15 days of Bobath/NDT). Subjects showed a marked increase in stride length, cadence and speed during the first phase A, but showed decreases or remained stable during phase B. Increases occurred again in the final A (treadmill/FES) phase. At the end of the study all patients could walk independently.

The findings of two systematic reviews examining the use of FES to improve muscle strength and walking in individuals following stroke were inconclusive (van Peppen et al 2004; Pomeroy et al 2006). However, problems encountered in reviewing the literature on electrical stimulation included small numbers of participants, lack of homogeneity in hemiplegic subjects, and differences in dose and outcome measures used (Pomeroy et al 2006) and, as a result, the findings of the review are meaningless. Pomeroy and colleagues (2006) point out that there is a general reduction in functional capacity in skeletal muscle after stroke, unrelated to the severity of paresis but related to the absence of daily physical activity (Potempa et al 1996; Hachisuka et al 1997). FES therefore may be a potentially effective means of maintaining the functional integrity of muscle when it is combined with task-oriented training.

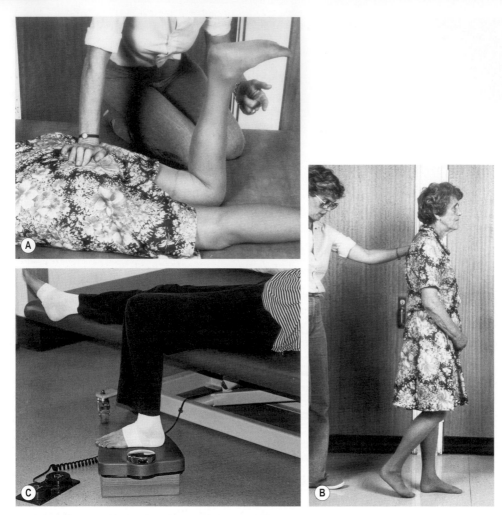

Figure 5.12 Simple exercises to elicit and gain control over muscle activity during movement of one joint or several. (A) Training control of hamstrings. Therapist flexes the knee to 90° and the patient attempts to lower the foot (eccentric contraction) then immediately flex the knee (concentric contraction) without rotating at the hip. As she gets more control she can practise stopping and starting in various parts of range. (B) She is now getting the idea of walking backward (extending her hip as she flexes the knee to take a step). (C) This exercise involves complex action by mono- and bi-articular muscles that cross the hip, knee and ankle. The goal is to raise the hip off the bed (hip extension) by pushing down through the heel. Poor limb control is evident if the foot slides forward (quadriceps action unopposed by knee flexors) and if the heel is lifted (plantarflexors unopposed by anterior tibials).

Gluteal taping on the paretic side (Fig. 5.14) as a training aid can lead to an immediate short-term improvement in hip extension at the end of single stance, with an increase in step length on the non-paretic side and an overall increase in stride length (Kilbreath et al 2006). McConnell (2002) has hypothesized that this taping technique may alter the orientation of muscle fibres, increasing the overlap between the actin and myosin filaments and therefore the possible cross-bridge interactions.

Preservation of soft tissue extensibility

Due to weakness and subsequent inactivity, soft tissues are likely to become stiffer and shorter. Muscle flexibility and length must be maintained since muscle shortening restricts movement and imposes abnormal segmental alignment throughout the walking cycle. For example, a contracted or stiff soleus muscle not only prevents ankle

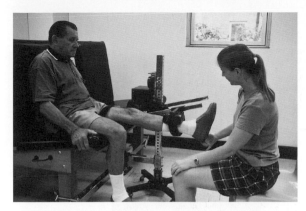

Figure 5.13 Activating the quadriceps initially with an eccentric contraction followed immediately with a concentric contraction. The therapist assists with knee extension and the patient attempts to control the weight of the shank while lowering the foot. This can also be performed without the dynamometer.

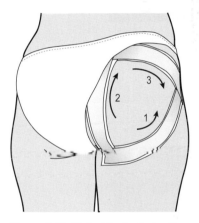

Figure 5.14 Gluteal taping helps the person get the idea of extending the hip at the end of stance phase. *(Reproduced from SL Kilbreath et al 2006 with permission).*

dorsiflexion and hip extension in standing but also interferes with progression forward of the body mass over the foot in stance phase, and dorsiflexion for heel contact at the end of swing.

Preservation of functional length, in particular of soleus and hip flexors, requires active stretch during walking and other activities that make similar length demands. Practice of standing up and sitting down with feet positioned behind the knee puts an active stretch on soleus as the person stands up. Passive methods may be necessary in the early acute phase (see Fig 2.10A). However, it is active stretch that preserves functional length (see Ch. 2). A patient who already has reduced or limited joint mobility due to calf muscle contracture may require prolonged stretching using serial casting with follow-up exercises and training (Moseley 1997).

MAXIMIZING SKILL, SPEED, ENDURANCE AND FITNESS FOR GAIT COMPETENCY

On average, 'normal' walking speed is approximately 1.2 m/s (Olney et al 1986). Not surprisingly, walking speeds have been found to vary in able-bodied subjects depending on location and intention (strolling for pleasure vs hurrying to work), with women reaching the same velocity as men by shortening their steps and increasing cadence. The literature suggests that an average walking speed of 1.1–1.5 m/s is probably fast enough to be functional as a pedestrian in different environmental and social contexts. Walking speed required to cross a street safely using pedestrian lights varies considerably depending on many factors, including whether in rural or urban settings. Walking speeds compatible with stepping on or off a moving footway, crossing a street with and without pedestrian lights, getting in or out of a lift, walking up and down a kerb all need to be practised to enable the individual to walk in the community. Distances required for independence in an urban area are far greater than those typically used as criteria in rehabilitation for assessing independence in community walking (Lerner-Frankiel et al 1986; Lord & Rochester 2005).

An increase in walking speed has been found to be associated with an improved walking pattern. An increase in speed is associated with greater hip extension in late stance and a larger burst of work by the hip flexors at the initiation of swing (Olney et al 1991). In a subsequent study, the greater the angle of hip extension in late stance, the greater was the speed of walking and a strong relationship existed between walking speed and maximum hip flexion moment (Olney et al 1994). These findings support the suggestion that the hip muscles play a major role in balancing the upper body segment over the legs (Winter 1987).

The criteria for gait competency in the community include the ability to:

- walk at speeds fast enough to cross streets safely: at least 1.1–1.5 m/s
- walk for a long enough time and far enough to accomplish daily tasks – about 500 m
- turn the head while walking
- use anticipatory strategies to avoid or accommodate obstacles
- react quickly enough to slips and trips and avoid a fall by stepping
- negotiate stairs, kerbs, ramps, moving footways, and carry objects.

Verbal encouragement and external cues are given to increase gait speed. A recent study demonstrated that individuals after stroke can increase their overground walking speed two to three times beyond comfortable levels given

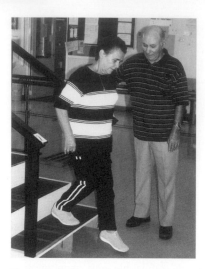

Figure 5.15 Her husband supervises as she practises stair walking in a circuit class. *(Courtesy of F Mackey and colleagues, Illawarra Area Health Service, Australia).*

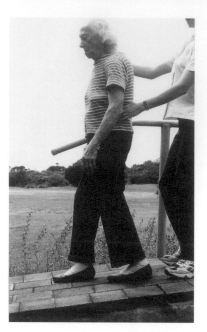

Figure 5.16 Walking up and down a ramp. She needs to be reminded to use her calf muscles for push-off when walking up.

instructions to 'Walk as fast as you can, as if you are trying to catch the bus', and encouragement. Faster walking was associated with bilateral increases in joint range and muscle activation, as well as improvement in some spatio-temporal variables, for example, increased step length and decreased double support phase. Quality of life scales completed by the participants indicated that increasing speed resulted in a greater behavioural repertoire in every-day life (Lamontagne & Fung 2004).

Intensive practice of ascending and descending stairs (Fig. 5.15) is necessary to increase strength and familiarity with this and other similar activities such as stepping up a kerb. It has been reported that more falls occur on stairs than in level walking, indicating the importance of training this activity. Walking up and down ramps (Fig. 5.16), hills, around obstacles, squatting to pick up an object (Fig. 5.17), stepping over objects (Fig. 5.18), marching on the spot (Fig. 5.19), carrying parcels, stopping and turning, and stepping quickly in all directions are introduced, to prepare the patient for dealing with the complexities of walking in the built and natural environments (Fig. 5.20).

ENVIRONMENTAL MODIFICATION

The rehabilitation environment can be organized to facilitate flexibility of walking performance. Walking should not be a special event that occurs only with the physiotherapist in the safe physiotherapy environment. An early goal for the patient could be to walk to the next appointment, or at least part of the way, with the explicit aim of

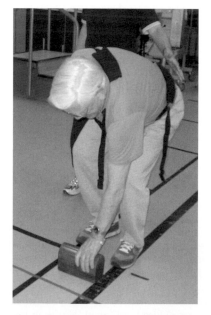

Figure 5.17 Squatting to pick up an object from the floor on a circuit walk. His narrow base is encouraged by lines on the floor. *(Courtesy of K Schurr and S Dorsch, Physiotherapists, Lidcombe-Bankstown Hospital, Sydney).*

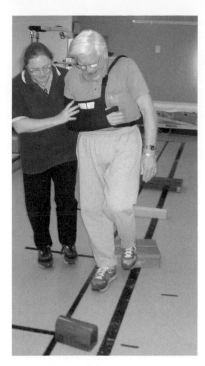

Figure 5.18 Walking over obstacles. He has caught his heel on the step with his trail leg and needs to lift his leg higher. Note he is wearing a belt with grab handles and is confined to a narrow base by lines on the floor. *(Courtesy of K Schurr and S Dorsch, Physiotherapists, Liverpool-Bankstown Hospital, Sydney).*

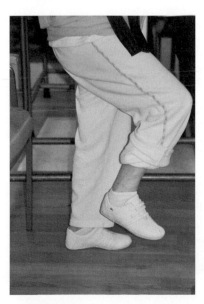

Figure 5.19 Marching on the spot – as one leg lifts the other leg loads. Hip flexors need to be able to generate sufficient power for pull-off.

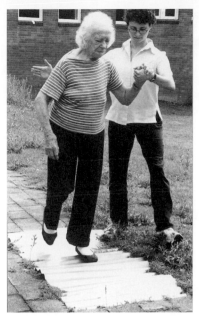

Figure 5.20 Walking on an uneven corrugated surface. Therapist gives support at the start.

walking further each day rather than being transported in a wheelchair.

The environment can be organized to facilitate a particular outcome or prevent unwanted adaptations from becoming habitual. A person who walks with a wide base can be encouraged to walk within a boundary outlined on the floor or on footprints.

As soon as the person achieves some independence, challenging and variable practice is introduced: judging the speed of people and objects moving while walking in a busy corridor; walking in different lighting conditions; walking under obstacles. This latter provides a challenge as it imposes the need for controlled flexion and extension of the lower limbs (squatting – eccentric contraction followed by extension).

The application of virtual reality technology in rehabilitation can provide walking practice in virtual environments in which simulated real-world objects and events can be sensed and reacted to. Virtual environments may be particularly useful when it is difficult to provide appropriate walking practice outdoors and in extreme weather conditions. The high-tech nature of the practice itself can be a further motivation for patients (Malouin & Richards 2005). The main benefit of environmental modification may come from provision of problem-solving tasks that challenge and drive changes in motor control.

Cueing. The significance of visual and auditory cues during walking training in individuals with Parkinson's disease is discussed in Chapter 13. Rhythmical auditory cueing versus non-cueing during walking trials in stroke subjects can increase the time spent in stance on the paretic leg and increase rhythmicity (Thaut et al 1993). Interestingly, rhythmic cueing not only modified the amplitude and timing of gastrocnemius muscle activation in the paretic leg with a high degree of task specificity, but also decreased the amplitude of muscle activity on the intact side, indicating 'cooperation' between both lower limbs. Variability in EMG amplitude also decreased, suggesting an improvement in motor unit recruitment. It would be interesting to explore whether the improved performance would carry over into other environments.

MEASURING TREATMENT EFFECTS AND RETENTION

Functional tests include:

- Motor Assessment Scale walking item
- 6–10-metre walk test (speed)
- 6-minute walk test (endurance)
- timed 'up-and-go' test
- step test
- obstacle course test (Means et al 1996).

Walking speed may be the most important clinical measure of functional ability. Several critical biomechanical parameters are speed dependent. For example, as push-off power and magnitude of hip flexion on the paretic side increase, so does speed. The 6–10-metre walk test is useful in the acute phase as a guide to progress. However, walking speed over a short distance may overestimate locomotor capacity (Dean et al 2001). Since distance, as well as walking speed, is important for independent mobility outside the house, both speed and endurance need to be trained and measured.

AIDS AND ORTHOSES

A recent synthesis of best evidence so far shows no support for the provision of orthoses such as ankle–foot orthoses (AFOs) or hand-held walking aids (van Peppen et al 2004). If a device is considered worth trying for a particular person, it is recommended that natural walking speed is measured while using the orthosis or aid, as the patient's preferred speed with and without the device gives a good indication of the relative merits of the device (Olney 2005).

Walking aids

Only recently have the effects of different types of sticks been compared. Walking aids including parallel bars, quadripod/tripod (three-/four-point) stick, walking frame and an assistant's arm all rely on support through the upper limb and unload the weightbearing structures of the lower limb (Winter et al 1993). A quadripod stick offers no advantage over a standard stick in terms of standing balance (Milczarek et al 1993) or in spatiotemporal variables. Although all walking aids impose some mechanical constraint, a simple walking stick may interfere least with balance and walking yet provide some assistance and increase confidence (Kuan et al 1999).

Ankle–foot orthoses

The most commonly prescribed orthosis with a view to improving gait is an AFO. Research into the potential of an AFO to improve ankle/foot mechanics during walking has produced equivocal results and the issue of whether or not to prescribe some form of AFO remains controversial.

A major consideration in determining the use of an AFO is the evaluation from a mechanical and muscular perspective. Constraint of any joint necessitates mechanical adaptation in both the ipsilateral and contralateral limbs and may reduce the need for muscles to contract at appropriate times and with appropriate intensity throughout the gait cycle. Although a rigid AFO holds the foot in some dorsiflexion, it imposes a mechanical resistance to plantarflexion for push-off. An orthosis that provides mediolateral stability at the subtalar joint, without unduly limiting plantarflexion or dorsiflexion, may hold the foot in a balanced position if it inverts or everts on contact.

More recently, the addition of hinged joints allows freer or controlled ankle movement. The effect of this modification needs to be studied further to establish the imposed mechanical and muscular adaptations in both the ipsilateral and contralateral legs. A systematic review of the impact of AFOs on gait and on leg muscle activity in stroke reported that there was a lot of variability among studies and small subject numbers. The impact on muscle activity remains unclear but there may be some beneficial effects on gait speed. The review highlights the need for well-designed randomized controlled studies (Leung & Moseley 2003). The use of 'smart' orthoses to enable walking practice and to 'force' a segmental alignment appropriate for the activation of certain critical muscle groups remains for future development (Shepherd 1997).

One-arm wheelchair

Propelling a one-arm wheelchair with the non-paretic arm and leg may promote a form of early independence in getting from one place to another. However, the physical actions involved focus attention on the non-paretic side and would contribute to learned non-use of both inactive limbs. It should be avoided.

In conclusion, if physiotherapists are to be part of neurological rehabilitation in the twenty-first century, it is time for a paradigm shift to more scientifically-based walking rehabilitation. One of the major goals of biomechanical research is for findings to be transferred into guidelines designed to improve rehabilitation outcomes (Olney et al 1988; Sutherland 2002; Carr & Shepherd 2003). We would add that such guidelines, having been enunciated and shown to be effective, need to be implemented and evaluated on both a short- and long-term basis.

REFERENCES

Ada L, Dean CM, Bampton J et al 2003 A treadmill and overground walking program improves walking in persons residing in the community after stroke: a placebo-controlled randomized trial. Arch Phys Med Rehabil 84:1486–1491.

Ada L, Dorsch S, Canning CG 2006 Strengthening interventions increase strength and improve activity after stroke: a systematic review. Aust J Physiother 52:241–248.

Agahari I, Shepherd RB, Westwood P 1996 A comparative evaluation of lower limb forces in two variations of the step exercise in able bodied subjects. In: Lee M, Gilleard W, Sinclair P et al (eds) Proceedings of 1st Australasian Biomechanics Conference. University of Sydney, NSW, Australia:94–95.

American College of Sports Medicine 2002 Progression models in resistance training for healthy adults. Med Sci Sports Exerc 34:364–380.

Andriacchi TP, Andersson GBJ, Fermier RW et al 1980 A study of lower-limb mechanics during stairclimbing. J Bone Joint Surg 62A:749–757.

Barbeau H, Rossignol S 1967 Recovery of locomotion after chronic spinalization in the adult cat. Brain Res 412:84–95.

Barbeau H, Visintin M 2003 Optimal outcomes obtained with body-weight support combined with treadmill training in stroke subjects. Arch Phys Med Rehabil 84:1458–1465.

Bernstein N 1967 Coordination and regulation of movement. Pergamon, New York.

Boakes JL, Rab GT 2006 Muscle activity during walking. In: Rose J, Gamble JG (eds) Human walking 3rd edn. Lippincott Williams & Wilkins, Philadelphia:103–118.

Bohannon RW 1986 Strength of lower limb related to gait speed and cadence in stroke patients. Physiother Can 38:204–206.

Bohannon RW, Andrews AW 1990 Correlation of knee extensor muscle torque and spasticity with gait speed in patients with stroke. Arch Phys Med Rehabil 71:330–333.

Bortz WM 1982 Disuse and aging. J Am Med Assoc 248:1203–1208.

Bradford J, McFadyen BJ, Winter DA 1988 An integrated biomechanical analysis of normal stair ascent and descent. J Biomech 21:733–744.

Brown TG 1914 On the nature of the fundamental activity of the nervous centres; together with an analysis of the conditioning of rhythmic activity in progression, and a theory of the evolution of function in the nervous system. J Physiol Lond 48:18–46.

Buchner DM, Larson EB, Wagner EH et al 1996 Evidence for a non-linear relationship between leg strength and gait speed. Age Ageing 25:386–391.

Carlsoo S, Dahllof A, Holm J 1974 Kinetic analysis of gait in patients with hemiparesis and in patients with intermittent claudication. Scand J Rehabil Med 6:166–179.

Carr JH, Shepherd RB 1987 A motor relearning programme for stroke, 2nd edn. Butterworth Heinemann, Oxford.

Carr JH, Shepherd RB 2003 Stroke rehabilitation. Guidelines for exercise and training to optimize motor skill. Butterworth Heinemann, Oxford.

Cress ME, Schechtman KB, Mulrow CD et al 1995 Relationship between physical performance and self-perceived physical function. J Am Geriatr Soc 43:93–101.

Crosbie J, Vachalathiti R, Smith R 1997 Age, gender and speed effects on spinal kinematics during walking. Gait Posture 5:13–20.

Dean CM, Richards CL, Malouin F 2000 Task-related training improves performance of locomotor tasks in chronic stroke. A randomized controlled pilot trial. Arch Phys Med Rehabil 81:409–417.

Dean CM, Richards CL, Malouin F 2001 Walking speed over 10 metres overestimates locomotor capacity after stroke. Clin Rehabil 15:415–421.

Duysens J, van de Crommert HWAA 1998 Neural control of locomotion. Part 1: the central pattern generator from cats to humans. Gait Posture 7:131–141.

Eastlake ME, Arvidson J, Snyder-Mackler L et al 1991 Interrater reliability of videotaped observational gait-analysis assessment. Phys Ther 71:465–472.

Eberhart HD, Inman VT, Bresler B 1965 The principal elements in human locomotion. In: Klopstag PF, Wilson DP (eds) Human limbs and their substitutes. McGraw-Hill, New York:437–471.

Eng JJ, Tang P-F 2007 Gait training strategies to optimize walking ability in people with stroke: a synthesis of the evidence. Expert Rev Neurother 7:1417–1436.

Eng JJ, Winter DA 1995 Kinetic analysis of the lower limbs during walking: what information can be gained from a three-dimensional model? J Biomech 28:753–758.

Eng JJ, Chu KS, Kim CM et al 2003 A community-based group exercise program for persons with chronic stroke. Med Sci Sports Exerc 35:1271–1278.

Engardt M, Knutsson E, Jonsson M et al 1995 Dynamic muscle strength training in stroke patients: effects of knee extension torque. Arch Phys Med Rehabil 76:419–425.

Finch L, Barbeau H 1985 Influences of partial weight-bearing on normal human gait: the development of a gait retraining strategy. Can J Neurol Sci 12:183.

Finch L, Barbeau H, Arsenault B 1991 Influence of body weight support on normal human gait: development of a gait retraining strategy. Phys Ther 71:842–856.

Forssberg H 1982 Spinal locomotor functions and descending control. In: Sjolund B, Bjorklund A (eds) Brain stem control of spinal mechanisms. Elsevier Biomedical Press, New York.

Gabell A, Nayak VSC 1984 The effect of age on variability in gait. J Gerontol 39:662–666.

Gordon J 1991 Spinal mechanisms of motor coordination. In: Kandel E, Schwartz JH, Jessell TM (eds) Principles of neural science, 3rd edn. Appleton and Lange, Norwalk, CT:582–595.

Gracies J-M 2005 Pathophysiology of spastic paresis. 1: Paresis and soft tissue changes. Muscle Nerve 31:535–551.

Grillner S, Shik ML 1973 On the descending control of the lumbosacral spinal cord from the 'mesencephalic locomotor region'. Acta Physiol Scand 87:320–333.

Hachisuka K, Umezu Y, Ogata H 1997 Disuse muscle atrophy of lower limb in hemiplegic patients. Arch Phys Med Rehabil 78:13–18.

Haines RF 1974 Effect of bed rest and exercise on body balance. J Appl Physiol 36:323–327.

Hamel KA, Okita N, Higginson JS et al 2005 Foot clearance during stair descent: effects of age and illumination. Gait Posture 21:135–140.

Harris-Love ML, Macko RF, Whitall J et al 2004 Improved hemiparetic muscle activation in treadmill versus overground walking. Neurorehabil Neural Repair 18:154–160.

Hausdorff JM, Rios DA, Edelberg HK 2001 Gait variability and fall risk in community-living older adults: a 1-year prospective study. Arch Phys Med Rehabil 82:1050–1056.

Herbert RD, Sherrington C, Maher C et al 2001 Evidence-based practice – imperfect but necessary. Physiother Theory Pract 17:201–211.

Hesse S, Bertelt C, Jahnke MT et al 1995a Treadmill training with partial body weight support compared with physiotherapy in nonambulatory hemiparetic patients. Stroke 26:976–981.

Hesse S, Malezic M, Schaffrin A et al 1995b Restoration of gait by combined treadmill training and multichannel electrical stimulation in non-ambulatory hemiparetic patients. Scand J Rehabil Med 27:199–204.

Hesse S, Helm B, Krajnik J et al 1997 Treadmill training with partial body weight support: influence of body weight release on the gait of hemiparetic patients. J Neurol Rehabil 11:15–26.

Hesse S, Konrad M, Uhlenbrock D 1999 Treadmill walking with bodyweight support versus floor walking in hemiplegic subjects. Arch Phys Med Rehabil 80:421–427.

Hesse S, Schmidt H, Werner C 2006 Machines to support motor rehabilitation after stroke: 10 years of experience in Berlin. J Rehabil Res Dev 43:671–678.

Inman VT, Ralston HJ, Todd F 1981 Human walking. Williams and Wilkins, Baltimore, MD.

Jansen EC, Vittas D, Hellberg S, et al 1982 Normal gait of young and old men and women. Acta Orthopaed Scand 53:193–196.

Jorgensen L, Engstad T, Jacobsen BK 2002 Higher incidence of falls in long-term stroke survivors than in population controls: depressive symptoms predict falls after stroke. Stroke 33:542–547.

Kilbreath S, Perkins S, Crosbie J et al 2006 Gluteal taping improves hip extension during stance phase of walking following stroke. Aust J Physiother 52:53–56.

Kim CM, Eng JJ 2003 The relationship of lower-extremity muscle torque to locomotor performance in people with stroke. Phys Ther 83:49–57.

Kim CM, Eng JJ 2004 Magnitude and pattern of 3D kinematic and kinetic gait profiles in persons with stroke: relationship to walking speed. Gait Posture 20:140–146.

Kuan T, Tsou J, Fong-Chin S 1999 Hemiplegic gait of stroke patients: the effect of using a cane. Arch Phys Med Rehabil 80:777–784.

Lamontagne A, Fung J 2004 Faster is better: implications for speed-intensive gait training after stroke. Stroke 35:2543–2548.

Lerner-Frankiel MB, Vargas S, Brown M et al 1986 Functional community ambulation: what are the criteria? Clin Manag 6:12–15.

Leung J, Moseley A 2003 Impact of ankle–foot orthoses on gait and leg muscle activity in adults with hemiplegia: systematic literature review. Physiotherapy 89:39–55.

Liu MQ, Anderson FC, Pandy MG et al 2006 Muscles that support the body also modulate forward progression during walking. J Biomech 39:2623–2630.

Lord SR, Fitzpatrick RD 2001 Choice stepping reaction time: a composite measure of falls risk in older people. J Gerontol 56A:M627–M632.

Lord S, Sherrington C, Menz H et al 2007 Falls in older people: risk factors and strategies for prevention, 2nd edn. Cambridge University Press, Cambridge.

Lord SE, Rochester L 2005 Measurement of community ambulation after stroke: current status and future developments. Stroke 36:1457–1461.

Luft AR, Macko RF, Forrester LW et al 2009 Treadmill exercise activates subcortical neural networks and improves walking after stroke: a randomized controlled trial. Stroke 39:1–8.

McConnell J 2002 Recalcitrant chronic low back and leg pain – a new theory and different approach to management. Man Ther 7:183–192.

McFadyen BJ, Winter DA 1988 An integrated biomechanical analysis of normal stair ascent and descent. J Biomech 21:733–744.

Macko RF, Ivey FM, Forrester LW et al 2005 Treadmill exercise rehabilitation improves ambulatory function and cardiovascular fitness in patients with chronic stroke: a randomized controlled trial. Stroke 36:2206–2211.

Malouin F 1995 Observational gait analysis. In: Craik RL, Oatis CA (eds) Gait analysis. Theory and applications. Mosby, St Louis:112–124.

Malouin F, Richards CL 2005 Assessment and training of locomotion after stroke: evolving concepts. In: Refshauge K, Ada L, Ellis E (eds) Science-based rehabilitation: theories into practice. Elsevier, Oxford:185–222.

Marigold DS, Patla AE 2008 Age-related changes in gait for multi-surface terrain. Gait Posture 27:689–696.

Marks M 1953 Gait studies of the hemiplegic patient and their clinical applications. Arch Phys Med Rehabil 34:9–25.

Means KM, Rodell DE, O'Sullivan PS 1996 Use of an obstacle course to assess balance and mobility in the elderly. Am J Phys Med Rehabil 75:88–95.

Mehrholz J, Werner C, Kugler J et al 2007 Electromechanical-assisted gait training for walking after stroke. Cochrane Database Syst Rev, Issue 4. Art. No.: CD006185. DOI: 10.1002/14651858.CD006185.pub2.

Milczarek JJ, Lee Kirby R, Harrison ER et al 1993 Standard and four-footed canes: their effect on the standing balance of patients with hemiparesis. Arch Phys Med Rehabil 74:281–285.

Morris SL, Dodd KJ, Morris ME 2004 Outcomes of progressive resistance strength training following stroke: a systematic review. Clin Rehabil 18:27–39.

Moseley A 1997 The effect of casting combined with stretching on passive ankle dorsiflexion in adults with traumatic head injuries. Phys Ther 77:240–247.

Moseley A, Stark A, Cameron ID et al 2005 Treadmill training and body weight support for walking after stroke. Cochrane Database Syst Rev 2005, Issue 4. Art. No.: CD002840. DOI: 10.1002/14651858.CD002840. pub2.

Murray MP, Drought AB, Kory RC 1964 Walking patterns of normal men. J Bone Joint Surg 46A:335–360.

Murray MP, Kory RC, Clarkson BH 1969 Walking patterns in healthy old men. J Gerontol 24:169–178.

Murray MP, Kory RC, Sepic SB 1970 Walking patterns of normal women. Arch Phys Med Rehabil 51:637–650.

Musacchia XJ, Deavers DR, Meininger GA et al 1980 A model for hypokinesia: effects on muscle atrophy in the rat. J Appl Physiol 48:479–486.

Nadeau S, McFadyen BJ, Malouin F 2003 Frontal and sagittal plane analyses of the stair climbing task in healthy adults aged over 40 years: what are the challenges compared to level walking? Clin Biomech 18:950–959.

Newham DJ, Hsiao S-F 2001 Knee muscle isometric strength, voluntary activation and antagonistic co-contraction in the first six months after stroke. Dis Rehabil 23:379–386.

Olney SJ 2005 Training gait after stroke: a biomehanical perspective. In: Refshauge K, Ada L, Ellis E (eds) Science-based rehabilitation: theories into practice. Elsevier, Oxford:159–184.

Olney SJ, Richards C 1996 Hemiparetic gait following stroke. Part 1: characteristics. Gait Posture 4:136–148.

Olney SJ, Monga TN, Costigan PA 1986 Mechanical energy of walking of stroke patients. Arch Phys Med Rehabil 67:92–98.

Olney SJ, Jackson VG, George SR 1988 Gait re-education guidelines for stroke patients with hemiplegia using mechanical energy and power analyses. Physiother Can 40:242–248.

Olney SJ, Griffin MP, Monga TN et al 1991 Work and power in gait of stroke patients. Arch Phys Med Rehabil 72:309–314.

Olney SJ, Griffin MP, McBride ID 1994 Temporal, kinematic, and kinetic variables related to gait speed in subjects with hemiplegia: a regression approach. Phys Ther 74:872–885.

Pavol MJ, Owings TM, Foley KT et al 1999 The sex and age of older adults influence the outcome of induced trips. J Gerontol 54A:M103–M108.

Perry J 1992 Gait analysis. Normal and pathological function. Slack, Thorofare, NJ.

Pohl M, Mehrholz J, Ritschel C et al 2002 Speed-dependent treadmill training in ambulatory hemiparetic stroke patients: a randomized controlled trial. Stroke 33:553–558.

Pollock M, Foster C, Knapp D et al 1987 Effect of age and training on aerobic capacity and body composition of master athletes. J Appl Physiol 62:725–731.

Pomeroy VM, King LM, Pollock A et al 2006 Electrostimulation for promoting recovery of movement or functional ability after stroke. Cochrane Database Syst Rev, Issue 2. Art. No.: CD003241. DOI: 10.1002/14651858.CD003241.pub2.

Potempa K, Braun LT, Tinknell T et al 1996 Benefits of aerobic exercise after stroke. Sports Med 21:337–346.

Potter JM, Evans AL, Duncan G 1995 Gait speed and activities of daily living function in geriatric patients. Arch Phys Med Rehabil 76:997–999.

Richards CL, Malouin F, Wood-Dauphinee S et al 1993 Task-specific physical therapy for optimization of gait recovery in acute stroke patients. Arch Phys Med Rehabil 74:612–620.

Richards CL, Malouin F, Dean C 1999 Gait in stroke: assessment and rehabilitation. Clin Geriatr Med 15:833–855.

Rogers MW, Johnson ME, Martinez KM et al 2003 Step Training improves the speed of voluntary step initiation in aging. J Gerontol 58A:46–51.

Rose J, Gamble JG eds 2006 Human walking, 3rd edn. Lippincott Williams & Wilkins, Philadelphia.

Rossignol S, Barbeau H, Julien C 1986 Locomotion of the adult chronic spinal cat and its modifications by monoaminergic agonists and antagonists. In: Golberger M, Gorio M, Murray M (eds) Development and plasticity of the mammalian spinal cord. Liviana Editrice Spat, Padua:323–346.

Rutherford OM 1988 Muscular coordination and strength training: implications for injury rehabilitation. Sports Med 5:196–202.

Said CM, Goldie PA, Patla AE et al 1999 Obstacle crossing in subjects with stroke. Arch Phys Med Rehabil 80:1054–1059.

Salbach NM, Mayo NE, Wood-Dauphinee S et al 2004 A task-orientated intervention enhances walking distance and speed in the first year post stroke: a randomized controlled trial. Clin Rehabil 18:509–519.

Scarborough DM, Krebs DE, Harris BA 1999 Quadriceps muscle strength and dynamic stability in elderly persons. Gait Posture 10:10–20.

Sharp SA, Brouwer BJ 1997 Isokinetic strength training of the hemiparetic knee: effects on function and spasticity. Arch Phys Med Rehabil 78:1231–1236.

Shepherd RB 1997 Optimising motor performance following brain lesions. In: Proceedings of the Annual Scientific Meeting of ISPO, Australia.

Shiavi R 1985 Electromyographic patterns in adult locomotion: a comprehensive review. J Rehabil Res Devel 22:85–98.

Smith A 1990 The measurement of human motor performance. In: Ada L, Canning C (eds) Key issues in neurological physiotherapy. Butterworth Heinemann, Oxford:51–79.

Startzell JK, Owens DA, Mulfinger LM et al 2000 Stair negotiation in older people: a review. J Am Geriatr Soc 48:567–580.

Strandberg L, Lanshammar H 1981 The dynamics of slipping accidents. J Occup Accid 3:153–162.

Sutherland DH 2001 The evolution of clinical gait analysis. Part I: kinesiological EMG. Gait Posture 14:61–70.

Sutherland DH 2002 The evolution of clinical gait analysis. Part II: kinematics. Gait Posture 16:159–179.

Teixeira-Salmela LF, Olney SJ, Nadeau S et al 1999 Muscle strengthening and physical conditioning to reduce impairment and disability in chronic stroke survivors. Arch Phys Med Rehabil 80:1211–1218.

Teixeria-Salmela LF, Nadeau S, McBride I et al 2001 Effects of muscle strengthening and physical conditioning training on temporal, kinematic and kinetic variables during gait in chronic stroke survivors. J Rehabil Med 33:53–60.

Thaut MH, McIntosh GC, Prassas SG et al 1993 Effect of rhythmic auditory cuing on temporal stride parameters and EMG patterns in hemiparetic gait of stroke patients. J Neurol Rehabil 7:9–16.

Vandervoort AA, Chesworth BM, Jones M et al 1990 Passive ankle stiffness in young and elderly men. Can J Aging 9:204–212.

van Peppen RPS, Kwakkel G, Wood-Dauphine S et al 2004 The impact of physical therapy on functional outcomes after stroke: what's the evidence? Clin Rehabil 18:833–862.

van Vliet P 1988 Kinematic analysis of videotape to measure walking following stroke: a case study. Aust J Physiother 34:48–51.

von Schroeder HP, Coutts RD, Lyden PD et al 1995 Gait parameters following stroke: a practical assessment. J Rehabil Res Dev 32:25–31.

Weerdesteyn V, Rijken H, Geurts ACH et al 2006 A five-week exercise program can reduce falls and improve obstacle avoidance in the elderly. Gerontology 52:131–141.

Whipple RH, Wolfson LI, Amerman PM 1987 The relationship of knee and ankle weakness to falls in nursing home residents: an isokinetic study. J Am Geriatr Soc 35:13–20.

Whittle MW 2007 Gait analysis: an introduction, 4th edn. Butterworth Heinemann, Oxford.

Winter DA 1980 Overall principle of lower limb support during stance phase of gait. J Biomech 13:923–927.

Winter DA 1983 Biomechanical motor patterns in normal walking. J Mot Behav 15:302–330.

Winter DA 1984 Kinematic and kinetic patterns of human gait: variability and compensating effects. Hum Mov Sci 3:51–76.

Winter DA 1987 The biomechanics and motor control of human gait, University of Waterloo Press, Waterloo, Ontario.

Winter DA 1989 Coordination of motor tasks in human gait. In: Wallace SA (ed.) Perspectives on the coordination of movement. North-Holland, New York:329–363.

Winter DA 1991 Biomechanics and motor control of human gait: normal, elderly and pathological. University of Waterloo Press, Waterloo, Ontario.

Winter DA, Eng P 1995 Kinetics: our window into the goals and strategies of the central nervous system. Behav Brain Res 67:111–120.

Winter DA, Patla AE, Frank JS et al 1990 Biomechanical walking pattern changes in the fit and healthy elderly. Phys Ther 70:340–347.

Winter DA, McFadyen BJ, Dickey JP 1991 Adaptability of the CNS in human walking. In: Patla AE (ed.) Adaptability of human gait. Elsevier Science, Amsterdam:127–143.

Winter DA, Deathe AB, Halliday S et al 1993 A technique to analyse the kinetics and energetics of cane-assisted gait. Clin Biomech 8:37–43.

Witte US, Carlsson JY 1997 Self-selected walking speed in patients with hemiparesis after stroke. Scand J Rehabil Med 29:161–165.

Zachazewski JE, Riley PO, Krebs DE 1993 Biomechanical analysis of body mass transfer during stair ascent and descent of healthy subjects. J Rehabil Res Dev 30:412–422.

Chapter |6|

Reaching and manipulation

INTRODUCTION

For several decades there has been extensive scientific investigation of the motor control and biomechanical characteristics of reaching actions and hand use in monkeys and humans (e.g., Jeannerod 1990). The information gathered provides the scientific basis of many of the recent developments in clinical practice.

The upper limb functions principally for reaching, grasping and manipulation, sometimes for lifting the body mass, and, at periods of postural instability, for preserving balance. The arm transports the hand according to task, context and goal. It places the hand in the appropriate position and orientation in space to enable interaction with the environment and to achieve a specific goal, whether it is combing the hair or opening a door. Reaching is, therefore, the major purposive action of the arm, and interaction with the environment the major purpose of the hand. The distance we can reach is a function of arm length. If the object to be reached is beyond arm's length, movement of the body mass over the lower limbs in sitting and standing extends the distance that can be reached. If the object is judged out of reach, we take a step. Postural adjustments are part of the functional unit and are also specific to task and context.

The upper limb is involved in a large variety of tasks which require the limb to produce different joint configurations and different timing and sequencing of joint movements. Nevertheless, it is evident from research findings that the arm and hand function as a single unit in reaching and manipulation. In many activities involving reaching, the upper body or the entire body also become part of the single coordinated unit (Ada et al 1994). The individual both responds to environmental demands and imposes intentions upon the environment.

The fact that the arm and hand function as a single unit is remarkable given the number of components in the unit and the complexity of human manipulative actions. The unit is made up of many joints and muscles (mono-articular, bi-articular and multi-articular), with many degrees of freedom which must be constrained or utilized if reaching and manipulative activities are to be coordinated.

The function of the hands is as much sensory as it is motor (Hogan & Winters 1990). Tactile and pressure sensors give us information that helps us to identify objects, to classify them according to properties such as texture and density, and to gauge the potential for slippage. Although hand use is possible with diminished cutaneous afferent information, accuracy can be severely disturbed as cutaneous input appears critical for skilled object manipulation. In a study by Witney and colleagues in which the fingers were anaesthetized to prevent cutaneous feedback, participants showed an increase in grip force (Witney et al 2004). This may have been an attempt to obtain feedback by increasing pressure on the fingers but the coordination between grip and load forces was also poor. Subjects had difficulty sustaining the appropriate level of force.

In addition, due to the important informational role of vision in reaching and manipulation, eye and head movement play a critical part in enabling a coordinated movement to take place (Biguer et al 1982; Jeannerod 1990). Coordination between eye and hand movements has been described in pointing and in other actions (Biguer et al 1982; Beaubaton & Hay 1986). Vision is obviously critical to the locating of an object and the gathering of information related to the object, particularly its distance from the body and orientation. Vision enables precision. However, in the dark we can still manipulate objects successfully by substituting tactile senses, although reaching and grasping movements are slower and less precise.

The arms are also yoked into the postural system (Gentile 1987). When balance is compromised, the arms play a stabilizing and supportive function, and if balance is lost, the hands are used to form a new base of support. If an object is beyond arm's length, body movement toward the object provides an extension of the reach, effectively enlarging the attainable part of the surroundings. Unless the body is in a fully supported position, any reaching action in sitting or standing is preceded and accompanied by postural adjustments. These ensure that the body's segment alignment is appropriate to preserve stability during the upcoming perturbation caused by movement of the arm.

Postural adjustments occurring prior to and during arm movement are brought about by muscle activation and usually result in some alteration in segmental alignment (e.g., Bouisset & Zattara 1981). As well as numerous studies performed in standing, postural activity before and during arm movement has also been reported in sitting, during fast pointing (Crosbie et al 1995), in self-paced reaching to pick up an object (Dean & Shepherd 1997) and in standing (Cordo & Nashner 1982; Wing et al 1997).

Most commonly performed tasks are carried out not with one hand but with two. In bimanual actions, the two upper limbs have to function in concert, and since the object being grasped and manipulated becomes the connection between the two limbs, the interactions are complex. The requirement for coordination of the two limbs needs to be kept in mind in clinical practice, particularly during rehabilitation of individuals with hemiplegia, and training must involve the practice of bimanual actions as well as exercises to regain muscle activity in the affected limb.

The dilemma for the patient in rehabilitation is the large number of actions that must be relearned in order to return to an independent life. He or she must regain the ability to move many body segments as a coordinated unit in functional actions with many different goals, and with a damaged system. There is one particular problem to be solved in clinical practice – how to drive the person to use the affected limb when it feels more natural to use the stronger limb to accomplish the goals of daily life.

REACHING TO GRASP: DESCRIPTION OF THE ACTIVITY

Many of the early studies of reaching were of one- or two-joint movements carried out in the horizontal plane and under highly constrained conditions (e.g., Karst & Hasan 1990; Flanagan et al 1993). There have been, however, an increasing number of studies of more 'natural' reaching or pointing movements in which the individual interacts with an everyday object. It is these studies which are of particular relevance to clinical practice since they provide essential information from which analysis and intervention can be planned and carried out.

According to Jeannerod's investigations, reaching to grasp an object can be divided into two components: *a transportation component* in which the hand moves quickly to the vicinity of the target, and a slower *manipulation component* when, under visual control, final adjustment to the grasp apertures is made just prior to grasp (Jeannerod 1984). The relationship between these two components has also been investigated (e.g., Jeannerod 1981, 1984; Marteniuk et al 1990; Hoff & Arbib 1993).

Evidence that the arm and hand function as a single unit comes from the finding that the hand starts to open for grasp at the start of the reaching action (Jeannerod 1981; Marteniuk et al 1990; Hoff & Arbib 1993). Jeannerod (1981) filmed his subjects as they reached for objects of various sizes lying on the surface of a table. The grasp aperture (the distance between thumb and index finger) increases throughout the transport phase, reaching a maximum before contact and around the time the transport movement starts to decelerate. The grasp size then decreases as the hand nears the object (Fig. 6.1). When under visual control, the distance between the two grasp components (thumb and index finger), although a little greater than necessary for the size of the object, reflects the size of the object. The aperture is greater when visual control is removed. Once the hand is in contact with the object to be grasped, guidance comes from tactile and pressure receptors.

A study of a single subject (Wing & Fraser 1983) suggests that the thumb plays a role in guiding the transport component of reaching (Fig. 6.2). The investigators noted that during the final approach phase in a reaching task, closing of the hand from peak aperture was largely due to movement of the index finger with little thumb movement. The authors suggested that, since the position of the thumb relative to the line of approach to the object remained invariant, thumb stabilization may provide a focus for visual monitoring of the relationship between grasp aperture and object size. It is critical in rehabilitation that time is spent training grasp and release involving the radial side of the hand as the thumb and forefinger are major contributors to grasp.

Although the arm and hand are controlled as a single unit, details vary according to the task and the context in which it is performed. For example, the task affects temporal aspects of coordination. In a simple action such as reaching to press a switch, the reach component is carried out faster than in a more complex task, reaching to take a glass of water (Dean et al 1999). The relative durations of

the acceleration and deceleration phases differ for different types of task (Marteniuk et al 1987).

It also makes a difference to the organization of both transport and manipulation components of the movement whether subjects reach to grasp with the whole hand or with a precision grip (Castiello et al 1992). The object and what is to be done with it affect the shaping of the grasp. In reaching to grasp a mug, for example, the hand is pre-shaped into a configuration suitable for grasping the handle.

Evidence of the effect of both the object and the individual's goal on reaching and grasping also comes from a study in which the orientation of the hand was shown to vary according to what was to be done with the object once it was grasped (Iberall et al 1986). When subjects were asked to tap the end of a cylinder on the table top, approach and grasp were different from when they were asked to shake the cylinder up and down (Fig. 6.3). The grasp and hand orientation that develops during transportation of the hand toward the object also reflects the final position desired for the object (Rosenbaum 1991; van Vliet 1993; van Vliet et al 1995), that is, whether the mug is to be raised to the lips or moved from table to floor. Knowledge of the properties of the object to be grasped (e.g., degree of fragility) can affect the transport phase, that is, the reach itself, with an increase in length of the deceleration phase when the object is perceived to be fragile compared to when it is not (Marteniuk et al 1987); that

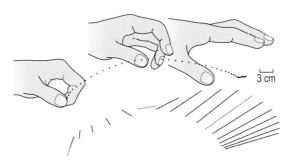

Figure 6.1 A cinematographic study by Jeannerod of reaching toward an object. Dots represent successive positions of the hand every 20 ms and illustrate fast movement of the hand toward the object, slowing down on approach. Lines represent the size of the grasp aperture (between thumb and index finger tip) every 40 ms. Note that aperture formation starts when movement starts and that the aperture reaches a maximum of 3 cm then decreases until it is the size necessary for grasping. *(Reproduced Long and Baddeley 1981, with permission from the International Association for the Study of Attention and Performance).*

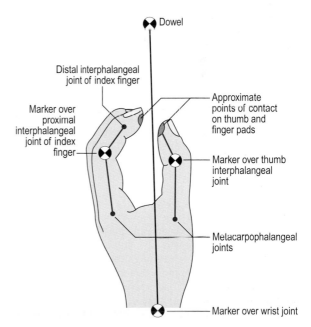

Figure 6.2 Drawing to illustrate position of markers used in digitizing transport and grasp components of reaching to an object. *(From Wing AM, Fraser C (1983) The contribution of the thumb to reaching movements. Quart J Exper Psychol 35A, 297–309. Taylor and Francis Ltd., http://www.informaworld.com).*

125

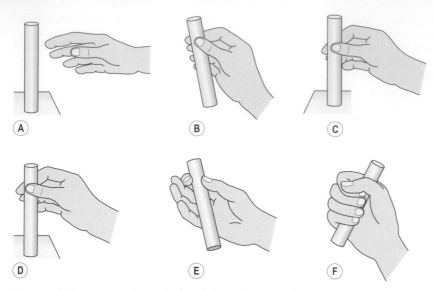

Figure 6.3 The two grasping tasks, (A–C) show the approach, grasp and place components of the task 'Place Cylinder', (D–F) show the grasp and lift, the transition from initial to a firmer grasp and the shake components of the task 'shake cylinder'. *(From Iberall et al, 1986. Opposition space as a structuring concept for the analysis of skilled hand movements. Exper Brain I5, 158–173. "With kind permission of Springer Science & Business Media.")*

is, we approach an object we perceive to be fragile more slowly and carefully.

The spatial and temporal relationships between trunk, lower limbs and arm movement in reaching are complex and reflect the degrees of freedom available, the task and the environmental context (Seidler & Stelmark 2000; Kuzoffsky et al 2001). Reaching out in standing involves preparatory postural adjustments and appropriate temporal coordination between leg and arm muscles. Kuzoffsky and colleagues (2001) examined a small group of people after stroke, reaching at shoulder height to pick up a milk carton on a shelf and place it nearby. Subjects showed preparatory postural adjustments (recorded on force plates and with electromyography (EMG) to gastrocnemius). The greatest difficulty was in timing and coordinating hand trajectory as the paretic limb moved through space.

Reaching to various parts of the workspace can be achieved by a great variety of movement combinations. For example, reaching to an object placed within arm's length involves principally the shoulder, elbow, wrist, forearm and hand joints, although the upper body, if it is not supported, may also move to a small extent at the hips (Dean & Shepherd 1997). Reaching beyond arm's length, however, involves movement at all these joints and, theoretically, with a multitude of possible configurations, as shown in Figure 6.4. The magnitude of trunk and shoulder movement increased and elbow movement decreased as reaching distance was increased in a study carried out in sitting by Dean and colleagues (1999). Overall it seems that the upper body plays a general transport role and the

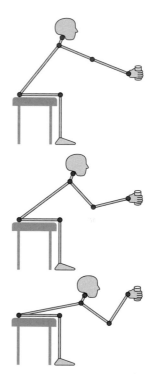

Figure 6.4 Different patterns of the reach action made to a target in the same part of the workplace by a stick figure with 3 degrees of freedom. *(From Rosenbaum el al 1993, with permission).*

arm a more corrective role, countering any variability in movement as the hand approaches the target (Seidler & Stelmark 2000).

In reality, however, it is likely that only the most cost-efficient (parsimonious) options are used (Kelso et al 1994), the hip, glenohumeral and shoulder girdle joints functioning as a multisegmental linkage (Kaminski et al 1995). Two studies have shown a remarkable consistency in movement pattern both for individuals and groups of individuals when they reached forward in sitting to an object beyond arm's reach (Kaminski et al 1995; Dean & Shepherd 1997).

Normally the system learns to use the most efficient options or 'simplifying strategies' to control complex multisegmental movements. These are made possible by anatomical configurations, neuronal connectivity and biomechanical characteristics of linked segments (see Zatsiorsky et al 1998, 2000; Zong-Ming et al 1998a,b for discussion). The concept of simplification is of considerable interest in physiotherapy practice as it enables the development of exercises that have the best chance of transfer to improved performance of a number of different (but similar) tasks.

The upper limbs are also involved in *throwing and striking actions*. These actions have their own patterns of coordination, reflecting the different interactions required, the intentions of the performer and the type of object. Most of these actions are characterized by sequential motions of the segments comprising the linkage, with movements of proximal segments preceding more distal segments (Zajac & Winters 1990, Putnam 1993). Such a sequence maximizes the speed of the distal segment as it releases the ball or swings the bat.

As arm movements are linked into postural support mechanisms, postural adjustments vary with the task and environment, and the demands of stability can affect the speed and accuracy of upper limb movements. Stability of the upper body in sitting and standing is critical to the performance of daily actions and the lower limbs play a significant role in supporting and balancing the body mass as demonstrated in biomechanical studies in sitting (Dean et al 1999). It should therefore be clear that early training of challenging reaching actions in sitting and standing is important for promoting both postural stability and functional performance of actions involving the upper limb.

Bimanual reaching actions. The spatiotemporal organization of limb movement varies according to whether one or both hands are used (Castiello et al 1992). It takes into account the physical characteristics of the object, for example, its shape and fragility, and what is to be done with it (van Vliet 1993; Smeets & Brenner 1999). There has been considerable experimental interest in bimanual actions which illustrate the cooperative manner in which the two hands interact with objects to achieve a goal (e.g.,

Marteniuk et al 1984; Castiello et al 1993). Cooperation between the two hands and the predictive nature of some tasks are shown in an experiment in which the subject drops a ball into a cup held by the other hand. The grip force of the cup hand increased *in anticipation of* the ball's impact, that is before the ball hit the cup (Johansson & Westling 1988). The role of the cerebellum in anticipatory control was noted in other similar bimanual loading–unloading tasks (Diedrichsen et al 2005).

Speed of hand movement is also affected when both hands are used. If a task requires that one limb has to perform a more complex action than the other, which requires a longer movement time, the other limb slows down also so that both hands arrive at the target simultaneously (Kelso et al 1979). In many bimanual reaching-to-grasp tasks, the two hands perform different actions in order to achieve the goal. Nevertheless, both limbs tend to be constrained as a single unit while engaged in the task. For example, in using the hands to open a can, one hand holds the can to stabilize it while the fingers of the other grasp the ring in order to pull. In the former, the whole hand forms the grasp; in the latter, only the tips of the fingers and thumb are used.

A kinematic study of this task (Castiello et al 1993) illustrates very well the difference between unimanual and bimanual reaching to grasp and between grasping with the whole hand or with fine precision grasp. The results showed that, in unimanual reaching, reaches to the ring (the more complex precision task) are performed more slowly than reaches to the can (the whole-hand task). However, in bimanual reaching to grasp the can with one hand and pull the tab to open it with the other, although the kinematic details differed according to the task, there was no difference in movement duration between the two limbs (Fig. 6.5). The speed–accuracy trade-off would suggest that the accuracy requirement of the more precise task requires the decrease in speed. In this bimanual task, the accuracy requirement of one hand's contribution therefore demands that both hands slow down so that they reach the target at the same time. A similar result was found for a task in which one hand opened a drawer and the other took out a rod from the drawer (Wiesendanger et al 1996).

Due to the complexity of bimanual tasks, it is necessary for a person with upper limb dysfunction to have the opportunity to be trained and to practise such tasks. It is clear that without specific practice of bimanual actions, regaining the use of both hands together in the same task may not occur.

Information about the nature of the action of reaching and how it changes and why provides the rationale for the task-oriented training of reaching actions in people with dysfunction of motor control mechanisms. Reaching practice should always involve objects of different types or a target in different parts of the workspace, and different goals. Attempts are made in training to increase the speed

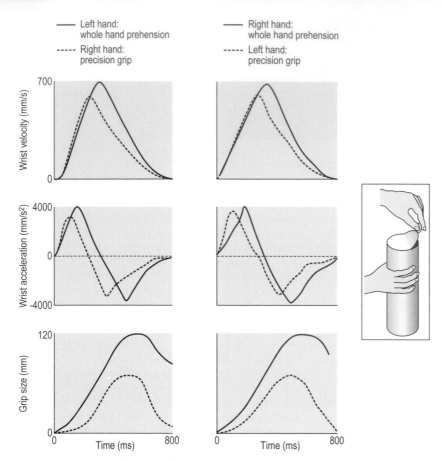

Figure 6.5 A single trial of the bilateral task. Three traces on Right: wrist velocity (top), wrist acceleration (middle) and grip size (lower) during the reach to grasp (R hand) and pull tab (L hand) tasks. Traces on Left are for a trial in which the tasks for each hand were reversed. Note that in both cases peak velocity, acceleration and deceleration occur earlier for the precision grip hand. The 'can' (inset) used in the experiment. *(Reprinted from Castiello et al (1993) with kind permission of Elsevier Science, Amsterdam, The Netherlands).*

of reaching actions as well as the control of the limb. A major aim in rehabilitation is to restore, as far as possible, the flexibility of arm and hand use.

THE UPPER LIMBS IN WEIGHTBEARING

We bear weight through one or both arms when we push a drawer shut, push up out of a low chair and push ourselves up from the floor. Movement takes place principally at the joints of the shoulder complex and elbows. The shoulder and elbow extensor muscles (particularly triceps brachii) must be able to generate enough force to lift a proportion of our body weight or overcome the resistance of the drawer. The wrist must be flexible enough to allow

the necessary extension so that the pushing force acts through the palm of the hand.

MANIPULATION: DESCRIPTION OF THE ACTIVITY

The hand is the principal means by which the individual interacts with people and objects in the external environment. The anatomical structure of the hand and the nature of corticomotor-neuronal connections to hand muscles (Landsmeer 1976; Smith 1981; Muir 1985; Lemon et al 1990, 1991) allow a large number of combinations of joint rotations and of movement possibilities. Even in relatively simple tasks, there may be a variety of different configurations of hand segments. It has been shown that the intention as well as the object itself, its physical characteristics and what is to be done with it affect approach and grasp as well as manipulation (Iberall et al 1986; Rosenbaum et al 1992; van Vliet 1993; Smeets & Brenner 1999) (see Fig. 6.3). Organization of corticomotor neuronal input involves axons directly facilitating motor neurons supplying hand muscles. These axons diverge intraspinally, making functional contact with a small number of different target muscles making up the 'muscle field' of the corticomotor-neuronal cell (Lemon et al 1991).

Lemon and colleagues (1991) have pointed out that during natural manipulative or prehension tasks, many different muscles are active. When the fingers move to manipulate an object, the dominant pattern is one of fractionation of muscle activity. When force is required in gripping, a pattern of co-contraction emerges, with the number of muscles involved depending on the degree of force exerted.

Grip is typically categorized as either precision or power (Napier 1956), the former involving pads of digits and sometimes only thumb and index finger, the latter the whole hand. This general distinction between accuracy and power remains despite the more recent acknowledgement of the task and object relatedness of grasp configurations (Iberall & Lyons 1984; Castiello et al 1993) (Fig. 6.6).

The hand takes on various configurations in order to perform grasping and manipulative tasks. The large number of small bones which make up the hand are moulded into the necessary shapes by an interplay between passive and active properties of hand and forearm muscles. Despite the tendency for interaction between the components of the hand due to its articulated anatomy, the various components can also function relatively

independently, producing more fractionated movement of individual fingers or thumb when the task demands (as in playing a musical instrument, typing on a keyboard or pressing a button).

Many tasks involve interactions between an object and thumb and index finger as the object is grasped and manipulated. These actions require the thumb to abduct and rotate and the index finger to flex so that their palmar surfaces contact the object. Force is effectively exerted on the object primarily by long flexor muscles of the thumb and index finger, and stabilization of each bone is achieved by a combination of joint geometry and intrinsic musculature (Spoor 1983; Lemon et al 1991). The force produced on the index finger by the thumb, for example, is countered by the first dorsal interosseus muscle. The force produced on the mobile carpometacarpal joint of the thumb is constrained by activity of all the thenar muscles (Chao et al 1989).

As in any other part of the body's segmental linkage, force applied to one segment can affect segments at some distance from the original force, and motor control mechanisms must take these segmental interactions into account. With the hand, the combination of small mobile segments and a rich array of muscles means that the complexity of these interactional forces, even though they may be small, is considerable. The lumbrical and interossei muscles, for example, exert axial rotary moments of force which are balanced by other appropriate muscles (Lemon et al 1991). Not surprisingly, it appears that, for a given task, although similar muscle groups are active, the degree of activity and the relative contributions of muscles differ and are task related. At the cortical level also, the contributions of neurons varies; some cortical neurons that are active during fine movements (precision grips)

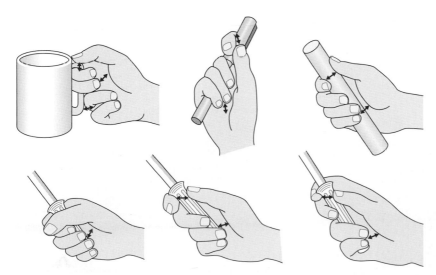

Figure 6.6 Task-related grasps showing the different 'oppositions' used. *(From Iberall et al, 1986. Opposition space as a structuring concept for the analysis of skilled hand movements. Exper Brain I5, 158–173. "With kind permission of Springer Science & Business Media.")*

become inactive during a power grip (Muir & Lemon 1983).

The fifth metacarpal and little finger, together with the fourth metacarpal and finger, are particularly significant in some grasping tasks. Tasks such as eating with a knife and fork or carrying a tray or a plate require these lateral segments of the hand, in the first example to lock the implement into the palm to allow manipulation, in the second and third examples to provide a support surface. These two grasps have been characterized as the locking and the supporting grip (Bendz 1993) (Fig. 6.7). Bendz has described these in some detail. In the *supporting grip*, flexion of the fifth metacarpal enables the little finger to prop up the plate and keep it horizontal. The metacarpals are flexed at the carpometacarpal joints, actively in the case of the fifth metacarpal, passively for the fourth because of the intercapitular ligament's attachments. For the *locking grip*, the tool is locked into the palm of the hand by the fourth and fifth fingers, flexed and rotated at the metacarpophalangeal (MCP) joints. The fifth metacarpal is flexed at the MCP joint by the hypothenar muscles. Opponens digiti minimi acts directly on the metacarpal, while the abductor digiti minimi and flexor brevis act indirectly to flex the metacarpal indirectly through their common attachment to the proximal phalanges of the little finger (Forrest & Basmajian 1965). Flexor brevis and the abductor also flex the little finger at the MCP joint and the abductor also rotates the finger at this joint. The fourth interosseus and long finger flexors act similarly on the fourth finger (Eyler & Markee 1954).

Bendz (1993) stresses that the major function of the abductor digiti minimi is in the application of flexing and rotational force to the proximal phalanx of the fifth finger at the MCP joint. The force provided by this muscle is augmented by the action of the flexor carpi ulnaris (FCU) via their common attachment to the pisiform bone. Using electrogoniometry and electromyography in two tasks, holding a knife and a plate, Bendz showed the effect of a loaded (grip knife firmly; lift plate) and an unloaded condition on the action of hypothenar muscles and FCU. Only in the loaded conditions, when more strength was required, was the FCU strongly active, illustrating this muscle's augmenting effect on hypothenar muscle activity.

This work by Bendz is particularly interesting as it reminds the physiotherapist of the importance of knowing the functional anatomy of the hand. It is clear also that these grasps need specific training with practice of holding, manipulating and carrying different objects.

There are several grip variations used by individuals when they manipulate food with cutlery. Most involve some interaction with the implement of the fourth and fifth fingers. For example, in the grip used in Figure 6.7A the wrist is held flexed and deviated to the ulnar side. Since the long finger extensors are fully lengthened in this position, it is likely that the muscles flexing the fourth and fifth fingers to hold the base of the knife and fork firmly in the palm also act to counteract some extending force. FCU would also be acting in this position, not only to augment the action of abductor digiti minimi but also to flex the wrist and deviate the hand to the ulnar side.

Shaping the hand to an object is critical for manipulation of that object. The carpal and metacarpal bones take on a concave shape through the combined actions of thenar, hypothenar and interossei muscles. It is suggested that such shaping constitutes a 'postural set' for the promotion of precision movements (Lemon et al 1991). A similar concept, that of a 'virtual finger' (Arbib et al 1985; Li et al 1998a,b), is that a group of fingers acts as a single functional unit. When an object is gripped strongly between fingers and thumb, forces are shared cooperatively between

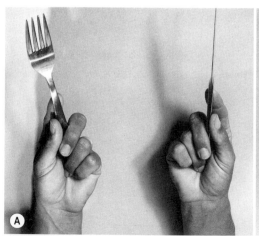 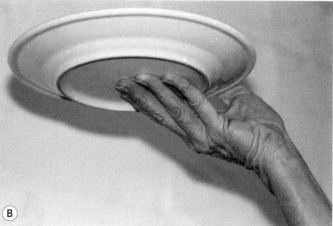

Figure 6.7 Ulnar grasps. (A) A locking grasp: 4th and 5th fingers exert force to stabilize the cutlery in the palm. (B) A supporting grasp: 4th and 5th fingers support the plate and keep it level. *(From Carr & Shepherd 1987, 2003, with permission).*

the four fingers of the functional unit (Li et al 1998a). When holding a mug, for example, three functional units, each producing force in different directions, cooperate to ensure a stable grasp (see Fig. 6.6). Shaping the hand for manipulating an object is therefore in part a function of the anatomy of the hand and in-hand manipulation of objects is associated with complex interactions between fingers in order to isolate motion appropriately (Hagar-Ross & Schreiber 1995).

These are useful simplifications when it comes to evaluating patient performance on manipulative tasks and planning intervention. However, it is also important from early after an acute lesion such as stroke to work toward the preservation of the integrity of the natural bony relationships of the hand, by preserving joint flexibility, soft tissue length and whatever contractility of muscle is possible.

While reaching for an object appears to be carried out under visual control, once the hand comes into contact with the object, major sensory inputs contributing to movement control have been shown to come from tactile and pressure inputs. The role of tactile receptors in glabrous (non-hairy) skin of the palm has been studied in detail. *Tactile cutaneous inputs* in the skin of the palm give information critical to our ability to localize stimuli and appreciate fine details. It is clear that motor commands are precisely tuned to relevant physical properties of objects. Johansson & Westling (1984) found that tactile signals are used to monitor the weight of an object (*vertical lifting force*) and the frictional characteristics of the object in relation to slip (*slip-triggered grip force*) enabling motor output (muscle force) to be adjusted accordingly. Moving the hand while holding an object produces inertial forces and these are compensated for by simultaneous changes in grip force (Westling & Johansson 1984; Johansson & Westling 1984, 1990; Johansson et al 1992a,b,c).

While perceived fragility can affect the reaching phase of the reach-to-grasp action, object weight affects only the time after hand contact. As object weight increases, the time spent in contact with the object prior to lifting it increases (Weir et al 1991). The pause before lift probably reflects the time needed to generate functionally effective forces. As the friction offered by an object decreases, grip force decreases. Reaching to grasp a slippery object (Flanagan & Wing 1993) results in slower movement times (Fikes et al 1994). A general function of all reaching-to-grasp tasks is that, once grasped, the object should not be dropped, whether it is light or heavy, slippery or not.

It can be seen therefore that sensory inputs from cutaneous touch and pressure receptors in the palm of the hand contribute to movement control. They help us to identify objects and classify them according to properties such as texture, shape, weight and potential for slipping, and enable motor output (muscle force) to be adjusted as necessary. Changes in grip force also occur in response to inertial forces produced by the movement occurring while the object is being moved. It is quite common in many neurological conditions for people to lack this adaptive force control and to have difficulty therefore in maintaining grasp while moving the limb. This ability may need to be emphasized in training and specifically practised.

Understanding these details of hand function provides information of value in designing an intensive exercise programme, in particular for a person who has sufficient muscle activity to move the wrist, fingers and thumb but insufficient motor control to use the hand effectively or spontaneously. As both the object itself and the goal of the person carrying out a task drives the control of the hand, the importance of individuals practising real tasks with real objects is quite evident. Practising real tasks, emphasizing the 'feel' of the object, may also aid the individual who has sensory impairment, although some individuals after stroke may also benefit from practice of more specific sensory recognition tasks.

RECOVERY OF UPPER LIMB FUNCTION

Perhaps the most serious consequence after an acute brain lesion, and particularly after stroke, is paresis of an upper limb. The effects of rehabilitation of functional recovery of the upper limb remain, in general, poor. Nevertheless there are increasing numbers of studies that indicate that a more task-oriented and intensive training from therapists with the scientific knowledge and skills in training movement can be effective.

There is evidence that recovery is minimal in individuals with a severely paralytic limb that persists over the first few weeks (Nakayama et al 1994a; Coote & Stokes 2001; Kwakkel et al 2003). These people after stroke may not, because of the site and extent of the lesion and co-morbidities, regain effective functional use of the paretic limb. The results of a study that tested motor-evoked potentials in response to transcortical magnetic stimulation (Pennisi et al 1999) suggested that individuals with paralysis of hand muscles in the first 48 hours after stroke with an absence of motor potentials were likely to have a poor prognosis for hand function. Absence of a measurable grip 1 month after a stroke may also be associated with poor functional recovery (Sunderland et al 1989). The potential of severely affected individuals is not understood.

Reports of recovery of upper limb function after stroke are not always helpful. Attitudes toward upper limb intervention and methods of treatment are going through a period of considerable change but many reports of outcome data are from studies carried out several decades ago, when treatment offered was more passive and less intensive than it is today in up-to-date units with well-trained staff and appropriate facilities. A more accurate picture of recovery potential and, in particular, of the potential effects of intervention for those with marked impairments is still to come. Studies of clinical outcomes and treatment effects so far have been heterogeneous, with patients not grouped according to severity of impairments. Measurement tools vary greatly in terms of what is measured and only recently have measures of actual arm use, a real indicator of functional ability, been reported (Liepert et al 1998; Kunkel et al 1999; Kwakkel et al 2003) Therapy methods may not be described in detail, although this too is gradually changing. Tests of treatment effects are now increasingly been carried out to investigate whether or not treatment effects are retained over time.

Details such as type and intensity of exercise and training are important since it is critical to know the details, the *process* of rehabilitation itself, that is, the methods used, in order to understand what it is that can affect brain reorganization and result in improved functional motor performance (Liepert et al 2001).

The complex nature of hand use, requiring coordination of many muscles and segments, and the nature of the lesion itself may be significant factors in recovery. However, there are other factors which may impact negatively upon outcome following stroke. One is the profoundly negative view that all recovery of arm function is intrinsic (Wade et al 1983; Heller et al 1987), that infers that what a person does, what happens to the person after an acute lesion, including therapy, has little effect on recovery processes (but see Ch. 1). Early studies suggested that most potential recovery of the upper limb takes place within 3 months (Wade et al 1983; Nakayama et al 1994b). However, more recent studies of task-related training and of active practice with forced use of the affected limb commenced more than 6 months after stroke have shown that substantial recovery is possible, considerably beyond the 3-month period (e.g., Ostendorf & Wolf 1981; Whitall et al 2000; Byl et al 2003; McCombe Waller & Whitall 2004). Although the most rapid recovery may take place very early as a result of spontaneous reparative processes within the brain, functional improvement goes on for much longer in those with active movement of the limb.

Today it is accepted that brain reorganization continues throughout life in response to learning and to the demands made on the system. A study of individuals several years after stroke (Liepert et al 1998) showed enlargement of the hand muscle area in the affected hemisphere, suggesting recruitment of adjacent brain areas. These changes had remained when examined 6 months later (Liepert et al 2000). Specific task-oriented training of simple repetitive thumb movements has been shown to elicit reorganization of cortical representations of the thumb that encoded kinematic details of the practice movement. These findings provide a link between active training and exercise, imposed use of the affected limb, brain reorganization and improvements in functional performance. After a training protocol involving increased task-oriented use of the paretic arm and enhanced sensory feedback from

repetitive exercise, Nelles and colleagues (2001) found increased activation of the contralateral sensorimotor cortex.

Turton (1998) described the implications for therapy that can be derived from the early brain imaging studies being carried out at that time. Reorganization (motor learning) may be a function of synaptic plasticity. Synapses are strengthened by repetitive afferent inflows. Hummelsheim and colleagues (1995) showed that voluntary activation of muscle had a greater effect on corticospinal input to motor neurons than passive sensory stimulation. The implications encourage a much more active exercise and training programme, particularly for those who have some muscle activation and functional use of the limb early post-lesion. Even in individuals with virtually no muscle activation, repetitive practice of simple movements may have a positive effect upon eventual recovery.

Tasks that make greater attentional demands, involve the need to learn a particular pattern of coordination or demand a high level of accuracy may in particular drive neural reorganization. Some have been shown to be associated with enlargement of sensory or motor body part representations in the cortex (Pascuol-Leone et al 1995). Evidence is gradually emerging that particular rehabilitation methods can induce lasting changes within the motor cortex (Liepert et al 2000, 2001; Nelles et al 2001) and probably elsewhere in the brain. These changes may be linked to positive outcomes or negative outcomes. What happens to the individual after an acute lesion, and this includes the details of rehabilitation, probably does matter.

The process of rehabilitation can have positive effects on recovery processes, but it may have no positive effect at all and this depends to quite a large extent on the effectiveness of methods used. Guidelines for training of reaching and manipulation developed from scientific developments in biomechanics, motor control and motor learning, and in mechanisms underlying impairments, have been available in the clinical literature for some time (e.g., Carr & Shepherd 1987a,b, 1998, 2003; Ada et al 1990; Shumway-Cook & Woollacott 2005). There is increasing evidence of positive effects, particularly in those whose impairments are in the mild-to-moderate range.

Clinical studies of the effects of upper limb rehabilitation that show the most positive results (e.g., Dean & Mackey 1992; Butefisch et al 1995; Mudie & Matyas 1996; Byl et al 2003; Pang et al 2006) were carried out with patients whose rehabilitation was active and task-related. In the Dean and Mackey study (1992), the extent of functional recovery at discharge was indicated by the highest score in the upper limb items of the Motor Assessment Scale (Carr et al 1985). According to this criterion, 52% of all stroke patients seen over a 1-year period were able to take a spoonful of fluid to the mouth and drink, use a pen, and comb their hair at the back of the head using the affected hand by the time of discharge.

It is not known how well patients with a less severely affected limb recover if they are given the best possible opportunity for training and exercise, and what part in driving neural reorganization and recovery active training and exercise can play. However it is quite common to see individuals after stroke whose spontaneous functional use of the limb is worse than would be anticipated given that they have active muscles and a degree of motor control. There is increasing evidence of positive effects from training programmes that involve early implementation of intensive task-oriented training of functional actions, with repetitive practice of meaningful actions, in an enriched learning environment with, where necessary, emphasis on compelling use of the paretic limb (van Vliet 1993; Platz et al 2001b; van Vliet & Turton 2001; van Peppen et al 2004; Winstein et al 2004; Davis 2006; Wolf et al 2006). Effective training programmes also involve group work and circuit training (Blennerhassett & Dite 2004; Pang et al 2006) and may function in community settings. These programmes appear to be most effective in those participants with the capacity for active limb use.

Attempts are increasingly being made to make such exercise and training programmes available to those who need ongoing opportunities for physical activity. One exercise programme, carried out in a group in a community hall, used a circuit training model, and provided strengthening exercises using elastic bands of various strengths for the upper limb, upper limb weightbearing exercises, weight lifting and practice of functional activities. Participants improved their upper limb functional performance on the Wolf Motor Function Test (WMFT) and expressed satisfaction in their improved daily activities (Pang et al 2006). The authors of this study categorized their subjects as mildly, moderately and severely impaired so it was possible to see the differential effects of the programme.

In general, those patients with mild-to-moderate functional impairment are most likely to benefit from exercise programmes. This is not surprising, but it illustrates how important it is for clinical studies to group patients according to some measure of disability. If group results stem from heterogeneous groups of patients, demonstrable benefits to the less severely handicapped are washed out and effective treatments may not be obvious. Recent studies are attempting to categorize participants. Winstein and colleagues (2004) divided their subjects into less severe and more severe. They found that patients who had task-specific training on upper limb tasks and those who had progressively resisted strength training improved their functional performance significantly more than a standard therapy group (neurodevelopmental therapy), with the task-specific training group gaining the greater long-term benefits. Treatment benefit was primarily in the less impaired people.

Poor recovery may therefore reflect not only the direct effects of the lesion itself but also inappropriate and insufficient therapeutic intervention for the upper limb, the ease with which patients manage their limited responsibilities with one hand when they are in hospital and rehabilitation centre, and the negative effects of inactivity and disuse on soft tissue adaptability. Therapy methods must play a significant part in results, and when more patients have access to newer more effective methods, outcomes should improve for many individuals.

MOTOR DYSFUNCTION

This section considers the major impairments and movement dysfunctions associated with vascular and traumatic brain injury (see also Ch. 8). Specific aspects of upper limb dysfunction in cerebellar ataxia and Parkinson's disease are discussed in Chapters 9 and 13.

Depressed motor output, decreased rate of neural activation, poor timing and coordination of limb segments and sensory deficits can impact severely on functional performance. Several papers have reported significant relationships between muscle weakness and poor functional performance (Boissy et al 1999; Mercier & Bourbonnais 2004). Muscle weakness and loss of manual dexterity are often compounded by the development of soft tissue changes, joint pain and, if there is a hemiplegic distribution, the natural tendency for the patient to focus on the non-paretic limb for their daily activities. A recent study (Harris & Eng 2007) found a significant relationship between isometric upper limb muscle strength, including grip strength, and measures of functional use.

Muscle weakness, impaired coordination and dexterity

The major impairments underlying the functional disability of the upper limb following an acute cortical lesion are muscle paralysis and/or weakness due to impaired muscle activation and reduced motor unit recruitment, and loss of intersegmental coordination (Burke 1988). The neurophysiological evidence (Colebatch & Gandevia 1989) is supported by clinical studies (Bourbonnais et al 1989; Gowland et al 1992), and by biomechanical and EMG studies.

Muscle weakness and impaired motor control affect motor performance according to the extent and distribution of paresis. An early study by Colebatch & Gandevia (1989) investigated the muscle strength of a group of patients with hemiplegia from stroke. The authors reported partial sparing of shoulder and elbow muscles, particularly of shoulder adductors, which were minimally affected. Inactivity of shoulder abductor muscles is typically observed. Another study of corticospinal influences on deltoid and pectoralis major confirmed a bilaterally distributed cortical motor outflow with inputs from both hemispheres to the shoulder adductors (Colebatch et al 1990). Overall, wrist and finger muscles, particularly the flexors, were the most affected. In the patients studied, there was no evidence that extensor muscles were weaker than flexor muscles. In other studies, reduced EMG activity was more evident in some muscles (biceps brachii) than in others (triceps brachii) (Colebatch et al 1986; Bourbonnais et al 1989).

The early belief that direct (monosynaptic) corticospinal projections exist only to hand muscles and not to more proximal muscles has been used to provide an explanation for the relatively poor recovery of distal movements compared to proximal. However, the above study provides evidence that there are also direct corticospinal projections to proximal muscles. The findings further suggest that these projections may be muscle-specific, and help to explain the severe involvement of deltoid muscle in some patients following stroke and the relative ease with which many people can be trained to activate the adductor muscles.

Muscle weakness may also vary according to the length at which the muscle is contracting. In one study, weakness was greatest in elbow flexor and extensor muscles when these muscles were at their shortened lengths (Ada et al 2003). Reduced grip-force control during grasping and lifting objects is a common problem and has been described in association with cerebral and cerebellar lesions and Parkinson's disease by several authors (Jeannerod 1984; Wing 1988; Muller & Dichgans 1994; Hermsdorfer & Mai 1996; Fellows et al 1998). This may also be due to sensory deficits.

Force produced when gripping can be slow to build up, difficult to stabilize at the required level for a particular task, and characterized by irregular force change (Hermsdorfer & Mai 1996). Sustaining and controlling grip force while grasping and lifting objects is a common problem that interferes with limb use. Slower recruitment times of flexor and extensor carpi radialis longus, biceps and triceps brachii, and difficulty sustaining a contraction have also been reported (Sahrmann & Norton 1977). These findings help to explain the slow movements commonly observed.

In addition to muscle weakness, a disturbance of motor unit activation patterns has been reported (Tang & Rymer 1981). However, whether or not this is directly the result of the lesion or of the development of maladaptive motor patterns is not clear. Co-activation of muscles is often observed clinically and has been reported in several studies (Chae et al 2002). This seems to reflect poor control of synergic muscle activity as well as a tendency to stiffen a limb to compensate for poor control.

It should be noted that there is increasing evidence that individuals with hemiplegia also have some impairment of the ipsilateral upper limb (Colebatch & Gandevia 1989; Newham & Hsiao 2001), with less force production than in age-matched able-bodied subjects. These findings may reflect the fact that between 10% and 30% of fibres in the lateral corticospinal tract are uncrossed (Haaland et al 2004).

Lack of coordination between limb segments has been investigated in many studies. In reaching forward, for example, a common problem is difficulty coordinating shoulder flexors and elbow extensors. Bi-articular biceps brachii is both a shoulder and an elbow flexor. Lack of coodination between synergic muscles (i.e., biceps and triceps brachii) in this two-joint movement can result in flexion of the shoulder and elbow when the person attempts to reach forward (Fig. 6.8A).

Muscle stiffness, muscle length changes, contracture

Secondary adaptations occurring post-lesion, principally due to immobility and disuse, include length-associated changes in muscles and other soft tissues. Muscles held short for long periods of immobilization (Fig. 6.8B) shorten and become stiffer, and when these muscles are activated they generate tension at shorter lengths. A paretic limb rests naturally in internal rotation and adduction at the glenohumeral joint, flexion at the elbow, forearm pronation, thumb adduction, and finger and wrist flexion and it is these muscles that can quickly become stiff and develop contracture.

Adaptive movement patterns reflect paresis, imbalance between muscles acting over a joint, and soft tissue inflexibility (Carr & Shepherd 1996). The person's adaptive movement appears to represent the best attempt possible given the impairments and the biomechanical possibilities of a multisegment system. For example, if it is difficult to flex the shoulder and extend the elbow to reach forward for an object, reaching distance is typically increased by moving the upper body forward at the hips. When shoulder flexors (deltoid, supraspinatus) are paretic, an attempt to reach may involve lateral flexion of the spine and elevation of the shoulder girdle (see Fig. 2.11).

The relationship between spasticity (stretch reflex hyperactivity) and upper limb dysfunction has until recently been considered to be strong, however the effects of spasticity on functional movement are unclear. For example, there is some evidence that spasticity (reflex hyperactivity) does not have a major impact on function, particularly following stroke (O'Dwyer et al 1996). With this group of patients, and with other individuals with central lesions, resistance offered to passive movement that may be perceived by the clinician as spasticity is not necessarily due to reflex hyperactivity but due in part to increased muscle stiffness and muscle contracture. This is a critical point since the belief that spasticity is the dominant impairment has resulted in relatively passive interventions involving inhibition of spastic muscle contractions. On the other hand, when it is clear that weakness and incoordination

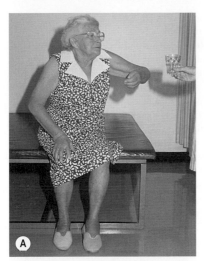

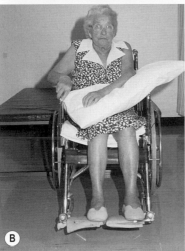

Figure 6.8 Post-stroke. (A) An attempt at reaching to take a glass. The 2-joint muscle, biceps brachii, flexes the shoulder but also flexes the elbow in the absence of triceps brachii activation. (B) A common resting posture with the paretic limb supported on a pillow in GH joint internal rotation and adduction, elbow flexion, forearm pronation and wrist flexion. In the absence of movement the muscles held short will develop adaptive changes including contracture. This position must be avoided.

are the major impairments interfering with function, therapy shifts to more active exercise and training. For example, instead of inhibiting spastic muscle activity, active exercise and training aim to develop greater efficiency of muscle activity in the performance of simple everyday tasks.

Muscles that typically develop contracture are shoulder adductors and internal rotators, elbow flexors, pronators, wrist and finger flexors and thumb adductors (see Fig.

6.8B). When muscles become shorter and stiffer, hypersensitivity of stretch receptors may develop (see Ch. 8). These adaptations to muscle paralysis and disuse may be prevented or at least minimized by intensive active exercise of the limb and, while muscles remain paralysed, by positioning of the limb carried out during the day.

Muscle activation and some active use of the limb are critical and must be a priority from the earliest stage post-lesion. For people who do not recover effective active limb use, muscle contracture is likely to develop. Methods of minimizing contracture and preventing a stiff, immobile and painful limb need further development. Failure to recover the ability to use the limb can result in depression and withdrawal (Balliet et al 1986). When one limb is affected, the very large number of tasks usually performed bimanually can only be attempted with difficulty, if at all.

Motor Performance

There is an increasing number of investigations of reaching performance and manipulation in brain-injured individuals. Kinematic analyses of reaching tasks and analyses of force production between hand segments and the object being manipulated provide the basis of our understanding of poor functional performance. The use of non-invasive methods of examining brain function has also resulted in findings which help clarify issues raised in the clinic about the nature of impairments.

Reaching. After an acute lesion, reaching and pointing movements may be slower, less accurate, more segmented and poorly coordinated (Levin 1996; Cirstea et al 2003). Disruption of elbow–shoulder coordination and decreased range of joint movement compared to able-bodied individuals have been reported (Cirstea & Levin 2000). As a result, the trunk's contribution to the movement was increased as individuals took advantage of the degrees of freedom available. Deficits in interjoint coordination are evident during many reaching actions, with difficulty making smooth and continuous movements (Trombly 1992, 1993; Cirstea & Levin 2000). Problems coordinating the limb are illustrated by lack of synchronized movement at the glenohumeral and elbow joints (Levin 1996). Excessive and unintended movements can occur between linked segments, for example difficulty extending the elbow while simultaneously flexing the shoulder (Lang & Schieber 2004; Zachowski et al 2004; McCrea et al 2005) (see Fig. 6.8A).

Observable problems with reaching to an object include deviations in hand path and inability to pre-shape the hand prior to grasp. The hand may not open until it reaches the object and may not be oriented to grasp the object appropriately in terms of its characteristics (e.g., shape) or what is to be done with it. Hand path deviations may be caused by inability to combine, for example, glenohumeral joint flexion with external rotation plus a deficiency in supination. Poor timing of hand contact may result in the hand knocking into the object or closing before the object is reached.

In bimanual reaching actions, the movement is typically performed more slowly than when the task is performed unimanually and this has also been reported from studies of people with stroke (Platz et al 2001a) with additional findings of some dyssynchrony between limbs in the bimanual tasks. Many of the studies of reaching after stroke have involved non-functional tasks. A recent biomechanical study examined a functional reaching task in which the two limbs worked collaboratively to achieve the goal (Kilbreath et al 2006). The task was to reach forward, grasp, transport and put down, with one hand or both hands, either a large or two small trays (grasping them by their handles). Participants with stroke in general took longer than the unaffected individuals and timing parameters showed less synchronicity, and these two findings were particularly evident with the two small trays. Interacting with the two trays is a more complex task than with one tray. The authors suggested that the slower movement duration might have reflected the greater complexity of this part of the task compared with the transport phase. Participants may have had particular difficulty coordinating the two hands as they moved to grasp the trays. They may also have been controlling the two arms separately, turning the single task into a dual task. The results and the authors' interesting speculations support the importance of including bimanual training even in patients who have moderate functional recovery of the affected limb.

In cerebellar ataxia, reaching is characterized by delayed movement times, particularly when reaching toward moving objects, and delayed reaction times. Movement trajectories are typically characterized by under- and overshooting the target (dysmetria) and decomposition of movement (Bastian et al 1996, 2000).

There may also be impaired multijoint coordination, and decreased ability to coordinate wrist and finger movements in association with Parkinson's disease (Bertram et al 2005). In this case, medication can improve the speed of reaching but not the modulation of movement.

Grasping and manipulation. Some individuals may demonstrate impaired modulation of grip force during manipulation of objects and release (Quancy et al 2005). After stroke, difficulty overcoming the mechanical coupling that exists naturally among fingers affects the ability to move fingers independently (Raghaven et al 2006). In Parkinson's disease, difficulty with release and releasing an object too slowly have been found (Gordon et al 1997).

Difficulty using the hand may include greater ability to flex the fingers and wrist than to extend them (although finger flexors are typically weak); a tendency for finger flexion to be associated with wrist flexion rather than extension (reflecting lack of synergistic wrist extensor activity); thumb extension instead of abduction in releasing a grip; and inability to cup the hand by rotating the thumb and little finger inwards. Muscle contracture also interferes with hand use, for example a contracted thumb adductor muscle with a decreased web space makes it difficult to grasp objects (Fig. 6.9).

Clumsiness of fine finger control is commonly reported and people with some ability to activate hand muscles may still have great difficulty gaining the ability to move fingers independently, as in finger tapping (Prigatano & Wong 1997; McCombe Waller & Whitall 2004). Problems with fine motor control in finger tapping have been noted also in the non-paretic hand (McCombe Waller & Whitall 2004).

Abnormal posturing of the hand (Fig. 6.10) is seen in a few people some time after stroke, and may represent dystonic movement or an acquired motor pattern. Unusual posturing of the hand is described by Jeannerod (1986), with palmar grasping of an object rather than grasping with finger tips. He ascribes this to a mismatch between visual and proprioceptive inputs.

An individual with hemiplegia may not use the affected hand, even when active use of the limb is possible, unless the other hand is immobilized (Taub et al 1993). There is evidence from monkey experiments and from studies and observations of adults and children with hemiplegia that compelling active participation of the affected limb by constraining the more effective limb can lead to increased use of the affected arm in certain individuals. Forced use is discussed below as a training strategy in patients with a hemiplegic distribution of muscle weakness.

TRAINING OF REACHING AND MANIPULATION

Rehabilitation for motor disorders of the upper limb is a challenge for patients and therapists. In the last few decades, however, a number of biomechanical and physiological studies have taught us more about the organization of various reaching actions, of grasping and manipulating objects. We are gaining more insight into the complexity of upper limb control and of the factors driving neural reorganization and motor learning after a brain lesion affecting the motor system. Out of this increase in scientific understanding, new methods are being developed and tested in the clinic. We have outlined below a group of rehabilitation strategies based on our current scientific understanding, most of which have been shown to be effective at certain levels of effectiveness and in certain individuals.

Effective functional use of the upper limb is absolutely dependent on functional hand grasp and release. Movements of the upper limb are driven by the hand and the

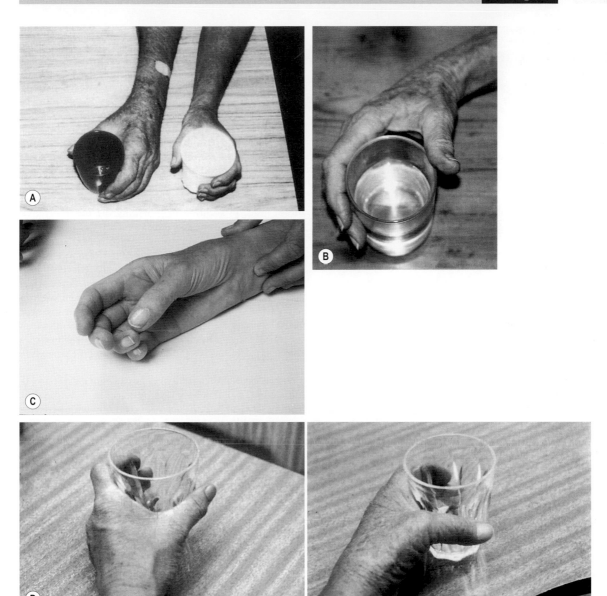

Figure 6.9 (A) It is difficult to hold and manipulate objects if wrist extension and forearm supination are absent. Note the difference in hand and forearm alignment between the arm with weak muscles and short long finger flexors and pronators compared to normal (on Right). (B) Thumb extension to release the glass takes the place of thumb abduction when abductor pollicis brevis is weak. (C) Weakness of hand muscles means the hand is unable to assume a cupping posture of palm and fingers and the thumb and 4th and 5th digits cannot be opposed. (D) Grasping the glass is normally made possible by the extensible web space between thumb and index metacarpals (Left). Shortening of web space soft tissues (including thumb adductor muscle) forces an abnormal posture at the MCP joint (Right).

placement of the hand in the person's close environment or workspace. Consequently, reaching practice should always involve a target or an object for the hand, and intensive and repetitive practice of finger and wrist exercises and simple tasks should begin from the time therapy is initiated.

Training of active movements of the arm and hand, based on task practice but including isolated joint movements if necessary, starts early, with the patient sitting at a table. When muscle weakness is severe, emphasis is on eliciting activity in key muscles plus repetitive practice of simple movements. Reaching and finger movements

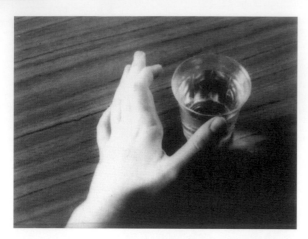

Figure 6.10 Dystonic movement is evident after a stroke as the hand reaches to pick up the glass. Note that grasp aperture is formed by thumb and side of index finger.

involved in grasp and release are emphasized. The focus is on promoting activity of the limb for different tasks, preventing contracture of at-risk muscles and stimulating and preserving muscle contractility.

Chapter 2 describes research findings on motor learning that make clear how important the actual techniques of training can be. For example, *verbal instructions* are an important part of training yet there may be little emphasis placed on how instructions are given during clinical practice. A study of training reaching tasks in people after stroke found that how instructions were given by the therapist made a marked difference to outcome in terms of motor performance (Fasoli et al 2002). The occupational therapists involved in the study gave externally-focused (task-related) or internally-focused (movement-related) instructions. Participants performed three tasks: 1) moving a can from shelf to table; 2) moving an apple from shelf to basket; and 3) moving a mug from table to saucer. As they did these tasks they were instructed to pay attention to the object's characteristics or to their arm and the movements at the elbow, wrist and fingers. Participants with stroke increased peak velocity and decreased movement time when they paid attention to the objects. On the can task they reduced the number of movement units, that is they moved more smoothly. Similar effects were found in the able-bodied subjects. The externally-focused instructions directed visual attention toward the 'affordances' of objects, the possibilities for interaction raised by the objects, while the internally-focused instructions emphasized proprioceptive feedback. It is apparent that people spontaneously attend more to visual than to proprioceptive feedback (Weiss & Jeannerod 1998).

In addition to motor impairments, sensory and visuospatial impairments may also affect recovery. Both have been shown to benefit from specific retraining (e.g., Yekutiel & Guttman 1993; Carey et al 2002; Byl et al 2003;

Sullivan & Hedman 2004). However, implicit in the concept of task-related training is the manipulation of objects with different characteristics (shapes, sizes, textures) for a variety of different purposes. It is likely that intensive task-related training encourages the interaction of somatosensory and visual information relevant to the task, in addition to stimulating an increase in attention span. Task-related training provides the possibility of improving the person's ability to select, attend to and respond to relevant sensory inputs and to use the information to control muscle force and the coordination of limb segments.

Feedback can be augmented in the training process to aid learning. Practice of simple active movements and of motor tasks, in addition to providing the internally-generated feedback from the movement that is part of the mechanism of motor control, also involves external feedback from: 1) watching the effects of performance – 'Was the goal achieved?' (see Fig. 6.8A); 2) the effects of grip force – 'Is the object squashable, slippery, hard?' (Fig. 6.11); and 3) from the path of the hand or configuration of the hand – 'Can I pick it up?' The therapist can augment visual feedback by helping the person focus their attention on critical features in the environment when walking; specific sensations such as the sense of loading the feet while standing up.

Verbal feedback from the therapist, while it can provide motivation, can also have disadvantages as it can be misleading, unclear and, if given concurrently with performance, probably counterproductive (Winstein et al 1996; Schmidt & Wulf 1997). Instructions and feedback appear most effective when given before performance and when pointing out an external focus rather than an internal body focus.

Visual inputs are critical to reaching and manipulation. A study of stroke found that reaching to a moving object could result in better performance (smoother, faster movement, with better timing) than reaching to the same object when stationary (Lee et al 1984). The authors suggested that recovery may be aided by such exercises designed to visually drive the system. Over the years other research findings have pointed to a dominance of vision over touch. Work being done currently on virtual environments is indirectly exploring the relationship between vision and performance.

The results of some early studies suggested that EMG feedback can assist stroke patients to regain some active function in the upper limb. For example, an early investigation involving specific exercise for triceps brachii (Wolf et al 1994) showed that, in the group that received EMG feedback, activity in triceps increased significantly. However, information regarding a transfer to improved functional performance or increased use of the limb, due to the incorporation of EMG feedback into a training programme, is lacking. EMG can be useful in giving the patient and therapist information about underlying capacity for voluntary muscle activity (Fig. 6.12). The advantage

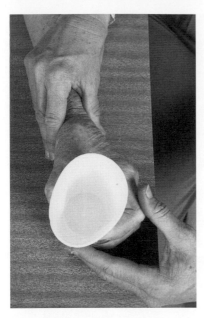

Figure 6.11 Grasping and lifting a polystyrene (deformable) cup gives feedback about excessive force generation. Therapist is temporarily holding her wrist in some extension to restrain a tendency to flex as she grasps the cup – focus of attention is preserving the shape of the cup.

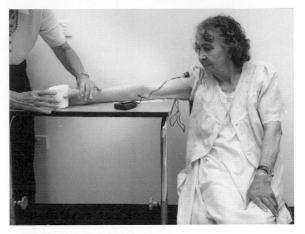

Figure 6.12 Using an EMG device to monitor activity in deltoid muscle during attempts at reaching forward on the table.

of electronic training and a feedback device is that the patient can be encouraged to use it during the day as part of simple task practice and it is more interesting and likely to be effective than simple feedback from muscle activity. The use of EMG-triggered electrical stimulation is described later in the chapter.

Task modification. A major factor in early training of the upper limb is the need to modify what is to be practised in order to take into account the individual's motor impairments. For example, a person may appear to have a paralysed limb under certain circumstances (e.g., when asked to lift the arm). However, when conditions have been modified (the arm supported on a table) so that the amount of muscle force that needs to be generated in order to achieve movement is minimal, the person may be able to achieve some movement of the limb (Fig. 6.13). Practice of simple actions using muscles that can be activated may have a positive motivational effect on the initially severely impaired patient.

Constraint of a body segment can be used to train better control between other segments. When one reaches for objects within arm's length, the upper body is relatively still. When reaching beyond arm's length, the trunk plays an active role and the action begins with trunk flexion at the hips. However, when an individual has poor coordination between shoulder and elbow movement in reaching, flexion of the trunk at the hips may increase as a means

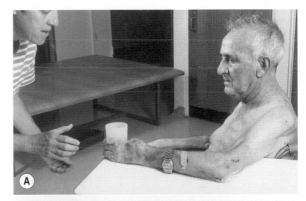

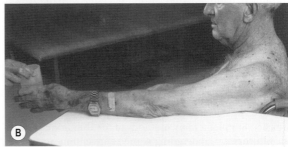

Figure 6.13 He is able to reach forward and pass the glass by sliding his arm over the table. Weak activation of the deltoid muscle, which would normally be the response to friction from the table, is evident. He should be able to raise his arm above the table after many repetitions – then he would practise without it.

Box 6.1 **Task-oriented training method**

- Simple repetitive exercises
- Task-specific training and practice (reaching and manipulative tasks with objects), to achieve effective functional performance, focus on speeding up, hand dexterity
- Training to increase functional muscle strength and endurance
- Bimanual training and practice
- Task training and practice plus constraint

Supplementary methods

- Electrical stimulation
- Mental practice
- Robotic and non-robotic training devices
- Computerized training
- Virtual environments

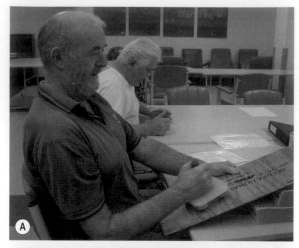

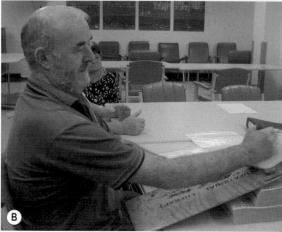

Figure 6.14 Hand class: repetitive shoulder flexion and elbow extension in the sagittal plane to train interjoint coordination – he is aiming for continuous smooth rhythmic movement (up/down, up/down). A metronome can be used to help him focus on timing rather than the movement itself. *(Courtesy of S. Dorsch & K Schurr, Physiotherapy Dept, Bankstown-Lidcombe Hospital, Sydney).*

of reaching the target, in order to compensate for reduced elbow or shoulder motion (Levin et al 2002). This adaptation or compensation, if persistent, may limit potential recovery (Ada et al 1994). Studies of reaching training in which trunk movement is constrained have found increased elbow movement and decreased trunk movement after training (Michaelsen et al 2001; Michaelsen & Levin 2004; Michaelsen et al 2006). These studies show that multijoint coordination and functional improvement can result from simple strategies to force a reorganization of interjoint relationships.

The absence of sitting balance should not be a deterrent to early training of upper limb function. Practice of reaching to objects or pointing in sitting and standing is also a means of improving a person's balance in these positions. Similarly, absence of, or poor control of, the shoulder for reaching should not be considered a deterrent to early training of hand function. Sitting at a table with the arm(s) supported enables the person to practise hand tasks and reaching exercises even when control over reaching and balance are poor (Fig. 6.14). In lying and with the arm supported in sitting, reaching and pointing can also be practised before the individual is able to raise the arm actively to the horizontal.

Methods of rehabilitation that are science-based and found to be effective under certain conditions are listed in Box 6.1. Supplementary methods of rehabilitation include an old therapy undergoing some re-invention and novel methods that take advantage of latest technological developments, such as virtual environments and robotic and non-robotic training devices. Novel methods of stimulating hand function early after stroke in patients with marked impairments include drug therapies and low-frequency repetitive transcranial magnetic stimulation

(rTMS) to the contralesional motor cortex (Liepert et al 2007) or transcranial direct current stimulation (tDCS) (Hummel et al 2005). rTMS was shown in a single case study to improve hand dexterity in the short term. A study of small-amplitude vibration to the bellies of several small finger muscles, tested using motor-evoked potentials and TMS, has been shown to alter the excitability of motor pathways controlling the stroke-affected hand (Wang et al 2006). The authors hypothesize that individualized muscle vibration might potentially be used to increase excitability of the motor pathway controlling an agonist muscle during voluntary movement. The next step is to test the effects of such stimulation on functional performance in an intensive task-specific hand-use training programme.

Task-oriented training and practice

In developing control over the linked segments of the upper limb, individuals with motor impairments must regain the ability to match their motor performance to the characteristics of objects, the goal and the environment in which the action is being performed. They learn again to judge how the hand should be oriented to match the object and what is to be done to it; whether all or only some of the fingers are needed in order to grasp the object; and how much force to apply. In reaching, individuals have to learn to control for direction and distance. They have to regain the ability to judge the distance over which they can successfully reach, which means knowing the length of the arm and the distance over which other body segments can extend the reach. This means that the individual must learn to incorporate the necessary postural adjustments into reaching and manipulation in upright positions such as sitting and standing.

As in all task-oriented training, the patient is given a goal, an object or target is always involved, and, where possible, the object and the task itself should be meaningful, attract attentional focus and give feedback (particularly tactile and visual feedback, and knowledge of results). The presence of an object enhances the performance of reaching in both able-bodied and stroke individuals. In biomechanical studies, Wu and colleagues (2000, 2004) showed that reaching was smoother and more coordinated when subjects reached towards coins in order to sweep them off the table into the other hand, compared with reaching to sweep the table with no functional purpose. Another investigation of patients practising a simple grasp, lift and move a cup from one place to another found significantly improved limb coordination and maximum grip strength (Woldag & Hummelsheim 2002).

For the person with minimal or moderate loss of function, training proceeds immediately to intensive and repetitive task practice with emphasis on particular aspects of the action that are difficult. For example, a person may need to practise speeding up performance to maximize skill and dexterity; task difficulty may need to be varied, including more challenging tasks that require great accuracy; load carried, lifted or manipulated may be increased to improve strength and endurance of the limb.

Training addresses each individual's functional limitations, and feedback and instructions with a specific focus is provided by the therapist. Tasks are varied to encourage the effectiveness of muscle contractility at particular muscle lengths. Providing concrete knowledge of progress by presenting a weekly chart of scores on a functional scale (e.g., Motor Assessment Scale) or specific task (e.g., nine-hole peg test) helps to motivate and instruct. For patients with muscle paralysis or severe deficits in muscle activation, however, they must first regain the ability to activate their muscles. After an acute lesion such as stroke or traumatic brain injury, voluntary activation of muscles even for simple one-joint movements may be very difficult. The first step in intervention, therefore, is to engage the person in simple exercises that stimulate muscle activation and the ability to generate force and move a limb or segment of a limb. People who initially have severe muscle weakness may have the potential to make some degree of functional recovery. It is therefore necessary that they also make an early start on an intensive and active training process.

A warm-up before the serious business of intensive exercise and training can help a person to relax, move and become more flexible, particularly at an early stage of treatment. A warm-up might include shoulder shrugging (unilateral and bilateral) and shoulder circling, and in sitting, upper body rotation at the thoracolumbar spine and trunk side bends.

Several studies, including randomized controlled trials, show that a task-oriented training programme that includes specific practice of a variety of meaningful, interesting tasks can be effective, with the greatest effects occurring in those people who have a moderate degree of voluntary muscle activation but are relatively weak, uncoordinated, slow in performance and clumsy (Platz et al 2001b; Winstein et al 2004; Pang et al 2006).

Simple repetitive exercises

Part of the complexity of hand movement arises out of the large number of degrees of freedom potentially available in the multisegmental physical structure of the hand and from the different possibilities inherent in the physical interaction between intention and object. Without the ability to activate a muscle and control the required forces, it may, however, be impossible to practise specific functional tasks. Simple repetitive exercises, that may need to be directed toward one muscle group (Box 6.2), EMG-triggered electrical stimulation, or practice with a non-robotic or robotic trainer, may enable the patient to

---

Box 6.2 **Simple repetitive exercises**

- Reaching forward (shoulder flexion, elbow extension)
- Shoulder external rotation plus forearm supination, elbow flexed
- Opening/closing of hand aperture (thumb and finger extension/flexion)
- Wrist flexion and extension in mid-rotation of forearm
- Finger flexion/extension
- Grasping, releasing and placing different objects

activate muscles and do simple movements (see Fig. 6.21). This simplification of complex actions is designed to help the person to activate muscles in tasks such as grasping and releasing objects of different size and shape leading into more complex interactions of the hand(s) with objects. Several studies show that repetitive practice of simple exercises can lead to improved functional performance even in the chronic phase after stroke (Butefisch et al 1995; Hummelsheim et al 1996; Mudie & Matyas 1996; Carey et al 2002).

These simple actions are essential at some stage and in varying degrees in many tasks. Despite the limitless variety of tasks we perform daily with our hands, different tasks involve the putting together in various combinations of a relatively small number of configurations used for specific grasps and actions (see the different grips in Figs 6.6 and 6.7; see also Kapandji 1992 on thumb oppositions).

Simple exercises may be useful in training a complex task such as cutting with a knife or manipulating a fork to pick up food. The index finger presses down on the implement, directing force downward. The wrist is flexed and a palmar view of the grasp makes it clear that crucial to any pressure downward through the knife and fork with the index finger is the ability to hold the implement firmly into the palm. Cooperation between functional groupings of fingers normally produces appropriate levels of opposing forces. Critical to effective use of this grip is the ability of long finger flexors to generate force at a shortened length, a length at which the muscle's capacity to generate force is limited by its structure and by the need to counteract the extending force produced by the stretched finger extensors. Practice with knowledge of the main features of the grip may enable the person to develop effective control over these grip components and the tasks involved, although the person's focus may initially be on exercises in which they repetitively generate muscle force to push down on the implement with the index finger, or press the implement firmly into the palm with wrist flexed, and so on. When they practise cutting food with the knife or picking up food with the fork, the focus then shifts to the task and the goal of the task. Of course, using chopsticks involves another set of grips and finger configurations.

Motor performance in manual tasks is governed to a considerable extent by objects and their 'affordances' (Gibson 1977). That is to say, objects offer possibilities for interaction. When we reach out for an object, the movement pattern reflects its position in relation to the body and its orientation, as well as what we are intending to do with it (Iberall et al 1986; Rosenbaum et al 1990). Objects for practice should be chosen not only for their inherent interest and usability but also for the options they offer for hand orientation. For example, in Figure 6.15, if a person has difficulty controlling the orientation of the hand and limb during reach, and reaches persistently with the shoulder internally rotated and the forearm pronated, an object is chosen that demands a relatively externally rotated and supinated approach. Objects are chosen and computer and other games played that actively encourage the action with which the person has difficulty

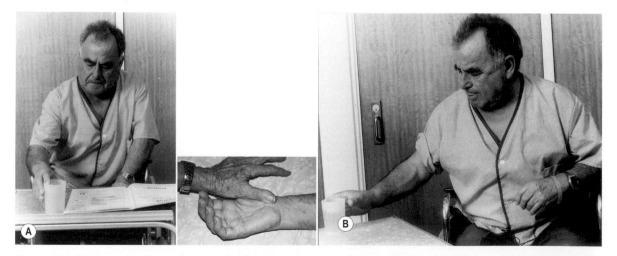

Figure 6.15 (A) He reaches forward to take the glass. As he cannot supinate his forearm enough to take hold in the usual way he tries to pick it up with his hand on top of the glass. The problem is compounded by reduced GH external rotation (B) After some simple repetitive pronation/ supination and external rotation practice and brief passive stretching of his stiff pronators, he can overcome the stiffness and although the glass is placed out to the side he can shape his hand appropriately for picking it up.

(Fig. 6.16). Objects should enable practice to take place without too big a struggle – tasks should on the whole be challenging but not impossible.

One of the few clinical studies of specific task-oriented training of simple actions examined a programme of repetitive and intensive finger tracking with a group of participants on average 5 years after their stroke. Significant improvement was found in task performance and transfer to improved performance scores on the box and block test (grasp, transport and place wooden blocks) (Carey et al 2002). The experimenters focused on finger

movement as its loss is a major functional problem after acute brain lesion. All participants had at least 20° of MCP joint extension but slower than normal hand opening from a fist. Significant motor performance changes were accompanied by brain reorganization imaged by functional magnetic resonance imaging (fMRI). At pretest, cortical activation was ipsilateral to the training hand; after finger tracking training, activation had shifted to the contralateral side. An untrained stroke group did not make any of these changes. Training involved tracking of a target on a computer screen using reciprocal flexion and extension movements of the index finger. Training methods were based on motor learning principles, including presentation of a variety of target waveforms that required problem solving, and encouraged flexibility of performance. Hand position varied between pronation, supination and mid-position. Participants performed 60 tracking trials several times a week for 18–20 sessions altogether.

This important study demonstrates that training needs to be of a meaningful and challenging task, repetitive and intensive, and that, for the effects to be understood, details of the programme (the methods used and dosage) must be documented in detail. Another study of repetitive finger movement is described below (Butefisch et al 1995). The results of both studies emphasize the importance of getting the fingers and thumb moving, and of concentrating on flexion and extension exercises since they, in all their different configurations, are the major movements of the hand (Fig. 6.17).

Functional strength training

There is increasing clinical research support for repetitive practice of task-related strengthening exercises and for their generalization into more functional activities. The emphasis in strength training research is now on the specificity of such training, for example on the need for training to be specific to particular sporting activities (kicking a football, hitting a tennis ball). In clinical neurological practice also, the need for strength training to take account of poor interjoint coordination and the need to relearn the specific action patterns of effective task performance are now generally recognized.

It is likely that all patients who regain the ability to generate muscle force after an acute lesion can benefit from strength training for the upper limbs, particularly for muscles used in tasks performed at shoulder height and above, pushing and pulling tasks, and tasks involved in gripping, holding and lifting objects. Winstein and colleagues (2004) found that patients in a less severe group improved significantly in functional performance as well as isometric strength after a strength training programme. However, these participants showed longer lasting benefits after a task-specific training programme.

Hand grip strength has been found to correlate significantly with upper extremity functional tests more than 1

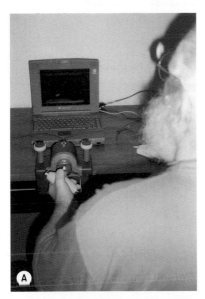

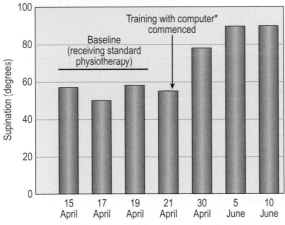

Figure 6.16 (A) Independent practice of forearm supination/pronation on the Upper Limb Exerciser. The computer game linked to the manipulandum provides motivation and quantitative feedback. *(Courtesy of Biometrics Ltd, Ladysmith, VA, USA).* (B) The results after 6 weeks training. *(Unpublished data courtesy of Dr S Kilbreath).*

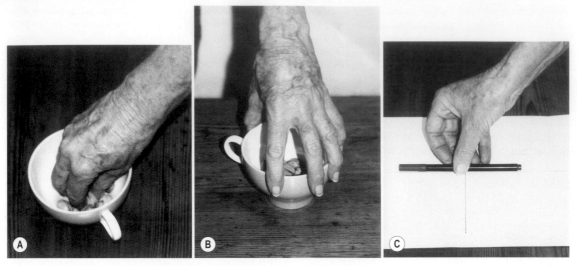

Figure 6.17 Some examples of actions that require different finger groupings.

year post-stroke (Boissy et al 1999). Hand grip strength is critical to many everyday tasks such as undoing a jar lid or lifting a saucepan, and a significant relationship between hand grip force and a saucepan task has been reported (Turner & Ebrahim 1992). Few clinical studies have examined strength training for the arm and hand.

A report of a randomized and controlled clinical trial 15 years ago described the effect of specific training of hand exercises (squeezing two metal bars together, rapid resisted wrist extensions performed both isotonically and isometrically) in 27 patients following stroke (Butefisch et al 1995). Patients showed a significant increase in grip strength, and in peak force of isometric hand extension and peak acceleration. Most interesting, however, was the carryover to improvement of functional performance as measured on the Rivermead Motor Assessment Scale. The biomechanical parameters improved in parallel with the functional improvement. Subjects showed no increase in spasticity or in associated movements: specifically there was a decrease in Ashworth Scale scores (reduced resistance to passive movement) and in associated movements during the training period. The design of the study supports the investigators' view that the positive treatment effect was due to the training and not to 'spontaneous recovery'. Many of the patients who improved most already had some muscle activity before training.

It is likely that strength training is most effective at improving functional performance when built into task practice. This is done by gradually increasing load in order to increase force-generating capacity and the timing of peak forces. In task practice, load is increased by increasing the weight of objects lifted. Some examples of exercises are shown in Box 6.3 and in Figure 6.18.

> **Box 6.3 Strength training**
>
> - Gripping exercises using grip-force dynamometer, spring-resisted gripping device or plastic putty, pouring water from vessel to vessel (increasing weight of one, decreasing weight of the other); various types of grip are practised with different objects
> - Use of progressively heavier objects in reaching, lifting and manipulating tasks
> - Elastic band exercises, using progressively tighter bands
> - Pushing, pulling exercises, using body weight or elastic bands
> - Arm cycling (bimanual or unimanual)

As a guide, a maximum number of repetitions up to 10 should be attempted, performed in sets of three. Progressive resistance elastic band exercises can be effective, with a carryover to improved functional performance (Thielman et al 2004). Many of the exercises above, including arm cycling, can be practised independently.

Bimanual training and practice

It is important to train bimanual actions specifically since the two upper limbs work cooperatively in most everyday functions. For example, unscrewing a jar involves coordinating opposing forces between lid and jar and the two hands. The non-dominant hand reaches to hold the jar steady, gripping with the whole hand, while the dominant hand reaches with hand pre-shaped to grasp the lid and unscrew it.

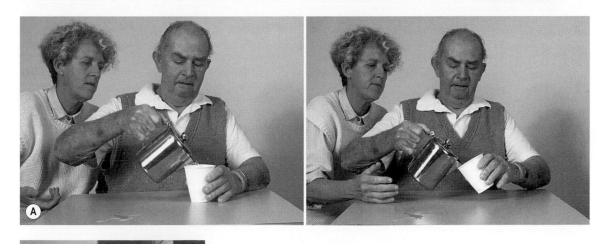

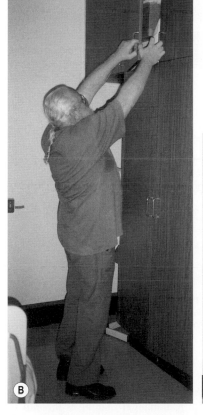

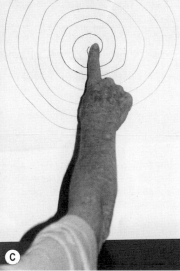

Figure 6.18 A selection of exercises while holding arm(s) raised. (A) Pouring water from one vessel to the other. He is living at home and wants to improve dexterity and avoid clumsiness with kitchen equipment. (B) It is important to organize practice of actions performed with arms reaching above the head. Even when arm elevation can be achieved, muscles often lack the endurance to keep them elevated longer. (C) Tracing the circle requires smooth controlled action. Arm elevation increases endurance of active muscles.

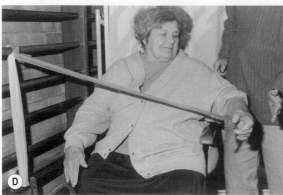

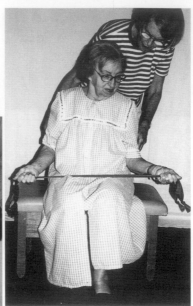

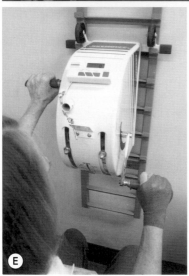

Figure 6.18 *continued* (D) Some examples of elastic band exercises. This exercise to strengthen external rotator muscles is particularly important and can be started early in rehabilitation with the easiest of the bands. (E) Arm cycling is useful for independent practice.

In everyday life, actions performed bimanually are more common than unimanual actions (Kilbreath & Heard 2005). In patients with a predominantly unilateral pattern of dysfunction it is likely that training needs initially to emphasize muscle activation and task practice using the affected limb. 'Forced' use of the affected limb by constraint of the less affected limb may be critical to maximizing recovery of function in individuals who have muscle activation and some use of the affected limb. However, it should be expected that, even with potentially useful recovery of this limb, functionally effective bilateral hand use will not be automatically acquired without bimanual practice (Fig. 6.19).

Bimanual training should therefore begin early, as soon as the patient has the ability to control simple movements with the affected limb. Bimanual training is thought to permit interhemispheric facilitation of the limbs (Parlow & Dewey 1991). From an early stage, the patient practises simple tasks in which both hands work cooperatively to hold and manipulate an object, using each hand to perform a different action (open a can, dial a telephone) and to work together in tasks in which the two hands do the same action either in the same direction (using a rolling pin or rolling up a towel), or in opposite directions (using gardening shears) or in rhythmical sequential actions like arm cycling. Other exercises to stimulate active

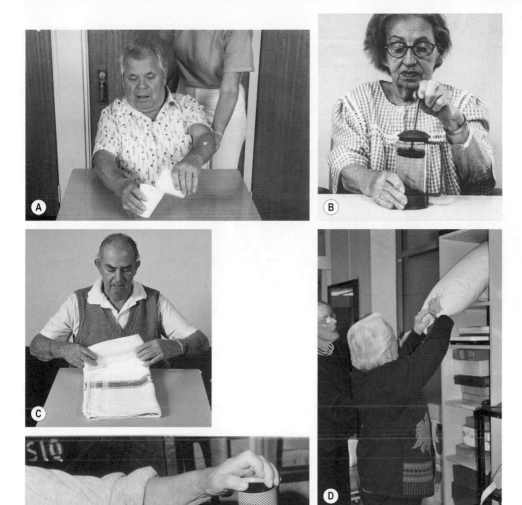

Figure 6.19 Practice of bimanual actions gives opportunity to regain the ability to time movement and coordinate actions of both limbs. (A) It is an effort pouring accurately while holding arms at shoulder height. (B) Exerting the appropriate amount of force takes practice. (C) When folding a towel the two hands work together. (D) Reaching above the head. (E) Lifting the lid.

use of the limbs include push-ups against the wall, folding a towel, scooping coins off a tabletop into the other hand, removing lids from jars and cans, pouring from one polystyrene cup to another without deforming the cup, progressing to pouring from jug to cup, reaching up to a cupboard, using a screwdriver and so on.

Patients also need intensive practice of tasks which require the two limbs to time their movements to an external event (e.g., catching a ball) and which require the ability to make sensitive responses to environmental demands (Fig. 6.20).

There is some research interest in bilateral activation as a possible means of enhancing movement of the impaired limb after stroke. Two small studies reported by Mudie & Matyas (1996) demonstrated that it is possible to improve unilateral movements of a moderately severely affected

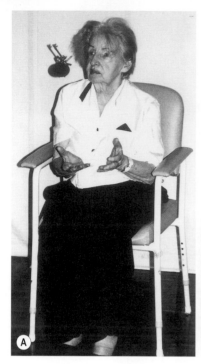
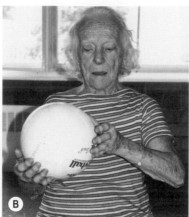
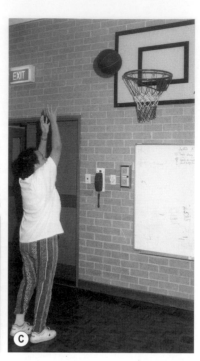

Figure 6.20 Tasks requiring external timing control or precision are also practised in an upper limb training class. (A) Catching keys. (B) Rolling a ball between hands. (C) Basketball.

upper limb after stroke by using bimanual simultaneous practice. Three tasks were practised – block placement, simulated drinking and peg targeting. Performance of these tasks was tested with emphasis on accuracy of end-point location. Kinematic parameters including joint angles and temporal aspects of movement were also measured. It was suggested that practice in which the two hands perform the same action might result in permanent reorganization of the normal process of unimanual activation, resulting in improved performance not only in the bimanual actions but also in unilateral actions performed by the affected limb. There is some evidence from patient self-report that there was a transfer into other actions and that patients maintained their gains over a 6-month no-training period.

The authors suggested that improvement in unimanual actions by the affected limb after bilateral practice may be due to an unmasking of existing redundant connections, including uncrossed ipsilateral connections. The positive effects reported by Mudie & Matyas (1996) support the view that the influence of the ipsilateral cortex may be stronger when its function is specifically required (Tanji et al 1988). In a further study, showing improvements in functional use of the affected limb, Mudie & Matyas (2000) proposed that bilateral simultaneous movement might promote interhemispheric disinhibition allowing

reorganization, including the construction of new task-relevant neural networks.

Findings from several other clinical studies report positive effects of structured bimanual training. Whitall and colleagues (2000) combined principles of forced use and task specificity in bimanual repetitive upper limb training with rhythmic auditory cueing using a training device (BATRAC). Participants were more than 6 months following a stroke. They sat with upper body constrained, held two handles and performed pushing/pulling movements of both arms. Movements were simultaneous and alternating, the metronome cueing at their preferred speed. Significant improvements were found in functional performance, isometric strength and actual daily arm use, and benefits were retained for 8 weeks after completion of the study.

In another study of BATRAC training (McCombe Waller & Whitall 2004) using similar methodology and subjects, participants were tested on a repetitive finger tapping task. They tapped with the index finger of both hands, either in phase or antiphase. Deficits in fine motor control were noted in both paretic and non-paretic hands, with some generalization from the repetitive reaching training to improved repetitive finger movement in some participants. When BATRAC training was tested against a standardized dose-matched programme based on neurodevelopmental principles, significant changes in brain activation were seen in contralesional sensorimotor areas and ipsilesional cerebellum (via fMRI) in six of the nine patients who had BATRAC training, and these six individuals also showed significantly greater improvement in functional outcome compared to the neurodevelopmental group (Luft et al 2004).

In some studies of complex bimanual tasks in individuals with brain lesions, however, the impaired limb seemed to constrain the less impaired limb, the movement pattern of the less impaired limb degrading to match the impaired limb's performance (Lewis & Byblow 2004). More research is needed on the contribution of bimanual upper limb training in individuals with unilateral brain lesions. However, enough is understood about the control of interlimb coordination both to encourage greater use of bimanual task-oriented training in various forms and to make obvious the need for repetitive practice.

Forced use of a limb

In the 1980s, Taub showed, with both deafferented and hemiplegic monkeys, that a paralysed or insensate arm would be left to hang by the side when there was one effective upper limb (Taub 1980). He referred to this behaviour as 'learned non-use', suggesting that the monkeys learned *not* to use the affected limb, that non-use was a conditioned suppression of movement. However, when the intact limb was restrained and the monkey was trained to use the affected limb with feedback rewards, the affected limb became functional.

Promising results in humans have also been reported in adults after stroke (Taub et al 1993; Morris et al 1997; Miltner et al 1999; Wolf et al 2002; Alberts et al 2004; Page et al 2004). Some studies of task-oriented training that report positive findings included in their programme constraint of the non-paretic limb. A combination of meaningful and intensive task training, practice in using the affected arm and a strategy to force use of that limb can be effective in individuals who can at the very least actively extend wrist and fingers. Constraint prevents the non-paretic limb from taking over and may overcome this conditioned response by creating a real necessity to use the limb. Contrast this with a hospital and rehabilitation setting that makes only limited demands on the person, providing little incentive to use the impaired limb. Added to this, therapists may provide a sling in order to prevent glenohumeral joint subluxation or for comfort. The results of the early experiments with monkeys suggest that holding the paretic limb in a sling may encourage learned non-use of the limb, contrary to the best intentions of the rehabilitation team.

In hemiplegia, some patients, although they regain active use of the affected limb, prefer to use the other limb. Although it may appear that the hand has useful function, it is unlikely to be used if movement is too slow, takes too much effort or if sensation is impaired. Preferring the unaffected hand may be more likely in those whose non-dominant hand is affected, although this has not been tested. Constraint-induced movement therapy (CIMT), developed by Edward Taub and colleagues out of his experiments with monkeys, may be particularly effective in this group of people, who may benefit greatly from a period of intensive task-oriented training and practice. In CIMT, the non-impaired limb is usually constrained by a sling or a mitt for several hours of the day, with the need to use the impaired limb exclusively for all daily tasks. This is in addition to a time being set aside for practice of specific tasks. Most studies of the effects of CIMT have involved patients with minimal to low upper limb functional ability (Miltner et al 1999; Bonifer et al 2005; Dettmers et al 2005; Uswatte et al 2006).

Benefits can last for as long as 24 months (Miltner et al 1999; Wolf et al 2008). Some studies have shown considerable improvement in the actual amount of use of the limb in the real world (Taub et al 1993; Kunkel et al 1999). Studies of brain reorganization show an association between increased use of the affected limb, improved motor performance and brain reorganization (Liepert et al 1998, 2000, 2001). Individuals appear to tolerate the constraint well (Dromerick et al 2000).

The first results of a multicentre trial (EXCITE) were published in 2006 and show significant improvements in functional performance and paretic arm use compared to control groups (Wolf et al 2006, 2007, 2008). This trial studied the effects of intervention in individuals with stroke occurring 3 to 9 months earlier. Participants wore a restraining mitt on the non-paretic hand for 90% of the waking day, and carried out a standardized programme of repetitive task practice of functional activities and training of the paretic limb every week day for up to 6 hours per day for 2 weeks. Change was measured using the Wolf Motor Function Test, the Motor Activity Log, a measure of real-time use of the limb, and the Stroke Impact Scale. The results show that a combination of intensive, repetitive, meaningful task training, practice and a strategy that creates a real necessity to move the affected limb can be effective in individuals who can actively extend the wrist and fingers. Constraint prevents the unaffected limb from taking over and may overcome the conditioned response.

Guidelines for a procedure to use in the clinic can be gathered from the studies cited above. Taub and colleagues (1993), in their randomized controlled trial, restrained their subjects (a median of 4 years post-stroke) during waking hours (except during certain activities: excretory functions, activities where balance might be compromised, when sleeping) for 14 days. The unaffected limb was constrained in a resting hand splint and sling. Each week day, patients spent 7 hours at the rehabilitation centre. They were given a variety of tasks to be carried out over 6 hours while movement of the unaffected limb was constrained. The constrained group achieved marked change, from an initially severe motor impairment to improved motor function and lifestyle. Furthermore, this group maintained their improvement over a 2-year period. It is important to note that, to be eligible to be included in the study, patients had to be able to extend their fingers (MCP and interphalangeal joints) at least 10° and their wrist at least 20°.

A biomechanical study of arm movement (reaching forward to a target and taking the hand to the mouth) illustrated the kinematic effects of motor recovery associated with constraint-induced training (Caimmi et al 2008). The results showed that increased use of the limb was a consequence of improved speed of movement and better coordination between shoulder and elbow. A study that examined muscle force production after a period of CIMT (Alberts et al 2004) found a reduction in variability of muscle forces suggesting that increased control of muscle forces and increased speed of task completion explained the improvements in dexterity.

In the protocol shown in Box 6.4 we have outlined a methodology similar to that used in testing CIMT outcomes and using methodology developed by Taub and Wolf. This protocol could be followed for 2 weeks initially and objectively tested before and after the completion of the contraint programme. Task practice should be continued for longer if necessary.

Note that it is important to ensure the individual's understanding of and compliance with the constraint. Therefore:

- teach the person how to put on and take off the constraint independently
- in making a behavioural contract with each person, work from their daily routine to decide which activities to carry out with constraint and which require two hands
- request a diary be filled in to enable monitoring of the activities outside therapy time.

Supplementary methods

Mental practice

Mental practice has been used for many years as part of sports training and is currently of general interest in rehabilitation (see Ch. 2). Mental practice, in which simple physical actions are rehearsed in the mind, may assist some patients by focusing attention on the action to be performed (Page et al 2001). This may be particularly useful for the person who is unable to practise reaching and manipulative actions physically, and can be carried out by the person independently once they can visualize performance clearly. There is some evidence that it may play a part in improving task performance after stroke (Page 2000; Page et al 2001; Crosbie et al 2004; Dijkerman et al 2004; Liu 2004). A systematic review (Zimmerman-Schlatter et al 2008) concluded that there is

---

> **Box 6.4 Protocol for task-specific training plus constraint**
>
> *Criteria for inclusion*
> - Wolf's Minimum Motor Criteria: ability to extend wrist at least 20°, interphalangeal and MCP finger joints at least 10°
> - Willingness of patient to attend initially for a training programme 5 days per week for 2 weeks
>
> *Constraint*
> - Hand splint with wrist of non-paretic arm in some extension + sling, or mitt/glove + reminders not to use the non-paretic limb
> - Wear splint for a prescribed number of hours on each week day for 2 weeks
>
> *Behavioural contract*
> - Seek agreement with patient about activities to be performed without constraint: e.g., bathing, parts of dressing, activities where balance may be an issue and, with constraint: e.g., eating, grooming, toileting, some domestic tasks
>
> *Programme of exercises*
> - Prescribed number of hours of task-oriented training and practice for the paretic limb + home practice
>
> *Measurement*
> - Performed before and after 2-week programme and after a few weeks (for retention)

---

modest evidence to support the benefits of motor imagery for patients with upper limb dysfunction.

In the first edition we referred to the relationship between mental practice and brain reorganization. In early work on mental simulation or imagery of motor actions, cerebral blood flow studies suggested that the same central structures that are involved in the physical performance are part of the network involved (Salford et al 1995). Mental practice can promote modulation of neural circuits during the early stage of learning a complicated finger exercise and cortical motor output maps showed that mental practice could lead to the same plastic changes in the motor system as those occurring with repetitive physical practice (Pascuol-Leone et al 1995). More recent brain imaging studies confirm these findings (Gerardin et al 2000; Hanakawa et al 2003).

Electrical stimulation

Successful rehabilitation of upper limb function is dependent on the patient being able to regain the ability to activate muscles and to control segmental movements necessary for functional actions. It is also critical to minimize the secondary disuse changes that occur as a result of immobility. There has been renewed interest in the potential for newer electrostimulation technologies to stimulate motor learning (Chae & Yu 1999).

When modern scientific scrutiny is applied to various means of applying electrical stimulation (ES), the effects on muscle and nerve are not clear, although this modality has been used in physiotherapy for decades. Although it is used to stimulate muscle activity, its effect on the re-establishing of voluntary muscle activation is not known.

Various forms of neuromuscular ES, including functional electrical stimulation (FES), and the use of multiple contraction sites to evoke a particular pattern of muscle activity have been shown to have positive effects. These effects have included improved performance of active wrist and finger extension (Dimitrijevic et al 1996; Glanz et al 1996; Pandyan et al 1996; Hummelsheim et al 1997; Chae et al 1998; Powell et al 1999). ES to the hand via mesh-glove afferent stimuli (Dimitrijevic et al 1996) demonstrated increased EMG activity in wrist extensors, and increased amplitude of active wrist extension. All participants had some volitional control of wrist extension prior to the ES. A few studies have reported a carryover to improved functional performance. A study of a home-based programme of FES after stroke (Alon et al 2003) reported subjects were able to move faster on dexterity tests such as the Jebsen-Taylor, box and block and nine-hole peg tests. Although upper limb function may improve in the short term, there may be no long term retention (Sonde et al 2000). As Yu and colleagues (2001) have pointed out, it is likely that beneficial effects of ES will be retained only in patients who have regained some functional use of the limb.

Some investigations have examined, with positive functional outcomes, the effects of coupling intent with stimulation, that is combining active voluntary exercise for specific muscles and ES (Kraft et al 1992; Hummelsheim et al 1996; Francisco et al 1998; Sullivan & Hedman 2004). One study that has done this has shown that *EMG-triggered ES*, where the patient's voluntary muscle contraction is assisted by ES, can produce positive effects on functional motor performance more than 1 year after a stroke (Cauraugh et al 2000). This study set out to train wrist and finger extension because absence of controlled wrist and finger extension is recognized as a common cause of disability in hand use and the ability to sustain extension is critical for use of the fingers in most hand activities. In addition, patients performed multiple repetitions, as many as 360 repetitions over the course of one training programme. The positive effects of combining active practice of simple but critical movements with the assistance of ES included improved performance on the box and block test (grasp, transport and place wooden blocks).

Some recent clinical practice guidelines (Duncan et al 2005) recommend FES for people with impaired muscle contraction, and for those with shoulder subluxation. There is some evidence in systematic reviews of an improvement in shoulder subluxation (Chae & Yu 2000; Price & Pandyan 2001). However, a meta-analysis of studies reporting the effects of FES on shoulder subluxation (Ada & Fongchomcheay 2002) showed that FES given early after stroke can minimize the development of inferior glenohumeral joint displacement, but not prevent subluxation from developing. A Cochrane systematic review (Pomeroy et al 2006) reported significant improvements in some aspects of muscle function and functional ability. It is possible that ES applied to specific task-related muscles in conjunction with a task-specific training programme may be more beneficial than stimulation in the absence of such active training.

The possibility of restorative effects resulting from ES to paretic muscles is not known. Asanuma & Keller (1991) hypothesized some time ago that proprioceptive and cutaneous impulses associated with repetitive movement can induce long-term potentiation in the motor cortex. There is some support for repetitive training of wrist and finger extensors using EMG-triggered ES in individuals with some voluntary muscle activation, but whether it offers any advantage over repetitive volitional and task-oriented training or the new electromechanical and robotic devices is yet to be explored.

Computer-aided, robotic and non-robotic mechanical training devices, virtual reality

Many new technological developments have the potential to augment the training by therapists, to increase time spent in practice of upper limb activities, number of repetitions, the intensity of practice and therefore stimulate motor learning. They may also lead to an increase in actual limb use. It has been suggested that technical aids might help focus a person's attention on critical aspects of training, enhance motivation and provide feedback (Platz 2004). Many devices are intrinsically interesting in themselves, providing novel and exciting ways of exercising mental and physical faculties. To be effective, such devices need to provide repetition and interest. The task being carried out should be challenging and engaging (Plautz et al 2000). It should also be meaningful for the individual.

Computer games. An early study of computerized training demonstrated the effectiveness of an interesting and interactive computer game (Krichevets et al 1995). The subject was a boy of 13 years with Erb's palsy who had virtually no voluntary movement in his arm. He interacted with the game by moving a cursor. Specially devised adjustable controls enabled the required movements to be changed. The game required accuracy in the control of spatial and temporal movement parameters At the end of training the boy could activate shoulder external rotator muscles that were previously inactive and he was able to raise the arm forward almost to shoulder height without adaptive movements. The findings supported the growing understanding that the most effective exercises are those in which the patient acts voluntarily, is an active participant and is motivated by the task itself and the desire to succeed.

Robotic and non-robotic devices. Devices are also being developed that enable increased repetitions of simple movements to be performed even by people with minimal muscle activity. The MIT-Manus robotic device (Hogan & Krebs 2004) provides graded assistance and as the person gains some control over the arm the assistance is decreased. Increasing challenges, including added resistance, can also be provided. A robot-assisted trainer, the Bi-Manu-Track (Hesse et al 2003), allows bilateral passive and active practice of forearm pronation/supination and wrist flexion/extension.

There is emerging evidence of the positive effects of various forms of robot-mediated training for upper limb function (Volpe et al 2000; Lum et al 2002a,b; Coote & Stokes 2005; Colombo et al 2008). For example, robot training can improve muscle activity during reaching. Automated arm movement training (Platz et al 2005) and robot-assisted therapy (Fasoli et al 2004; Hesse et al 2006; Wu et al 2006) are reported to reduce impairment and improve muscle activity and function. However, overall, the results of carryover into improved functional performance are equivocal so far (Krebs et al 2002; Gallichio & Kluding 2004; Hesse et al 2006; Lam et al 2006). Results may improve when robot-assisted training is placed within the context of an intensive task-focused exercise and training programme.

Non-robotic training device. A non-robotic training device has recently been developed for individuals with a severe upper limb paresis as a means of exercising the paretic limb, enabling the person with severe paresis to participate actively in intensive repetitive task-oriented practice (Barker et al 2008). The Sensorimotor Active Rehabilitation Training (SMART) Arm (Fig. 6.21) can be used in conjunction with EMG-triggered ES. The device was developed to train a reaching action made simple by decreasing both the available degrees of freedom and the resistance. The load can be increased to increase the force requirement. Two groups of participants at least 6 months post-stroke underwent three 60-minute training sessions per week for 4 weeks at home. The training dose was set at 60 repetitions per session (6 sets of 10) for the first three sessions, and at 80 repetitions for nine sessions. Subjects reached to a target and load was increased after 10 successful repetitions. One group also received EMG-triggered ES to the triceps brachii muscle. All participants scored 3 or less on the Motor Assessment Scale upper arm function item (unable to hold arm horizontal) at the start of the trial. Both groups that trained on the SMART trainer could reach further, were stronger, had better functional arm

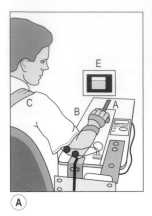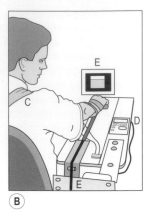

Figure 6.21 A non-robotic training device, the Sensorimotor Active Rehabilitation Training (SMART) Arm (NeuroTrac 5, Verity Medical Ltd). Note that positioning can be set up so that the reaching action includes external rotation of the GH joint as it is flexed forward. Shoulder movement can also be practised in standing by elevating the mechanism. *(Courtesy of Dr Ruth Barker, James Cook University, Townsville, Australia).*

movement (Motor Assessment Scale scores), decreased resistance to passive elbow movement (Modified Ashworth Scale), and improvements were retained for 2 months. The third group of control subjects showed no change.

Virtual reality. Virtual environments are also designed to aid motor learning. Enriched virtual environments have been developed that present a task requiring problem solving in order to acquire a skill (Deutsche et al 2004). This new technology is being investigated in clinical populations. Improvements in motor activity have been reported; for example, a decrease in hemispatial neglect after a training programme using a virtual hand (Castiello et al 2004). Improved limb control during pouring tasks was reported in an early study of four young subjects with traumatic brain injury who were trained on virtual pouring tasks (Holden & Dyar 2002). Training in virtual environments plus use of a haptic (tactile) device resulted in improved manual dexterity, grip force and motor control (Broeren et al 2004).

Developments of new technological devices is at the experimental stage and many are expensive. Nevertheless, the possibilities for future development of cheaper, effective trainers are exciting.

Orthoses and passive stretching

Slings and orthoses are frequently recommended as a means of holding a limb in what is considered an 'optimum' position in order to prevent soft tissue contracture and also to stretch already short muscles. However, splinting may not have the beneficial effects intended. In a randomized controlled trial, subjects within 6 months of stroke wore a hand splint, with the hand in 10–30° of extension, for up to 12 hours at night for 4 weeks (Lannin et al 2003). No significant effects were found. A systematic review in 2003 found insufficient evidence to support or refute the effectiveness of hand splinting after stroke (Lannin & Herbert 2003). However, in a later study by Lannin and colleagues (2007), individuals within 2 months of a stroke wore a hand splint either in a neutral position or with wrist and fingers fully extended in a protocol similar to the earlier study. Neither splint significantly increased extensibility of wrist and long finger flexors and patients showed 22° less extension compared to baseline. There is therefore no evidence so far in support of hand splints worn overnight.

Casting to prevent predictable muscle length changes following traumatic brain injury may be effective when the individual is unconscious. Serial casting to stretch shortened muscles may also become necessary. Most investigations of serial casting have been of the lower limb. However, casting can also be used to stretch muscles or reduce dystonic spasms in the upper limb (Kitson 1991). (For a description of casting, refer to Ch. 12.)

In individuals with problems activating and controlling hand muscles, the thumb typically lies in an adducted position and web space soft tissues rapidly become short. In training, it may be helpful to support the thumb in a small orthosis so that the carpometacarpal joint is maintained in some abduction and opposition. The splint serves to maintain passively the extent of the grasp aperture so that, in the absence of active thumb abduction, the soft tissues between thumb metacarpal and index metacarpal may not shorten. A small splint can allow hand use and encourage thumb participation in reaching and grasping tasks.

The need for a sling to support the paretic upper limb in stroke is questionable and raises the issue of whether a sling can be a potent factor in causing learned non-use of the limb and adaptive muscle shortening. The use of slings that hold the glenohumeral joint in internal rotation and adduction should be discontinued. The issue of shoulder supports is discussed in the Appendix to Chapter 11.

Passive stretching to paretic muscles, usually by positioning the limb, as a means of preserving muscle length and preventing contracture may be provided in the clinic for those people who cannot actively move the limb. Evidence from animal studies suggests that intermittent stretch for 30 minutes a day can prevent soft tissue adaptations that occur with immobility (Williams 1990). Ada and colleagues (2005) found that 30 minutes of positioning in glenohumeral joint external rotation reduced the development of contractures in the internal rotator muscles in patients after stroke. Since contracture of these muscles can occur so easily when the paretic limb is held immobile in the resting position, this positioning programme should be included for those with severe limb weakness (Fig. 6.22).

Although stretching may give some temporary relief to the patient, it is unlikely that length can be preserved in the absence of active movement and the evidence so far suggests that this may be so. Four weeks of daily stretch to wrist and finger flexors for 30 minutes to people after stroke with no active wrist extension resulted in no worthwhile effect (Horsley et al 2007). Similar discouraging results have been found in other studies (Turton & Britton 2005). Passive stretching via positioning may, however, have a beneficial effect if started early after stroke, in those with weak but active muscles, in preventing shortening and stiffness that develop quickly in shoulder muscles in particular but also in wrist muscles. Nevertheless, the only effective way to preserve muscle length is by active movements that stretch the muscles through their functional ranges.

The evidence suggests that critical features in training of the upper limb include the following:

- An early start to active and challenging exercise and task practice.
- Simple repetitive exercises to improve activation and control of weak muscles.
- Task-related training to improve functional strength, power, endurance, motor control and skill.
- Opportunity to practise intensively during the day, supervised, in groups and independently, with bi- and unimanual tasks.
- Prevention of soft tissue adaptations, particularly muscle shortening, loss of extensibility and stiffness.
- Forced use of the affected limb with constraint of the unaffected limb and intensive training and practice.
- Avoiding one-arm drive wheelchairs and slings that impose immobility on the limb.

Practice is likely to be enhanced and intensity increased by activities that provide motivation and incentive (meaningful, challenging and concrete tasks); use of games, exercise machines and robotic, electromechanical, virtual, computer-controlled devices to enable active practice, and mental practice.

In conclusion, the major impairments affecting the upper limb following an acute brain lesion are weakness due to diminished motor outflow to muscles, diminished sensory inputs and the secondary impairments resulting from disuse and immobility. The real picture of recovery of upper limb function after an acute brain lesion may reflect not only the level of initial impairment but also the amount and type of physical training and practice available to the person, and whether or not there is a compulsion to use the limb.

Major factors in poor recovery may be the minimal time spent in active training (10 minutes per day – Goldie et al 1992; Bernhardt et al 2004; Ada et al 2006) and the use of outdated therapy methods that are more often passive than active. The clinical literature on rehabilitation of

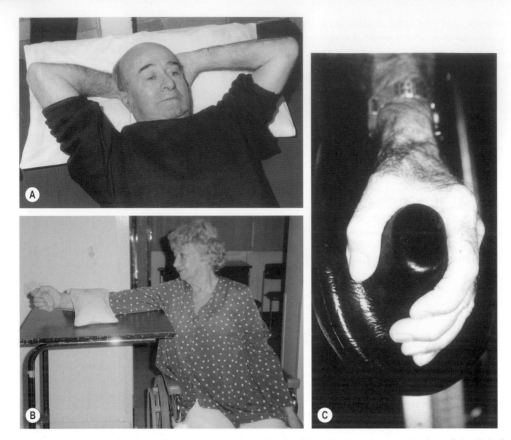

Figure 6.22 During the day, when the person is not involved in active practise, positioning of the limb for approximately 30 mins may prevent stiffness and contracture from developing in vulnerable muscles. (A) & (B) To stretch GH internal rotator and adductor muscles. (C) A gutter with thumb piece to prevent pronator and thumb adductor muscle shortening.

upper limb function suggests, however, that there are currently changes occurring in clinical practice with an increasing interest in the use of the more active and challenging methods that are task-related and involve specific training and repetitive exercise. These methods are based in science, specifically on findings in the movement sciences, including neuroscience, biomechanics and exercise science. There are promising signs that intensive task-oriented training is effective, and recent systematic reviews are providing us with some evidence.

It is also becoming obvious that rehabilitation units must work out ways to increase the amount of time people spend on task. In the case of post-stroke inpatient rehabilitation, for example, facilities should be available for people to spend a modified 'working day' concentrating on learning to use both upper limbs in essential daily tasks, as well as on learning to walk independently and regaining balance stability. The use of group circuit training at upper limb work stations enables more practice time than the traditional one-to-one mode of delivery favoured by many therapists. Aides and therapists can supervise practice, the therapist training individuals when necessary.

What the severely impaired person can accomplish with exercise and training is not known and how long such training should persist is not known, yet the methods for seeking the answer to this question currently exist. It may be that some patients with paralysed hand muscles early after stroke will recover little if any functional use. Those with some muscle activity in the wrist and hand may do well if intervention begins early, is active and intense and frequent through the day, and if training emphasizes repetitive exercise, meaningful task-oriented training, forced use of the affected limb(s) and bimanual exercise.

The process of therapy itself, the methods used, may be a major factor in reorganization of motor control systems, together with the rehabilitation environment. Some of the older therapies were relatively passive, lacking active participation of the patient. The focus was proximally, on the shoulder girdle and trunk, rather than on the hand (see comments by Butefisch et al 1995). It is also clear that a very small percentage of the day may be spent in activities related to the affected upper limb when the total time spent in therapy is examined. Although therapists may think they are addressing their interventions to the affected limb, the patient is still able to use the non-paretic limb for many functional activities both during and after therapy sessions, and most actions are, therefore, carried out by this limb. There is still too much emphasis on slings and splints and one-arm propelled wheelchairs, all of which constrain the affected limb, prevent its use and may mitigate against any potential for recovery of the affected limb. Too little time is spent in stroke rehabilitation in promoting active use of the upper limb, after stroke in particular, with intensive training in important tasks and in exercise.

The evidence from reading some current physiotherapy texts is that early, active and vigorous upper limb functional training is still neglected in rehabilitation (Turton 1998). Intervention may still consist of passive interventions, including passive or assisted movements focused on the trunk and shoulder girdle and splinting for the shoulder and hand. Fifteen years ago, Butefisch and colleagues (1995) commented that hand function, specifically voluntary activation of distal arm and hand musculature, was typically not addressed in commonly used physiotherapy approaches. It is time for change and we should make the opportunity to take the next step in improving the rehabilitation process and turn it into the active, intensive and challenging process it could be.

REFERENCES

Ada L, Fongchomcheay A 2002 Efficacy of electrical stimulation in preventing or reducing subluxation of the shoulder after stroke: a meta-analysis. Aust J Physiother 48:257–267.

Ada L, Canning C, Paratz J 1990 Care of the unconscious head-injured patient. In: Ada L, Canning C (eds) Key issues in neurological physiotherapy. Butterworth Heinemann, Oxford:249–288.

Ada L, Canning C, Kilbreath SL et al 1994 Task-specific training of reaching and manipulation. In: Bennett KMB, Castiello U (eds) Insights into the reach to grasp movement. Elsevier, Amsterdam:239–268.

Ada L, Canning CG, Low S-L 2003 Stroke patients have selective weakness in shortened range. Brain 126:724–731.

Ada L, Goddard E, McCully J et al 2005 Thirty minutes of positioning reduces the development of shoulder external rotation contractures after stroke: a randomized controlled trial. Arch Phys Med Rehabil 86:230–234.

Ada L, O'Dwyer N, O'Neill E 2006 Relation between spasticity, weakness and contracture of the elbow flexors and upper activity after stroke: an observational study. Disabil Rehabil 28:891–897.

Alberts J, Butler A, Wolf SL 2004 The effects of constraint-induced movement therapy on precision grip: a preliminary study. Neurorehabil Neural Repair 18:250–258.

Alon G, Sunnerhagen KS, Geurts AC et al 2003 A home-based self-administered stimulation program to improve selected hand functions in chronic stroke. Neurorehabilitation 18:215–225.

Arbib MA, Iberall T, Lyons D 1985 Coordinated control programs for control of the hands. In: Goodwin AW, Darian-Smith I (eds) Hand function and the neocortex. Exp Brain Res Suppl 10, Springer-Verlag, Berlin:111–129.

Asanuma H, Keller A 1991 Neuronal mechanisms of motor learning in mammals. Neuroreport 2:217–224.

Balliet R, Levy B, Blood KMT 1986 Upper extremity sensory feedback therapy in chronic cerebrovascular accident patients with impaired expressive aphasia and auditory comprehension. Arch Phys Med Rehabil 67:304–310.

Barker RN, Brauer SG, Carson R 2008 Training of reaching in stroke survivors with severe and chronic upper limb paresis using a novel nonrobotic device: a randomized clinical trial. Stroke 39:1800–1807.

Bastian AJ, Martin TA, Keating JG et al 1996 Cerebellar ataxia: abnormal control of interaction torques across multiple joints. J Neurophysiol 76:492–509.

Bastian AJ, Zachowski AM, Thach WT et al 2000 Cerebellar ataxia: torque deficiency or torque mismatch between joints. J Neurophysiol 83:3019–3030.

Beaubaton D, Hay L 1986 Contribution of visual information to feedforward and feedback processes in rapid pointing movements. Hum Mov Sci 5:19–34.

Bendz P 1993 The functional significance of the fifth metacarpus and hypothenar in two useful grips of the hand. Amer J Phys Med Rehabil 72:210–213.

Bernhardt J, Dewey HM, Thrift AG et al 2004 Inactive and alone: physical activity in the first 14 days of acute stroke unit care. Stroke 35:1005–1009.

Bertram CP, Lemay M, Stelmach GE 2005 The effect of Parkinson's disease on the control of multisegmental coordination. Brain Cogn 57:16–20.

Biguer B, Jeannerod M, Prablanc C 1982 The coordination of eye, head and hand movements during reaching at a single visual target. Exp Brain Res 46:301–304.

Blennerhassett J, Dite W 2004 Additional task-related practice improves mobility and upper limb function early after stroke: a randomized controlled trial. Aust J Physiother 50:219–224.

Boissy P, Bourbonnais D, Carlotti MM et al 1999 Maximal grip force in chronic stroke subjects and its relationship to global upper extremity function. Clin Rehabil 13:354–362.

Bonifer NM, Anderson KM, Arciniagas DB 2005 Constraint-induced movement therapy after stroke: efficacy for patients with minimal upper-extremity motor ability. Arch Phys Med Rehabil 86:1867–1873.

Bouisset S, Zattara M 1981 A sequence of postural movements precedes voluntary movement. Neurosci Lett 22:263–270.

Bourbonnais D, Vanden-Noven S, Carey KM et al 1989 Abnormal spatial patterns of elbow muscle activation in hemiparetic human subjects. Brain 112:85–102.

Broeren J, Rydmark M, Sunnerhagen KS et al 2004 Virtual reality and haptics as a training device for movement rehabilitation after stroke: a single case study. Arch Phys Med Rehabil 85:1247–1250.

Burke D 1988 Spasticity as an adaptation to pyramidal tract injury. Adv Neurol 47:401–423.

Butefisch C, Hummelsheim H, Mauritz K-H 1995 Repetitive training of isolated movements improves the outcome of motor rehabilitation of the centrally paretic hand. J Neurol Sci 130:59–68.

Byl N, Roderick J, Mohamed O et al 2003 Effectiveness of sensory and motor rehabilitation of the upper limb following the principles of neuroplasticity: patients stable poststroke. Neurorehabil Neural Repair 17:176–191.

Caimmi M, Carda S, Giovanzana C et al 2008 Using kinematic analysis to evaluate constraint-induced movement therapy in chronic stroke patients. Neurorehabil Neural Repair 2:31–39.

Carey JR, Kimberley TJ, Lewis SM et al 2002 Analysis of fMRI and finger tracking in subjects with chronic stroke. Brain 125:773–788.

Carr JH, Shepherd RB 1987a A motor relearning programme for stroke, Butterworth Heinemann, Oxford.

Carr JH, Shepherd RB (eds) 1987b Movement science. Foundations for physical therapy in rehabilitation. Aspen, Rockville, MD.

Carr JH, Shepherd RB 1996 'Normal' is not the issue: it is 'effective' goal attainment that counts. Behav Brain Sci 19:72–73.

Carr JH, Shepherd RB 1998 Neurological rehabilitation. Optimising motor performance. Butterworth Heinemann, Oxford.

Carr JH, Shepherd RB 2003 Stroke rehabilitation. Guidelines for exercise and training to optimize motor skill. Butterworth Heinemann, Oxford.

Carr JH, Shepherd RB, Nordholm L et al 1985 A motor assessment scale for stroke. Phys Ther 65:175–180.

Castiello U, Bennett KMB, Paulignan Y 1992 Does the type of prehension influence the kinematics of reaching? Behav Brain Res 50:7–15.

Castiello U, Bennett KMB, Stelmach GE 1993 The bilateral reach to grasp movement. Behav Brain Res 56:43–57.

Castiello U, Lusher D, Burton C et al 2004 Improving left hemispatial neglect using virtual reality. Neurol 62:1958–1962.

Cauraugh J, Light K, Dangbum K et al 2000 Chronic motor dysfunction after stroke: recovering wrist and finger extension by electromyography-triggered neuromuscular stimulation. Stroke 31:1360–1364.

Chae J, Yu D 1999 Neuromuscular stimulation for motor relearning in hemiplegia. Crit Rev Phys Rehabil Med 11:279–297.

Chae J, Yu D 2000 A critical review of neuromuscular electrical stimulation for treatment of motor dysfunction in hemiplegia. Assist Technol 12:33–49.

Chae J, Bethoux F, Bohinc T et al 1998 Neuromuscular stimulation for upper extremity motor and functional recovery in acute hemiplegia. Stroke 29:975–979.

Chae J, Yang G, Park BK et al 2002 Muscle weakness and cocontraction in upper limb hemiparesis: relationship to motor impairment and physical disability. Neurorehabil Neural Repair 16:241–248.

Chao EYS, An K-N, Cooney WP et al 1989 Biomechanics of the hand. World Scientific Publishing, Singapore.

Cirstea MC, Levin MF 2000 Compensatory strategies for reaching in stroke. Brain 123:940–953.

Cirstea MC, Mitnitski AB, Feldman AG et al 2003 Interjoint coordination dynamics during reaching in stroke. Exp Brain Res 151:289–300.

Colebatch JG, Gandevia SC 1989 The distribution of muscular weakness in upper motor neuron lesions affecting the arm. Brain 112:749–763.

Colebatch JG, Gandevia SC, Spira PJ 1986 Voluntary muscle strength in hemiparesis: distribution of weakness at the elbow. J Neurol Neurosurg Psychiatry 49:1019–1024.

Colebatch JG, Rothwell JC, Day BL et al 1990 Cortical outflow to proximal arm muscles in man. Brain 113:1843–1856.

Colombo R, Pisano F, Micera S et al 2008 Assessing mechanisms of recovery during robot-assisted neurorehabilitation of the upper limb. Neurorehabil Neural Repair 22:50–63.

Coote S, Stokes EK 2001 Physiotherapy for upper extremity dysfunction following stroke. Phys Ther Rev 6:63–69.

Coote S, Stokes EK 2005 Effect of robot-mediated therapy on upper extremity dysfunction post-stroke – a single case study. Physiotherapy 91:250–256.

Cordo PJ, Nashner LM 1982 Properties of postural adjustments associated with rapid arm movements. J Neurophysiol 47:287–302.

Crosbie J, Shepherd RB, Squires TJ 1995 Postural and voluntary movement during reaching in sitting: the role of the lower limbs. J Hum Mov Studies 28:103–126.

Crosbie JH, McDonough SM, Gilmore DH et al 2004 The adjunctive role of mental practice in the rehabilitation of the upper limb after hemiplegic stroke: a pilot study. Clin Rehabil 18:60–68.

Davis JZ 2006 Task selection and enriched environments: a functional upper extremity training program for stroke survivors. Top Stroke Rehabil 13:1–11.

Dean C, Mackey F 1992 Motor assessment scale scores as a measure of rehabilitation outcome following stroke. Aust J Physiother 38:31–35.

Dean C, Shepherd RB 1997 Task-related training improves performance of seated reaching tasks following stroke: a randomised controlled trial. Stroke 28:1–7.

Dean C, Shepherd R, Adams R 1999 Sitting balance 1: trunk–arm and the contribution of the lower limbs during self-paced reaching in sitting. Gait Posture 10:135–144.

Dettmers C, Teske U, Hamzei F et al 2005 Distributed form of constraint-induced movement therapy improves functional outcome and quality of life after stroke. Arch Phys Med Rehabil 86:204–209.

Deutsche JE, Merians AS, Adamovich S et al 2004 Development and application of virtual reality technology to improve hand use and gait of individuals post-stroke. Restor Neurol Neurosci 22:371–386.

Diedrichsen J, Verstynen T, Lehman SL et al 2005 Cerebellar involvement in anticipating the consequences of self-produced actions during bimanual movements. J Neurophysiol 93:801–812.

Dijkerman HC, Ietswaart M, Johnston M et al 2004 Does motor imagery training improve hand recovery in chronic stroke patients? A pilot study. Clin Rehabil 18:538–549.

Dimitrijevic MM, Stokic DS, Wawro AW et al 1996 Modification of motor control of wrist extension by mesh-glove electrical afferent stimulation in stroke patients. Arch Phys Med Rehabil 77:252–258.

Dromerick AW, Edwards D, Hahn M et al 2000 Does the application of constraint-induced movement therapy during acute rehabilitation reduce arm impairment after ischaemic stroke. Stroke 31:2984–2988.

Duncan PW, Zorowitz R, Bates B et al 2005 Management of adult stroke rehabilitation care. A clinical practice guideline. Stroke 36:e100–e143.

Eyler D, Markee J 1954 The anatomy and function of the intrinsic musculature of the fingers. J Bone J Surg 36A:1–10.

Fasoli SE, Trombly CA, Tickle-Degnen L et al 2002 Effect of instructions on functional reach in persons with and without cerebrovascular accident. Am J Occup Ther 56:380–390.

Fasoli SE, Krebs HI, Stein J et al 2004 Robotic therapy for chronic motor impairments after stroke: follow-up results. Arch Phys Med Rehabil 85:1106–1111.

Fellows SJ, Noth J, Schwarz M et al 1998 Precision grip and Parkinson's disease. Brain 121:1171–1184.

Fikes TG, Klatzky RL, Lederman SJ 1994 Effects of object texture on precontact movement time in human prehension. J Mot Behav 26:325–332.

Flanagan JR, Wing JM 1993 Modulation of grip force with load force during point-to-point arm movements. Exp Brain Res 95:131–143.

Flanagan JR, Ostry DJ, Feldman AG 1993 Control of trajectory modifications in target-directed reaching. J Mot Behav 25:140–152.

Forrest W, Basmajian J 1965 Function of human thenar and hypothenar muscles. J Bone Joint Surg 47A:1585–1594.

Francisco G, Chaie J, Shawla H et al 1998 Electromyogram-triggered neuromuscular stimulation for improving arm function of acute stroke survivors: a randomized pilot study. Arch Phys Med Rehabil 79:570–575.

Gallichio J, Kluding P 2004 Virtual reality in stroke rehabilitation: review of the emerging research. Phys Ther Rev 9:207–212.

Gentile AM 1987 Skill acquisition: action, movement, and neuromotor processes. In: Carr JH, Shepherd RB (eds) Movement science. Foundations for physical therapy in rehabilitation. Aspen, Rockville, MD.

Gerardin E, Sirigu A, Lehericy S et al 2000 Partially overlapping neural networks for real and imagined hand movements. Cereb Cortex 10:1093–1104.

Gibson JJ 1977 The theory of affordances. In: Shaw R, Bransford J (eds) Perceiving, acting and knowing: towards an ecological psychology. Erlbaum, Hillsdale, NJ:67–82.

Glanz M, Klawanski S, Stason W et al 1996 Functional electrostimulation in poststroke rehabilitation: a meta-analysis of the randomized controlled trials. Arch Phys Med Rehabil 77:549–553.

Goldie P, Matyas T, Kinsella G 1992 Movement rehabilitation following stroke. Research report to the Department of Health, Housing and Community Services, Victoria, Australia.

Gordon AM, Ingvarsson PE, Forssberg H 1997 Anticipatory control of manipulative forces in Parkinson's disease. Exp Neurol 145:477–488.

Gowland C, deBruin H, Basmajian JV et al 1992 Agonist and antagonist activity during voluntary upper-limb movement in patients with stroke. Phys Ther 72:624–633.

Haaland KY, Prestopnik JL, Knight RT 2004 Hemispheric asymmetries for kinematic and positional aspects of reaching. Brain 127:1145–1158.

Hagar-Ross CK, Schreiber MH 1995 Quantifying the independence of human finger movements: comparisons of digits, hands, and movement frequencies. J Neurosci 20:8542–8550.

Hanakawa T, Immisch I, Toma K et al 2003 Functional properties of brain areas associated with motor-execution and imagery. J Neurophysiol 89:989–1002.

Harris JE, Eng JJ 2007 Paretic upper-limb strength best explains arm activity in people with stroke. Phys Ther 87:88–97.

Heller A, Wade DT, Wood VA et al 1987 Arm function after stroke: measurement and recovery over the first three months. J Neurol Neurosurg Psychiatry 50:714–719.

Hermsdorfer J, Mai N 1996 Disturbed grip-force following cerebral lesions. J Hand Ther 9:33–40.

Hesse S, Schulte-Tigges G, Konrad M et al 2003 Robot-assisted arm trainer for the passive and active practice of bilateral forearm and wrist movements in hemiparetic subjects. Arch Phys Med Rehabil 84:915–920.

Hesse S, Schmidt H, Werner C 2006 Machines to support motor rehabilitation after stroke: 10 years of experience in Berlin. J Rehabil Res Dev 43:671–678.

Hoff B, Arbib MA 1993 Models of trajectory formation and temporal interaction of reach and grasp. J Mot Behav 25:175–192.

Hogan N, Krebs HI 2004 Interactive robots for neurorehabilitation. Restor Neurol Neurosci 22:349–358.

Hogan N, Winters JM 1990 Principles underlying movement organization: upper limb. In: Winters JM, Woo SL-Y (eds) Multiple muscle systems: biomechanics and movement organization, Springer-Verlag, New York.

Holden M, Dyar T 2002 Virtual training: a new tool for neurorehabilitation. Neurol Report 26:62–71.

Horsley SA, Herbert RD, Ada L 2007 Four weeks of daily stretch has little or no effect on wrist contracture after stroke: a randomized controlled trial. Aust J Physiother 53:239–245.

Hummel F, Celnik P, Giraux P et al 2005 Effects of non-invasive cortical stimulation on skilled motor function in chronic stroke. Brain 128:490–499.

Hummelsheim H, Hauptmaann B, Neumann S 1995 Influence of physiotherapeutic techniques on motor evoked potentials in centrally paretic hand extensor muscles. Electroencephalog Clin Neurophysiol 97:18–28.

Hummelsheim H, Amberger S, Mauritz KH 1996 The influence of EMG-initiated electrical muscle stimulation on motor recovery of the centrally paretic hand. Eur J Neurol 3:245–254.

Hummelsheim H, Maier-Loth ML, Eickhof C 1997 The functional value of electrical muscle stimulation for the rehabilitation of the hand in stroke patients. Scand J Rehabil Med 29:3–10.

Iberall T, Lyons D 1984 Towards perceptual robotics. Proceedings of

IEEE International Conference on Systems, Man and Cybernetics, Halifax, Nova Scotia:147–157.

Iberall T, Bingham G, Arbib MA 1986 Opposition space as a structuring concept for the analysis of skilled hand movements. Exp Brain Res 15:158–173.

Jeannerod M 1981 Intersegmental coordination during reaching at natural visual objects. In: Long J, Baddeley A (eds) Attention and performance, Vol 9. Erlbaum, Hillsdale, NJ:153–168.

Jeannerod M 1984 The timing of natural prehension movements. J Mot Behav 16:235–254.

Jeannerod M 1986 Mechanisms of visuomotor coordination: a study in normal and brain-damaged subjects. Neuropsychology 24:41–78.

Jeannerod M 1990 The neural and behavioral organization of goal-directed movement. Clarendon Press, Oxford.

Johansson RS, Westling G 1984 Roles of glabrous skin receptors and sensorimotor memory in automatic control of precision grip when lifting rougher or more slippery objects. Exp Brain Res 56:550–564.

Johansson RS, Westling G 1988 Programmed and triggered actions to rapid load changes during precision grip. Exp Brain Res 71:72–86.

Johansson RS, Westling G 1990 Tactile afferent signals in the control of precision grip. In: Jeannerod M (ed.) Attention and performance. Erlbaum, Hillsdale, NJ:677–713.

Johansson RS, Riso R, Hager C et al 1992a Somatosensory control of precision grip during unpredictable pulling loads. I. Changes in load force amplitude. Exp Brain Res 89:181–191.

Johansson RS, Hager C, Riso R et al 1992b Somatosensory control of precision grip during unpredictable pulling loads. II. Changes in load force rate. Exp Brain Res 89:192–203.

Johansson RS, Hager C, Backstrom L 1992c Somatosensory control of precision grip during unpredictable pulling loads. III. Impairments during digital anaesthesia. Exp Brain Res 89:204–213.

Kaminski TR, Bock C, Gentile AM 1995 The coordination between trunk and arm motion during pointing movements. Exp Brain Res 106:457–466.

Kapandji AI 1992 Clinical evaluation of the thumb's opposition. J Hand Ther 5:102–106.

Karst GM, Hasan Z 1990 Direction-dependent strategy for control of multi-joint arm movements. In: Winters JM, Woo SL-Y (eds) Multiple muscle systems: biomechanics and movement organization. Springer-Verlag, New York:268–281.

Kelso JAS, Southard DL, Goodman D 1979 On the coordination of 2-handed movements. J Exp Psychol Hum Percept Perform 5:229–238.

Kelso JAS, Buchanan JJ, Murata T 1994 Multifunctionality and switching in the coordination dynamics of reaching and grasping. Hum Mov Sci 13:63–94.

Kilbreath SL, Heard RC 2005 Frequency of hand use in healthy older persons. Aust J Physiother 51:119–122.

Kilbreath SL, Crosbie J, Canning CG et al 2006 Inter-limb coordination in bimanual reach-to-grasp following stroke. Disabil Rehabil 28:1435–1443.

Kitson A 1991 Inhibitive castings for the upper limb: a case study. Aust J Physiother 37:237–242.

Kraft GH, Fitts SS, Hammond MC 1992 Techniques to improve function of the arm and hand in chronic hemiplegia. Arch Phys Med Rehabil 73:220–227.

Krebs HI, Volpe BT, Ferraro M et al 2002 Robot-aided neurorehabilitation: from evidence-based to science-based rehabilitation. Top Stroke Rehabil 8:54–70.

Krichevets AN, Sirokina EB, Yevsevicheva IV et al 1995 Computer games as a means of movement rehabilitation. Disabil Rehabil 17:100–105.

Kunkel A, Kopp B, Muller G et al 1999 Constraint-induced movement therapy for motor recovery in chronic stroke patients. Arch Phys Med Rehabil 80:624–628.

Kuzoffsky A, Apel I, Hirschfeld H 2001 Reaching-lifting-placing task during standing after stroke: coordination among ground reaction forces, ankle muscle activity, and hand movement. Arch Phys Med Rehabil 82:650–660.

Kwakkel G, Kollen BJ, van der Grond J et al 2003 Probability of regaining dexterity in the flaccid upper limb. Stroke 34:2181–2186.

Lam YS, Man DWK, Tam SF et al 2006 Virtual reality training for stroke rehabilitation. Neurorehabilitation 21:245–253.

Landsmeer JMF 1976 Atlas of anatomy of the hand. Churchill Livingstone, Edinburgh.

Lang CE, Scheiber MH 2004 Reduced muscle selectivity during individuated finger movements in humans after damage to the motor cortex or corticospinal tract. J Neurophysiol 91:1722–1733.

Lannin NA, Herbert RD 2003 Is hand splinting effective for adults following stroke? A systematic review and methodological critique of published research. Clin Rehabil 17:807–816.

Lannin NA, Horsley SA, Herbert R et al 2003 Splinting the hand in the functional position after brain impairment: a randomized, controlled trial. Arch Phys Med Rehabil 84:297–302.

Lannin NA, Cusick A, McCluskey A et al 2007 Effects of splinting on wrist contracture after stroke. A randomized controlled trial. Stroke 38:111–116.

Lee DN, Lough F, Lough S 1984 Activating the perceptuo-motor system in hemiparesis. J Physiol 349:328.

Lemon RN, Mantel GWH, Rea PA 1990 Recording and identification of single motor units in the free to move primate hand. Exp Brain Res 81:95–106.

Lemon RN, Bennett KM, Werner W 1991 The cortico-motor substrate for skilled movements of the primate hand. In: Requin J, Stelmach GE (eds) Tutorials in motor neuroscience. Kluwer, Dordrecht:477–495.

Levin MF 1996 Interjoint coordination during pointing movements is disrupted in spastic hemiparesis. Brain 119:281–293.

Levin MF, Michaelsen SM, Cirstea CM et al 2002 Use of the trunk for reaching targets placed within and beyond the reach in adult hemiparesis. Exp Brain Res 143:171–180.

Lewis GN, Byblow WD 2004 Bimanual coordination dynamics in poststroke hemiparetics. J Mot Behav 36:174–188.

Li Z-M, Latash ML, Newell KM 1998a Motor redundancy during maximal voluntary contraction in four-finger tasks. Exp Brain Res 122:71–78.

Li Z-M, Latash ML, Zatsiorsky VM 1998b Force sharing among fingers as a model of the redundancy problem. Exp Brain Res 119:276–286.

Liepert J, Miltner WHR, Bauden H et al 1998 Motor cortex plasticity during constraint-induced movement therapy in stroke. Neurosci Lett 250:5–8.

Liepert J, Bauder H, Miltner W et al 2000 Treatment-induced cortical reorganisation after stroke in humans. Stroke 31:1210–1216.

Liepert J, Uhde I, Graf S et al 2001 Motor cortex plasticity during forced-use therapy in stroke patients: a preliminary study. J Neurol 248:315–321.

Liepert J, Zittel S, Weiller C 2007 Improvement of dexterity by single session low-frequency repetitive transcranial magnetic stimulation over the contralesional motor cortex in acute stroke: a double-blind placebo-controlled crossover trial. Restor Neurol Neurosci 25:461–465.

Liu KPY 2004 Mental imagery for relearning of people after brain injury. Brain Inj 18:1163–1172.

Luft AR, McCombe Waller S, Whitall J et al 2004 Repetitive bilateral arm training and motor cortex activation in chronic stroke. JAMA 292:1853–1861.

Lum P, Reinkensmeyer D, Mahoney R et al 2002a Robotic devices for movement therapy after stroke: current status and challenges to clinical acceptance. Top Stroke Rehabil 8:40–53.

Lum PS, Burgar CG, Shor PC et al 2002b Robot-assisted movement training compared with conventional therapy techniques for the rehabilitation of upper-limb motor function after stroke. Arch Phys Med Rehabil 83:952–959.

McCombe Waller S, Whitall J 2004 Fine motor control in adults with and without chronic hemiparesis: baseline comparison to nondisabled adults and effects of bilateral arm training. Arch Phys Med Rehabil 85:1076–1083.

McCrea PH, Eng JJ, Hodgson AJ 2005 Time and magnitude of torque generation is impaired in both arms following stroke. Muscle Nerve 28:46–53.

Marteniuk RB, MacKenzie CL, Baba DM 1984 Bimanual movement control: information processing and interaction effects. Q J Exp Psychol 36A:335–365.

Marteniuk RB, MacKenzie CL, Jeannerod M et al 1987 Constraints on human arm movement trajectories. Can J Psychol 41:365–378.

Marteniuk RB, Leavitt J, MacKenzie CL et al 1990 Functional relationships between grasp and transport components in a prehension task. Hum Mov Sci 9:149–176.

Mercier C, Bourbonnais D 2004 Relative shoulder flexor and handgrip strength is related to upper limb function after stroke. Clin Rehabil 18:215–221.

Michaelsen SM, Levin MF 2004 Short-term effects of practice with trunk restraint on reaching movements in patients with chronic stroke. A controlled trial. Stroke 35:1914–1919.

Michaelsen SM, Luta A, Robi-Bramy A 2001 Effect of trunk restraint on the recovery of reaching movements in hemiparetic patients. Stroke 32:1875–1883.

Michaelsen SM, Dannenbaum R, Levin MF 2006 Task-specific training with trunk restraint on arm recovery in stroke: randomized control trial. Stroke 37:186–192.

Miltner W, Bauder H, Sommer M et al 1999 Effects of constraint-induced movement therapy on patients with chronic motor deficits after stroke: a replication. Stroke 30:586–592.

Morris DM, Crago JE, DeLuca SC et al 1997 Constraint-induced movement therapy for motor recovery after stroke. Neurorehabil 9:29–43.

Mudie MH, Matyas TA 1996 Upper extremity retraining following stroke: effects of bilateral practice. J Neurol Rehabil 10:167–184.

Mudie MH, Matyas TA 2000 Can simultaneous bilateral movement involve the undamaged hemisphere in reconstruction of neural networks damaged by stroke? J Disabil Rehabil 22:23–37.

Muir RB 1985 Small hand muscles in precision grip. In: Goodwin AW, Darian-Smith I (eds) Hand function and the neocortex. Exp Brain Res Suppl 10, Springer-Verlag, Berlin:155–174.

Muir RB, Lemon RN 1983 Corticospinal neurons with a special role in precision grip. Brain Res 261:312–316.

Muller F, Dichgans J 1994 Impairments of precision grip in two patients with acute unilateral cerebellar lesions: a simple parametric test for clinical use. Neuropsychology 32:265–269.

Nakayama H, Jorgensen HS, Raaschou HO et al 1994a Recovery of upper extremity function in stroke patients: the Copenhagen stroke study. Arch Phys Med Rehabil 75:394–398.

Nakayama H, Jorgensen HS, Raaschou HO et al 1994b Compensation in recovery of upper extremity function after stroke: the Copenhagen stroke study. Arch Phys Med Rehabil 75:852–857.

Napier JR 1956 The prehensile movement of the human hand. J Bone Joint Surg 38:902–913.

Nelles G, Jentzen W, Jueptner M et al 2001 Arm training induced brain plasticity in stroke studied with serial positron emission tomography. Neuroimage 31:1146–1154.

Newham DJ, Hsiao S-F 2001 Knee muscle isometric strength, voluntary activation and antagonistic co-contraction in the first six months after stroke. Disabil Rehabil 23:379–386.

O'Dwyer N, Ada L, Neilson PD 1996 Spasticity and muscle contracture following stroke. Brain 119:1737–1749.

Ostendorf CG, Wolf SL 1981 Effect of forced use of the upper extremity of a hemiplegic patient on changes in function. Phys Ther 61:1022–1028.

Page SJ 2000 Imagery improves upper extremity motor function in chronic stroke patients: a pilot study. Occup Ther J Res 20:200–215.

Page SJ, Levine P, Sisto SA et al 2001 Mental practice combined with physical practice for upper-limb motor deficit in subacute stroke. Phys Ther 81:1455–1462.

Page SJ, Sisto S, Levine P et al 2004 Efficacy of modified constraint-induced therapy in chronic stroke: a single blinded randomized controlled trial. Arch Phys Med Rehabil 85:14–18.

Pandyan AD, Power J, Futter C et al 1996 Effects of electrical stimulation on the wrist of hemiplegic subjects. Physiotherapy 82:184–188.

Pang MY, Harris JE, Eng JJ 2006 A community-based upper-extremity group exercise program improves motor function and performance of functional activities in chronic stroke: a randomized controlled trial. Arch Phys Med Rehabil 87:1–9.

Parlow SE, Dewey D 1991 The temporal locus of transfer of training between hands: an interference study. Behav Brain Res 46:1–8.

Pascuol-Leone A, Dang N, Cohen LG et al 1995 Modulation of muscle responses evoked by transcranial magnetic stimulation during the acquisition of new fine motor skills. J Neurophysiol 67:1037–1045.

Pennisi G, Rapisarda R, Bella R et al 1999 Absence of response to early transcranial magnetic stimulation in ischaemic stroke patients: prognostic value for hand motor recovery. Stroke 30:2666–2700.

Platz T 2004 Impairment-oriented training (IOT) – scientific concept and evidence-based treatment strategies. Restor Neurol Neurosci 22:301–315.

Platz T, Bock S, Prass K 2001a Reduced skilfulness of arm motor behaviour among motor stroke patients with good clinical recovery: does it indicate reduced automaticity? Can it be improved by unilateral or bilateral training? A kinematic motion analysis study. Neuropsychology 39:687–698.

Platz T, Winter T, Muller N et al 2001b Arm ability training for stroke and traumatic brain injury patients with mild arm paresis: a single-blind, randomized, controlled trial. Arch Phys Med Rehabil 82:961–968.

Platz T, Eickhof C, Nuyens G et al 2005 Clinical scales for the assessment of spasticity, associated phenomena, and function: a systematic review of the literature. Disabil Rehabil 27:7–18.

Plautz EJ, Miliken GW, Nudo RJ 2000 Effects of repetitive motor training on movement representations in adult squirrel monkeys: role of use versus learning. Neurobiol Learn Mem 74:27–55.

Pomeroy VM, King LM, Pollock A et al 2006 Electrostimulation for promoting recovery of movement or functional ability after stroke. Cochrane Database Syst Rev, Issue 2. Art. No.: CD003241. DOI: 10.1002/14651858.CD003241.pub2.

Powell J, Pandyan AD, Granat M et al 1999 Electrical stimulation of wrist extensors in post-stroke hemiplegia. Stroke 30:1384–1389.

Price CI, Pandyan AD 2001 Electrical stimulation for preventing and treating post-stroke shoulder pain: a systematic Cochrane review. Clin Rehabil 15:5–19.

Prigatano GP, Wong JL 1997 Speed of finger typing and goal attainment after unilateral cerebral vascular accident. Arch Phys Med Rehabil 78:847–852.

Putnam CA 1993 Sequential motions of body segments in striking and throwing skills: descriptions and explanations. J Biomech 26(Suppl 1):125–135.

Quancy RBM, Perea S, Maletsky R et al 2005 Impaired grip force modulation in the ipsilateral hand after unilateral middle cerebral artery stroke. Neurorehabil Neural Repair 19:338–349.

Raghaven P, Petra E, Krakmauer JW et al 2006 Patterns of impairment in digit dependence after subcortical stroke. J Neurophysiol 95:369–378.

Rosenbaum DA 1991 Human motor control. Academic Press, San Diego, CA.

Rosenbaum DA, Vaughan J, Barnes HJ et al 1990 Constraints on action selection: overhand versus underhand grips. In: Jeannerod M (ed.) Attention and performance. Erlbaum, Hillsdale, NJ:321–342.

Rosenbaum DA, Vaughan J, Barnes HJ et al 1992 Time course of movement planning: selection of handgrips for object manipulation. J Exp Psychol Learn Mem Cog 18:1058–1073.

Rosenbaum DA, Engebrecht SE, Bushe MM et al 1993 Knowledge model for selecting and producing reaching movements. J Mot Behav 25:217–227.

Sahrmann SA, Norton BJ 1977 The relationship of voluntary movement to spasticity in the upper motor neuron syndrome. Ann Neurol 2:460–465.

Salford E, Ryding E, Rosen I et al 1995 Motor performance and motor ideation of arm movements after stroke: a SPECT rCBF study. In: Proceedings of the World Confederation of Physical Therapy Congress, Washington, DC:793.

Schmidt RA, Wulf G 1997 Continuous concurrent feedback degrades motor skill learning: implications for training and simulation. Hum Factors 39:509–525.

Seidler RD, Stelmark GE 2000 Trunk-assisted prehension: specification of body segments with imposed temporal constraints. J Mot Behav 32:379–389.

Shumway-Cook A, Woollacott M 2005 Motor control. Translating research into clinical practice 3rd edn. Lippincott, Philadelphia.

Smeets JBJ, Brenner E 1999 A new view on grasping. Motor Control 3:237–271.

Smith AM 1981 The coactivation of antagonist muscles. Can J Physiol Pharmacol 59:733–747.

Sonde L, Kalimo H, Fernaeus SE et al 2000 Low TENS treatment on post-stroke paretic arm: a three-year follow-up. Clin Rehabil 14:14–19.

Spoor C 1983 Balancing a force on the finger tip of a two-dimensional finger without intrinsic muscles. J Biomech 16:497–504.

Sullivan JE, Hedman LD 2004 A home program of sensory and neuromuscular electrical stimulation with upper-limb task practice in a patient 5 years after a stroke. Phys Ther 84:1045–1054.

Sunderland A, Tinson D, Bradley L et al 1989 Arm function after stroke. An evaluation of grip strength as a measure of recovery and a prognostic indicator. J Neurol Neurosurg Psychiatry 52:1267–1272.

Tang A, Rymer WZ 1981 Abnormal force-EMG relations in paretic limbs of hemiparetic human subjects. J Neurol Neurosurg Psychiatry 44:690–698.

Tanji J, Okano K, Sato K 1988 Neuronal activity in cortical motor areas related to ipsilateral, contralateral and bilateral digit movement of the monkey. J Neurophysiol 60:325–343.

Taub E 1980 Somatosensory deafferentation in research with monkeys: implications for rehabilitation medicine. In: Ince LP (ed.) Behavioural psychology and rehabilitation medicine. Williams and Wilkins, Baltimore, MD:371–401.

Taub E, Miller NE, Novak TA et al 1993 A technique for improving chronic motor deficit after stroke. Arch Phys Med Rehabil 74:347–354.

Thielman GT, Dean CM, Gentile AM 2004 Rehabilitation of reaching after stroke: task-related training versus progressive resistance exercise. Arch Phys Med Rehabil 85:1613–1618.

Trombly CA 1992 Deficits of reaching in subjects with left hemiparesis: a pilot study. Am J Occup Ther 46:887–897.

Trombly CA 1993 Observations of improvement of reaching in five subjects with left hemiparesis. J Neurol Neurosurg Psychiatry 56:40–45.

Turner DP, Ebrahim S 1992 Relation between handgrip strength, upper limb disability and handicap among elderly women. Clin Rehabil 6:117–123.

Turton A 1998 Mechanisms for recovery of hand and arm function after stroke: a review of evidence from studies using non-invasive investigative techniques. Br J Occup Ther 61:359–364.

Turton AJ, Britten E 2005 A pilot randomized controlled trial of a daily muscle stretch regime to prevent contractures in the arm after stroke. Clin Rehabil 19:600–612.

Uswatte G, Giuliani C, Winstein C et al 2006 Validity of accelerometry in patients with sub-acute stroke; evidence from the extremity constraint-induced therapy evaluation trial. Arch Phys Med Rehabil 87:1340–1345.

van Peppen RPS, Kwakkel G, Wood-Daupinee S et al 2004 The impact of physical therapy on functional outcomes after stroke: what's the evidence? Clin Rehabil 18:833–862.

van Vliet P 1993 An investigation of the task-specificity of reaching: implications for re-training. Physiother Theory Pract 9:69–76.

van Vliet PM, Turton A 2001 Directions in retraining reaching. Crit Rev Phys Rehabil 13:313–338.

van Vliet P, Kerwin DG, Sheridan M et al 1995 The influence of goals on the kinematics of reaching following stroke. Neurol Report 19:11–16.

Volpe BT, Krebs HI, Hogan N et al 2000 A novel approach to stroke rehabilitation: robot-aided sensorimotor stimulation. Neurology 54:1938–1944.

Wade DT, Langton Hewer R, Wood VA et al 1983 The hemiplegic arm after stroke: measurement and recovery. J Neurol Neurosurg Psychiatry 46:521–524.

Wang B-S, Settle K, Perreault EJ 2006 Vibratory afferent inputs modulated motor pathway excitability and hand function following stroke. 15th International Conference on Mechanics in Medicine and Biology, Singapore:296–299.

Weir P, MacKenzie CL, Marteniuk RG et al 1991 The effects of object weight on the kinematics of prehension. J Mot Behav 23:192–204.

Weiss P, Jeannerod M 1998 Getting a grasp on coordination. News Physiol Sci 13:70–75.

Westling G, Johansson RS 1984 Responses in glabrous skin mechanoreceptors during precision grip in humans. Exp Brain Res 66:128–140.

Whitall J, McCombe Waller S, Silver KHC 2000 Repetitive bilateral arm training with rhythmic auditory cueing improves motor function in chronic hemiparetic stroke. Stroke 31:2390–2395.

Wiesendanger M, Kazennikov O, Perrig C et al 1996 Two hands – one action. In: Wing AM, Haggard P, Flanagan R (eds) Hand and brain neurophysiology and psychology of hand movements. Academic Press, Orlando, FL.

Williams PE 1990 Use of intermittent stretch in the prevention of serial sarcomere loss in immobilised muscle. Ann Rheum Dis 49:316–317.

Wing AM 1988 A comparison of the rate of pinch grip force increases and decreases in Parkinsonian bradykinesia. Neuropsychology 26:479–482.

Wing AM, Fraser C 1983 The contribution of the thumb to reaching movements. Q J Exp Psychol 35A:297–309.

Wing AM, Flanagan JR, Richardson J 1997 Anticipatory postural adjustments in stance and grip. Exp Brain Res 116:122–130.

Winstein CJ, Schmidt RA, Nicholson DE et al 1996 Learning a partial-weight-bearing skill: effectiveness of two forms of feedback. Phys Ther 76:985–993.

Winstein CJ, Rose DK, Lewthwaite R et al 2004 A randomized controlled comparison of upper-extremity rehabilitation strategies in acute stroke: a pilot study of immediate and long-term outcomes. Arch Phys Med Rehabil 85:620–628.

Witney A, Wing A, Thonnard JL et al 2004 The cutaneous contribution to adaptive precision grip. Trends Neurosci 27:637–643.

Woldag H, Hummelsheim H 2002 Evidence-based physiotherapeutic concepts for improving arm and

hand function in stroke patients. J Neurol 249:518–528.

Wolf SL, Catlin PA, Blanton S et al 1994 Overcoming limitations in elbow movement in the presence of antagonist hyperactivity. Phys Ther 74:826–835.

Wolf SL, Blanton S, Baer H et al 2002 Repetitive task practice: a critical review of constraint induced movement therapy in stroke. Neurologist 8:325–338.

Wolf SL, Winstein CJ, Miller JP et al 2006 Effect of constraint-induced movement therapy on upper extremity function 3 to 9 months after stroke. JAMA 296:2095–2104.

Wolf SL, Newton H, Maddy D et al 2007 The EXCITE trial: relationship of intensity of constraint induced movement therapy to improvement in the Wolf Motor Function Test. Restor Neurol Neurosci 25:549–562.

Wolf SL, Winstein CJ, Miller JP et al 2008 Retention of upper limb function in stroke survivors who have received constraint-induced movement therapy: the EXCITE randomized trial. Lancet Neurol 7:33–40.

Wu C, Trombly CA, Lin K et al 2000 A kinematic study of contextual effects on reaching performance in persons with and without stroke: influences of object availability. Arch Phys Med Rehabil 81:95–101.

Wu C, Trombly CA, Lin K et al 2004 Effects of object affordances on reaching performance in persons with and without cerebrovascular accident. Am J Occup Ther 52:447–456.

Wu Z-W, Ju M-S, Lin C-CK 2006 Motor learning of normal subjects in tracking with rehabilitation robot. 15th International Conference on Mechanics in Medicine and Biology, Singapore.

Yekutiel M, Guttman E 1993 A controlled trial of the retraining of the sensory function of the hand in stroke patients. J Neurol Neurosurg Psychiatry 56:241–244.

Yu D, Chae J, Walker ME et al 2001 Percutaneous intramuscular electric stimulation for the treatment of shoulder subluxation and pain in patients with chronic hemiplegia: a pilot study. Arch Phys Med Rehabil 82:20–25.

Zachowski KM, Dromerick AW, Sahrmann SA et al 2004 How do strength, sensation, spasticity and joint individuation relate to the reaching deficits of perople with chronic hemiparesis? Brain 127:1035–1046.

Zajak FE, Winters JM 1990 Modeling musculoskeletal movement systems: joint and body-segment dynamics, musculotendinous actuation and neuromuscular control. In: Winters JM, Woo SL-Y (eds) Multiple muscle systems: biomechanics and movement organization. Springer-Verlag, New York:121–148.

Zatsiorsky VM, Zong-Ming L, Latash ML 1998 Coordinated force production in multi-finger tasks: finger interaction and neural network modeling. Biol Cybern 79:139–150.

Zatsiorsky VM, Zong-Ming L, Latash ML 2000 Enslaving effects in multi-finger force production. Exp Brain Res 131:187–195.

Zimmerman-Schlatter A, Schuster C, Puhan MA et al 2008 Efficacy of motor imagery in post-stroke rehabilitation: a systematic review. J Neuroeng Rehabil 5:8.

Zong-Ming L, Latash ML, Zatsiorsky VM 1998a Force sharing among fingers as a model of the redundancy problem. Exp Brain Res 119:276–286.

Zong-Ming L, Latash ML, Newell KM et al 1998b Motor redundancy during maximal voluntary contraction in four-finger tasks. Exp Brain Res 122:71–78.

Chapter | 7 |

Balance

INTRODUCTION

Balance can be defined as the ability to control the body mass relative to the base of support (Ghez 1991). Whether we are stationary or moving, we are unaware of the complex neuromuscular and mechanical processes that control our balance. The forces that disturb balance are gravitational and other forces arising from muscle contractions and interactions between segments during movement, or from disturbances as a result of an unexpected perturbation such as a push, a trip or a collision.

Balance (postural control) only becomes obvious to us when we feel unsteady, or accidentally trip or fall, or when disease or trauma damages sensorimotor systems.

Balance dysfunction, particularly on our feet, is a devastating sequel to a neurological lesion since balancing the body mass over the base of support under different task and environmental conditions is one of the most critical motor control factors in daily life. Training balanced movement may be the most significant part of neurorehabilitation.

In attempting to define balance, many different terms are used in the literature to describe the fact that we live in a gravitational environment, where no matter what we do we must learn to take account of its effects (Fig. 7.1). The term *postural stability* describes the ability to maintain the position of the body's centre of body mass (COM) within specific boundaries of space, or stability limits. Maintenance of stability is a dynamic process that involves establishing an equilibrium between all the forces (stabilizing and destabilizing) acting on the body so that the body remains in an intended position or is able to progress through an intended movement without losing balance (Melvill-Jones 2000). The term *postural control* typically refers to the mechanisms by which we control our balance. Control is maintained by *postural adjustments* that consist of muscle activations and segmental movements. It is muscle activity and joint movement that directly ensure balance is preserved or restored. The term *posture* describes the alignment of body segments in relation to one another and to the environment.

Ghez (1991) described a 'family of adjustments' needed to maintain a posture and to move. These adjustments have three goals: to support the head and body against gravity and other external forces; to maintain the COM aligned and balanced over the base of support; and to stabilize parts of the body while other parts are moved. The postural system must meet three main challenges

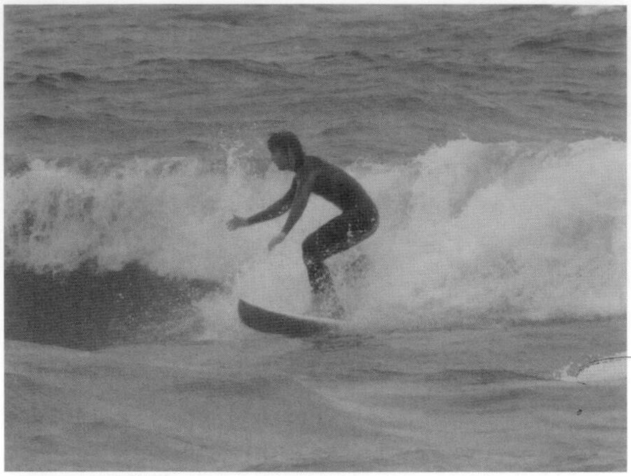

Fig. 7.1 Balance is learned during practice of a task and ongoing practice of a skilled activity.

according to Melvill-Jones (2000). It must maintain a *steady state* (balance) in the presence of gravity, it must generate adjustments that *anticipate* self-initiated goal-directed movements and it must be *adaptive* during these movements and in response to external perturbations. The ability to balance is integral to the execution of most movements and cannot be separated from the action or the environment in which it is performed. The functionally significant components of balance are maintenance of a stable posture, postural adjustments in anticipation of and during a self-initiated movement, and postural adjustments made in response to an external perturbation. Balance, therefore, forms the foundation for all voluntary motor skills (Massion & Woollacott 1996).

The mechanical problem of maintaining balance is particularly challenging for the central nervous system (CNS). For humans in standing, two-thirds of the body mass is some distance from the base of support (Winter et al 1990). Even when stationary, the body must do work to remain upright against the force of gravity. The standing human frame, flexible and multisegmented, with its small base of support and its many degrees of freedom, requires highly developed postural control to ensure that the body remains upright and balanced.

The body is considered stable when the COM is maintained over the base of support. The term COM refers to a point in the total body mass calculated by finding the weighted average of the COM of each body segment. Central to balance control is the need to keep the line of gravity* within the perimeter of the base of support, or on track to a new base of support as in walking or running (Winter 1995a); that is, within the limit of stability. This is not a fixed boundary but changes according to task, to

skill level and the environment. It is the point beyond which we cannot preserve balance without making a new base of support, which we do by stepping, holding onto a stable object, or by over-balancing, reaching out or falling. An appropriate relationship must be maintained between the body and the environment for effective performance of any task.

The adjustments we make in order to preserve equilibrium are flexible and varied due to the potential for dynamic interactions offered by the segmental linkage. Postural adjustments are the muscle activation patterns and segmental movements that enable us to control this linkage in relation to the base of support. Movement of a body segment, whether as part of a self-initiated movement or in response to an unexpected externally-imposed movement, perturbs postural stability. Even the smallest actions such as taking a deep breath(Gurfinkel & Elner 1988) or turning the head are characterized by oscillations of the centre of gravity (COG) which are counteracted by muscle activity and small, barely detectable segmental movements (Bouisset & Duchenne 1994). The simple act of raising the arm to reach for an object destabilizes balance unless precisely timed anticipatory muscle activity and small joint movements are initiated before the start of arm movement. These small adjustments minimize potential disturbances to balance that movement may cause. Similar responses enable us to cope with unexpected disturbances. Therefore, since postural control must be integrated with volitional movement, the postural control processes must also be capable of adaptive learning. The current view is that postural control involves the behaviourally meaningful integration of many different neural systems, including those associated with cognition (Melvill-Jones 2000).

Maintenance of balance requires attentional resources even in able-bodied young subjects. Sustaining attention to a task and avoiding distraction were found to be related to the ability to balance in a study of individuals post-stroke (Stapleton et al 2001). Paying attention to environmental cues is particularly important when balance is threatened or likely to be threatened. Focusing on an external visual cue rather than on postural control itself is likely to lead to better performance, enabling balance to self-regulate and adapt (Guadagnoli et al 2002).

In the past, postural stability was explained by the action of postural reflexes controlled at a relatively low level of the nervous system. Based on experimental work on decerebrate cats and dogs (Magnus 1926; Sherrington 1961) and observational studies of human infants in the early twentieth century, it was concluded that postural control in humans could be explained by these simple righting and equilibrium, or tilting, reflexes. These ideas formed the basis of the methods of clinical practice developed by the Bobaths in the 1950s.

However, there is now a considerable body of research indicating that control of balance cannot be considered

---

*The vertical projection of the COM is often described as the line of gravity.

automated and controlled by postural reflexes (Woollacott & Shumway-Cook 2002). Today, we recognize that postural control is more complex, that it is task and context dependent, involving all levels of the neuromuscular system. Simple postural reflexes cannot account for the complexity of postural control during skilled, purposeful movements (Melvill-Jones 2000). Balance is therefore not based on a set of reflexes but is an integral part of the task and is learned (both intrinsically and extrinsically) along with the task and becomes more effective with training. Recently developed physiotherapy methods reflect this knowledge (e.g., Carr & Shepherd 1998, 2003; Shumway-Cook & Woollacott 2001, 2007). However, despite evidence to the contrary, the belief that postural reflexes (e.g., righting and equilibrium reactions) form the basis of postural control via postural reflex mechanisms lingers on in physiotherapy, in spite of lack of scientific support and clinical evidence, and has diverted attention in clinical practice away from the preparatory and task-specific nature of balance.

SENSORIMOTOR INTERACTION

Balance emerges from a complex interaction between sensory and musculoskeletal systems modified within the CNS in response to changing internal and external conditions. Sensory systems (vestibular, visual and somatosensory) provide information about where the body is in space and whether it is stationary or in motion. The vestibular system provides information about the position of the head in relation to gravity as well as information about motion through linear and angular acceleration of the head. The proprioceptive system, consisting of muscle, joint and cutaneous (tactile and pressure) receptors, provides information about the state of the effector system of muscles and joints, such as length and force output of muscles, our position in space and information about the environment such as surface conditions. It provides information about movement of the body in relation to the base of support, and movement and orientation of body segments in relation to each other. Plantar cutaneous mechanoreceptors have been shown to play a significant role in balance regulation when the feet form the base of support (Do et al 1990; Duysens et al 2000). Cutaneous mechanoreceptors in the soles of the feet and proprioceptors in leg muscles provide information about load (Dietz et al 1992; Kavounoudias et al 2001). The visual system provides information about where we are in relation to our surroundings and is interpreted in light of experience.

Our sensitivity to visual information appears particularly important to skill in balancing the body while walking, since it specifies the relationship between ourselves and the properties of the environment (Owen 1985). Visual inputs tell us the position of relevant objects in the environment, our distance from them and whether they are stationary or moving. We scan the environment as we move, and visual information enables us to judge when a moving object will reach us, or when we will land on the floor in a jump. We can predict time-to-contact very accurately (Dietz & Noth 1978), and this enables us to change our stride appropriately so we correctly time when to place our foot on the kerb in crossing the street. Time-to-contact information also helps us to walk through a crowded hall, judge the closing doors of a lift (elevator), and step onto an escalator or moving walkway.

Visual information provides a reference for verticality since many things in the built environment (e.g., window and door frames, legs of a table) are aligned vertically, providing what Gibson (1979) called 'exproprioceptive information'. Under certain conditions, the information we receive may not be helpful. For example, in a dark room, adults have been shown to alter their standing alignment to fit with the alignment of a luminous rod, even when it was angled away from the vertical (De Wit 1972).

Another type of visual information comes more indirectly from our surroundings (see Gibson 1979). As we walk, our surroundings move past us in an expanding optic array. Moving room experiments have shown that subjects sway inappropriately when the walls of the room move toward them or away from them (Lee & Lishman 1975). The movement of the walls away from subjects presented similar information (from peripheral vision) as would be present if they had swayed backward. They responded to this perceived sway (an illusion of self-motion) by swaying forward. It appeared therefore that they were paying more attention to the visual (in this case misleading) inputs than to the more accurate (in this case) proprioceptive inputs. Adult subjects did not fall in this experiment, however toddlers who took part in a similar experiment did fall (Lee & Aronsen 1974).

The narrower the support base and the lower the skill level of the individual, the more critical vision seems to be for balance, suggesting a critical interaction between base of support, the availability of visual inputs and skill level (Slobounov & Newell 1994). Elderly people report difficulty moving about in the dark when visual judgements cannot be made about their position in space. Standing with eyes closed can be difficult and one-legged standing with eyes closed may be impossible.

The role of different sensory inputs is controversial, but it is likely that they are integrated and coordinated in a task-relevant manner that is dependent on the environment. For example, when the support surface is perturbed, able-bodied subjects rely primarily on somatosensory information under normal sensory conditions when all sensory inputs are available (Nashner & Berthoz 1978). When support surface information is unreliable, for example when standing on a narrow beam, visual information increases in importance (Lishman & Lee 1973). Redundancy of sensory inputs and the ability of the CNS to modify the relative importance of any one sense for postural control enables able-bodied individuals to maintain balance in a variety of environments and to improve balance as part of learning a new motor skill. Redundancy within the sensory system can have functional advantages. It may enable not only verification of inputs that may be conflicting, but also allows for compensation when one system is dysfunctional (Winter et al 1990).

BIOMECHANICAL DESCRIPTION

The human body presents an interesting and unique structure from a biomechanical perspective. In the standing position, multiple linked segments must be maintained in a stable position on a narrow support base. Linked-segment dynamics play an important role in the control of the gravitational and other forces that arise from interaction between these segments as we move (Yang et al 1990).

Quiet standing

Although we do not often stand quite still, when we do, small movements of the body mass about the base of support, called *postural sway*, occur. These can be observed in force platform measures and in measures of body movement taken with a sway meter (Fig. 7.2). Sheldon (1963) described postural sway as the constant small deviations from the vertical and their subsequent correction to which all human beings are subject when standing upright. Although passive elastic restoring forces are involved in these small movements, standing still is an active process, involving changes in muscle activity (Day et al 1993) and small joint rotations (segmental movements).

Control of balance when standing requires an integrated response to visual, vestibular and somatosensory inputs. The relative contribution of each of these systems has been studied by experimentally blocking each of these inputs and measuring the subsequent changes in postural sway. The amount of sway in quiet standing varies according to a number of factors, including environmental events, whether the eyes are open or closed, and even how deeply we breathe (Gurfinkel & Elner 1973). Sway also varies according to foot position and width of base of support (Kirby et al 1987). In general, the magnitude of postural sway is said to be greatest in the very young and the very old. Factors found to be highly correlated with increased sway in the elderly include reduced muscle strength, reduced peripheral sensation, poor near vision acuity and slowed reaction time (Lord et al 2007).

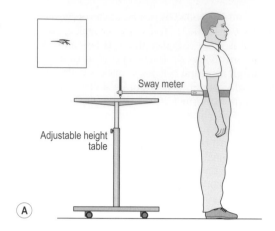

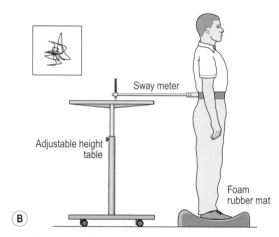

Fig. 7.2 A portable 'sway meter' used to measure body displacement at the level of the waist. (A) Standing on the floor. (B) Standing on a foam rubber mat. *(Reprinted from Lord et al 2007 with permission of Cambridge University Press, Cambridge, UK).*

The extent of postural sway as a clinical measure of balance provides only limited information about the ability to respond to the changing demands of a particular task, and gives no information about the movements occurring within the segmental linkage above the base of support (Kuo & Zajac 1993). Its functional relevance is unclear. Postural sway is poorly related to dynamic actions such as walking (Gill-Body & Krebs 1994; Colle 1995), and limiting body sway does not necessarily lead to improved stability. It may be that the number of fluctuations is more important than the extent of sway.

Several authors (Horak 1987; Massion 1992) have pointed out that decreased postural sway should not be confused with stability. There is considerable variability among able-bodied individuals, and ballet dancers and athletes may have a relatively large extent of sway, while highly skilled pistol shooters (Arutyunyan et al 1969) have a minimal degree of sway as they prepare to pull the trigger. In clinical practice, the focus should be on regaining the ability to move freely without losing balance, rather than on controlling postural sway.

Balance during self-initiated movements

The performance of all self-initiated actions, even simple acts such as raising an arm in standing, are preceded by precisely timed *anticipatory or preparatory postural adjustments*. These occur before the action is initiated, as well as during movement, in order to minimize the destabilizing effects on balance caused by the movement itself (Eng et al 1992). Preparatory leg muscle activity (Belenkii et al 1967) and small segmental movements (Zattara & Bouisset 1988) form part of the action, and are highly specific to and an integral part of that action. They vary with speed and support conditions. Anticipatory and ongoing postural adjustments ensure the body's COM stays within the base of support. When the arm is raised, reactive forces produced by the arm movement affect the rest of the body (the segmental linkage), while at the same time the displacement of the arm (the arm's mass) alters the position of the COM (Eng et al 1992).

Preparatory muscle activity seems to be an integral and implicit part of the action in that it prevents destabilization of the COM due to limb or trunk movement. A study of rising onto tip-toes provides a good example of the efficiency of the underlying mechanism. The prime mover is triceps surae. However, triceps activity is preceded by preparatory activation of tibialis anterior, quadriceps and biceps femoris. Activation of triceps (a two-joint muscle) without this preparatory activity would lead to a backward shift of the COM and to flexion of the knee; the subject would fall backward. The task can be achieved only if the body mass is shifted forward by tibialis anterior, with quadriceps holding the knee extended before the heels are raised (Diener et al 1992).

Postural muscle activity is remarkably adaptable and varies according to task and environmental demands. This point is illustrated in Figure 7.3. Subjects interacted with the handle in four different ways: (A) The subject stands on a firm platform and pulls on a fixed handle as soon as possible after an auditory cue. To maintain position, contraction of a leg muscle (gastrocnemius) occurs before the arm muscle (biceps brachii) contracts to pull the handle.

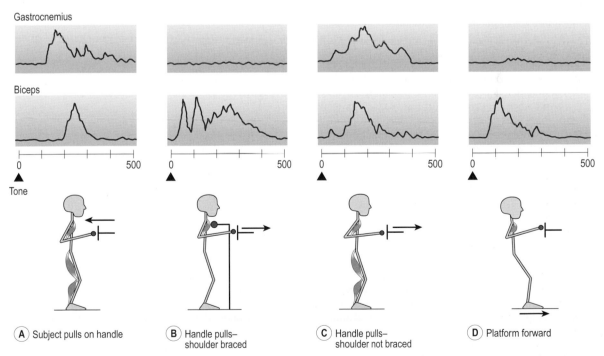

Fig. 7.3 An example of specificity of muscle activity. An arm muscle (biceps brachii) and a leg muscle (gastrocnemius) were monitored during different task requirements. (A) Subject pulls on the handle. (B) Unexpected movement of the handle when the subject leans against chest support. (C) As in B but subject is free standing. (D) Unexpected forward movement of the platform. (*Adapted from Nashner LM 1983, with permission*).

(B) When the chest is supported and the handle is unexpectedly pulled away from the subject, there is an early response in biceps brachii, and gastrocnemius remains silent. However, (C) when the handle unexpectedly pulls the free-standing subject forward, the early biceps brachii response is suppressed so that the counter-balancing arm and leg muscles can act simultaneously. (D) When the support surface unexpectedly moves forward, tilting the subject back, there is an early biceps brachii response, and the gastrocnemius is silent since its contraction would tilt the subject further back. These experiments illustrate the extreme sensitivity of postural adjustments to the demands of context.

Shifting from two legs to one leg

Consider what actually happens when one leg is actively lifted while we remain supported and balanced on the other. It is more complex than one would imagine and requires a particular type of anticipatory postural adjustment since the moving limb forms part of the support base. The point to be noted is that both limbs are involved in the preparatory lateral shift of body mass. This enables the optimum postural set for the leg raise and is an integral part of the action (Lee et al 1995; Mercer & Sahrmann 1999; Kirker et al 2000).

Several studies have examined a group of actions in which the body mass is shifted laterally to free one leg from support. Examples of actions that involve this adjustment are moving to a one-legged stance, taking the first step in walking (Kirker et al 2000) and placing one foot on a step (Mercer & Sahrmann 1999). Milliseconds before the foot is lifted from the floor, the centre of pressure† (COP) shifts briefly over to this foot, providing the necessary ground reaction force to shift the COP across to the support limb. The postural adjustments in the mediolateral direction occur primarily in the shank/foot and thigh/pelvis linkage (Winter 1995). The dynamic role of hip abductor muscles in contributing to the initiation and performance of the weight shift to one side is in addition to their role in stabilizing the pelvis at the hip during single leg stance (Pai et al 1994). For a patient to re-establish this mechanism requires practice of single limb support and stepping with both lower limbs.

Walking

To walk without veering to one side or increasing the base of support requires ongoing postural adjustment. The rhythm and speed of walking mean that the actual amount of muscle activity involved is minimal. If we stop mid-stride, however, it may be difficult not to over-balance.

---

†Centre of foot pressure is measured as ground reaction forces under the foot or feet with a force plate/s.

Walking in a busy street increases the need to control balance against unexpected pushes and to control the body's path through the crowd.

Sensory inputs in general and visual inputs in particular provide information that makes it possible for us to walk in cluttered environments and on uneven terrain. Vision provides information almost instantaneously about both static and dynamic features of the near and far environment. This information is used to plan adjustments to the basic walking pattern (Patla 1997) as we think about other things.

The challenges to stability during walking are of greater complexity than during quiet standing. During normal human gait the line of gravity falls outside the boundaries of the base of support for 80% of the stride (Fig. 7.4), a situation of potential instability (Winter et al 1991). The upper body is balanced over the lower limbs during

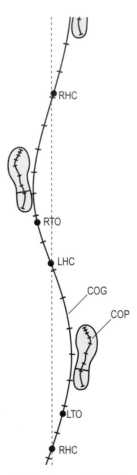

Fig. 7.4 A translational plot showing the body's COG and foot COP for one walking stride. Note the COG never passes over the foot indicating that walking is essentially an inherently unstable activity. HC, heel contact; TO, toe-off.
(Reproduced from Winter et al 1991, with permission.)

walking primarily by hip flexors and extensors in the plane of progression and hip abductor and adductor muscles in the frontal plane, to counteract the imbalance of the upper body in single support (Winter et al 1993). Trunk muscles perform a balancing function together with muscles linking the upper body with the lower limbs. Foot placement also plays a role in balancing the body mass.

Investigations into the responses to anticipated and unexpected perturbations during walking have demonstrated that they are context specific and phase dependent (Nashner 1980; Dietz et al 1986; Figura et al 1986; Patla 1986). When subjects are asked to pull or push on a handle while walking, the results indicate that they tend to time the push or pull to coincide with heel contact, with postural muscle activity preceding the onset of arm activity and directionally specific (Nashner & Forssberg 1986). When Patla (1986) had subjects flex the arm rapidly at the shoulder in response to a visual cue during gait, postural leg muscle activity preceded arm activity in stance phase and occurred after arm movement during swing. Thus, we can see how actions that are potentially destabilizing are timed to occur in the gait cycle at an optimal time to preserve stability.

Sitting

Anticipatory and ongoing postural adjustments are not isolated to tasks we perform while standing. However, compared with the number of investigations of postural control in standing, postural control in sitting has not been studied to the same extent. Reaching in sitting involves not only movement of the arm but also movement of the trunk at the hips to extend our reaching distance, with active use of the lower limbs to aid in balancing the body mass by providing an 'active' base of support.

Sitting does not present the same threat to stability as standing due to the larger base of support. In contrast to standing, where the feet provide a small base of support, in sitting with feet on the floor, the thighs and feet make up a relatively large base of support. However, when sitting with the legs hanging free, such as over the side of a bed, only the thighs are supported. We cannot reach as far forward or sideways in this position (Chari & Kirby 1986) since the limit of stability is reached sooner. In this relatively less supported position, activity in muscles that link the trunk segment with the thighs enables us to move the body mass a limited distance in different directions over the hips. Whether or not the feet are on the floor, muscles linking the pelvis and trunk (e.g., spinal flexors and extensors) also ensure appropriate alignment and stability of the trunk and head during activities performed in sitting.

Postural control in sitting requires the ability to balance on different types of seats while performing a variety of tasks, frequently at more than arm's length, in both sagittal and frontal planes. Lower limb muscles play an active role in supporting and balancing the body mass when we move about in sitting. In studies of reaching forward beyond arm's length, leg muscles were active before the arm moved both at fast and slow speeds (Crosbie et al 1995; Dean et al 1999a,b). Tibialis anterior was activated and ground reaction forces under the feet occurred before the start of arm movement. Toward the end of the reach, calf and knee muscle activity brakes the forward movement of the body mass (Fig. 7.5). Shank and thigh muscles play a less active role when reaching is self-paced and within arm's length than when movement is fast and the target is at a greater distance (Dean et al 1999a,b).

In general, trunk muscles act as postural stabilizers during movements in sitting that involve the upper limbs. However, when reaching involves moving beyond arm's length in order to transport the hand to a target, the trunk also plays a role in extending the reach distance. That is, movement of the trunk by flexion and extension at the hips is an integral part of the reaching movement (Kaminski et al 1995; Dean et al 1999a,b). The distance we can reach is also affected by the extent of thigh support (Dean et al 1999a,b).

Reaching sideways in sitting is more destabilizing than reaching forward in the sagittal plane since the body mass shifts onto one leg and the perimeter of the base of support is reached earlier. Few studies have examined lateral movements in sitting. In one study, young able-bodied men sat with arms folded across the chest and feet on two force plates. They were asked to move their body mass as far to the right as possible. The findings were similar to leg raising studies in standing – the lower limbs were active in a coordinated manner in the preparatory phase. Before weight was shifted over the right leg, the left leg loaded and the right leg unloaded (Sekiya & Takahashi 2001). Practising tasks that involve reaching sideways in sitting should be incorporated into balance and upper limb training programmes. Impaired ability to perform this action has a negative effect on many functional tasks including dressing and reaching to pick up objects.

Standing up and sitting down

Standing up from a seated position is one of the most commonly performed human actions and is an important prerequisite for the performance of many tasks. It is of particular interest in the study of balance since it involves considerable displacement of the COM during the transition from a relatively stable base of support (thighs and feet) to a dynamically unstable one (the feet). Propelling the body mass forward and upward represents a self-generated disturbance of postural stability, the effect of which must be adequately compensated for by neuromotor and musculoskeletal mechanisms throughout the movement. The timing of the change from propulsion to braking in the horizontal direction is particularly critical to balance control.

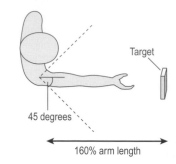

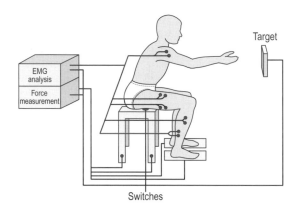

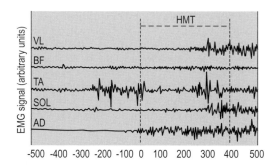

Fig. 7.5 Fast reaching to a target. *(Top)* Laboratory set-up; *(lower)* trial from one subject showing typical EMG traces from ipsilateral vastus lateralis (VL), biceps femoris (BF), tibialis anterior (TA), soleus (Sol) and anterior deltoid (AD) in a forward reach. Note, TA is the first muscle to turn on and it turns on before the focal arm muscle AD. Fast reaching beyond arm's length is an effective way to activate TA. *(Adapted from Crosbie J et al 1995, with permission).*

Both standing up and sitting down are achieved with large angular displacement at the hips resulting from forward flexion of the erect trunk segment (head, arms and trunk). In standing up, the first phase of the action occurs while the person remains seated and relatively stable. It is characterized by the generation of trunk/hip angular momentum. Trunk angular displacement must be far

enough and fast enough to accelerate the body mass forward from movement initiation, but it must also be constrained in order to maintain stability as standing is reached.

Conversely, the hip angular displacement required to sit down is also potentially destabilizing as it is superimposed on upright standing. Difficulty initiating sitting down and controlling movement of the COM backward can result in a rapid descent to sitting comparable to a fall (Dubost et al 2005).

Difficulty standing up from a chair is common in elderly people for many reasons but particularly if ability to balance the body is impaired. Schultz and colleagues (1992) compared sit-to-stand performance in young and elderly adults, some of whom in the latter group could not stand up without using their arms. Older adults had significantly increased angular displacements at the hip and knee joints compared with the young, but only moderate differences in peak joint moments of force at thighs-off. The larger joint displacements resulted in a more anterior position of the COM at thighs-off. This strategy provides more stability at thighs-off, since the COM would be within the foot support area before the extension phase begins.

Individuals with a neurological deficit and the frail elderly are at risk of losing independence if unable to stand up safely from a seated position. The possibility of falling and the inability to react quickly enough to prevent a fall while standing up and sitting down is well documented (Tinetti et al 1988; Nyberg & Gustafson 1995; Cheng et al 2001). Both actions require complex coordination of body segments while preserving balance. Lower limb muscle strength and balance both play a role in standing up. Lower limb muscle force production generally correlates with dynamic stability and is a strong predictor of the ability to stand up (Schenkman et al 1996).

Postural responses to perturbations

Unexpected perturbations are typically experienced when sitting or standing on a supporting surface that moves (on a train or a boat), when tripping over an obstacle or walking on a slippery surface, or when pushed in a crowd. Under these circumstances, postural adjustments occur in response to perturbations that are more threatening to our balance than those associated with self-initiated movements. Even under changing demands, however, we may use experience and visual information to predict an upcoming perturbation and to make preparatory adjustments accordingly. That is why we grab hold of a stable object if we are perturbed or if we suspect we will be thrown off balance. We step around or over perceived obstacles, and maintain a high degree of alertness in potentially hazardous conditions.

A number of investigations have been performed in order to assess an individual's ability to react to unexpected perturbations. In these experiments, subjects are mechanically disturbed by applying a direct force to the body or by moving the supporting surface on which they are standing. Experiments with a moveable platform that produces a postural perturbation in standing were first investigated by Nashner (1982) and were subsequently developed into a sensory organization test that involves sensory manipulation to identify the contribution of different sensory systems to stability (e.g., Nashner & Berthoz 1978; Nashner et al 1982). These tests are thought to provide useful information about how efficiently the person's sensory and motor systems respond to external perturbation.

Investigations have identified three postural muscle synergies that may be used to maintain standing balance during different support surface perturbations. Postural muscle activations in response to unexpected movements are specific both to the action and to the context in which that action takes place. These rapid muscle activations are not, however, like reflexes, since they are appropriately scaled to achieve the goal of stability (Ghez 1991). The most common response to minor anteroposterior translation of the supporting surface is a response, called an *ankle strategy*, in which postural adjustments are made principally at the ankle joint. Muscles are activated in a distal-to-proximal sequence, either anterior lower limb muscles to correct posterior destabilization or posterior limb muscles for anterior destabilization (Nashner & McCollum 1985). A stronger perturbation or a narrower support surface may require a *hip strategy* in which larger multijoint movements are used to bring the COM back within the base of support. Postural adjustments in this situation are made principally at the hip.

A *stepping response* is characterized by rapid steps, hops or stumbles that are made to form a new base of support for the body's COM when ankle or hip strategies have failed to compensate for very large or rapid perturbations. Originally it was thought that the stepping strategy only occurred with very marked instability or strong and rapid perturbations. However, earlier investigations had actually constrained the foot position, either implicitly or explicitly. More recent research suggests that a step strategy may often be preferred for even minor perturbations (Maki & McIlroy1997). The role of the fixed-support hip strategy appears to be limited to conditions that preclude the options of stepping or grasping. While these responses can be observed in simple clinical and laboratory settings, it appears to be more accurate to consider that adjustments that bring about balanced movement are task and context specific. The mechanical constraints of the segmental linkage and its dynamics are major factors in the muscle activation patterns that emerge during action.

Adaptive learning of postural control is illustrated in investigations of support surface movements. During unexpected support surface perturbations, the motor system can adapt according to stability needs (Fig. 7.6). In this

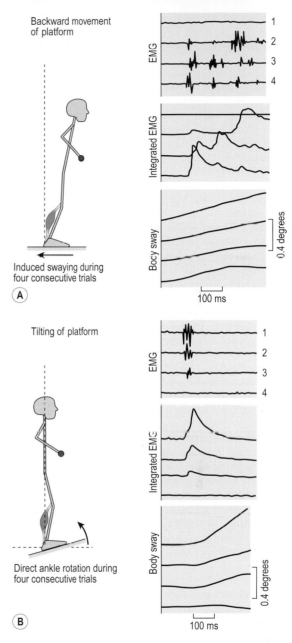

Fig. 7.6 Muscles that contract during unexpected support surface perturbations adapt to counteract the disturbance, i.e. appropriate anticipatory responses to postural disturbance can be learned. (A) Movement of the platform backward tilts the body forward. This stretches gastrocnemius triggering a reflexive response that stabilizes posture and prevents a fall forward. In successive trials the muscle response occurs progressively earlier. (B) When the feet are unexpectedly tilted toes-up, action by gastrocnemius is attenuated (i.e. it gradually disappears) since it would have a destabilizing effect. *(From Ghez C 1991, with permission).*

experiment the subject stands erect on a platform that can slide backward (A) or tilt toes-up (B). Both manoeuvres stretch the gastrocnemius. However, while forward sway induced by unexpected backward movement of the platform requires contraction of gastrocnemius to prevent a fall forward, backward sway that occurs when the platform is unexpectedly tilted toes-up requires that this muscle be inactive. Contraction of anterior leg muscles prevents the subject losing balance backward. In both conditions there is clear evidence that the subject learns to adapt the muscular response. Patients with cerebellar disorders, however, may be unable to make adaptive changes to postural control, suggesting an important role for the cerebellum in this type of motor learning (Horak & Diener 1994).

Occasionally when walking, we may trip and stumble. The source of tripping is often an uneven pavement, a misjudged step or an unseen or unexpected obstacle. A trip can occur in the swing phase of walking if toe clearance is insufficient. When this occurs, knee flexors of the swing leg and hip abductors and ankle plantarflexors of the stance leg have a shorter latency when a trip is induced early in swing (Eng et al 1994). When the trip occurs later in swing, however, the muscle response is different (Winter 1995b). A critical factor for recovery of balance after a trip is how quickly restorative forces can be generated. The rate of torque development (the time taken to generate peak force) rather than the available strength may be critical to balance recovery (Chen 1993). Divided attention increases the risk of tripping when negotiating obstacles in both young and old subjects and is likely to increase the risk of tripping in older subjects.

Studies of postural responses to stumbling while walking provide information about the mechanisms of these compensatory or *reactive balance responses*. The visual system plays an important part in identifying and avoiding potential threats to balance (Patla 1997). Avoidance of over-balancing or losing balance requires the ability to interpret afferent information to keep the COM within the base of support (Marigold et al 2004a) and depends to a large extent on the ability to pay attention to our surroundings, to identify and act quickly enough upon potential threats to stability. Support and stepping limbs both play an important role in protective stepping. Ineffective use of either the support or stepping limb can lead to a fall. The support limb serves to slow the body's 'fall' and provide time for an effective protective step (Pavol et al 2004).

To avoid threats to balance we may walk around obstacles, adapt our step length, width and height, increase ground clearance to avoid hitting an obstacle on the ground, bend down to increase head clearance to avoid hitting an obstacle, change direction or stop. These strategies are adaptive and are implemented for protection to ensure stability of the moving body. Kinaesthetic, tactile and vestibular inputs play an important role, particularly in the reactive control of balance during walking.

Reactive postural control by definition is a last resort or back-up in regaining balance and relies upon triggering quick responses (Patla 1993, 1997). As well as visually evaluating the external environment, an accurate internal representation of the forces acting on and within the body maintains stability both within the body and between the body and the supporting surface, steadying body parts for movement and stabilizing the body against gravity (Massion 1992). It is only when unexpected events occur and we fail to respond quickly enough that the emergency back-up system or reactive balance response is called in (Patla 1995; Huxham et al 2001). Both stepping and grasping reactions are the preferred options and can be initiated early, before the COM is near the limit of the base of support (Maki & McIlroy 1997). The responses are rapid and directionally specific. We lose balance only when unexpected events occur and we fail to respond quickly enough. Training programmes should include practice of rapid stepping, in particular of crossover stepping (see Figs. 7.21 & 7.22).

Compensatory stepping and grasping reactions are normally initiated and executed rapidly. The reaction to lateral destabilization is more complicated than antero-posterior destabilization due to the musculoskeletal restrictions on lateral lower limb movement. Crossover stepping appears to predominate in young able-bodied adults but is likely to cause problems for individuals with poor balance. Sensory feedback appears to become increasingly important in unpredictable conditions. Evidence suggests that plantar pressure feedback is an important source of feedback for the control of compensatory stepping (Do et al 1990).

In daily life, we are often required to remain balanced in standing while *withstanding the application of external forces*, for example picking up a heavy object or standing in a crowd. Such forces may be applied in a sagittal or frontal plane or diagonally. There has, however, been relatively little investigation of this aspect of balance in either able-bodied or disabled individuals (Lee et al 1988; Wing et al 1993). Lee and colleagues (1988) found little difference between healthy older (48–78 years) and younger (20–40 years) subjects in the maximal load they could withstand. Both groups, however, found posteriorly directed loads twice as destabilizing as loads applied from the side or in an anterior direction. The authors found no relationship between subjects' ability to withstand a load and their scores on timed tests of standing in regular, tandem and single-leg stance. These results illustrate the specificity of balance tests.

AGE-RELATED CHANGES

In spite of a large body of literature that has attempted to characterize the effect of ageing on balance, the issue remains complex, multifactorial and unclear. Increasing age is associated with a reduction in muscle strength and an increasing risk of developing pathologies that lead to degeneration in neural and/or musculoskeletal systems (Horak et al 1989). These authors draw attention to different definitions of elderly in research reports, and the relatively unselected populations typically investigated. There is no consistency among studies as to what demographic group constitutes 'older people'. It is also difficult to sort out whether physical deterioration is due to an ageing process or to a relatively inactive lifestyle. Inactivity may itself result in disuse changes in the neuromuscular system, including muscle weakness and slowed response time, and results in a reluctance to put balance under threat.

There are numerous reports of *loss of isometric and dynamic muscle strength* that may have been exacerbated by physical inactivity associated with a sedentary lifestyle. Overall muscle strength decreases only marginally in men aged between 20–40, whereas in women muscle strength declines from an earlier age than men and at a greater rate. In both men and women, however, muscle strength declines significantly after 60 (Lord et al 2007). Leg extensor power (the product of force and the rate of force generation) appears to decline at an even greater rate than isometric strength (Skelton et al 1994).

Lower limb muscle weakness has significant implications for older people and is a major risk factor for falling. Reduced strength is also reflected in difficulty standing up from a seated position without use of the arms. Inability to stand up without using the hands for steadying oneself is a significant factor in falls in both community- and institutional-dwelling groups of older people (Campbell et al 1989; Lord et al 2003). Use of hands to aid balance is only possible for the initial phase of standing up and the individual has to be able to balance while raising the body over a small base of support.

Loss of ankle joint mobility and reduced strength in the dorsi- and plantarflexor muscles are particularly significant for balance control (Vandervoort et al 1992). Severe weakness of muscles crossing the ankle, particularly ankle dorsi- and plantarflexors, has been reported in older individuals with a history of falls (Whipple et al 1987) and illustrates the critical role in postural stability of muscles that link the shank segment to the foot. Limited ankle mobility (particularly dorsiflexion) may also provoke tripping and falling. Decreased ankle mobility is particularly evident in women and is associated with increased and stiffer connective tissue and reduced strength of dorsi- and plantarflexor muscles (Vandervoort et al 1992).

Although postural sway has been reported to increase with advancing age, measurement of sway alone is not a good predictor of falls since performance on this test is variable (Lord et al 2007). A common observation in elderly people after a period of bed rest is loss of balance backward that may reflect a perceptual bias away from the erect position provoked by prolonged positioning in supine (Bohannon 1999). A major cause of postural instability and falls in older adults may also be related to central and peripheral visual impairments, to visual perceptual impairments and impairments in vestibular function. Defective visual perception of horizontal and vertical has been implicated in falling in older adults (Tobis et al 1981). One study of postural stability in standing during active body movement showed that elderly individuals may have difficulty balancing in standing when turning the head (Koceja et al 1999), which may reflect deficits of vestibular function. Several investigations utilizing sensory organization tests have shown that older subjects are less able to adapt to altered visual and support surface conditions compared to younger individuals (Whipple et al 1993).

There have been substantial gains in the evidence base over the last decade that have increased our understanding of the epidemiology and risk factors for falls by elderly individuals and strategies for prevention. Table 7.1 shows that aspects of vision and reduced functioning of peripheral sensation, muscle strength and reaction time are major contributors to falls. Reaction time has been consistently found to decline with age, even allowing for factors such as physical health, mode of response and level of motivation. Individuals with slowed reaction time may be susceptible to falls as a result of an inability to correct postural imbalance quickly enough. Medication side-effects are also implicated as risk factors for falling.

IMPAIRED POSTURAL CONTROL AND FUNCTIONAL LIMITATIONS

Any disruption to the ability to control the body's position in space as a consequence of a lesion to the CNS compromises postural stability. Laboratory and clinical investigations of postural control in patients with neurological conditions (stroke, traumatic brain injury, Parkinson's disease, multiple sclerosis) provide insights into the sensory and motor impairments that contribute to postural instability and are described in more detail in Chapters 11–14.

Impairments in physical function affecting balance and mobility include reduced muscle strength, power and endurance, reduced coordination, and disordered sensory and perceptual processes and cognitive dysfunction. These impairments all contribute to an increased incidence of falls. Executive functions such as cognitive flexibility or self-regulation, that is the ability to suppress reactive behaviour in favour of planned behaviour, and working memory, incorporate complex attentionality. Any of these functions may be impaired when the brain is lesioned, and problems such as risk taking and impaired selective attention may result.

Table 7.1 Sensory and neuromuscular factors associated with falls in the elderly

Factor	Strength of association
Vision	
Poor visual contrast sensitivity	***
Decreased depth perception	***
Poor visual acuity	**
Visual field loss	*
Increased visual field dependence	*
Poor hearing	–
Reduced vestibular function	*
Peripheral sensation	
Reduced vibration sense	***
Reduced tactile sensitivity	***
Reduced proprioception	**
Muscle strength	
Reduced muscle strength	***
Reduced muscle power	*
Reduced muscle endurance	*
Reaction time	
Poor simple reaction time	***
Poor choice reaction time	***

(Reprinted from Lord et al 2007, with permission).

Prolonged immobility and disuse imposed by an acute neural lesion, the relatively static nature of rehabilitation and an inactive lifestyle in individuals with chronic neural lesions living in the community all lead to adaptive changes in the musculoskeletal and cardiorespiratory systems. The resulting decrease in muscle strength and endurance, length-associated changes in soft tissues restricting joint range, decreased sensory receptiveness and deconditioned aerobic capacity can have significant effects on the individual, augmenting the postural dyscontrol and cognitive dysfunction.

Impairments affecting motor control and underlying poor balance may include a decrease in rate and frequency of motoneuron activation (loss of muscle strength) and poor timing of muscle activations (loss of coordination). These deficits affect all movement and interfere with the effective performance of everyday actions. The impairments lead to inability to control dynamic interactions between segments to maintain a relatively stable posture, to control segmental movement and balance during task performance and to respond rapidly both to anticipated and to unexpected perturbations.

Visual, tactile, proprioceptive and vestibular impairments can interfere with the processing of afferent inputs from the environment and from movement itself. Injury to or disease of higher centres may disrupt neural processing centres making it difficult to resolve conflicts among the senses. If one system is dysfunctional, redundancy in the system allows for compensation (Winter et al 1990). However, the ability to balance decreases when the functional redundancy between the sensory systems is reduced. The ability to re-weight sensory information requires cognitive processing and is therefore attention demanding. Vision is particularly important to balance, more so when standing on a compliant surface (Di Fabio & Badke 1991). Although individuals following stroke, for example, may be able to perform well in a well-lit environment on a firm, flat surface, they may have difficulty walking on carpet or in the dark (Shumway-Cook & Woollacott 2001). The clinical test, Sensory Interaction in Balance, provides a way of examining redundancy. The test provides a clinical method to evaluate somatosensory, visual and vestibular function for maintenance of upright posture (Nashner et al 1982) by modifying visual and support surface conditions.

Various biomechanical studies have examined individuals with neurological dysfunction performing self-initiated functional actions such as walking, standing up and sitting down, reaching to grasp or point in standing. Other studies have examined people's responses to unexpected perturbations. In these studies, balance dysfunction is inferred from evidence of slow movement times compared to age-matched able-bodied subjects, increased base of support, use of hands for support and balance and a tendency to lose balance while being tested. The findings are summarized in Box 7.1.

In response to these functional limitations, certain predictable adaptations to poor balance can be observed which reflect a range of adaptations that are mechanically possible (Box 7.2). If adaptive behaviours are allowed to persist, they may become habitual, preventing the individual from regaining flexibility in different contexts and environments. Fear of falling in the elderly and disabled population is a significant barrier to physical, social and recreational participation.

There is no single test that can measure all aspects of balance since balance is an integral part of all our daily actions. Tests that measure aspects of mobility, endurance and balance during task performance, such as the 6–10-metre walk test (speed, cadence, step length), 6-minute walk test (endurance), step test, repetitive sit-to-stand test, timed up-and-go test, are simple and reliable. A test is selected for its relevance to the specific information needed. They are described in Chapter 3.

Box 7.1 **Some experimental findings**

- Delayed or absent anticipatory and ongoing postural adjustments (Horak et al 1984; Di Fabio et al 1986; Lee et al 1988; Di Fabio & Badke 1990; Marigold et al 2004b) resulting in an inability to move without swaying, staggering and over-balancing
- Quiet stance – co-activation of muscles in the lower limb, resulting in a stiffening of the limb, rather than activation of muscles in a directionally-specific manner (Horak et al 1988)
- Walking – reduced speed and increased time spent in double support (von Schroeder et al 1995; Olney & Richards 1996)
- Stepping over obstacles – difficulty balancing on one leg to step (Said et al 1999) and decreased obstacle clearance (Said et al 2005)
- Reaching forward in sitting – reduced ground reaction forces under the feet limit the distance and speed of reaching (Dean & Shepherd 1997)
- Standing up – increased movement times (Engardt & Olsson 1992; Cheng et al 2001)
- Unexpected support surface perturbations – delayed or absent responses (Duncan & Badke 1987; Shumway-Cooke & Olmscheid 1990). Muscle onset latencies may be delayed and decreased in amplitude
- Difficulty withstanding force applied to the waist (Lee et al 1988) or to the hip (Wing et al 1993) and coping with release in both sagittal and frontal planes. Subjects were not obviously more affected by force applied to the paretic compared with the non-paretic side
- Slowed rate of force production (Canning et al 1999)
- Delayed stepping response (Marigold et al 2004b)
- People over 65 years of age may fall at least once annually (Lord et al 2003)

Box 7.2 **Adaptations to instability**

- Favouring the stronger and more rapidly responsive lower limb in sitting, standing, standing up and walking
- Increasing the base of support in sitting, standing (Fig. 7.7) and walking
- Restricting movement of the body mass (stiffening the body) to limit movement of the COM, for example not reaching beyond arm's length in sitting and standing
- Using and reliance on the hands/arms for support and balance (Fig. 7.8), even a constant grabbing onto something stable
- Avoiding threats to balance. Individuals with poor balance may avoid certain actions and restrict their physical and social activities for fear of falling. They align limb segments in ways that enable them to avoid moving the body mass too close to their limit of stability (Fig. 7.9). In sitting, for example, the individual may bend the trunk forward to reach for an object rather than sideways, since the latter involves shifting over a narrower base of support (Fig. 7.10)
- Prolonged immobility and lack of active stretch may lead to soft tissue adaptations, limiting joint range

performed with sufficient dosage and without reliance on upper limbs (Sherrington et al 2008a).

Mobility requires an accurate sense of balance and lower limb muscles that are strong enough to support and transport the body mass, capable of producing force quickly enough and at the appropriate time to respond to expected and unexpected events. Extensibility of soft tissue and joint flexibility are also important (see Ch. 2) and must be preserved (Fig. 7.11).

A shift in understanding of the functional significance of impaired muscle strength in patients with CNS lesions has led to a growing emphasis on functional, that is task-related, strength training. It is now recognized that lower limb muscle weakness and slowed force build-up are associated with functional disability, immobility, difficulty standing up and reduced gait speed, and are a major risk factor in falling in older and disabled people (e.g., Cheng et al 1998; Hyndman et al 2002; Marigold et al 2004a; Lord et al 2007). Training programmes should also include exercises that require a fast build-up of muscle force and propulsive (i.e., powerful) bursts of muscle activity.

The increasing proportion of elderly people in many countries has prompted a major research focus on risk factors and prevention of falls. It is becoming increasingly clear that although there are many different types of exercise available, some are more likely to result in improvement in balance and prevent falls than others. Lord and

BALANCE TRAINING

Balance is trained simultaneously as part of functional motor actions. Control and stability of the body mass is specific to each task and the conditions in which it is carried out – developing skill in any action involves in large part the acquisition of balance control. Laboratory investigations of both self-initiated actions and responses to expected and unexpected perturbations have repeatedly demonstrated the task- and context-specificity of postural adjustments. There is increasing evidence that challenging balance exercises in standing, with the aim of standing with feet close together and practising controlled movements of the COM, is the optimal way to improve balance during the performance of everyday actions when

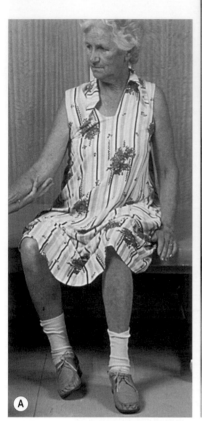

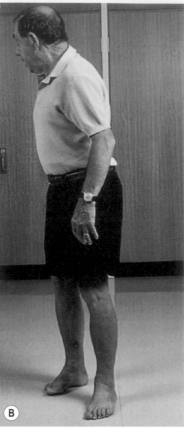

Fig. 7.7 (A) No active support through paretic R lower limb – it falls out sideways at the hip. (B) He increases the base of support by externally rotating the R paretic leg when he turns to speak to his wife. Notice how 'stiff' he is.

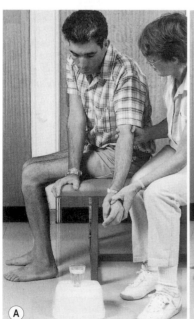

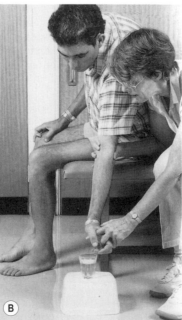

Fig. 7.8 This man has a paralysed L arm and leg and has just started exercising. (A) It is difficult for him to move sideways away from a stable position. He uses his R arm for support and balance and is reluctant to move further to the L in case he falls. (B) He is able to move further to the L as he gets the idea of loading his L leg which gives him more stability.

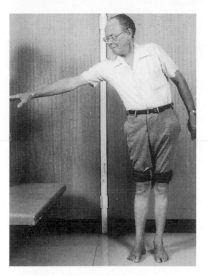

Fig. 7.9 He avoids movement sideways over the weak R leg as he reaches laterally to touch a target.

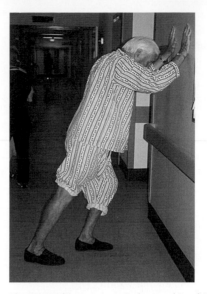

Fig. 7.11 This man is actively stretching his R calf muscle as he practises push-ups against the wall to improve control of his R arm.

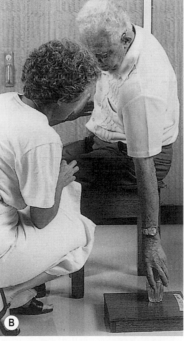

Fig. 7.10 Reaching sideways. (A) He moves the body forward and reaches back to the glass. (B) Note, he can move his body sideways when the reach distance is decreased.

colleagues (2007), summarizing the current evidence from 44 randomized controlled trials, point out that effective exercise programmes for preventing falls comprise challenging and progressive balance exercises performed in weightbearing positions that minimize the use of upper limbs for support. These factors seem to discriminate between effective and non-effective interventions. As Lord and colleagues (2007) point out, exercise programmes are likely to be more effective if targeted to the person's particular deficits and lifestyle.

Further research is needed to provide evidence of efficacy for balance-focused task-specific exercise programmes in neurological rehabilitation. Training everyday actions during rehabilitation also needs to take account of the complex environments outside the rehabilitation setting, the precarious nature of balance and the significance of fear of falling in the lives of the elderly and disabled. It is incumbent on clinicians to do better. The guidelines for training outlined below are based on contemporary theories and research, and provide a logical foundation for training. A recent Cochrane systematic review recommends that future research should investigate clearly described intervention methods including task-specific training (Pollock et al 2007).

Postural stability, whether in quiet standing or when moving, requires a sense of awareness of where one is in space and the ability to make adjustments by appropriately timed and scaled muscle activations. Practice, therefore, is designed to enable the individual to learn again how to control movements of the COM relative to the base of support, and even when the base of support is changing, for example in standing up and walking.

Normally we automatically set up the segmental (postural) alignment that best suits an action prior to the start of that action, for example we pull our feet back before standing up, an alignment that favours the necessary muscle activity and feels comfortable. Similarly, early after stroke or traumatic brain injury, postural stability in sitting can only be regained with the person sitting. The therapist may have to help the person into sitting as a prerequisite for getting the idea of balancing the body mass. However, self-initiated movements of the body mass over the base of support (thighs and feet) then provide the opportunity to regain the ability to cope with gravity and also to focus attention on the people and objects around the room. Re-establishing sitting balance without arm use very early after stroke and traumatic brain injury impacts positively on many critical functions (Johansson 2000). Achieving effective postural control in sitting is significantly related to mobility outcomes after stroke (Morgan 1994) and has been reported to be an important milestone in the rehabilitation/recovery process (Sandin & Smith 1990; Tsang & Mak 2004).

Reaching to a concrete goal in sitting and standing is task specific but also involves implicit training of balance. Initially, the target to reach or pick up can be placed at arm's length. It can then be moved further away so that the person is pushed near his or her limits of stability (Perennou & Bronstein 2005) (Fig. 7.12).

Loading the lower limbs. Patients with muscle weakness and poor motor control have difficulty shifting weight from one leg to the other and therefore lack effective and efficient anticipatory, ongoing and responsive postural adjustments. The ability to transfer weight from one leg to the other is critical for functional mobility and a prerequisite for walking and stair climbing (Eng & Chu 2002). However, one study showed that participants

post-stroke could shift only 55% of their body weight onto the paretic limb when standing with the paretic limb in front, and only 65% of their body weight in a lateral direction with the feet parallel (Goldie et al 1996a,b). It is also a common finding that stroke patients bear less weight on the paretic limb when standing up from a seated position (Engardt & Olsson 1992).

Loading the lower limb is critical for stimulating muscle activity – receptors sensitive to load have been shown to activate leg extensor muscles during locomotion in cats. Sensitivity to load has also been recorded in humans, with a high correlation between extensor muscle activity and limb loading. Load receptors are said to be particularly important in signaling COM position (Dietz et al 1992).

An *overhead harness* makes if possible for even a weak person to load a paretic limb in standing while controlling movements of the COM without grabbing for support and without fear of falling (Fig. 7.13). Reaching, stepping and step-up exercises can all be practised in a harness and should commence early after an acute lesion, since patients soon learn to adapt to poor stability by avoiding movement. Hill and colleagues (1994) reported a decrease in fear of falling and increased confidence in a group of elderly individuals wearing a harness. Their results indicate that dynamic and natural movements were unhindered despite being carried out in the harness.

Availability of external supports such as a harness or a *belt with grab handles* (Fig. 7.14) for walking practice increases confidence of both patient and therapist. Without such devices, standing actions and walking are likely to be deferred to some hypothetical time in the future, or if they are practised, patients may learn to rely on their hands and staff members to support them. Balance will not improve until the person has the opportunity to practise moving independently and hands free, creating the need to make active anticipatory postural adjustments and ongoing corrections. The therapist close by (but not holding on) can provide some emotional stability and inspiration although the task may demand physical instability. Holding on to a person eliminates the need for them to make active corrections. The base of support should be narrow and use of the hands must be avoided as even touching a support with a finger changes the underlying mechanisms of postural adjustment.

Some simple methods of retraining tasks with concrete goals are illustrated below. A concrete task rather than an abstract one takes the person's attention away from the need to balance by directing it toward the goal of the action itself. This is particularly useful for a person early after stroke who is frightened of falling if they move.

The following exercises involve weightbearing with quite small excursions of the COM. Actions may need to be modified initially so that adjustments required for successful performance are relatively small. This reduces balance demands, making the task potentially achievable in a simplified form while still presenting a challenge.

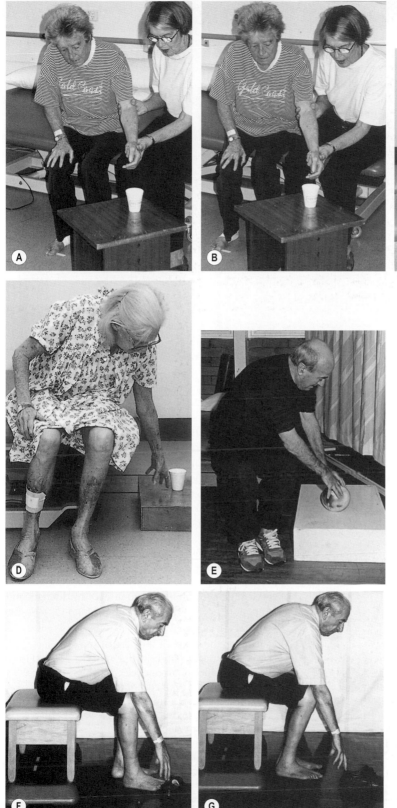

Fig. 7.12 Training sitting balance, i.e. the ability to move about in sitting without falling or holding on. (A) On her early attempt at reaching to the cup she is reluctant to move her body over to the L; (B) some improvement is evident after a few repetitions. She is able to reach further and is more confident in her ability to regain the upright position. The therapist is supporting the paretic arm, as she cannot move it herself, but she moves her body actively to the L side. (C) Using the L leg for support and balance she reaches forward. (D) Using the L leg for support and balance as she reaches to the side and back. (E) Reaching bimanually is practised also. (F, G) Moving the feet back forces loading through the paretic R leg. The further the object is from the foot, the more loading.

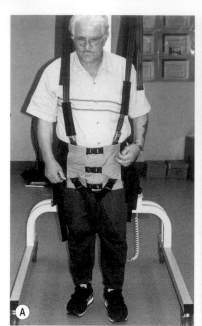
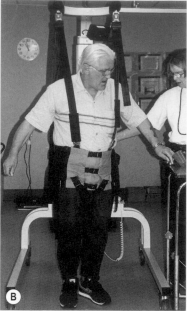
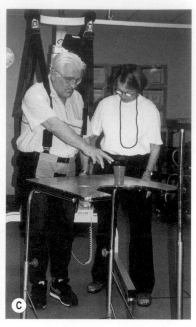

Fig. 7.13 Training balance in a harness. (A) Notice that he loads his R leg more than his paretic L leg. (B) Reaching to the cup on his L, his instability is evident as he tries to turn his hand and take the cup. (C) After several practices he is more confident and is reaching across the body to the L. Note that his attentional focus is on the cup (a concrete task) and not on his balance.

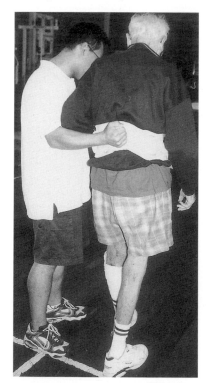

Fig 7.14 A belt with grab handles gives some reassurance to patient and therapist without interfering with the action. *(Handi-Lift/Walk Belt. Pelican Manufacturing, Osborne Park Western Australia 6017).*

These actions can be practised in both sitting and standing, and should target an individual's particular deficits:

- Looking up at the ceiling (Fig. 7.15A) (anticipatory activations of leg muscles ensure the COM does not move back when the head is tilted back).
- Turning to look over each shoulder, scanning the environment to pick out specified items, without moving her feet (Fig. 7.15B).
- Reaching forward, sideways, backwards, up and down to take an object (Fig. 7.15C–F).

Tasks are made progressively more challenging in terms of speed and predictability, postural stability, strength and coordination in both sitting and standing by the following:

- Changing the shape of the base of support (feet together, tandem standing, one foot on a step (Fig. 7.16), or standing on one leg). Sensory input can also be modified by incorporating an eyes-closed condition or a foam surface (Marigold et al 2005).
- Increasing and varying the object's weight and distance from the body.
- Increasing the object's size so both hands must be used (Fig. 7.17).
- Changing the location of the object – moving laterally is harder than moving forward.
- Increasing speed demands.
- Squatting to pick up an object on a box (Fig. 7.18), progressing to the floor.

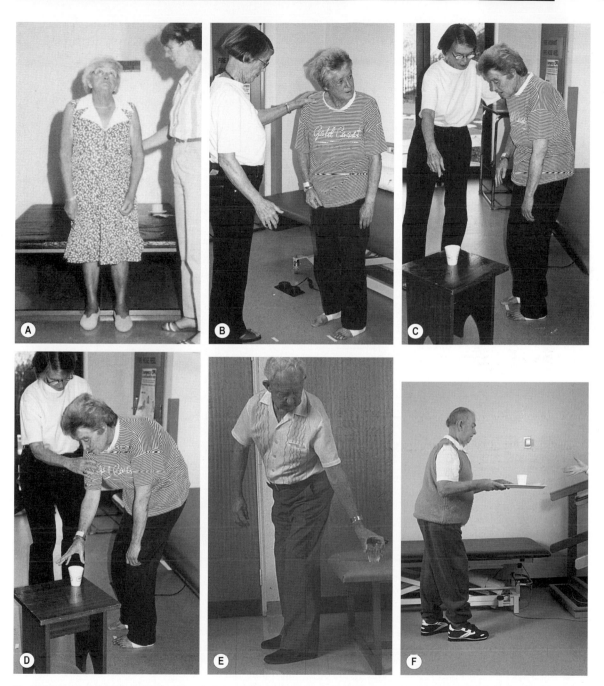

Fig 7.15 Getting the idea of balancing during small movements of the body mass. (A) Looking up at the ceiling to locate a target. (B) Turning to look over her shoulder to find out the time from the wall clock. She also practises turning to the R. As she becomes more confident the foot position can be changed to half tandem and the task can be changed. (C) She is not confident about picking up the cup as it means moving her weight over the L leg. (D) She reaches across her body. At first she is doubtful she can pick up the cup but with stand-by reassurance and instructions to bend her knees she succeeds. (E) He is practising moving about in standing. He turns to put the glass down on the bench behind without losing balance backward. (F) Holding himself stiffly with flexed hips in step standing – he is plucking up courage to pass the tray to the assistant.

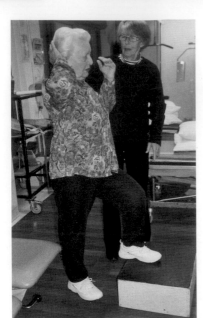

Fig 7.16 Once she gets a sense of balance in this position of considerable instability, she reaches toward her head.

- Touching blocks or marks on the floor with the toes to challenge mediolateral stability (Fig. 7.19).
- Responding to external demands, as in catching a ball (Fig. 7.20).
- Challenging the individual's weak spots, for example in directions that are particularly hard to control.

These actions are self-initiated and train postural adjustments, anticipatory, ongoing and reactive as part of the actions themselves. In general, however, focus of the learner is on the task, not on the need to balance. In this way, the person develops the ability to cope with the interactive forces set up by segmental movement. Movement excursions are increased with the COM moving closer to the perimeter of the base of support.

There is increasing research evidence that balance can be improved by paying attention to the task itself, that is, the effects of movement, rather than to balancing (Stoffregen et al 2000; Wulf et al 2001). For example, holding a glass of water while reaching to place it on a table may seem too difficult, but is made easier by an external focus on not spilling the water, rather than on balance itself. Wulf and colleagues (2004) suggest that the motor system is a smart system that optimizes control processes on the basis of movement effect relative to what the performer wants to achieve (the intention or goal) (see Ch. 2). The patient can be taught the technique of focusing the eyes on a point ahead to maximize stability in difficult balancing situations. Fixing the gaze in this way or on the object to be reached keeps the head and eyes steady and can increase the sense of being balanced.

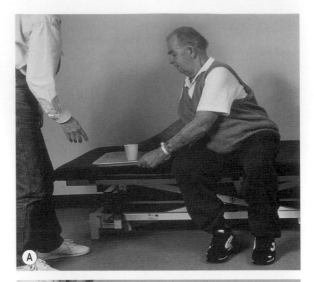

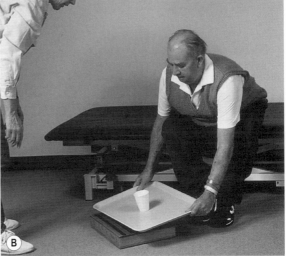

Fig 7.17 The task is to move the tray from bench to floor without spilling the water or dislodging the cup, i.e. the focus is on concrete goals.

By practising varied actions in different environments, the person has the opportunity to regain the skill of balancing without thinking about *how* they do it. It is always important that the task is concrete so the success or otherwise of the person's action is immediately knowable.

Functional strength training

There is now considerable evidence that strength relates directly to functional motor control and that both can be improved by intensive and functionally based training that is challenging for the individual. Training is progressed to extend the capabilities of each individual.

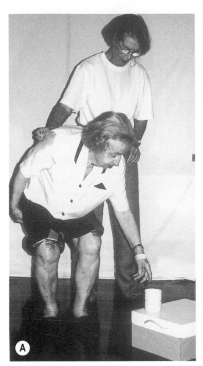
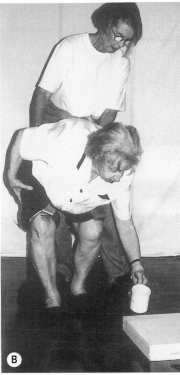

Fig 7.18 Squatting practice: (A) practising with the cup on a box develops confidence to reach even lower (B).

Multiple repetitions are required and load is increased to increase strength and power (see Ch. 2).

For most daily tasks, such as standing up from a chair, walking, squatting and stair climbing, the feet are in contact with the ground and muscles work to support, balance and propel the body mass over the feet. The basic pattern of intersegmental coordination of these actions consists of flexion and extension at the hips, knees and ankles, the three joints acting as a single unit as the body mass is raised and lowered over the base of support (see figures in Ch. 2). These exercises strengthen weak muscles concentrically and eccentrically using body weight resistance and provide practice of segmental limb control, and they are familiar actions to the individual. In addition, these exercises require coordination of muscles that make postural adjustments. Soft tissue extensibility must be preserved in order to allow the necessary joint displacements. Reduced joint range has a negative effect on the mechanics of an action.

Exercise intensity is increased by increasing the number of repetitions (see Ch. 2), the height of the blocks for step-ups, lowering the height of the chair for standing up and decreasing hand support. Several studies have added weight resistance with good effect – for example, marching with 0.5-kg ankle weights to strengthen hip flexor muscles for pull-off in walking (Eng et al 2003), wearing weights around the torso during repetitive standing up and sitting

down in children with cerebral palsy (Liao et al 2007) or practising sit-to-stand with weighted vests.

Strength training for neurological patients should have as its main effect improved function in actions necessary for wellbeing and participation. However, strength training itself may not generalize into improved functional performance. Several authors have noted greater benefit from lower limb weightbearing exercise programmes (Krebs et al 2007; Olivetti et al 2007; Sherrington et al 2008b) compared with non-weightbearing strength training in elderly individuals, some of whom had a neurological lesion. In these studies, the activities practised showed greater improvement illustrating the specificity principle in exercise (see Ch. 2). The results of these studies illustrate the neural component of strength adaptation (Sale 1988) since functional strength is a neuromuscular phenomenon and an increase in strength occurs earlier than an increase in muscle mass. It is noted by the authors that these studies carried out in an inpatient rehabilitation setting or in community programmes were both feasible and safe.

Maximizing skill

Activities are made progressively more challenging according to their destabilizing effects (depending on the individual's level of ability), with more complex environments

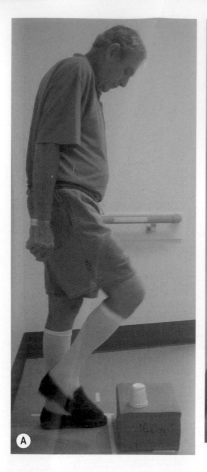
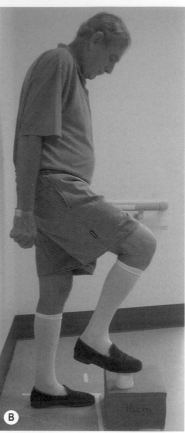

Fig 7.19 Stepping to touch a plastic cup requires careful foot placement while loading and balancing on one leg then changing to the other leg. *(Courtesy of K Schurr and S Dorsch, Physiotherapy Department, Bankstown-Lidcombe Hospital, Australia).*

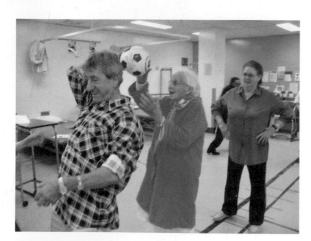

Fig 7.20 Having fun in an exercise class: passing the ball. Focus is on the ball. *(Courtesy of K Schurr and S Dorsch, Physiotherapy Department, Bankstown-Lidcombe Hospital, Australia).*

and with unpredictable demands. The following activities involve dynamic loading and unloading of lower limbs:

- Stepping to pick up an object placed beyond the person's limit of stability, making it necessary to take a step.
- Crossover stepping to marks on the floor (Fig. 7.21).
- Lunges in different directions.
- Stepping or dancing in time with music.
- Responding to external timing demands: playing games that require a rapid response and make it imperative to take a step, such as catching and throwing a ball, bouncing a ball, kicking a ball, computer-controlled games played in standing (e.g., Nintendo Wii).
- Coping with complexity and uncertainty in the environment. For example, negotiating an obstacle course, under and over objects, automatic lift doors, making sudden stops and turns, tandem walking (Fig. 7.22A), crossover walking (Fig. 7.22B), stepping over objects (Fig. 7.22C), marching on the spot with hips flexing to 90° and simultaneously performing

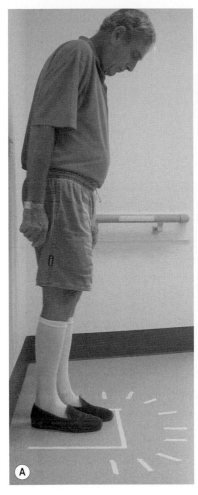 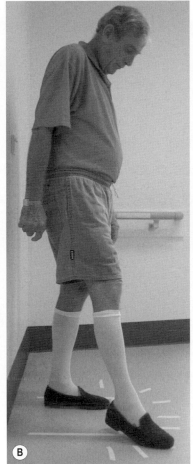 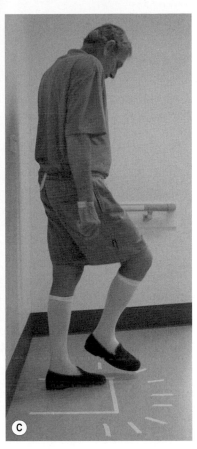

Fig 7.21 Stepping out and stepping across the supporting leg are difficult actions for someone with poor balance when asked to do it quickly but are normally critical responses to prevent a fall from a stumble. *(Courtesy of K Schurr and S Dorsch, Physiotherapy Department, Bankstown-Lidcombe Hospital, Australia).*

two actions, such as walking and talking, or carrying an object.

Feedback devices. Visual or auditory feedback has been suggested to provide an additional means of training balance. Computerized devices and force platforms give visual feedback of the position of the COP on a screen as the person attempts to control the extent of postural sway or shifts the body mass to a specific target. A Cochrane systematic review concluded that although force platform feedback in standing improved stance symmetry, it did not improve clinical balance outcomes (Berg Balance Scale, timed up-and-go test) nor did it improve overall independence (Barclay-Goddard et al 2004). Similarly,

another review was unable to confirm any carryover from increased stance symmetry to improved performance in gait performance tests. That is, although an individual may increase stance symmetry, it did not generalize into functional improvement (van Peppen et al 2004). The issue of specificity is a particularly complex one in balance, both in training methods and in measurement.

Visual feedback may, however, provide a diversion to overcome a reluctance to move and get the idea of balancing the body mass over the base of support and be both interesting and fun for a while (Fig. 7.23). However, the individual must have the opportunity to move on and learn to use naturally occurring feedback in the practice of real-life tasks.

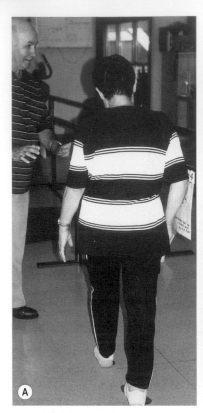

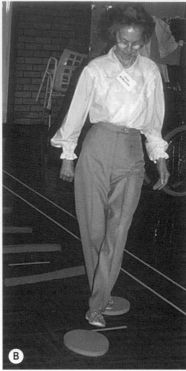

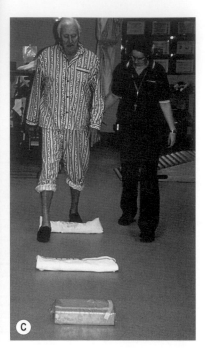

Fig 7.22 Stepping on markers on the floor. (A) Tandem walking (Courtesy of F Mackey and colleagues, Illawarra Area Health Service, Australia.) (B) Cross-over stepping. (C) Walking on an obstacle course – stepping over objects. Attention is directed toward height or width of objects, i.e. focus is on the obstacles rather than on body movement and balance.

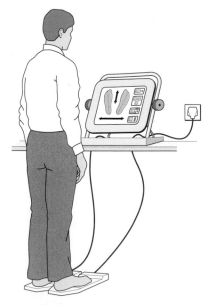

Fig 7.23 Computerized devices such as the Balance Performance Monitor (SMS Healthcare) can be used to give feedback about postural sway.

SUMMARY

Given that the ability to balance underlies all our actions, rehabilitation programmes should emphasize sitting, standing and body transport with opportunities to regain a sense of balance. Fear on the part of the rehabilitation team that the patient may fall should not hold staff back from intensive and challenging training that may help the patient regain the ability to balance independently. The use of a harness enables even a weak person to control small movements of the COM without fear of falling. An understanding of the importance of lower limb muscle strength to balance increases the likelihood that rehabilitation will be effective in improving balance and preventing falls, particularly in elderly individuals.

We would urge a change in attitude to balance training giving greater priority to challenging balance in different contexts while building up the individual's confidence in their ability to recover balance by moving their feet rather than grabbing onto the nearest solid structure.

REFERENCES

Arutyunyan GA, Gurfinkel VS, Mirskii M 1969 Organization of movements on execution by man of an exact postural task. Biofizika 14:1103–1107.

Barclay-Goddard RE, Stevenson TJ, Poluha W et al 2004 Force platform feedback for standing balance training after stroke. Cochrane Database Syst Rev, Issue 4. Art. No.: CD004129. DOI: 10.1002/14651858.CD004129.pub2.

Belenkii V, Gurfinkel VS, Paltsev YI 1967 Elements of control of voluntary movement. Biofizika 12:135–141.

Bohannon RW 1999 Observations of balance among elderly patients referred to physical therapy in an acute care hospital. Physiother Theory Pract 15:185–189.

Bouisset S, Duchene J-L 1994 Is body balance more perturbed by respiration in seating than in standing posture? Neuroreport 5:957–960.

Campbell AJ, Borrie MJ, Spears GF 1989 Risk factors for falls in a community based prospective study of people 70 years and older. J Gerontol 44A:M112–117.

Canning CG, Ada L, O'Dwyer N 1999 Slowness to develop force contributes to weakness after stroke. Arch Phys Med Rehabil 80:66–70.

Carr JH, Shepherd RB 1998 Neurological neurorehabilitation: optimizing motor performance. Elsevier, Oxford.

Carr JH, Shepherd RB 2003 Stroke rehabilitation: guidelines for exercise and training to optimize motor skill. Elsevier, Oxford.

Chari VR, Kirby RL 1986 Lower-limb influence on sitting balance while reaching forward. Arch Phys Med Rehabil 67:730–733.

Chen HC 1993 Factors underlying balance restoration after tripping: biomechanical model analyses. Doctoral Dissertation, University of Michigan.

Cheng PT, Liaw MY, Wong MK et al 1998 The sit-to-stand movement in stroke patients and its correlation with falling. Arch Phys Med Rehabil 79:1043–1046.

Cheng P, Wu S, Liaw M et al 2001 Symmetrical body-weight distribution training in stroke patients and its effect on fall prevention. Arch Phys Med Rehabil 82:1650–1654.

Colle FM 1995 The measurement of standing balance after stroke. Physiother Theory Pract 11:109–118.

Crosbie J, Shepherd RB, Squire T 1995 Postural and voluntary movement during reaching in sitting: the role of the lower limbs. J Hum Mov Studies 28:103–126.

Day B, Steiger MJ, Thompson PD et al 1993 Effect of vision and stance width on human body motion when standing: implications for afferent control of lateral sway. J Physiol 46:479–499.

Dean CM, Shepherd RB 1997 Task-related training improves performance of seated reaching tasks following stroke: a randomised controlled trial. Stroke 28:722–728.

Dean C, Shepherd R, Adams R 1999a Sitting balance I: trunk–arm and the contribution of the lower limbs during self-paced reaching in sitting. Gait Posture 10:135–144.

Dean C, Shepherd RB, Adams RD 1999b Sitting balance II: reach direction and thigh support affect the contribution of the lower limbs when reaching in sitting. Gait Posture 10:147–153.

De Wit G 1972 Optic versus vestibular and proprioceptive impulses measured by posturometry. Agressologie 13:75–79.

Diener H-C, Dichgans B, Guschlbauer M et al 1992 The coordination of posture and voluntary movement in patients with cerebellar dysfunction. Mov Disord 7:14–22.

Dietz V, Noth J 1978 Pre-innervation and stretch responses of triceps brachii in man falling with and without visual control. Brain Res 142:576–579.

Dietz V, Quintern J, Boos G et al 1986 Obstruction of the swing phase during gait: phase-dependent bilateral leg muscle coordination. Brain Res 384:166–169.

Dietz V, Gollhofer A, Kleiber M et al 1992 Regulation of bipedal stance: dependency on 'load' receptors. Exp Brain Res 89:229–231.

Di Fabio RP, Badke MB 1990 Extraneous movement associated with hemiplegic postural sway during dynamic goal-directed weight distribution. Arch Phys Med Rehabil 71:365–371.

Di Fabio RP, Badke MB 1991 Stance duration under sensory conflict conditions in patients with hemiplegia. Arch Phys Med Rehabil 72:292–295.

Di Fabio RP, Badke MB, Duncan PW 1986 Adapting human postural reflexes following a localized cerebrovascular lesion: analysis of bilateral long latency responses. Brain Res 363:257–264.

Do MC, Bussel B, Breniere Y 1990 Influence of plantar cutaneous afferents on early compensatory reactions to forward fall. Exp Brain Res 79:319–324.

Dubost V, Beauchet O, Manckiyoundia P et al 2005 Decreased trunk angular displacement during sitting down: an early feature of aging. Phys Ther 85:404–412.

Duncan PW, Badke MB 1987 Stroke rehabilitation: the recovery of motor control. Year Book Medical Publishers, Chicago.

Duysens J, Clarac F, Cruse H 2000 Load regulating mechanisms in gait and posture: comparative aspects. Physiol Rev 80:83–133.

Eng JJ, Chu KS 2002 Reliability and comparison of weight-bearing ability during standing tasks for individuals with chronic stroke. Arch Phys Med Rehabil 83:1138–1144.

Eng JJ, Winter DA, Patla AE et al 1992 Role of the torque stabilizer in postural control during rapid voluntary arm movements. In: Woollacott M, Horak F (eds) Posture and gait: control of mechanisms. 11th International Symposium of the Society for Postural and Gait Research, University of Oregon, Portland, OR.

Eng JJ, Winter DA, Patla AE 1994 Neuromuscular strategies for recovery from a trip in early and late swing during human walking. Exp Brain Res 102:339–349.

Eng JJ, Chu KS, Kim M et al 2003 A community-based group exercise program for persons with chronic stroke. Med Sci Sports Exerc 35:1271–1278.

Engardt M, Olsson E 1992 Body weight-bearing while rising and sitting down in patients with stroke. Scand J Rehabil Med 24:67–74.

Figura F, Felici F, Macellari V 1986 Human locomotion adjustments during perturbed walking. Hum Mov Sci 5:313–332.

Ghez C 1991 Posture. In: Kandel ER, Schwartz JH, Jessell TM (eds) Principles of neural science, 3rd edn. Appleton and Lange, Norwalk, CT:596–608.

Gibson JJ 1979 The ecological approach to visual perception. Houghton Mifflin, Boston.

Gill-Body K, Krebs D 1994 Usefulness of biomechanical measurements approaches to rehabilitation. Top Geriatr Rehabil 10:82–96.

Goldie PA, Matyas TA, Evans OM et al 1996a Maximum voluntary weight-bearing by the affected and unaffected legs in standing following stroke. Clin Biomech 11:333–342.

Goldie PA, Evans O, Matyas T 1996b Performance in the stability limits test during rehabilitation following stroke. Gait Posture 4:315–322.

Guadagnoli M, McNevin N, Wulf G 2002 Cognitive influences to balance and posture. Orthoped Phys Ther Clin N Am 11:131–141.

Gurfinkel VS, Elner AM 1973 On two types of static disturbances in patients with local lesions of the brain. Agressologie 14D:65–72.

Gurfinkel VS, Elner AM 1988 Participation of secondary motor area of the frontal lobe in organization of postural components of voluntary movements in man. Neurophysiology 20:7–14.

Hill KM, Harburn KL, Kramer JF et al 1994 Comparison of balance responses to an external perturbation test, with and without an overhead harness safety system. Gait Posture 2:27–31.

Horak F 1987 Clinical measurement of postural sway in adults. Phys Ther 67:1881–1885.

Horak FB, Diener HC 1994 Cerebellar control of postural scaling and central set in stance. J Neurol Sci 72:479–493.

Horak FB, Esselman P, Anderson ME et al 1984 The effects of movement velocity, mass displaced and task certainty on associated postural adjustments made by normal and hemiplegic individuals. J

Neurol Neurosurg Psychiatry 48:1020–1028.

Horak FB, Nashner LM, Nutt JG 1988 Postural instability in Parkinson's disease: motor coordination and sensory organization. Neurol Report 12:54–55.

Horak FB, Shupert CL, Mirka A 1989 Components of postural dyscontrol in the elderly: a review. Neurobiol Aging 10:727–738.

Huxham FE, Goldie PA, Patla AE 2001 Theoretical considerations in balance assessment. Aust J Physiother 47:89–100.

Hyndman D, Ashburn A, Stack E 2002 Fall events among people with stroke living in the community: circumstances of falls and characteristics of fallers. Arch Phys Med Rehabil 83:165–170.

Johansson B 2000 Brain plasticity and stroke rehabilitation: the Willis lecture. Stroke 31:223–230.

Kaminski T, Bock C, Gentile AM 1995 The coordination between trunk and arm motion during pointing movements. Exp Brain Res 106:457–466.

Kandel ER, Schwartz JH, Jessel TM 1991 Principles of neural science, 3rd edn. Appleton and Lange, Norwalk, CT.

Kavounoudias A, Roll R, Roll JP 2001 Foot sole and ankle muscle inputs contribute jointly to human erect posture regulation. J Physiol 532:869–878.

Kirby RL, Price NA, MacLeod DA 1987 The influence of foot position on standing balance. J Biomech 20:423–427.

Kirker SGB, Simpson S, Jenner JR et al 2000 Stepping before standing: hip muscle function in stepping and standing balance after stroke. J Neurol Neurosurg Psychiatry 68:458–464.

Koceja DM, Allway D, Earles DR 1999 Age differences in postural sway during volitional head movements. Arch Phys Med Rehabil 80:1537–1541.

Krebs DE, Scarborough DM, McGibbon CA 2007 Functional vs. strength training in disabled elderly outpatients. Am J Phys Med Rehabil 86:93–103.

Kuo AD, Zajak FE 1993 A biomechanical analysis of muscle strength as a limiting factor in standing posture. J Biomech 26(Suppl 1):137–150.

Liao H, Liu Y, Liu W et al 2007 Effectiveness of loaded sit-to-stand resistance exercise for children with mild spastic diplegia: a randomized clinical trial. Arch Phys Med Rehabil 88:25–31.

Lee DN, Aronson E 1974 Visual proprioceptive control of standing in human infants. Percept Psychophys 15:529–532.

Lee DN, Lishman JR 1975 Visual proprioceptive control of stance. J Hum Mov Sci 1:87–95.

Lee WA, Deming L, Sahgal V 1988 Quantitative and clinical measures of static standing balance in hemiparetic and normal subjects. Phys Ther 68:970–976.

Lee RG, Tonolli I, Viallet F et al 1995 Preparatory postural adjustments in Parkinsonian patients with postural instability. Can J Neurol Sci 22:126–135.

Lishman JR, Lee DN 1973 The autonomy of visual kinaesthesis. Perception 2:287–294.

Lord SR, March LM, Cameron ID et al 2003 Differing risk factors for falls in nursing home and intermediate-care residents who can and cannot stand unaided. J Am Geriatr Soc 51:1645–1650.

Lord SR, Sherringon C, Menz H et al 2007 Falls in older people. Cambridge University Press, Cambridge.

Magnus R 1926 Some results of studies in the physiology of posture. I. Lancet 221:531–536.

Maki BE, McIlroy WE 1997 The role of limb movements in maintaining upright stance: the 'change in support' strategy. Phys Ther 77:488–507.

Marigold DS, Eng JJ, Tokuno CD et al 2004a Contribution of muscle strength and integration of afferent input to postural instability in persons with stroke. Neurorehabil Neural Repair 18:222–229.

Marigold DS, Eng JJ, Inglis JT 2004b Modulation of ankle muscle postural reflexes in stroke: influence of weight-bearing load. Clin Neurophysiol 115:2789–2797.

Marigold DS, Eng JJ, Dawson AS et al 2005 Exercise leads to faster postural reflexes, improved balance, and mobility and fewer falls in older persons with stroke. J Am Geriatr Soc 53:416–423.

Massion J 1992 Movement, posture and equilibrium: interaction and coordination. Prog Neurobiol 38:35–56.

Massion J, Woollacott M 1996 Normal balance and postural control. In: Bronstein AM, Brandt T, Woollacott M (eds) Clinical aspects of balance and gait disorders. Edward Arnold, London:1–18.

Melvill-Jones G 2000 Posture. In: Kandel ER, Schwartz JH, Jessell TM (eds) Principles of neuroscience, 4th edn. McGraw-Hill, New York:816–831.

Mercer VS, Sahrmann SA 1999 Postural synergies associated with a stepping task. Phys Ther 79:1142–1152.

Morgan P 1994 The relationship between sitting balance and mobility outcome in stroke. Aust J Physiother 40:91–95.

Nashner LM 1980 Balance adjustments of humans perturbed while walking. J Neurophysiol 44:650–664.

Nashner LM 1982 Adaptation of human movement to altered environments. Trends Neurosci 5:358–361.

Nashner LM 1983 Analysis of movement control in man using the moveable platform. In: Desmedt JE (ed.) Motor control mechanisms in health and disease. Raven Press, New York:607–619.

Nashner LM, Berthoz A 1978 Visual contribution to rapid motor responses during posture control. Brain Res 150:403–407.

Nashner LM, Forssberg H 1986 Phase-dependent organisation of postural adjustments associated with arm movements while walking. J Neurophysiol 55:1382–1394.

Nashner LM, McCollum G 1985 The organisation of human postural movements: a formal basis and experimental synthesis. Behav Brain Sci 8:135–172.

Nashner LM, Black FO, Wall C 1982 Adaptation to altered support and visual conditions during stance: patients with vestibular deficits. J Neurosci 2:536–544.

Nyberg L, Gustafson Y 1995 Patient falls in stroke rehabilitation. A challenge to rehabilitation strategies. Stroke 26:838–842.

Olivetti L, Schurr K, Sherrington C et al 2007 A novel weight-bearing strengthening program during rehabilitation of older people is feasible and improves standing up more than a non-weight-bearing strengthening program: a

randomised trial. Aust J Physiother 53:147–153.

Olney SJ, Richards C 1996 Hemiparetic gait following stroke, Pt 1: characteristics. Gait Posture 4:136–148.

Owen DH 1985 Maintaining posture and avoiding tripping. Clin Geriatr Med 1:581–599.

Pai Y-C, Rogers MW, Hedman LD et al 1994 Alteration in weight-transfer capabilities in adults with hemiparesis. Phys Ther 74:647–657.

Patla AE 1986 Adaptation of postural response to voluntary arm raises during locomotion in humans. Neurosci Lett 68:334–338.

Patla AE 1993 Age-related changes in visually guided locomotion over different terrains: major issues. In: Stelmach GE, Homberg V (eds) Sensori-motor impairments in the elderly. Kluwer, Dordrecht:231–252.

Patla AE 1995 A framework for understanding mobility problems in the elderly. In: Craik RL, Otis CA (eds) Gait analysis: theory and application. Mosby, St Louis:436–449.

Patla AE 1997 Understanding the roles of vision in the control of human locomotion. Gait Posture 5:54–69.

Pavol MJ, Runtz EF, Pai Y-C 2004 Diminished stepping responses lead to a fall following a novel slip induced during a sit-to-stand. Gait Posture 20:154–162.

Perennou DA, Bronstein AM 2005 Balance disorders and vertigo after stroke: assessment and rehabilitation. In: Barnes MP, Dobkin BH, Bogousslavsky J (eds) Recovery after stroke. Cambridge University Press, Cambridge:320–396.

Pollock A, Baer G, Pomeroy VM et al 2007 Physiotherapy treatment approaches for the recovery of postural control and lower limb function following stroke. Cochrane Database Syst Rev, Issue 1. Art. No.: CD001920. DOI: 10.1002/14651858.CD001920. pub2.

Said CM, Goldie PA, Patla AE et al 1999 Obstacle crossing in subjects with stroke. Arch Phys Med Rehabil 80:1054–1059.

Said CM, Goldie PA, Culham E et al 2005 Control of lead and trail limbs during obstacle crossing following stroke. Phys Ther 85:413–427.

Sale DG 1988 Neural adaptation to resistance training. Med Sci Sports Exerc 20:S135–145.

Sandin KJ, Smith BS 1990 The measure of balance in sitting in stroke rehabilitation prognosis. Stroke 21:82–86.

Schenkman M, Hughes MA, Samsa G et al 1996 The relative importance of strength and balance in chair rise by functionally impaired older individuals. J Am Geriatric Soc 44:1441–1446.

Schultz AB, Alexander NB, Ashton-Miller JA 1992 Biomechanical analyses of rising from a chair. J Biomech 25:1383–1391.

Sekiya N, Takahashi M 2001 Control of lateral weight-transfer initiation during sitting. Percept Mot Skills 99:291–304.

Sherrington C 1961 The integrative action of the nervous system, 2nd edn. Yale University Press, New Haven, CT.

Sherrington C, Whitney JC, Lord SR et al 2008a Effective exercise for the prevention of falls: a systematic review and meta-analysis. J Am Geriatr Soc 56:2234–2243.

Sherrington C, Pamphlett PI, Jacka JA 2008b Group exercise can improve participants' mobility in an outpatient rehabilitation setting: a randomized controlled trial. Clin Rehabil 22:493–502.

Shumway-Cook A, Olmscheid R 1990 A systems analysis of postural dyscontrol in traumatically brain-injured patients. J Head Trauma Rehabil 5:51–62.

Shumway-Cook A, Woollacott MH 2001, 2007 Motor control theory and practical application, 2nd and 3rd edns. Lippincott Williams & Wilkins, New York.

Skelton DA, Greig CA, Davies JM et al 1994 Strength, power and related functional ability of healthy people aged 65–89 years. Age Ageing 23:371–377.

Slobounov S, Newell KM 1994 Postural dynamics as a function of skill level and task constraints. Gait Posture 2:85–93.

Stapleton T, Ashburn A, Stack E 2001 A pilot study of attention deficits, balance control and falls in the acute stage following stroke. Clin Rehabil 15:437–444.

Stoffregen TA, Pagualayan RJ, Bardy BG et al 2000 Modulating postural control to facilitate visual performance. Hum Mov Sci 19:203–220.

Tinetti ME, Speechley M, Ginter SF 1988 Risk factors for falls among elderly persons living in the community. N Engl J Med 319:1701–1707.

Tobis JS, Nayak L, Hoehler F 1981 Visual perception of verticality and horizontality among elderly fallers. Arch Phys Med Rehabil 62:619–622.

Tsang YL, Mak MK 2004 Sit-and-reach test can predict mobility of patients recovering from acute stroke. Arch Phys Med Rehabil 85:94–98.

Vandervoort AA, Chesworth BM, Cunningham DA et al 1992 Age and sex effects on mobility of the human ankle. J Gerontol Med Sci 47:M17–M21.

van Peppen RPS, Kwakkel G, Wood-Dauphinee S et al 2004 The impact of physical therapy on functional outcomes after stroke: what's the evidence? Clin Rehabil 18:833–862.

von Schroeder HP, Courts RD, Lyden PD 1995 Gait parameters following stroke: a practical assessment. J Rehabil Res Dev 32:25–31.

Whipple RH, Wolfson LI, Amerman PM 1987 The relationship of knee–ankle weakness to falls in nursing home residents: an isokinetic study. J Am Geriatr Soc 35:13–20.

Whipple R, Wolfson C, Derby C et al 1993 Altered sensory function and balance in older persons. J Gerontol 48:71–76.

Wing AM, Goodrich S, Virji-Babul N et al 1993 Balance evaluation in hemiparetic stroke patients using lateral forces applied to the hip. Arch Phys Med Rehabil 74:292–299.

Winter DA 1995a ABC (anatomy, biomechanics and control) of balance during standing and walking. Waterloo Biomechanics, Waterloo, Ontario.

Winter DA 1995b Total body kinetics: our window into the synergies of human movement. Wartenweiler Memorial Lecture. Proceedings of XVth Congress of ISB, Jyvaskyla, Finland:8–9.

Winter DA, Patla AE, Frank JS 1990 Assessment of balance control in humans. Med Prog Technol 16:31–51.

Winter DA, McFadyen BJ, Dickey JP 1991 Adaptability of the CNS in human walking. In: Adaptability of human gait. Elsevier Science, Amsterdam:127–143.

Winter DA, Prince F, Stergiou P et al 1993 M/L and A/P motor responses associated with COP changes in quiet standing. Neurosci Res Comm 12:141–148.

Woollacott M, Shumway-Cook A 2002 Attention and control of posture and gait: a review of an emerging area of research. Gait Posture 16:1–14.

Wulf G, McNiven N, Shea CH 2001 The automaticity of complex motor skill learning as a function of attentional focus. Q J Exp Psychol 54A:1143–1154.

Wulf G, Mercer J, McNevin N et al 2004 Reciprocal influences of attentional focus on postural and suprapostural task performance. J Mot Behav 36:189–199.

Yang JF, Winter DA, Wells RP 1990 Postural dynamics in the standing human. Biol Cyber 62:309–320.

Zattara M, Bouisset S 1988 Chronometric analysis of the posturo-kinetic programming of voluntary movement. J Mot Behav 18:215–225.

Part | 3 |

Body function and structure, limitations in activities and participation

Chapter | 8 |

Upper motor neuron lesions

INTRODUCTION

It is common for both acute and chronic brain injury to involve the cortically originating motor system: the cortical neuron, its pathways and connections. Lesions involving the corticospinal pathways can occur at any level: in the cortex, internal capsule, brain stem or spinal cord. Such lesions may result from stroke, traumatic brain injury or tumour, multiple sclerosis, cerebral palsy or spinal cord injury.

In the neurosciences, it has been typical since Hughlings Jackson (Walshe 1961) to consider the dyscontrol characteristics associated with the upper motor neuron (UMN) syndrome as either *negative features* such as impaired muscle activation, weakness or paralysis and loss of dexterity, or *positive features*, the newly emerging phenomena, such as stretch-sensitive muscle overactivity or spasticity (Burke 1988; Gracies 2005a,b). In the earlier edition we proposed a third group of *adaptive features* since it was likely that adaptive changes to the neural system, muscles and other soft tissues, and adaptive motor behaviours underlie many clinical signs and could also affect functional recovery (Fig. 8.1). It is now clear that these are additional insults to the neuromusculoskeletal structures involved in movement (Gracies 2005a). After an acute lesion, recovery processes commence and the neuromotor systems involved in movement begin to adapt both to the effect of the lesion and to subsequent events. While the adaptations to motor behaviour that occur as people attempt to carry out motor tasks are easily observable, adaptive changes in soft tissues (particularly muscles), occurring as a result of disuse imposed by weakness or paralysis, may go unnoticed.

The negative and positive features have appeared to be relatively independent phenomena and related to the site and amount of tissue damage and spontaneous recovery processes (Landau 1980). Positive features were seen as exaggerations of normal phenomena or release phenomena, and included increased sensitivity of proprioceptive and cutaneous reflexes (spasticity). They were thought to be due to involvement of parapyramidal fibres (Burke 1988), and possibly related to secondary functional disturbances in surviving tissue.

Recent technological developments and scientific findings enable some clarification of the disordered mechanisms underlying impairments and of the extent and effect of post-lesion adaptations to the neural and musculoskeletal systems that compound the disability. These advances

©2010 Elsevier Ltd
DOI: 10.1016/B978-0-7020-4051-1.00017-5

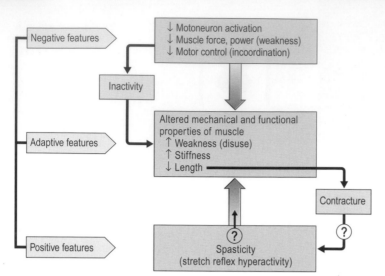

Figure 8.1 The positive, negative and adaptive features of the upper motor neuron syndrome.

are driving a re-evaluation of the functional significance of different clinical signs (Gracies 2005a,b; Dietz & Sinkjaer 2007).

It is now generally accepted that the negative features of paralysis or weakness, slowness of movement, loss of coordination or dexterity in particular, together with secondary adaptive changes in muscle properties, such as increased stiffness and length-associated changes, provide the major obstacles to recovery of functional motor performance. These features are more disabling to the patient than hyperactive stretch reflexes (Burke 1988; Landau 1988; Sheean 2002). Spasticity may be an adaptive phenomenon, occurring post-lesion in response to changes in muscle that lead to contracture (Gracies 2005b). Oversensitive muscle stretch receptors (hyperreflexia) appear to make a relatively minor contribution to dysfunctional motor performance (Dietz & Sinkjaer 2007). Patients themselves are usually more preoccupied with their loss of strength, their inability to walk and loss of dexterity in hand use, and with stiffness associated with muscle changes, than with the manifestations of hyperactive reflexes.

Nevertheless, the nature of what is called in the clinic 'spasticity' has been and remains, although to a lesser extent in the 21st century, a controversial issue. Although Hughlings Jackson in the 19th century considered the positive and negative features to be different in mechanism, it is still assumed that the movement disability is directly related to hyperactive reflexes and that improved movement function will occur after modification of reflex hyperactivity (Jackson 1958). However, there is no clinical or experimental evidence to support this view (Thach & Montgomery 1990; Richards et al 1991; Sheean 2002), and the last decade has seen considerable re-interpretation. These assumptions are no longer common.

In the first edition we attempted to clarify the nature of the controversy. We argued that rehabilitation should be directed toward the so-called negative impairments and subsequent adaptations. In this new edition we refer to more recent research findings that confirm this direction and give new insights into underlying mechanisms of impairments and adaptations. We make recommendations for clinical intervention based on current understanding of how the system works and how this is affected by an acute brain lesion. The emerging evidence base also helps to clarify what might be the most effective methods to use in rehabilitation. Vigorous active movement training, task specific and repetitive, and prevention of contracture development appear the most likely methods to be effective in optimizing functional recovery. In those individuals who recover little or no motor function, the development of contracture and spasticity is an ever-present threat and drug therapy may be necessary to decrease pain and discomfort.

NEGATIVE FEATURES: PRIMARY IMPAIRMENTS FOLLOWING CENTRAL LESIONS

Following an UMN lesion, there may be insufficient descending fibres converging on the final motor neuron population either to shape complex movements by graded activation of coordinating muscles or to bring motor neurons to the high-frequency discharges necessary for tetanic contraction strength (Landau 1988). This insufficiency results in weakness (decreased voluntary motor unit activation), slowness of movement, decreased motor unit recruitment and loss of dexterity and coordination. It is apparent that some disorganization of motor output at the segmental level arises which also contributes to the weakness (Tang & Rymer 1981).

When the system is in a state of shock after a lesion of acute onset, there may be a profound depression of motor function in which all muscles of the affected limb(s) are involved. In this state, tendon reflexes may be decreased (hyporeflexia) or absent (areflexia). Clinically, the terms hypotonus, flaccidity, flaccid paralysis and paresis have been used interchangeably to indicate a low state of 'tone'. It is more useful to regard the absence of muscle activation as a state of paralysis and reduced muscle force generation as weakness, since these terms are more clearly descriptive of the state of affairs.

The concept of tone itself is vague. Normal resting muscle tone does not depend on neural mechanisms and any active resistance felt on passive movement is due to mechanical factors (Burke 1988). There is no electrical activity (reflex activation) in resting muscle or when a muscle is passively stretched in a relaxed subject (Fig. 8.2). Twenty years ago, van der Meche & van der Gijn (1986) pointed out that if a person's limb feels flaccid, it is the result of weakness preventing the voluntary activity that normally occurs. They suggested that the use of the terms 'normal tone' and 'hypotonus' should be discontinued, and early in the 21st century they are much less in evidence.

The use of terms related to the state of tone distracts the clinician from a clear understanding of the characteristics of the negative features which should usually be the focus of rehabilitative training. Such discussion of terminology is therefore not trivial, since the clinician's knowledge of underlying mechanisms guides treatment planning. If it is understood that the patient has difficulty activating muscles, generating and timing appropriate forces and coordinating muscle forces to produce effective and efficient motor performance, and has a strong likelihood of developing secondary muscle changes, the clinician is more likely to use methods designed to address these issues during training and practice.

Paralysis and paresis (muscle weakness)

The corticospinal tract is the executive pathway for volitional goal-directed movement (Phillips & Porter 1977) and any interruption to that pathway can produce considerable movement deficit. Muscle weakness and its distribution after stroke has been described in several reports (Colebatch & Gandevia 1989; Gandevia 1993; Canning et al 1999, 2004; Ng & Shepherd 2000). Newham & Hsiao (2001) investigated and tracked voluntary isometric strength of quadriceps and hamstring muscles for the first 6 months in a small group of individuals after stroke. They found that maximum voluntary contraction (MVC) of these muscles in the paretic leg was approximately half that of healthy age-matched subjects. The non-paretic muscles were also weaker than healthy subjects.

There is now general agreement that the major clinical signs following stroke and resulting from motor cortex and corticospinal tract lesion are muscle weakness and motor dyscontrol. Weakness is defined as decreased maximum voluntary force (or torque) compared with normal age-matched values. In addition, patients have difficulty generating and timing muscle forces, controlling these and other forces generated by segmental movement and gravity, in order to produce effective motor performance. It is interesting that, although discussion of spastic reflex activity has produced a large body of literature, the mechanisms underlying muscle weakness and movement dyscontrol after brain lesion have been the subject of relatively less interest. Considerable investigative work has been done, however, on mechanisms underlying normal muscle function.

The mechanisms of muscle activation. Normally, the muscle force produced when muscles are active is dependent upon the number and type of motor units recruited, the characteristics of motor unit discharge and of the muscle itself (e.g., its cross-sectional area). We increase muscle force by increasing the number of active motor units and increasing the firing rates and frequencies of those active motor units. Firing of a motor unit results in a twitch (contraction) of the innervated muscle fibres. With an increase in firing rate, these twitches sum in order to increase and sustain force output.

Motor units are classified according to fatigue resistance and twitch tension into fast fatiguable (FF), fast fatigue resistant (FR) and slow fatigue resistant (S). Motor units

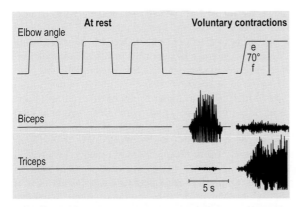

Figure 8.2 The effects of passive stretch of biceps and triceps brachii in a normal subject. (*Left*) Abrupt stretches of 70° amplitude do not evoke any reflex activity in either muscle. (*Right*) The degree of amplification of the EMG trace when the muscles are contracted strongly by the subject (biceps in flexion; triceps in extension) is provided for comparison. (*From Burke 1988, with permission*).

are normally recruited in an orderly pattern: those which produce low forces are recruited first, followed by higher force-producing units as force requirements increase. Amount of force generated is matched to task demands, and takes account of (is modified by) gravitational and interactional forces. The tension output of a skeletal muscle is defined by its length, its contraction velocity and the level of activity (Whitehead et al 2001). **Strength is therefore a neuromuscular phenomenon.** It is activity dependent, that is, relative to the action/task we are performing, not absolute (i.e., we are 'strong enough' to carry out certain tasks effectively or not). As an example, the quadriceps strength required to stand up from a chair or climb stairs is many times greater than in walking along a flat surface.

Weakness arises from two sources after a lesion of the neuromotor system – primarily from the brain lesion itself as a result of a decrease in descending inputs from corticospinal pathways converging on the final motoneuron population and, as a result, reduction in the number of motor units available for recruitment. Decreased motor unit recruitment results in difficulty voluntarily activating and sustaining skeletal muscle to generate movement (Bourbonnais & Vanden Noven 1989; Newham et al 1996; Gracies 2005a). Since skeletal muscle adapts to the level of use imposed on it (Lieber 1988), secondary sources of weakness arise as a consequence of lack of muscle activity and immobility (Farmer et al 1993). It is well known that major anatomical, mechanical and functional changes in skeletal muscles, including changes in properties of motor units, occur post-stroke in response both to the lesion and to post-lesion inactivity or disuse. Lieber and colleagues (2004) point out that these changes can impact on the neural system and on functional motor performance.

It has been known for several decades that decreased central input resulting from the lesion results in impaired regulation of force due to reduction in the firing rate of motor units* (Rosenfalck & Andreassen 1980; Gemperline et al 1995; Frontera et al 1997). These impairments reduce the efficiency of muscle contractions, contribute to slowness of movement, perception of increased effort and fatigue and, with impaired motor unit synchronization, contribute to disorganized motor control.

Central voluntary activation failure. Few studies have investigated muscle weakness early after the lesion, before the onset of adaptive effects of immobility and disuse. In one of these studies, significant voluntary activation failure of muscles (measured by twitch superimposition) was found after stroke, probably due to failure of motor unit recruitment or decreased firing rates in active units (Newham & Hsiao 2001; Riley & Bilodeau 2002). Activation failure affecting both limbs reflects the direct effects

on skeletal muscle of the neural lesion and the inputs to muscle from both cerebral hemispheres. Inability to recruit the entire motor unit population has been reported by others (Tang & Rymer 1981; Bourbonnais & Vanden Noven 1989; Gowland et al 1992; Newham et al 1996). It has been particularly noted that there is a failure to recruit high-threshold motor units and to modulate or increase motor unit discharge rates when attempting to increase voluntary force (Gemperline et al 1995; Frontera et al 1997; Gracies 2005a). Although decreased amplitude of force affects function, it is also the slow speed of peak force generation (power**) that is a most critical parameter for effective motor performance.

Decreased motor unit firing rates have been reported in intrinsic hand muscles (Rosenfalck & Andreassen 1980) and in tibialis anterior (Dietz et al 1986). An apparent adaptation to decreased motor neuron firing rates can be seen in elbow flexor muscles of patients with hemiplegia (Tang & Rymer 1981), with increased levels of electromyographic (EMG) activity produced per unit force. Since a decrease in firing rate results in decreased tension generated by the active motor units, additional motor units have to be recruited to counter the firing rate impairment and enable a greater development of force. This results in an increased sense of effort at low levels of activation, since a stronger central input would be required to generate a given level of force (Tang & Rymer 1981). An increased sense of effort has been reported elsewhere under similar conditions (Gandevia & McCloskey 1977).

McComas and colleagues (1973) reported a 50% *decrease in functioning motor units* between the second and sixth month after stroke. They suggested that this was due to trans-synaptic changes in motor neurons following degeneration of corticospinal fibres and the tendency for surviving motor units to change to type 1 fibres (slow twitch). An increase in slow-twitch and decrease in fast-twitch muscle fibres has been confirmed (Dattola et al 1993; Toffola et al 2001), with reduced firing rate during contraction. Evidence of denervation (e.g., Cruz-Martinez 1984), atrophy of some muscle fibres (especially fast-contracting fibres associated with FF and FR motor units) (Dietz et al 1986) and hypertrophy of other fibres (slow-contracting fibres associated with slow motor units) (Edstrom 1970) has also been reported.

Prolonged contraction times, particularly in fast-contracting motor units (Young & Mayer 1982; Visser et al 1985), may be related to *changes in motor unit type*. In individuals within a month after stroke, a unique class of motor units, which are slow contracting and fatiguable and not present in normal muscles, were identified by Young & Mayer (1982). The authors suggested that these motor units originated from fast-fatigable units. It appears, therefore, that an increase in the proportion of

---

*Motor units normally fire at the rate necessary for fusion of twitches.

**Power = force × angular velocity.

functionally slow motor units may be responsible in part, along with loss or reduction in motor unit synchronization (Farmer et al 1993), for the relatively slow rise to maximum tension of muscles, particularly those muscles with a high proportion of slow motor units. The fatigability of the slow fatigable motor units may help explain the poor endurance in sustaining muscle force output which is a common clinical observation. It is important to note that changes to muscle and motor unit may occur as an adaptive result of disuse following the brain lesion as well as due to diminished neural activation caused by the lesion and may therefore be preventable or remediable.

Distribution of muscle weakness. Lesion site and extent probably determine the distribution and degree of muscle weakness and there should not be an expectation that individuals after acute brain lesion are a homogeneous group. Several studies have commented on the high variability in the weakness distribution pattern (Colebatch et al 1986; Colebatch & Gandevia 1989; Mercier & Bourbonnais 2004) (Fig. 8.3). Furthermore, the degree of weakness differs for different muscle groups in the same individual.

Distal muscles commonly appear to be more affected than proximal (Andrews & Bohannon 2000), and the

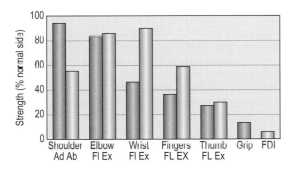

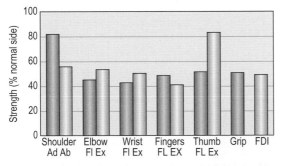

Figure 8.3 Distribution of muscle weakness in two subjects with hemiparesis. Note that the subject shown in the top bar chart (infarct of corona radiata) shows greater distal than proximal muscle weakness; the subject in the lower chart (distal occlusion of basilar artery) shows a similar degree of involvement in all muscles tested. *(From Colebatch and Gandevia 1989, with permission).*

greatest weakness is said to be in intrinsic hand muscles. Since corticospinal innervation is denser for the distal muscles of the hand (including muscles which cross the wrist), there may be considerably more deficit in manipulation and prehension than is evident elsewhere. It has been proposed that the differential effects of the lesion on the proximal and distal muscles appear to be associated with the strength of the corticospinal pathway (Mima et al 2001). Increased use of brain scanning techniques and of motor-evoked potentials using transcranial magnetic stimulation (TMS) should provide a clearer picture of the lesion and its effects on muscle innervation (Turton & Lemon 1999; Mima et al 2001).

Differential degrees of muscle weakness according to muscle length have been reported in clinical studies. After an acute lesion, a person may be able to generate sufficient muscle force to bear weight in standing without leg collapse when the knee is flexed a few degrees, but not be able to hold the knee extended at 0° (Winter 1985; Lomaglio & Eng 2008). Individuals in the early stages after stroke who can voluntarily contract and generate force with their quadriceps may need extra training to generate sufficient force with the knee from 0–10° in order to keep the knee extended when bearing load in standing. Ada and colleagues (2000, 2003) reported this differential effect of length on muscle strength in the upper limb, showing greater weakness of elbow flexors and extensors at shorter lengths. These findings are explained to some extent by the fact that muscles normally generate most torque at their mid-length and least torque at shorter lengths. Impaired activation of motor units would be expected therefore to exaggerate the phenomenon. Exercise and training should take this into account and include repetitive practice of actions (e.g., standing up and sitting down, step-ups, step-downs) that emphasize controlling the limb through the full range of movement (see Ch. 2).

Weakness is also, to some extent, task and context dependent. Beer and colleagues (1999) found that the extent of weakness of elbow flexors and extensors was strongly dependent on magnitude and direction of the torques generated at the shoulder. Exercises to build up strength in muscles should therefore emphasise a variety of different tasks with different movement patterns.

Weakness of an agonist muscle is not due to spasticity of its antagonist. Until recently, it has been assumed that apparent weakness in a muscle group (such as triceps brachii) is solely due to restraint by spastic antagonists (elbow flexors). However, several decades ago, Sahrmann & Norton (1977) found that the primary impairment during rapid voluntary flexion and extension movements at the elbow was a limited and prolonged recruitment of the agonist muscle and delayed cessation of agonist contraction at the end of the movement. Contrary to the common belief among clinicians at that time, they showed that the stretch reflex in the antagonist was not elicited in a way that would resist the agonist and, therefore, that antagonist stretch reflex hyperactivity was not a major contributor to the disability. These results showed that a major cause of poor motor performance after an acute central lesion is the ineffectiveness of muscle contractions; that is, impairments in muscle force generation and the timing of that force relative to the task at hand. Adaptive changes in muscle such as increased intrinsic stiffness of an antagonist may, however, provide resistance to agonist contraction in some patients (Dietz et al 1981), and this resistance may be incorrectly interpreted as due to spasticity.

Biomechanical and EMG studies of the timing and magnitude of muscle forces and the functional effects of muscle weakness help clarify the causes of dysfunctional performance. Several early investigations of walking showed diminished muscle (EMG) activity and impaired muscle activation patterns in the lower limb of patients with hemiparesis (e.g., Knutsson & Richards 1979). In investigations of the swing phase of gait, it was found that resistance to active dorsiflexion was provided by mechanical length-associated changes in muscle fibres in the calf muscles rather than hyperactivity in calf muscle stretch receptors.

Bilateral muscle weakness. Although a unilateral central lesion may produce motor impairments involving one side of the body, it has been shown that muscle activity of the other side may also be affected. For example, bilateral muscle activation failure has been reported after stroke (Newham & Hsiao 2001), and another study found significant weakness in muscles of the non-paretic lower limb (a 30% decrease in knee extensor strength) within the first week after stroke (Harris & Polkey 2001). These authors considered this reduction may be a secondary weakness, attributing it to the effects of disuse, specifically lack of exercise and nutritional support. One advantage of task-oriented training programmes is that the focus is on many functional actions that naturally involve both right and left limbs, for example standing up (Ch. 4), or walking on a treadmill (Ch. 5), or bimanual task practice (Ch. 6). In these exercises, the therapist ensures that both lower and upper limbs are exercised and muscles are trained to generate and control appropriate forces. Such a programme, modified to optimize performance of the paretic limb in particular, can provide a means of minimizing secondary weakness of both limbs but must start early since adaptive changes occur early.

Slowness of muscle activation and movement

Another consequence of impairments in neural activation of motor units and changes in muscle fibre type is slowness of movement and of initiating movement, to which weakness may contribute since the muscle forces needed for voluntary movement cannot rise to peak force fast enough to generate the power needed to move effectively. Slowness in standing up (Ada & Westwood 1992) and in walking (0.2–0.7 m/s for stroke subjects compared to 1.0–1.2 m/s for the able bodied) have been reported (Giuliani 1990; Lamontagne et al 2002), with reduced moments of force produced by calf muscles (Olney & Richards 1996; Lamontagne et al 2002), and longer time-to-peak force seen at push-off in stance phase (Olney et al 1991; Olney 2005). In a study of individuals more than 1 year after stroke, McCrea and colleagues (2005) found not only a significantly impairment of peak torque generation but also that participants took twice as long to reach peak torque with the paretic arm compared to their non-paretic arm and to able-bodied subjects. They also took significantly longer to reduce torque (Fig. 8.4). In other words, the ability to modulate force over time was impaired.

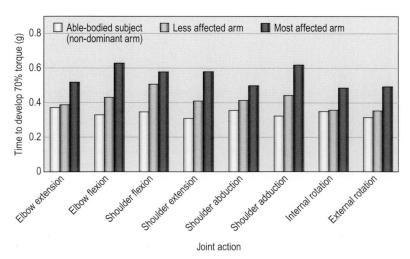

Figure 8.4 Time to develop peak joint torque. Clear column, able-bodied subject (non-dominant arm); cross-hatched column, less affected arm; filled column, most affected arm. *(From McCrea, Eng & Hodgson 2005, with permission).*

After stroke, when patients try to move fast, a similar problem occurs with a prolonged build-up to maximum tension at the initiation of the attempt at fast movement (Tsuji & Nakamura 1987). Slowing of the rate of voluntary muscle contraction appears to be due to loss of inputs from fast, large corticospinal tract neurons to peripheral motor neurons (see Burke 1988 for review). In attempts at fast alternating movements, slowness appears to be associated with reduction of motor unit synchronization (Farmer et al 1993). One of the earliest reports described deficient capacity to accelerate motion up to a pre-set speed for slow as well as fast movements, and the capacity to develop force for fast movement was more impaired than for slow movements (Knutsson & Martensson 1980).

In stroke subjects, it has also been found that the time taken for a single quadriceps twitch to relax to half its peak force may be significantly longer in the paretic than in the non-paretic limb (Newham et al 1996). Slow angular velocities have been reported in knee flexion and extension (Davies et al 1996). Several studies report that not only was the time taken to develop peak muscle force impaired, but also the time taken to decrease it.

Delayed contraction and relaxation times have been found to correlate significantly with physical disability (Chae et al 2002) since the action being performed is disorganized and therefore ineffective. There is some evidence that this problem can be overcome. Canning and colleagues (1999) reported from a study of 10 patients that 6 weeks after stroke, individuals took two to three times longer than able-bodied subjects to produce peak torque during isometric elbow flexor and extensor contractions. However, values were within normal limits by 25 weeks post-lesion. One subject could generate peak elbow flexor torque of 9 Nm, theoretically sufficient to lift her forearm and carry a small object. However, since it took her 7 seconds to reach peak torque, her arm at that stage was of limited functional use.

A few biomechanical studies have specifically examined power output after stroke. One study of quadriceps and hamstrings during leg cycling (Kautz & Brown 1998) found abnormal timing of EMG activity in both muscles, and less positive (concentric) work and more negative (eccentric) work than in able-bodied subjects. Olney (2005) investigated power output during gait and reported lower power amplitudes and decreased speeds of walking (see Ch. 5 for discussion).

Interventions that involve practise of actions with an early emphasis on performing at a near to normal speed and faster, and of actions that require a fast build up of force, may enable the system to improve the modulation and timing of muscle activation and functional performance.

Impaired coordination and loss of dexterity

The mechanisms that underlie weakness and slowness of force generation also produce a reduction in motor control, that is incoordination of limb segments during multisegmental actions. After an acute central lesion, motor output is both reduced and disorganized and muscle activity may no longer be well enough coordinated to meet task and environmental demands due to an impaired ability to fine-tune interactions between muscles (Kautz & Brown 1998).

There have been relatively few neurophysiological investigations of disordered motor control following stroke. However, kinematic and kinetic studies of reaching and hand function, walking and standing up are providing some insights. Training of motor control in the context of specific actions is a critical part of rehabilitation that aims to train an individual toward optimal (best possible) functional effectiveness. To implement this specific training, the clinician needs an understanding of biomechanics and the mechanisms of dyscontrol.

The term dexterity has been used to describe the ability to 'fractionate' movement, to make independent movements, particularly for fine manipulation (Burke 1988). Dexterity has also been described as adroitness or skill (O'Dwyer et al 1996), inferring the fine coordination of muscle activations that typifies the actions we confidently and skillfully perform in our daily lives. Bernstein (1991; cited in Latash & Latash 1994) defined dexterity as the ability to solve any motor task rationally, precisely, quickly and deftly. He suggested that dexterity, rather than being present in the motor act itself, is present in its interaction with the changing environment. Dexterity depends on a sustained and rapid transfer of sensorimotor information between intact cerebral cortex and spinal cord motor neurons (Darian-Smith et al 1996).

The relationship between relative strength (ability to generate and time sufficient muscle force for specific tasks and contexts) and dexterity (coordination of muscle activation) is unclear at the physiological level. In a functional sense, however, it is likely that they are linked, since the ability to generate force for a particular action depends on the ability to control many synergic muscles through concentric, eccentric and isometric actions, including antagonist muscles and muscles that stabilize the limb. It is probably the ability to control synergic muscle linkages during complex changes in direction and speed that underlies dexterity. This point may be illustrated by relationships reported between increased lower limb muscle strength and improved standing balance (Bohannon 1987, 1988).

The relationship between strength and dexterity may be more relevant (and therefore easier to show) in certain tasks. For example, a recent study used a novel laboratory tracking task designed to measure dextrous (controlled) motion at a single joint (elbow flexion and extension) in the transverse plane. Subjects were between 2 weeks and 24 months after stroke and there was a group of age-matched control subjects (Ada et al 1996). Performance on the tracking task deteriorated at the faster speed in all subjects, with a more pronounced decrease in accuracy for the stroke subjects, who also tended to move faster than was required to follow the targets. No statistical relationship was found between strength and dexterity in this task which required minimal muscle force generation since the motion was almost frictionless. The task, however, required the ability to brake forearm movement and to change direction. The relationship between dexterity and strength is highly likely to be task related. No studies were found that examined the strength/dexterity relationship in multijoint actions performed in more task-relevant planes of motion, such as reaching forward to an object.

The motor cortex and corticospinal tract are critical for the control of fine finger movements such as manipulating small objects in the palm (Porter & Lemon 1993). Control of finger movements gives us the ability to carry out a large repertoire of functions with our hands. A lesion of the motor cortex or corticospinal tract can affect the highly selective control of finger muscles and have a negative effect on dexterity (Kilbreath et al 2002). Limited independence of thumb and finger flexors has been reported (Kilbreath & Gandevia 1994), and recent work has shown a decrease in individuation of abduction–adduction movements of fingers that was correlated with decreased hand function (Lang & Schieber 2004). Detailed biomechanical descriptions of performance of major functional actions associated with brain lesions are given in Chapters 4–7, together with guidelines for functional retraining. These studies illustrate well the impaired coordination that can occur during actual performance of everyday tasks.

In summary, the negative clinical signs of weakness, slowness of movement and loss of fine motor control are due primarily to a decrease of descending inputs on motor units and impairments in coordination (synchronization) of motor unit activation. It is clear that these impairments are major causes of disability after acute brain lesion (Burke 1988; Fellows et al 1994; Carr et al 1995; Gracies 2005a). Inability to generate and time muscle forces in a task- and context-specific manner are major reasons for functional disability, together with the compounding effects of post-lesion disuse weakness and the adaptive changes that occur in soft tissues as a result of reduced muscle activation, immobility and disuse. Further investigations should clarify the underlying physiological mechanisms and enable the testing of the effects of specific exercises and training methods, not only on functional motor performance but also on the underlying mechanisms. The potential for specifically directed training to drive recovery and reorganization processes is as yet unknown.

POSITIVE FEATURES: NEWLY EMERGING PHENOMENA

Historically, the positive features of the UMN syndrome have been considered the result of abnormal excitability of proprioceptive and cutaneous reflexes (Burke 1988), that is reflex hyperactivity. The characteristic clinical signs of exaggerated proprioceptive reflexes are the clasp-knife phenomenon (a velocity-dependent build-up of reflex resistance), exaggerated tendon jerk (a synchronized reflex response generated by abrupt mechanical disturbance) and clonus (a sustained reflex response set in train by tendon percussion). Hyperactive cutaneous reflexes produce a flexor withdrawal reflex, extensor and flexor spasms, which are manifestations of a severely damaged spinal cord, and a Babinski (extensor plantar) response (toe extension evoked by a stimulus provided to the plantar surface of the foot). The positive features appear to be of extrapyramidal rather than pyramidal origin but the underlying pathophysiological mechanisms remain somewhat obscure. Other conditions associated with muscle overactivity are rigidity, tremor and dystonia (Gracies 2005b).

Spasticity has occupied a substantial amount of the neuroscience and rehabilitation literature for decades. It is the feature that most occupies the minds of clinicians whether they be from the therapy or the medical professions and it has been considered a major cause of functional disability. As pointed out by Landau (1980), there is a major problem inherent in the word itself since it is commonly used clinically to signify many different features associated with brain lesions. These range from loss of strength to increased tendon jerks, and include the resistance offered to passive movement of a limb (also called hypertonus) and disordered patterns of movement. The terms spasticity and spastic paresis are commonly used in a generic sense, and can cover several or all the phenomena seen following an UMN lesion.

This disparity in meaning has not made for ease of communication. In addition, it has become clear that there are other alternative explanations for some phenomena thought to be due solely to the 'positive' neural features. For example, what is called by clinicians 'spastic hypertonus' and described by patients as 'stiffness' are mainly due to mechanical, physiological and functional changes occurring in the muscles; that is, to secondary adaptations. Disorganized patterns of movement, as well as indicating neuromotor incoordination, may reflect behavioural adaptations to weakness and soft tissue changes rather than pathological patterns 'released' by the lesion.

The mechanisms producing the positive features are not understood. This is due to some extent to difficulties with neurophysiological and clinical testing, in interpreting results from heterogeneous groups of individuals with different lesion sites and sizes, and in determining the effect of post-lesion adaptations (Nielsen et al 2007). Many theories have been put forward over the decades (see Table 2 in Gracies 2005a), but scientific support is lacking. It has long been thought, for example, that increased dynamic fusimotor drive contributes to spasticity after stroke (e.g., Rushworth 1960). However, spindle behaviour has been shown to be similar in both patients and controls (Wilson et al 1999) and more recent research has concluded that fusimotor dysfunction contributes little if anything to the deficit (Nielsen et al 2007). Post-lesion adaptive muscle fibre contracture (including specialized spindle fibres) may, however, contribute to the development of spasticity and dysfunctional motor performance. A longitudinal study of 27 individuals charted the evolution of weakness, spasticity and contracture of elbow flexors over 12 months (Ada et al 2006). The major contributors to contracture were spasticity in the first months and weakness thereafter. The major and only contributor to functional limitations throughout the year was weakness.

There are currently signs of more discrimination with the increasing use of the definition formed by a consensus of neurologists and reported by Lance (1980). Whatever its pathophysiological mechanisms, spasticity reflects a disorder of motor control as suggested by this relatively narrow but widely accepted neurophysiological definition: a motor disorder characterized by a velocity-dependent increase in tonic stretch reflexes ('muscle tone') with exaggerated tendon jerks resulting from hyperexcitability of the stretch reflex as one component of the UMN syndrome (Lance 1980:485).

Gracies (2005b) differentiates between a stretch-sensitive and a non-stretch-sensitive form of muscle overactivity, the former occurring as a post-lesion adaptation

linked to adaptive muscle changes (increased intrinsic stiffness and contracture), with motor unit recruitment significantly affected by the response of stretch receptors. Non-stretch-sensitive muscle overactivity includes excessive cutaneous and nociceptive responses. Pandyan and colleagues (2005) describe spasticity as disordered sensorimotor control resulting from an UMN lesion, presenting as intermittent or sustained involuntary activation of muscles.

The Lance definition points out that the abnormality underlying spasticity is an adaptation of the stretch reflex, the response elicited when the limb is moved at particular velocities (Fig. 8.5). The stretch reflex is a contraction of muscle that occurs when the muscle is passively lengthened. Descending pathways from the brain normally modulate the strength of reflexes as we move. The stretch reflex consists of monosynaptic pathways which conduct afference from various receptors, mostly from muscle spindles, but also from Golgi tendon organs (see Pearson & Gordon 2001 for a review). The phasic component of the stretch reflex (of which the tendon jerk is a good example) responds to a rapid abrupt stretch of the muscle. On the other hand, the tonic component of the reflex responds to stretch of the muscle by slower movement, and produces a graded response. The tonic stretch reflex is modulated not only by the velocity of stretch but also by the length of the muscle at which the stretch occurs (Burke et al 1971a,b; Neilson & McCaughey 1982). This was confirmed recently by Mirbagheri and colleagues (2008) who reported that the contribution of intrinsic and reflex components of muscle stiffness may vary systematically with muscle length through passive range of motion. They found that reflex stiffness of calf muscles was greater in mid-range and intrinsic stiffness at the end of range. They pointed out that this means that clinicians' perceptions of

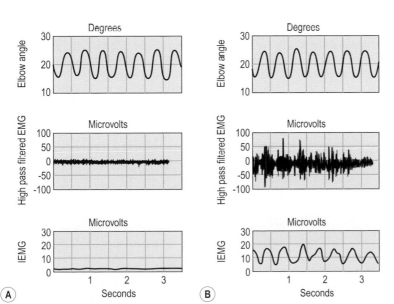

Figure 8.5 Response to passive stretch. (A) stroke subject with normal stretch reflex, (B) a stroke subject with hyperactive stretch reflex. Top traces: angle through which the elbow joint is moved. Middle traces: muscle response. Lower traces: IEMG on L illustrates no muscle response; IEMG on R shows the similar timing of the hyperactive response to the passive stretch of elbow flexors. *(From Ada & Canning 2005, with permission).*

increased tone during passive movement may have different origins depending on the length of the muscle.

The stretch reflex has a role in everyday activity and although the nature of that role is unclear it is gradually being elucidated. The system normally regulates the overall responsiveness of the tonic stretch reflex and even, to some extent, the phasic stretch reflex (e.g., the Jendrassik manoeuvre increases the response to the tendon tap). Dynamic modulation of muscle reflexes occurs during the performance of motor tasks. During a movement, the reflex can be tuned up or down so that a perturbation will result in an added amount of muscle activity or not, as the situation requires (Rothwell et al 1980). The stretch reflex may serve to add stiffness to a joint independently of central drive. Neural pathways enable the response to stretch to elicit activity in synergic muscles of the same segment as well as of adjacent segments (Cavallari & Katz 1989). Therefore, when holding a full glass of water while walking, the stretch reflexes may be tuned up to resist a possible perturbation. If the hand is knocked, not only the muscles of the forearm but also muscles of the upper arm (and of the lower limbs) will contract to resist tipping the glass and to preserve balance. The presence of both tonic and phasic components of the stretch reflex is, therefore, a normal phenomenon. The complexity of motor control during active performance is such that the need to train such actions specifically, and to have the patient practise specifically, is obvious.

Normally, during relaxation, there is no electrical response even to slow or moderate stretching of the muscle (Burke 1983). However, in the presence of spasticity, when the sensitivity of the reflex is exaggerated, the individual may be unable to control the reflex, which then responds to stretch of muscle, whether appropriate or not. How relevant this phenomenon is to the functional deficit is uncertain. There appears to be no evidence of a statistical relationship between stretch-sensitive reflex hyperactivity (as defined by passive testing) and functional activity (Katz et al 1992; Thilmann et al 1993; O'Dwyer et al 1996; Ada et al 1998; Sheean 2002). The results of tests of stretch reflexes at rest and during passive movement are unlikely to provide insights into the behaviour of these reflexes during active movement. Virtually all investigations of the mechanisms underlying spasticity in humans have examined reflex status during passive movement. Since there have been few studies of reflex activity during active voluntary movement, it is not surprising that we know so little about the effects of spasticity on functional motor performance.

It is only during active voluntary task performance that the potential functional effects of reflex hyperactivity can be analysed. Burne and colleagues (2005) point out that task performance is more likely to be limited by disturbed central modulation of reflex activity than by a persisting increase in reflex activity. Ada and colleagues (1998) compared the stretch-related activity of gastrocnemius in able-bodied and stroke subjects as the muscle was stretched through 20° into dorsiflexion as the subject voluntarily contracted the muscle. Both groups demonstrated similar amounts of reflex activity. However, deficits in dynamic reflex modulation have been reported in children with diplegic cerebral palsy during walking (Crenna 1998, 1999). In these studies, in which he collected EMG and biomechanical data, Crenna demonstrated that at push-off in stance phase the calf muscles were activated too early and with excessive amplitude. In other words, there was a lack of reflex modulation. In a study of arm movement after stroke, Levin and colleagues (2000) found limitations in regulating stretch-response thresholds in flexor and extensor muscles and in coordinating the regulation of thresholds in agonist and antagonist muscles. They pointed out that reflex hyperactivity may not be the problem, but rather the lack of modulation of stimulus–response thresholds as muscles are stretched during movement.

Increasing evidence suggests that in many patients stretch-sensitive muscle overactivity (spasticity) is adaptive and occurs in response to changes in muscle fibre length and intrinsic stiffness. Its role may be relatively minor in terms of its effects on performance, the major impairments interfering with movement dysfunction being decreased muscle activation, changes to muscle and impaired motor control. When spasticity is present after, for example, a stroke, it is usually mild (O'Dwyer et al 1996; Sommerfeld et al 2004). Excessive and persistent activity in paretic muscles called dystonia, defined as a stretch-sensitive tonic muscle contraction that occurs in the absence of voluntary input (Gracies 2005b), is sometimes seen after an acute lesion in patients with little or no recovery of muscle activation and function.

It is currently not clear from experimental findings to what extent spasticity (stretch reflex hyperactivity) is present in individuals after acute central lesion during active movement, or whether and in what way it may contribute to functional disability. If spasticity has no functional significance and is not a problem for the patient, which appears the case in many individuals after stroke, for example, then it need not be treated (Ada & Canning 2005; Nielsen et al 2007).

Evolution of spasticity (stretch-sensitive muscle hyperactivity)

In humans, both cerebral and spinal spasticity appear to have a slow time course of development following the initial insult, except in cases of high brainstem lesion (e.g., after traumatic brain injury), in which there may be an immediate increase in reflex state. Following stroke, reflex hyperactivity may be clinically evident a few weeks after the lesion (Gracies 2001). Chapman & Wiesendanger (1982) suggested that this slow time course is due to plastic or adaptive changes in synaptic connections occurring post-lesion, which may contribute to the development of spasticity. They pointed out that one response to denervation may be the formation of new synaptic connections through axonal sprouting. Since this sprouting has the same time course for development as that of hyperreflexia, the new, functional synaptic connections may actually mediate the hyperactive reflexes. Another possible response is an increase and abnormal sensitivity of pre- or post-synaptic elements to remaining afferent input, that is, an increased chemical sensitivity. A third possibility is that previously inactive synapses may become active. Hyperreflexia may, therefore, be the result of adaptations made by the neural system in response to neuronal disruption and post-lesion inactivity.

However, increased muscle stiffness, changes in muscle length and accumulation of connective tissue occurring post-lesion can also affect stretch receptor sensitivity (O'Dwyer et al 1996, Salazar-Torres et al 2004). Increased spindle sensitivity due to intrafusal shortening may cause the reflex to be elicited earlier in joint range because a given change of joint angle stretches the spindles more than normal. Stretch reflex hyperactivity may also be an adaptive response to non-functional, contracted muscles with increased intrinsic stiffness. It can develop very early in the presence of muscle inactivity and/or muscle imbalance (Burke & Gandevia 1988, Gracies et al 1997; Gracies 2005b). It is critical that the development of post-lesion muscle changes such as decreased length (contracture) are minimized by appropriate exercise, particularly in single-joint muscles such as shoulder internal rotators and soleus.

Of particular interest to clinicians is the evidence that the process of reorganization of remaining circuitry as well as structural changes within the CNS may be directly influenced, both positively or negatively, by certain external events (see Ch. 1) which could include the patient's post lesion experiences and patterns of use (including the rehabilitation process itself). Several studies support the view that hyperactive reflexes do not necessarily constitute a major impairment to functional movement in many patients with UMN syndrome. A low incidence of hyperreflexia has been reported in a group of 24 stroke patients within 13 months of stroke (O'Dwyer et al 1996). Others have reported that when hyperreflexia was decreased, there was no improvement in motor function (Landau 1980; Neilson & McCaughey 1982; Thach & Montgomery 1990: Sheean 2002); and others that exercises designed to increase muscle strength and functional performance are associated with increases in strength and function, with a decrease in spasticity (Levin & Hui Chan 1994; Butefisch et al 1995; Sharp & Brouwer 1997; Smith et al 1999; Teixeira-Salmela et al 1999).

Two signs that have been taken in the clinic to infer the presence of spasticity are resistance to passive movement and the appearance of abnormal patterns of movement. It is now evident that there may be alternative explanations for the mechanisms underlying these clinical signs. The following section examines this issue.

Resistance to passive movement (hypertonus). 'Tone' is typically tested in the clinic by passive movement of a joint or limb and by the Modified Ashworth Scale (Ashworth 1964). This test has in a sense contributed to the controversy which exists about the nature and significance of spasticity. Confusion arises from the fact that the test does not distinguish between the peripheral contribution due to muscle adaptations and the neural contribution due to increased stretch reflexes. The Modified Ashworth Scale, which grades tone according to the amount of resistance to passive movement, is an example of a scale that sets out to test one impairment (reflex activity) but really tests another (resistance to passive movement) (Bohannon & Smith 1987). The scale does not differentiate between neural factors and intrinsic muscle stiffness (Katz et al 1992).

Muscle tone is the force with which a muscle resists being lengthened (Pearson & Gordon 2001) and it depends on the intrinsic stiffness (elasticity) of the muscle. There is a neural component as the stretch reflex also resists lengthening of the muscle. Higher centres can adjust muscle tone under different task and contextual conditions. The term *hypertonus* is used by clinicians to describe an increased resistance to passive movement and hyperactive tendon jerks, reflecting an abnormal excitability of the components of the segmental stretch reflex arc (for discussion see Thilmann et al 1991b). It is evident, however, that resistance to passive movement is due principally to muscle morphology and mechanical factors. When a limb of an able-bodied person is moved passively by another individual, the response felt by the examiner may vary between total relaxation (the examiner takes the whole weight of the limb), some assistance (the movement is not really passive but has an active component), or some resistance or braking (the individual contracts a muscle at some time during the movement). If the passive movement is fast or abrupt, it will elicit the stretch reflex in an able-bodied subject. This is felt by the examiner as a 'catch' in the movement. However, although some resistance to passive movement may occur normally, there is no background motor unit activity in resting muscle in relaxed individuals (Burke 1988) and any resistance detected may represent a voluntary contraction by the individual. In individuals with a central lesion, resistance to passive movement may result from several factors (Katz & Rymer 1989), including:

- physical inertia of the extremity
- mechanical-elastic factors, particularly compliance of muscle, but also of tendon and connective tissue
- reflex muscle contraction.

Since inertia of the limb does not change, resistance to passive movement must represent changes in the musculotendinous unit, that is increased intrinsic muscle stiffness or contracture, and/or changes within the segmental reflex arc. Singer and colleagues (2003) concluded from their study of resistance to passive stretching of calf muscles that an important component of resistance was mechanical and unrelated to stretch-induced reflex muscle contraction. There is now a general consensus that adaptive morphological, mechanical and functional changes in soft tissues, occurring in response to diminished muscle contractility and physical inactivity, play the major role in resistance to both passive and active movement (Fig. 8.6).

Co-contraction/coactivation of agonist and antagonist muscles is commonly observed as the patient attempts to gain control over a limb. It is not itself abnormal. In able-bodied subjects, coactivation is evident in active movement and increases when speed is increased. Co-contraction can illustrate lack of skill in able-bodied adults attempting a new or difficult task, decreasing as skill level increases (Enoka 1997), and it has been observed in healthy individuals whose postural stability is challenged (Lamontagne et al 2000). Co-contraction increases as velocity of movement increases and is typically seen during isometric contractions. After an acute brain lesion it can also illustrate lack of skill in reorganizing action-specific muscle activation patterns in the presence of inadequate motor unit recruitment and muscle weakness. For example, a decrease in motor unit firing rate results in decreased muscle tension; additional motor units may be recruited to enable greater force development. Hence stiffening the lower limb in stance can prevent limb collapse but also restricts the flexibility of movement.

However, co-contraction can also occur to an excessive degree, resulting from prolonged and inappropriate muscle activation, for example, carried over from agonist to antagonist phase in a reciprocal movement such as flexion–extension of the elbow (Kamper & Rymer 2001). Whether an abnormal degree of co-contraction illustrates motor control dysfunction or reflex hypersensitivity or is an adaptation to motor control dysfunction may not be clear in the clinic. Antagonist co-contraction during active movement has been reported in several studies, during isometric torque generation (Dewald et al 1995) and during other actions such as walking (Gracies et al 1997). Chae et al (2002) reported a significant correlation between muscle weakness and the degree of co-contraction and motor disability in their group of patients.

Whether excessive co-contraction makes a major impact on functional motor performance is not clear. Some studies have shown that in the first few months after stroke, co-contraction may occur but not as a major feature (Sahrmann & Norton 1977; Gowland et al 1992). Newham and Hsiao (2001) found no excessive or unusual co-contraction between hamstrings and quadriceps during isometric testing after stroke. It is possible that the most disabling effects occur to individuals with poor recovery of function after an acute lesion. The development of disabling co-contraction may be minimized by a functional exercise and motor training programme designed to preserve the natural length of potentially short, stiff muscles (Gracies 2005b) and to train functional motor control in multisegmental movements.

Associated movements are unintended movements that accompany, but are not necessary for, volitional movement. They may result from irradiation of neuronal excitation across the cortex or spinal cord during voluntary movement. They are seen in the able bodied in complex tasks (Carey et al 1983), under stress and when generating maximum force levels, as well as illustrating lack of skill in attempts at a specific task. Using needle electrodes, experiments have shown that unnecessary muscle activation can be seen even when a movement is not present. It has been assumed that associated movements are a manifestation of spasticity (Bobath 1990), occurring clinically only in the presence of spasticity (Stevenson et al 1998). However, there is no evidence to support this theory (Ada & Canning 2005). No statistical relationship has been reported between associated movements and either stretch reflex activity or contracture (Ada & O'Dwyer 2001).

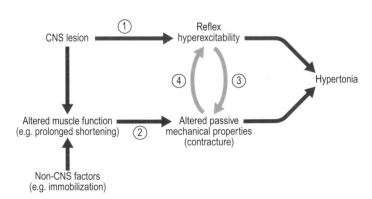

Figure 8.6 Two mechanisms considered to underlie hypertonus (1,2). Additional mechanisms (3,4) may relate to effects flowing between reflex hyperexcitability and altered passive mechanical properties. *(Reprinted from O'Dwyer and Ada 1996, with permission).*

ADAPTIVE FEATURES: SECONDARY PHYSIOLOGICAL, MECHANICAL AND FUNCTIONAL CHANGES IN MUSCLE AND OTHER SOFT TISSUE

The human system is highly adaptable and this underpins the natural flexibility of our movements. Adaptations to lack of muscle activity and joint movement can occur at all levels of the neuromuscular system from muscle fibre (including spindle) to motor cortex (McComas 1994). Changes in habitual levels of muscle activity and movement result in adaptive changes at any age and following any disruption to the system (Kleim et al 2003). When the level of physical activity involving a limb declines, the ensuing reduction in physiological demands further decreases capabilities of the limb (Duchateau & Enoka 2002). Severe paresis can result in inactivity of all muscles, not only those that are paretic, since it leads to immobilization of a limb, absence of weightbearing and general inactivity. Prolonged periods without weightbearing are known to have a significant effect on skeletal muscle of the lower limbs even in able-bodied individuals, and bed rest can lead to decreased strength, poor balance and increased fatigue, the extent depending on length of stay in bed (Berg & Tesch 1996). These conditions are reproduced after an acute lesion, and imposed immobility can be compounded by hospital procedures in the early stages post-stroke (Gracies 2005a).

It is becoming increasingly clear that major anatomical, metabolic, mechanical and functional changes within skeletal muscles occur post-lesion in response to the lesion and to post-lesion inactivity or disuse (for review see Lieber et al 2004). These peripheral changes can impact on the neural system itself and on functional motor performance. Adaptations include increased muscle stiffness, changes in the characteristics of skeletal muscle (e.g., in the elastic properties of muscle cells), structural and functional reorganization of muscle and connective tissue (McComas 1994; Sinkjaer & Magnussen 1994), changed motor patterns during functional activities and a habitual failure to use the paretic limbs and to substitute with the other. Inactivity leads to a decline in muscular endurance, and changes in the cardiorespiratory system increase the decline in physical fitness.

Experimental and clinical investigations of individuals with spasticity and rigidity have confirmed that resistance to passive movement is due not only to neural mechanisms but also to changes in mechanical fibre properties of muscle and in the tendon (Dietz et al 1981; Berger et al 1984; Thilmann et al 1991a; Carey & Burghardt 1993; Gracies 2005a), probably associated with immobility, inactivity and disuse. Perry, in 1980, was one of the first to point out that spasticity was usually accompanied by muscle contracture. Furthermore, it is a clinical observation that the prevention of soft tissue contracture results in decreased likelihood of spasticity developing (Perry 1980; Carr & Shepherd 1987, 1989; Ada & Canning 1990). Perry expressed the view that whether a patient's response to stretch remains just a diagnostic sign or becomes functionally obstructive is largely determined by the degree of contracture present.

In two separate studies carried out several decades ago, Dietz and colleagues (Dietz et al 1981; Berger et al 1982; Dietz & Berger 1983) investigated the ankle movement of adults with stroke and children with cerebral palsy during walking. During swing phase, ankle dorsiflexion range was decreased. EMG activity showed that, although there was activity in the anterior tibial muscles, activity in plantarflexors was minimal. The authors argued that the limited dorsiflexion was due not to heightened reflex responsiveness of the calf muscles but to changes in the mechanical properties of the muscles leading to stiffness.

Following further work, Dietz and colleagues (1991) argued that connective tissue stiffness may also contribute to the resistance. Berger and colleagues (1984) showed that while development of force in the stance phase of walking in able-bodied subjects was coupled to EMG activity in gastrocnemius, in subjects with spasticity (hyperreflexia and Babinski sign), force was coupled to muscle length and not to gastrocnemius EMG activity. These authors proposed that hypertonus was not related to exaggerated reflexes but to changes in muscle fibres. Work carried out by others more recently makes it clear that altered properties in soft tissues (muscle, tendon, connective tissue) are major contributors to stiffness.

Increased passive muscle stiffness, evident clinically when a muscle is passively or actively stretched, appears therefore to result from adaptive mechanical and morphological changes in muscle fibres and tendon and a build-up of connective tissue related to lack of contractile activity. Increased stiffness is well-documented after brain lesions (Thilmann et al 1991a; Sinkjaer & Magnussen 1994; Given et al 1995; Lamontagne et al 2000, 2002), and several studies help us to understand something of the functional impact of increased passive stiffness. For example, increases in stiffness of 43% have been reported in plantarflexor muscles on the paretic compared to the non-paretic side in stroke (Malouin et al 1997).

As a result of their experimental work, Hufschmidt & Mauritz (1985) proposed that the rapid rise in resistance to movement seen on passive stretch could be explained by reference to Hill's cross-bridge theory (Hill 1968); that is, abnormal cross-bridge connections in antagonist muscles could contribute to resistance to passive movement (Figs 8.7 and 8.8). These muscle changes would very likely occur in muscles which, in a relatively immobile limb, are subjected to prolonged positioning at a short length.

Muscle stiffness normally has an active component, caused by muscle contraction, and a passive component.

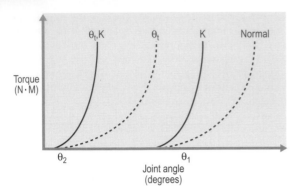

Figure 8.7 The relationship between muscle length and tension (muscle stiffness). Normal trace: normal state of reflex threshold and stiffness; θt,K: represents both decreased threshold and increased stiffness; θt: decreased threshold only; K: increased stiffness. *(From Rymer & Katz 1994, with permission).*

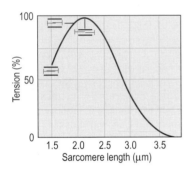

Figure 8.8 Normally the amount of contractile force a muscle can generate depends on its length, i.e., the degree of overlap of thick and thin filaments. Around the muscle's resting length, 2.0 μm, maximum force is attained and force is progressively reduced above and below this length. No active tension develops when sarcomeres are extended to 3.6–3.7 μm because cross bridges cannot form. *(Adapted from Edman KAP & Reggiani C 1987 The sarcomere length-tension relation determined in short muscle fibres of the frog. J Physiol **385**, 709–732, with permission).*

Passive stiffness reflects the viscoelastic properties of the muscle. One component of the resistance felt when a non-contracting muscle is passively lengthened is the inherent elasticity of the cross-bridges formed between actin and myosin filaments. Cross-bridge failure has also been suggested as a possible factor in the increased muscle stiffness found after a brain lesion (Carey & Burghardt 1993). In normal human muscle, stiffness due to cross-bridge attachment is partly dependent on the recent movement history of the muscle; that is, muscle 'memory'.

Contracture. Muscle represents a classic biological example of the relationship between structure and function (Lieber 1988). A muscle's length normally reflects the

typical lengths it is subjected to throughout our daily lives and is therefore subject to change. Immobility imposed on a patient by paralysis or severe weakness can result in soft tissue contracture and this has an adverse effect on both active and passive properties of muscle (Gossman et al 1982; Herbert 1988; Carey & Burghardt 1993; Herbert & Balnave 1993). Evidence from animal studies shows that muscles, when immobilized in their shortened position, lose sarcomeres and become shorter and stiffer† (Tabary et al 1972; Williams & Goldspink 1978; Witzmann et al 1982). It is similar in humans. A shorter than normal muscle is less extensible and physically restricts movement, and a muscle that develops contracture fatigues more rapidly (Arendt-Nielsen et al 1992). It should be noted that contracture of one muscle group, for example the hip flexors, can cause other muscles to shorten, for example the hip adductors and internal rotators.

Adaptive changes occurring after stroke can compound the effects of muscle weakness. The length of a muscle fibre is proportional to the speed at which a muscle can contract and relax (Jones & Round 1996). Any loss of length with changes to sarcomeres will result in reduced contractile speed. Changes in muscle stiffness also affect contractile speed (Newham 2005). In a normally activated muscle, the muscle's length affects its ability to generate force. Muscle length affects actin and myosin overlap and the length of the moment arm (Zajac 1989; Winters & Klewano 1993). Most torque is generated at mid-length and least torque at shortest length (Herzog et al 1991). For example, in able-bodied individuals, plantarflexor muscles generate less torque as ankle plantarflexion progressively increases. Several studies have illustrated this phenomenon.

Increased passive stiffness at the ankle joint in spastic patients has been reported even without marked clinical signs of contracture (Thilmann et al 1991a; Vattanasilp et al 2000), and it has been proposed that muscle stiffness associated with immobility may also be due to *thixotropy*, normally a minor behaviour of muscle. A thixotropic substance is one whose stiffness and viscosity is dependent upon the past history of movement (Hagbarth et al 1985). The term thixotropy describes tension which is almost independent of stretch velocity. Furthermore, muscle thixotropy, according to Proske and colleagues (1993), can exert a strong influence on reflexes either by changing the size of afferent input in response to a stimulus or by biasing spinal excitability levels through changes in maintained rates of afferent discharge. Some time ago, Williams (1980) reported changes in sensitivity of spindles in muscles immobilized at shorter lengths in animals.

---

†The property of muscle called stiffness is the force required to change the length of a resting muscle (see Sinkjaer & Magnussen 1994 for discussion of passive, intrinsic and reflex-mediated stiffness in patients with hemiparesis).

Spindles were activated at shorter lengths than in control animals. A similar finding was reported more recently in humans (Gioux & Petit 1993).

Connective tissue in muscle also undergoes remodelling as a result of immobility and probably contributes to the increased stiffness found in shortened muscle (Booth et al 2001). Connective tissue in an immobilized contracted muscle can therefore further decrease its compliance. This increases spindle stimulation and the spindle's response to stretch which is transmitted more efficiently in a less extensible muscle. Soft tissue adaptations provide, therefore, a mechanical cause for increased resistance to passive and active movement, in addition to forcing adaptive patterns of motor behaviours (Gracies 2005b).

Change in joints include proliferation of fatty tissue in the joint space, cartilage atrophy, weakening of ligament insertion sites, osteoporosis (Akeson et al 1987) and joint malalignment. Neural changes, including impaired motor (supraspinal) drive and secondary changes related to morphological plasticity (e.g., collateral sprouting) at the spinal cord level, can also result from post-lesion immobility and disuse (McComas 1994; Nielsen et al 2007). Studies in able-bodied individuals have shown decreased maximum firing rate of muscles and increases in recruitment threshold after a period of immobilization (Duchateau & Hainaut 1990). A larger number of motor units must be recruited to develop a submaximal contraction, since all motor units have lost part of their contractile tension.

In summary, Box 8.1 lists some of the adaptive physiological changes to muscle that may occur after acute brain lesion and associated with muscular inactivity and disuse. As a result of these changes, muscles become weaker, slower to contract and generate force, and stiffer. The individual loses cardiovascular fitness and is easily fatigued. Changes may occur quite quickly both in the able-bodied person and after brain lesion. Quadriceps atrophy has been reported as early as 3 days after immobilization in able-bodied individuals (Lindboe & Platou 1984), with 30% reduction in cross-sectional area reported as occurring within a month (Halkjaer-Kristensen & Ingemann-Hansen 1985). After stroke, changes in muscle length can occur as early as 2 months after stroke (Malouin et al 1997), and probably earlier.

Adaptive patterns of movement are evident following lesions involving the motor pathways. They are functional adaptations that become apparent when a person attempts to move in the presence of paresis of some muscles creating an imbalance between weaker and stronger muscle groups. Both muscle imbalance and contracture can affect the dynamics of the segmental linkage. When the person attempts a purposeful action, the movement pattern that emerges may be the best attempt under the circumstances, given the state of the neural and musculoskeletal systems and the dynamic possibilities inherent

---

Box 8.1 Summary points

- Loss of functional motor units (McComas 1994)
- Changes in muscle fibre type and size, e.g. severe atrophy of type II fibres with a predominance of slow-twitch type I fibres (Toffola et al 2001)
- Length-associated changes, including reduction in muscle fascicle length, with shortened muscle fibres and contracture
- Cellular atrophy that may be load dependent (Lieber et al 2004)
- Changes in muscle mechanical properties including increased muscle stiffness (Mirbagheri et al 2000)
- Increased sensitivity of muscle spindles in short, stiff muscles (Gracies 2005b)
- Proliferation of extracellular connective tissue (Booth et al 2001) with increased amount of collagen associated with resistance to passive stretch, muscle stiffness and contracture
- Increased connective tissue reduces muscle compliance and increases the spindles' responses to stretch (Williams 1980)
- Increased intramuscular fat (Ryan et al 2002)
- Changes in muscle metabolism such as reduced oxidative capacity (Potempa et al 1996)
- Reduced capillary density compatible with endurance de-training or inactivity (Sunnerhagen et al 1999)

---

in the multisegmental linkage (Shepherd & Carr 1991; Carr & Shepherd 1996). The observable movement pattern that emerges spontaneously as a person attempts to perform a task illustrates the imbalance between muscles that can generate force to move the limb and those which cannot. Knowledge of functional anatomy and biomechanics enables the therapist to plan training methods that can lead to improved strength and coordination, and more effective performance.

Movement is an effort for the patient as muscle weakness gives the perception of limb heaviness. Exaggerated force is generated by stronger muscles (including those muscles with bilateral innervation such as shoulder girdle elevators and glenohumeral adductors) as the individual struggles to perform an approximation of the action necessary to achieve the goal (see Fig. 2.11). In order to maintain extension of the lower limb in standing, for example, the patient may stiffen the knee by co-contracting muscles in order to prevent the limb from collapsing. Co-contraction of muscles or stiffening of a limb can therefore be a functional adaptation to motor impairments, illustrating the adaptive capacity of the system. In addition, adaptive shortening of soft tissues is a significant factor in the development of the restricted movements observed by clinicians, since movement is constrained by abnormally short tissues.

Holding the upper limb in flexion and lower limb in extension in standing has been considered to be the result of spasticity. However, there may be no evidence of spasticity (reflex hyperactivity) when it is tested. O'Dwyer and colleagues (1996) reported that many of the 24 post-stroke individuals they tested habitually held their elbow in some flexion even though they did not necessarily demonstrate reflex hyperactivity. Lance, in a letter to the Lancet in 1990, reminded us that spasticity does not include impaired voluntary movement and abnormal posture, but that these signs reflect adaptations to muscle weakness, changes in motoneuron firing patterns, soft tissue stiffness and contracture.

Changes in the properties of the muscle may lead to a new 'resting' position of the limb. Position sense in a paretic limb would be dependent on the muscle's history. In sitting, if there is severe muscle paresis, the arm may rest with the elbow flexed for long periods, defining, in the words of Proske and colleagues (1993), the muscle's recent history. This may help to explain why the resting posture for, say, the upper limb is so often with the elbow flexed when the limb is unsupported (e.g., in standing).

The mechanism underlying the resting length of muscle is not well understood. Holding a limb persistently in one position for prolonged periods may change muscle spindle sensitivity (Gioux & Petit 1993), and muscle contracture will 'fix' the position of the limb. The signal for limb position is provided by the resting discharge of muscle spindles (Gregory et al 1988). It is unlikely that a persistent limb position is due to spasticity although spasticity may be present.

CLINICAL INTERVENTION

While neuroscientists seek to understand the pathological mechanisms underlying the UMN lesion, the clinician needs also to identify what it is that most interferes with effective motor performance in order to plan appropriate rehabilitation. At the present state of knowledge, the major impairments interfering with functional motor behaviour are impaired muscle activation and weakness, impaired motor control including slowness of movement and a prolonged rise to peak force, and adaptive changes to muscles and other soft tissues. Given the nature of the adaptive changes occurring to both soft tissue and neural mechanisms and the rapidity of their development, encouraging the patient to be active and to exercise and practise for several periods throughout the day, starting as soon as possible after vital signs have stabilized, seems critical. The rehabilitation environment itself must encourage activity in sitting and standing.

Over the past three decades, much rehabilitation practice has operated from strong beliefs both about how the system functions and the neural consequences of the lesion – the impairments and adaptive muscle changes – many of which can no longer be supported. Some of these clinical beliefs have continued despite the publication of challenging new findings. However, neurological rehabilitation is making major changes, responding to recent scientific findings and seeking to develop and use an evidence base.

The major objective in rehabilitation is to train the individual to improve control over motor output during the performance of major functional actions using task-specific exercise and training. Training and exercise are aimed at stimulating muscle activation and muscle force generation (including the force and speed of muscle activation), increasing the amplitude and timing of muscle forces and intersegmental control. These neuromuscular abilities make up the strength of muscles. Training is directed overall to the behavioural or functional consequences, that is, the effectiveness of motor performance in meeting specific goals, and to the need for functional actions to be relearned. However, the specific effects of impairments are also addressed in training. For example, if a person is unable to activate quadriceps to hold the knee extended in standing (see p. 197), specific exercises are necessary to strengthen the muscles through the 0–10° range, both concentrically and eccentrically. The patient is encouraged to focus on this small movement. When active movement possibilities are limited, muscles at obvious risk of adapting to a shortened length should be positioned at full length for specified times during the day in order to avoid disabling contractures. There is some evidence that this can be effective (Ada et al 2005).

The functional consequences of task-specific training and exercise have the advantage of being readily identifiable with biomechanical and EMG examination, and may provide insight into the underlying pathophysiological mechanisms (Dietz 1992). Studies so far are producing encouraging results. Such an approach makes at least one major assumption: that directing movement training toward improved performance of everyday actions (sit-to-stand, walking, reaching for an object, manipulation) provides the system with the opportunity to re-adjust, to relearn a pattern of neuromotor activity which is relevant to the individual's goal. In other words, optimal recovery (neural reorganization) may best be stimulated by the patient practising motor tasks under similar conditions of strength, speed and accuracy as in real life and with similar cognitive demands.

It is likely that early, active and challenging rehabilitation may prevent or minimize adaptive musculoskeletal and behavioural changes associated with the negative features. Following an acute brain lesion, some muscle activity usually becomes evident after an initial period of shock, although output may be relatively uncontrolled. Lack of training in this early period may diminish the possibilities for return to optimal function. Furthermore, lack of use and prolonged immobility lead to soft tissue adaptation and 'learned non-use' (Taub 1980). Studies of neural recovery mechanisms in animals and humans suggest it is possible for intensive and meaningful task-oriented training to affect positively the recovery processes (see Ch. 1). Conversely, immobility and a non-challenging environment can negatively affect these processes.

Physical inactivity, which leads to a decline in physical endurance and physical fitness, decreased extensibility of soft tissue and contracture, is therefore a major consequence after a brain lesion and in chronic disease. Patients following stroke, for example, may spend long periods in sitting, inactive and relatively motionless (Bernhardt et al 2004; Smith et al 2008), and, following severe traumatic brain injury, immobility may be imposed by prolonged coma.

Active task-oriented exercise, in addition to its positive effects on functional performance, can also positively affect muscle morphology, mechanics and function, and can minimize or prevent muscle stiffness, inflexibility and contracture. Functional weightbearing exercises, following the principle of specificity and involving concrete tasks, with repetitive shortening and lengthening of muscles in concentric and eccentric contractions through full range (Fig. 8.9), are active functional ways of preserving soft tissue length.

Serial casting can be effective in maintaining and increasing length of at-risk muscles such as calf muscles (Moseley 1997) and may be required as a preventative measure when the patient is in coma and incapable of comprehending instructions (see Ch. 12). The major effect of casting is on the mechanics of muscle (Hummelsheim & Mauritz 1993). Manual stretching does not appear to be effective (Perry 1980; Herbert 1988; Horsley et al 2007).

Spasticity (reflex hyperactivity) is not typically a major obstacle to improved functional disability in people after acute central lesions who recover active movement. It is evident that active exercise can decrease reflex hyperactivity and muscle stiffness in people with a moderate increase in stretch reflex sensitivity who are capable of physical activity. However, for those who develop severe and intractable muscle hyperactivity, with a level of spasticity or spasms that interferes with functional activity or with personal care, drugs that modify transmitter release (e.g., baclofen, botulinum toxin) offer a means of damping down reflexive muscle activity to allow training and practice to proceed (Gracies et al 2007). Dynamic splinting using Lycra splints (Gracies et al 2000) may also have positive effects. However, consideration should be given to the possibility that efforts to decrease spastic muscle activity may decrease muscle activity needed for movement and such interventions should not be routinely provided.

Clinical testing. Since the major aim of neurological rehabilitation is to retrain motor function and prevent obstructive adaptations, clinical testing requires the measurement of motor performance by global functional scales

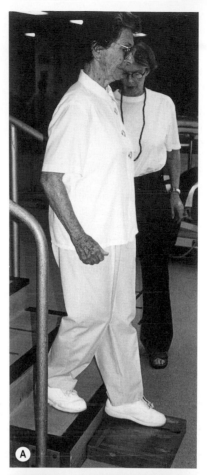

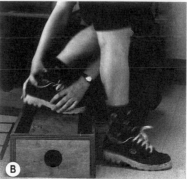

Figure 8.9 Task-specific functional exercise: (A) Practising step-downs as part of an exercise class. Note the active stretch to the soleus muscle (of the affected R leg) as it contracts eccentrically to lower the body mass. (B) Therapist holds the L foot steady as another person practises stepping up and down with the R leg. The step can be lowered if this height is too difficult. This exercise trains intersegmental control of the leg and balance, and also actively stretches the calf muscle.

such as the Motor Assessment Scale (Carr et al 1985) and tests of specific functions such as various parameters of gait performance. At times it may also be necessary to measure isometric and isokinetic muscle strength, functional strength, joint range of motion, muscle stiffness, length and spasticity. See Chapter 3 for examples.

In conclusion, we have set out in this chapter to describe clinically relevant information about the effects on functional motor performance of primary impairments and secondary adaptations following an acute lesion of the cortical motor system. Box 8.2 shows some summary points.

Rehabilitation should be directed toward training methods known to improve muscle strength and endurance and skill in motor performance. Emphasis is on intensive task-oriented training and functional strength training and practice to improve muscle contractility and extensibility (compliance), the amplitude, speed and timing of muscle force production, and intersegmental limb control. In addition to intensive training, a major focus in rehabilitation should be on preserving the length of muscle, of single-joint muscles such as shoulder internal rotators and soleus in particular, and encouraging the person to be physically and mentally active.

Box 8.2 Summary points

- Major primary impairments are failure to activate motor units due to disruption of the corticospinal pathway, resulting in reduced ability to generate and time muscle forces and to control synergic (intersegmental) muscle coordination. They are the major cause of functional disability
- Secondary adaptations to immobility and disuse are structural and functional changes to muscle, including increased intrinsic stiffness, reduced extensibility, contracture and increased sensitivity of muscle spindles
- The functional effects of spasticity (reflex hyperactivity) are unclear. No relationship has been found between spasticity and extent of motor disability. Decreasing hyperreflexia does not result in improved function. Strength training and exercise do not increase spasticity
- Repetitive active and task-specific exercise and functional strength training can increase functional strength and functional performance, decrease spasticity and muscle stiffness and actively preserve the length of muscle

---

REFERENCES

Ada L, Canning C 1990 Anticipating and avoiding muscle shortening. In: Key issues in neurological physiotherapy. Butterworth Heinemann, Oxford:219–236.

Ada L, Canning C 2005 Changing the way we view the contribution of motor impairments to physical disability after stroke. In: Refshauge K, Ada L, Ellis E (eds) Science-based rehabilitation. Butterworth Heinemann, Oxford 87–106.

Ada L, O'Dwyer N 2001 Do associated reactions in the upper limb after stroke contribute to contracture formation? Clin Rehabil 15:186–194.

Ada L, Westwood P 1992 A kinematic analysis of recovery of the ability to stand up following stroke. Aust J Physiother 38:135–142.

Ada L, O'Dwyer N, Green J et al 1996 The nature of the loss of strength and dexterity in the upper limb following stroke. Hum Mov Sci 15:671–687.

Ada L, Vattanasilp W, O'Dwyer N et al 1998 Does spasticity contribute to walking dysfunction after stroke. J Neurol Neurosurg Psychiatry 64:635–638.

Ada L, Canning C, O'Dwyer N 2000 Effect of muscle length on strength and dexterity after stroke. Clin Rehabil 14:55–61.

Ada L, Canning CG, Low S-L 2003 Stroke patients have selective muscle weakness in shortened range. Brain 126:724–731.

Ada L, Goddard E, McCully J et al 2005 Thirty minutes of positioning reduces the development of shoulder external rotation contractures after stroke: a randomized controlled trial. Arch Phys Med Rehabil 86:230–234.

Ada L, O'Dwyer N, O'Neill E 2006 Relation between spasticity, weakness and contracture of the elbow flexors and upper activity after stroke: an observational study. Disabil Rehabil 28:891–897.

Akeson WH, Amiel D, Abel MF et al 1987 Effects of immobilization on joints. Clin Orthop Relat Res 219:28–37.

Andrews AW, Bohannon RW 2000 Distribution of muscle strength impairments following stroke. Clin Rehabil 14:79–87.

Arendt-Nielsen L, Gantchev N, Sinkjaer T 1992 The influence of muscle length on muscle fibre conduction

velocity and development of muscle fatigue. Electroencephalogr Clin Neurophysiol 85:166–172.

Ashworth B 1964 Preliminary trial of carisoprodol in multiple sclerosis. Practitioner 192:540–542.

Beer RF, Given JD, Dewald PA 1999 Task-dependent weakness at the elbow in patients with hemiparesis. Arch Phys Med Rehabil 80:766–772.

Berg HE, Tesch PA 1996 Changes in muscle function in response to 10 days of lower limb unloading in humans. Acta Physiol Scand 157:63–70.

Berger W, Quintern J, Dietz V 1982 Pathophysiology of gait in children with cerebral palsy. Electroencephalogr Clin Neurophysiol 53:538–548.

Berger W, Horstmann G, Dietz V 1984 Tension development and muscle activation in the leg during gait in spastic hemiparesis: independence of muscle hypertonia and exaggerated stretch reflexes. J Neurol Neurosurg Psychiatry 47:1029–1033.

Bernhardt J, Dewey HM, Thrift AG et al 2004 Inactive and alone: physical activity in the first 14 days of acute stroke unit care. Stroke 35:1005–1009.

Bobath B 1990 Adult hemiplegia: evaluation and treatment, 3rd edn. Butterworth Heinemann, Oxford.

Bohannon RW 1987 Relative decreases in knee extension torque with increased knee extension velocities in stroke patients with hemiparesis. Phys Ther 67:1218–1220.

Bohannon RW 1988 Muscle strength changes in hemiparetic stroke patients during inpatient rehabilitation. J Neurolog Rehabil 2:163–166.

Bohannon RW, Smith MB 1987 Interrater reliability of a modified Ashworth Scale of muscle spasticity. Phys Ther 67:206–207.

Booth CM, Cortina-Borja MJ, Theologis TN 2001 Collagen accumulation in muscles of children with cerebral palsy and correlation with severity of spasticity. Dev Med Child Neurol 43:314–320.

Bourbonnais D, Vanden Noven S 1989 Weakness in patients with hemiparesis. Am J Occup Ther 43:313–319.

Burke D 1983 Critical examination of the case for and against fusimotor involvement in disorders of muscle tone. In: Desmedt JE (ed.) Advances in neurology, 39: motor control mechanisms in health and disease. Raven Press, New York:133–150.

Burke D 1988 Spasticity as an adaptation to pyramidal tract injury. In: Waxman SG (ed.) Advances in neurology, 47: functional recovery in neurological disease. Raven Press, New York:401–423.

Burke D, Gandevia SC 1988 Interfering cutaneous stimulation and the muscle afferent contribution to cortical potentials. Electroencephalogr Clin Neurophysiol 70:118–125.

Burke D, Andrews C, Ashby P 1971a Autogenic effect of static muscle stretch in spastic man. Arch Neurol 25:367–372.

Burke D, Gillies J, Lance J 1971b Hamstrings stretch reflex in human spasticity. J Neurol Neurosurg Psychiatry 34:464–468.

Burne JA, Carlton VL, O'Dwyer N J 2005 The spasticity paradox: movement disorder or disorder of resting limbs? J Neurol Neurosurg Psychiatry 76:47–54.

Butefisch C, Hummelsheim H, Mauritz K-H 1995 Repetitive training of

isolated movements improves the outcome of motor rehabilitation of the centrally paretic hand. J Neurol Sci 130:59–68.

Canning CG, Ada L, O'Dwyer N 1999 Slowness to develop force contributes to weakness after stroke. Arch Phys Med Rehabil 80:66–70.

Canning C, Ada L, Adams R et al 2004 Loss of strength contributes more to physical disability after stroke than loss of dexterity. Clin Rehabil 18:300–308.

Carey JR, Burghardt TP 1993 Movement dysfunction following central nervous system lesions: a problem of neurologic or muscular impairment. Phys Ther 73:538–547.

Carey LM, Allison JD, Mundale MO 1983 Electromyographic study of muscular overflow during precision handgrip. Phys Ther 63:505–511.

Carr JH, Shepherd RB 1987 A motor relearning programme for stroke, 2nd edn. Butterworth Heinemann, Oxford.

Carr JH, Shepherd RB 1989 A motor learning model for stroke rehabilitation. Physiother 75:372–380.

Carr JH, Shepherd RB 1996 'Normal' is not the issue: it is 'effective' goal attainment that counts. Behav Brain Sci 19:72–73.

Carr JH, Shepherd RB, Nordholm L et al 1985 A motor assessment scale for stroke. Phys Ther 65:175–180.

Carr JH, Shepherd RB, Ada L 1995 Spasticity: research findings and implications for intervention. Physiother 81:421–429.

Cavallari P, Katz R 1989 Pattern of projections of group I afferents from forearm muscles to motor neurones supplying biceps and triceps muscles in man. Exp Brain Res 78:465–478.

Chae J, Yang G, Park BK et al 2002 Muscle weakness and cocontraction in upper limb hemiparesis: relationship to motor impairment and physical disability. Neurorehabil Neural Repair 16:241–248.

Chapman CE, Wiesendanger M 1982 The physiological and anatomical basis of spasticity: a review. Physiother Can 34:125–136.

Colebatch JG, Gandevia SC 1989 The distribution of muscular weakness in upper motor neuron lesions affecting the arm. Brain 112:749–763.

Colebatch JG, Gandevia SC, Spira PJ 1986 Voluntary muscle strength in hemiparesis: distribution of

weakness at the elbow. J Neurol Neurosurg Psychiatry 49:1019–1024.

Crenna P 1998 Spasticity and 'spastic' gait in children with cerebral palsy. Neurosci Biobehav Rev 22:571–578.

Crenna P 1999 Pathophysiology of lengthening contractions in human spasticity: a study of the hamstring muscles during locomotion. Pathophysiology 5:283–297.

Cruz-Martinez A 1984 Electrophysiological study in hemiparetic subjects: electromyography, motor conduction and response to repetitive nerve stimulation. Electroencephalogr Clin Neurophysiol 23:139–148.

Darian-Smith I, Galea MP, Darian-Smith C 1996 Manual dexterity: how does the cerebral cortex contribute? Clin Exp Pharmacol Physiol 23:948–956.

Dattola R, Girlanda P, Vita G et al 1993 Muscle rearrangement in patients with hemiparesis after stroke. An electrophysiological and morphological study. Eur Neurol 33:109–114.

Davies JM, Mayston MJ, Newham DJ 1996 Electrical and mechanical output of the knee muscles during isometric and isokinetic activity in stroke and healthy adults. Disabil Rehabil 18:83–90.

Dewald JP, Pope PS, Given JD et al 1995 Abnormal muscle coactivation patterns during isometric torque generation at the elbow and shoulder in hemiparesis. Brain 118:495–510.

Dietz V 1992 Spasticity: exaggerated reflexes or movement disorder? In: Forssberg H, Hirschfield H (eds) On movement disorders in children. Karger, Basle:225–233.

Dietz V, Berger W 1983 Normal and impaired regulation of muscle stiffness in gait: a new hypothesis about muscle hypertonia. Exp Neurol 79:680–687.

Dietz V, Sinkjaer T 2007 Spastic movement disorder: impaired reflex function and altered muscle mechanics. Lancet Neurol 6:725–733.

Dietz V, Quintern J, Berger W 1981 Electrophysiological studies of gait in spasticity and rigidity. Evidence that altered mechanical properties of muscle contribute to hypertonia. Brain 104:431–449.

Dietz V, Ketelson UP, Berger W et al 1986 Motor unit involvement in spastic paresis: relationship between leg muscle activation and histochemistry. J Neurol Sci 75:89–103.

Dietz V, Trippel M, Berger W 1991 Reflex activity and muscle tone during elbow movements in patients with spastic paresis. Ann Neurol 30:767–779.

Duchateau J, Enoka RM 2002 Neural adaptations with chronic activity patterns in able-bodied humans. Am J Phys Med Rehabil 81:S17–S27.

Duchateau J, Hainaut K 1990 Effects of immobilization on contractile properties, recruitment and firing rates of human motor units. J Physiol 422:55–65.

Edman KAP, Reggiani C 1987 The sarcomere length–tension relation determined in short muscle fibres of the frog. J Physiol 385:709–732.

Edstrom L 1970 Selective changes in the sizes of red and white muscle fibers in upper motor lesions and Parkinsonism. J Neurol Sci 11:537–550.

Enoka RM 1997 Neural adaptations with chronic physical activity. J Biomech 30:447–455.

Farmer SF, Swash M, Ingram DA et al 1993 Changes in motor unit synchronization following central nervous lesions in man. J Physiol 463:83–105.

Fellows SJ, Kaus C, Thilmann AF et al 1994 Voluntary movement at the elbow in spastic hemiparesis. Ann Neurol 36:397–407.

Frontera WR, Grimby L, Larsson L 1997 Firing rate of the lower motoneuron and contractile properties of its muscle fibers after motoneuron lesion in man. Muscle Nerve 20:938–947.

Gandevia SC 1993 Strength changes in hemiparesis: measurements and mechanisms. In: Thilmann AF, Burke DJ, Rymer WZ (eds) Spasticity: mechanisms and management. Springer-Verlag, Berlin:111–122.

Gandevia SC, McCloskey DI 1977 Sensation of heaviness. Brain 100:345–354.

Gemperline JJ, Allen S, Walk D et al 1995 Characteristics of motor unit discharge in subjects with hemiparesis. Muscle Nerve 18:1101–1114.

Gioux M, Petit J 1993 Effects of immobilizing the cat peroneus longus muscle on the activity of its own spindles. J Appl Physiol 75:2629–2635.

Giuliani CA 1990 Adult hemiplegic gait. In: Smidt GL (ed.) Gait in rehabilitation. Churchill Livingstone, New York:253–266.

Given JD, Dewald JP, Rymer WZ 1995 Joint dependent passive resistance in paretic and contralateral limbs of spastic patients with hemispheric stroke. J Neurol Neurosurg Psychiatry 59:271–275.

Gossman MR, Sahrmann SA, Rose SJ 1982 Review of length-associated changes in muscle. Phys Ther 62:1799–1808.

Gowland C, deBruin H, Basmajian JV et al 1992 Agonist and antagonist activity during voluntary upper-limb movement in patients with stroke. Phys Ther 72:624–633.

Gracies JM 2001 Pathophysiology of impairment in spasticity: stretch as a treatment of spastic hypertonia. Arch Phys Med Rehabil 12:747–768.

Gracies J 2005a Pathophysiology of spastic paresis. I: paresis and soft tissue changes. Muscle Nerve 31:535–551.

Gracies JM 2005b Pathophysiology of spastic paresis. II: emergence of muscle overactivity. Muscle Nerve 31:552–571.

Gracies J-M, Wilson L, Gandevia SC et al 1997 Stretched position of spastic muscles aggravates their co-contraction in hemiplegic patients. Ann Neurol 42:438–439.

Gracies JM, Marosszeky JE, Renton R et al 2000 Short-term effects of dynamic Lycra splints on upper limb in hemiplegic patients. Arch Phys Med Rehabil 81:1547–1555.

Gracies JM, Singer BJ, Dunne JW 2007 The role of botulinum toxin injections in the management of muscle overactivity of the lower limb. Disabil Rehabil 29:1789–1805.

Gregory JE, Morgan DL, Proske U 1988 After-effects in the responses of cat muscle spindles and errors in limb position sense in man. J Neurophysiol 59:1220–1230.

Hagbarth K-E, Hagglund JV, Norkin M et al 1985 Thixotropic behaviour of human finger flexor muscles with accompanying changes in spindle and reflex responses to stretch. J Physiol 368:323–342.

Halkjaer-Kristensen J, Ingemann-Hansen T 1985 Wasting of the human quadriceps muscle after knee ligament injuries. 1. Anthrometric consequences. Scand J Rehabil Med Suppl 13:5–55.

Harris ML, Polkey MI 2001 Quadriceps muscle weakness following acute hemiplegic stroke. Clin Rehabil 15:274–281.

Herbert R 1988 The passive mechanical properties of muscle and their adaptations to altered pattern of use. Aust J Physiother 34:141–149.

Herbert RD, Balnave RJ 1993 The effect of position of immobilization on resting length, resting stiffness, and weight of the soleus muscle of the rabbit. J Orthop Res 11:358–366.

Herzog W, Koh T, Hasler E et al 1991 Specificity and plasticity of mammalian skeleton muscles. J Appl Biomech 16:98–109.

Hill DK 1968 Tension due to interaction between the sliding filaments in resting striated muscle: the effect of stimulation. J Physiol 199:637–684.

Horsley SA, Herbert RD, Ada L 2007 Four weeks of daily stretch has little or no effect on wrist contracture after stroke: a randomized controlled trial. Aust J Physiother 53:239–245.

Hufschmidt A, Mauritz K-H 1985 Chronic transformation of muscle in spasticity: a peripheral contribution to increased tone. J Neurol Neurosurg Psychiatry 48:676–685.

Hummelsheim H, Mauritz K-H 1993 Neurophysiological mechanisms of spasticity modification by physiotherapy. In: Thilmann AF, Burke DJ, Rymer WZ (eds) Spasticity: mechanisms and management. Springer-Verlag, Berlin:426–438.

Jackson JH 1958 Selected writings. In: Taylor J (ed.) John Hughlings Jackson. Basic Books, New York.

Jones DA, Round JM 1996 Skeletal muscle in health and disease; a textbook of muscle physiology. Manchester University Press, Manchester.

Kamper DG, Rymer WZ 2001 Impairment of voluntary control of finger motion following stroke: role of inappropriate muscle coactivation. Muscle Nerve 24:673–681.

Katz RT, Rymer WZ 1989 Spastic hypertonia: mechanisms and measurement. Arch Phys Med Rehabil 70:144–155.

Katz RT, Rovai GP, Brait C et al 1992 Objective quantification of spastic hypertonia: correlation with clinical findings. Arch Phys Med Rehabil 73:339–347.

Kautz SA, Brown DA 1998 Relationships between timing of muscle excitation and impaired motor performance during cyclical lower extremity movement in post-stroke hemiplegia. Brain 121:515–526.

Kilbreath SL, Gandevia SC 1994 Limited independent flexion of thumb and fingers in human subjects. J Neurophysiol 479:487–497.

Kilbreath SL, Gorman RB, Raymond J et al 2002 Distribution of the forces produced by motor unit activity in the human flexor digitorum profundus. J Physiol 543:289–296.

Kleim JL, Jones TA, Schallet T 2003 Motor enrichment and the induction of plasticity before or after brain injury. Neurochem Res 28:1757–1769.

Knutsson E, Martensson A 1980 Dynamic motor capacity in spastic paresis and its relation to prime mover dysfunction, spastic reflexes and antagonist co-activation. Scand J Rehabil Med 12:93–106.

Knutsson E, Richards C 1979 Different types of disturbed motor control in gait of hemiparetic patients. Brain 102:405–430.

Lamontagne A, Richards CL, Malouin F 2000 Coactivation during gait as an adaptive behavior after stroke. J Electromyogr Kinesiol 10:407–415.

Lamontagne A, Malouin F, Richards CL et al 2002 Mechanisms of disturbed motor control in ankle weakness during gait after stroke. Gait Posture 15:244–255.

Lance JW 1980 Symposium synopsis. In: Feldman RG, Young RR, Koella WP (eds) Spasticity: disordered motor control. Year Book Medical Publishers, Chicago:485–494.

Lance JW 1990 What is spasticity? Lancet 335:606.

Landau WM 1980 Spasticity: what is it? What is it not? In: Feldman RG, Young RR, Koella WP (eds) Spasticity: disordered motor control. Year Book Medical Publishers, Chicago:17–24.

Landau WM 1988 Parables of palsy, pills and PT pedagogy: a spastic dialectic. Neurology 38:1496–1499.

Lang CE, Schieber MH 2004 Reduced muscle selectivity during individuated finger movements in humans after damage to the motor cortex or cortsiospinal tract. J Neurophysiol 91:1722–1733.

Latash LP, Latash ML 1994 A new book by NA Bernstein: 'on dexterity and its development'. J Mot Behav 26:56–62.

Levin MF, Hui Chan C 1994 Ankle spasticity is inversely correlated with antagonist contraction in hemiparetic subjects. Electromyogr Clin Neurophysiol 34:415–425.

Levin MF, Selles RW, Verheul MH et al 2000 Deficits in the coordination of agonist and antagonist muscles in stroke patients: implications for normal motor control. Brain Res 853:352–369.

Lieber RL 1988 Comparison between animal and human studies of skeletal muscle adaptation to chronic stimulation. Clin Orthop Relat Res 233:19–24.

Lieber RL, Steinman S, Barash IA et al 2004 Structural and functional changes in spastic skeletal muscle. Muscle Nerve 29:615–627.

Lindboe CF, Platou CS 1984 Effect of immobilization of short duration on the muscle fibre size. Clin Physiol 4:183–188.

Lomoglio MJ, Eng JJ 2008 Nonuniform weakness in the paretic knee and compensatory strength gains in the nonparetic knee occur after stroke. Cerebrovasc Dis 26:584–591.

McComas AJ 1994 Human neuromuscular adaptations that accompany changes in activity. Med Sci Sports Exerc 26:1498–1509.

McComas AJ, Sica REP, Upton ARM et al 1973 Functional changes in motoneurones of hemiparetic patients. J Neurol Neurosurg Psychiatry 36:183–193.

McCrea PH, Eng JJ, Hodgson AJ 2005 Time and magnitude of torque generation is impaired in both arms following stroke. Muscle Nerve 28:46–53.

Malouin F, Bolleville C, Richards C et al 1997 Non-reflex mediated changes in plantarflexor muscles early after stroke. Scand J Rehabil Med 29:147–153.

Mercier C, Bourbonnais D 2004 Relative shoulder flexor and handgrip strength is related to upper limb function after stroke. Clin Rehabil 18:215–221.

Mima T, Toma K, Koshy B et al 2001 Coherence between cortical and muscular activities after subcortical stroke. Stroke 32:2597–2601.

Mirbagheri MM, Barbeau H, Kearney RE 2000 Intrinsic and reflex contributions to human ankle stiffness: variation with activation level and position. Exp Brain Res 135:423–436.

Mirbagheri MM, Alibiglou L, Thajchayapong M et al 2008 Muscle and reflex changes with varying joint angle in hemiparetic stroke. J Neuro Eng Rehabil 5:6.

Moseley AM 1997 The effect of casting combined with stretching on passive ankle dorsiflexion in adults with traumatic head injuries. Phys Ther 77:240–258.

Neilson PD, McCaughey J 1982 Self-regulation of spasm and spasticity in cerebral palsy. J Neurol Neurosurg Psychiatry 45:320–330.

Nielsen JB, Crone C, Hultborn H 2007 The spinal pathophysiology of spasticity – from a basic science point of view. Acta Physiol 189:171–180.

Newham DJ 2005 Muscle performance after stroke. In: Refshauge K, Ada L, Ellis E (eds) Science-based rehabilitation. Theory into practice. Elsevier, Oxford.

Newham DJ, Hsiao S-F 2001 Knee muscle isometric strength, voluntary activation and antagonist co-contraction in the first six months after stroke. Disabil Rehabil 23:379–386.

Newham DJ, Maystone MJ, Davies JM 1996 Quadriceps isometric force, voluntary activation and relaxation speed in stroke. Muscle Nerve 4:S53.

Ng S, Shepherd RB 2000 Weakness in patients with stroke: implications for strength training in neurorehabilitation. Phys Ther Rev 5:227–238.

O'Dwyer NJ, Ada L 1996 Reflex hyperexcitability and muscle contracture in relation to spastic hypertonia. Curr Opin Neurol 9:451–455.

O'Dwyer NJ, Ada L, Neilson PD 1996 Spasticity and muscle contracture following stroke. Brain 119:1737–1749.

Olney SJ 2005 Training gait after stroke: a biomechanical perspective. In: Refshauge K, Ada L, Ellis E (eds) Science-based rehabilitation. Theories into practice. Butterworth Heinemann, Oxford.

Olney SJ, Richards C 1996 Hemiparetic gait following stroke. Pt 1: characteristics. Gait Posture 4:136–148.

Olney SJ, Griffin MP, Monga TN et al 1991 Work and power in gait of stroke patients. Arch Phys Med Rehabil 72:309–314.

Pandyan AD, Gregoric M, Barnes MP et al 2005 Spasticity: clinical perceptions, neurological realities and meaningful measurement. Disabil Rehabil 27:2–6.

Pearson K, Gordon J 2001 Spinal reflexes. In: Kandel ER, Schwartz JH, Jessell TM (eds) Principles of neuroscience, 4th edn. McGraw-Hill, New York:713–735.

Perry J 1980 Rehabilitation of spasticity. In: Feldman RG, Young RR, Koella WP (eds) Spasticity: disordered motor control. Year Book Medical Publishers, Chicago.

Phillips CG, Porter R 1977 Corticospinal neurones. Their role in movement. Academic Press, New York.

Porter R, Lemon R 1993 Corticospinal function and voluntary movement. Oxford University Press, New York.

Potempa K, Braun LT, Tinknell T et al 1996 Benefits of aerobic exercise after stroke. Sports Med 21:337–346.

Proske U, Morgan DL, Gregory JE 1993 Thixotropy in skeletal muscle and in muscle spindles: a review. Prog Neurobiol 41:705–721.

Richards CL, Malouin F, Dumas F et al 1991 New rehabilitation strategies for the treatment of spastic gait disorders. In: Patla AE (ed.) Adaptability of human gait. Elsevier, New York:387–411.

Riley NA, Bilodeau M 2002 Changes in upper limb joint torque patterns and EMG signals with fatigue following a stroke. Disabil Rehabil 24:961–969.

Rosenfalck A, Andreassen S 1980 Impaired regulation of force and firing pattern of single motor units in patients with spasticity. J Neurol Neurosurg Psychiatry 43:907–916.

Rothwell JC, Traub MM, Marsden CD 1980 Influence of voluntary intent on the human long latency stretch reflex. Nature 286:496–498.

Rushworth G 1960 Spasticity and rigidity: an experimental study and review. J Neurol Neurosurg Psychiatry 23:99–118.

Ryan AS, Dobrovolny MA, Smith GV et al 2002 Hemiparetic muscle atrophy and increased intramuscular fat in stroke patients. Arch Phys Med Rehabil 83:1703–1707.

Rymer WZ, Katz RT 1994 Mechanisms of spastic hypertonia. Phys Med Rehabil 8:441–454.

Sahrmann SA, Norton BS 1977 The relationship of voluntary movement to spasticity in the upper motor neuron syndrome. Ann Neurol 2:460–465.

Salazar-Torres JJ, Pandyan AD, Price CIM et al 2004 Does spasticity result from hyperactive stretch reflexes? Preliminary findings from a stretch reflex characterization study. Disabil Rehabil 26:756–760.

Sharp SA, Brouwer BJ 1997 Isokinetic strength training of the hemiparetic knee: effects on function and spasticity. Arch Phys Med Rehabil 78:1231–1236.

Sheean G 2002 The pathophysiology of spasticity. Eur J Neurol Suppl 1:3–9.

Shepherd RB, Carr JH 1991 An emergent or dynamical systems view of movement dysfunction. Aust J Physiother 37:4–5.

Singer BJ, Dunne JW, Singer KP et al 2003 Velocity dependent plantarflexor resistive torque in patients with acquired brain injury. Clin Biomech 18:157–165.

Sinkjaer T, Magnussen I 1994 Passive, intrinsic and reflex-mediated stiffness in the ankle extensors of hemiparetic patients. Brain 117:355–363.

Smith GV, Silver KHC, Goldberg AP et al 1999 'Task-oriented' exercise improves hamstring strength and spastic reflexes in chronic stroke patients. Stroke 30:2112–2118.

Smith P, Galea M, Woodward M et al 2008 Physical activity by elderly patients undergoing inpatient rehabilitation is low: an observational study. Aust J Physiother 54:209–213.

Sommerfeld DK, Eek EU, Svensson AK et al 2004 Spasticity after stroke: its occurrence and association with motor impairments and activity limitations. Stroke 35:134–139.

Stevenson R, Edwards S, Freeman J 1998 Associated reactions: their value in clinical practice? Physiother Res Int 3:69–75.

Sunnerhagen KS, Svantesson U, Lonn L et al 1999 Upper motor neurone lesions: their effect on muscle performance and appearance in stroke patients with minor motor impairment. Arch Phys Med Rehabil 80:155–161.

Tabary JC, Tabary C, Tardieu G et al 1972 Physiological and structural changes in the cat soleus muscle due to immobilization at different lengths by plaster casts. J Physiol 224:231–244.

Tang A, Rymer WZ 1981 Abnormal force-EMG relations in paretic limbs of hemiparetic human subjects. J Neurol Neurosurg Psychiatry 44:690–698.

Taub E 1980 Somatosensory deafferentation research with monkeys: implications for rehabilitation medicine. In: Behavioral psychology in rehabilitation medicine: clinical applications, Williams and Wilkins, Baltimore:371–401.

Teixeira-Salmela LF, Olney SJ, Nadeau S et al 1999 Muscle strengthening and physical conditioning to reduce impairment and disability in chronic stroke survivors. Arch Phys Med Rehabil 80:1211–1218.

Thach WT, Montgomery EB 1990 Motor systems. In: Pearlman AL, Collins RC (eds) Neurobiology of disease. Oxford University Press, Oxford:168–196.

Thilmann AF, Fellows SJ 1991 The time-course of bilateral changes in the reflex excitability of relaxed triceps surae muscle in human hemiparetic spasticity. J Neurol 238:293–298.

Thilmann AF, Fellows SJ, Garms E 1991a The mechanism of spastic muscle hypertonus: variation in reflex gain over time course of spasticity. Brain 114:233–244.

Thilmann AF, Fellows SJ, Ross HF 1991b Biomechanical changes at the ankle joint after stroke. J Neurol Neurosurg Psychiatry 54:134–139.

Thilmann AF, Burke DJ, Rymer WZ 1993 Preface. In: Thilmann AF, Burke DJ, Rymer WZ (eds) Spasticity: mechanisms and management. Springer-Verlag, Berlin:v–vi.

Toffola ED, Sparpaglione D, Pistorio A et al 2001 Myoelectric manifestations of muscle changes in stroke patients. Arch Phys Med Rehabil 82:661–665.

Tsuji I, Nakamura R 1987 The altered time course of tension development during the initiation of fast movement in hemiplegic patients. Tohoku J Exp Med 151:137–143.

Turton A, Lemon RN 1999 The contribution of fast corticospinal input to the voluntary activation of proximal muscles in normal subjects and in stroke patients. Exp Brain Res 129:559–572.

van der Meche FGA, van der Gijn J 1986 Hypotonia: an erroneous clinical concept? Brain 109:1169–1178.

Vattanasilp W, Ada L, Crosbie J 2000 Contribution of thixotropy, spasticity, and contracture to ankle stiffness after stroke. J Neurol Neurosurg Psychiatry 69:34–39.

Visser SL, Oosterhoff E, Hermans HJ et al 1985 Single twitch contraction curve in patients with spastic hemiparesis in relation to EMG findings. Electromyogr Clin Neurophysiol 25:63–71.

Walshe FMR 1961 Contributions of John Hughlings Jackson to neurology. Arch Neurol 5:119–131.

Whitehead NP, Weerakkody NS, Gregory JE et al 2001 Changes in passive tension of muscle in humans and animals after eccentric exercise. J Physiol 533:593–604.

Williams RG 1980 Sensitivity changes shown by spindle receptors in chronically immobilized skeletal muscle. J Physiol 306:26P–27P.

Williams PE, Goldspink G 1978 Changes in sarcomere length and physiological properties in immobilized muscle. J Anat 127:459–468.

Wilson LR, Gandevia SC, Inglis JT et al 1999 Muscle spindle activity in the affected upper limb after a unilateral stroke. Brain 122:2079–2088.

Winter DA 1985 Concerning the scientific basis for the diagnosis of pathophysiological gait and for rehabilitation protocols. Physiother Can 37:245–252.

Winters JM, Klewano DG 1993 Effect of initial upper-limb alignment on muscle contributions to isometric strngth curves. J Biomech 26:143–153.

Witzmann FA, Kim DH, Fitts RH 1982 Hindlimb immobilization: length–tension and contractile properties of skeletal muscle. J Appl Physiol 53:335–345.

Young JL, Mayer RF 1982 Physiological alterations of motor units in hemiplegia. J Neurol Sci 54:401–412.

Zajac FE 1989 Muscle and tendon: properties, models, scaling, and application to biomechanics and motor control. Crit Rev Biomed Eng 17:359–411.

Chapter | 9 |

Cerebellar ataxia

Written with Phu Hoang

Ataxia (from the Greek, meaning 'not ordered') is a term used to describe a number of abnormal movements that may occur during the execution of voluntary movements including incoordination, delay in movements, dysmetria (inaccuracy in achieving a target), dysdiadochokinesia (inability to perform movements of constant force and rhythm) and tremor. In this chapter, discussions focus mainly on the role of the cerebellum in relation to its possible contribution to the control of movement, the aetiology and pathology of cerebellar lesions and the clinical signs considered to reflect cerebellar dysfunction. The results of biomechanical studies of movement in patients with cerebellar lesion are examined and described. Since underlying mechanisms of the observable deficits from cerebellar lesions or dysfunction are often not well understood, these descriptions are particularly helpful in planning motor training interventions.

INTRODUCTION

Control of movement is distributed throughout the central nervous system (CNS). The cerebellum has a part to play within this distributed system by functioning closely with other parts of the CNS including the motor cortex, basal ganglia, vestibular system and spinal motor system (Guberman 1994). The role of the cerebellum is concerned with the timing, coordination and integration of movements, including eye movements and speech. Therefore, lesions affecting the cerebellum would result in a disorder of movement coordination often termed as cerebellar ataxia. This is a descriptive term used to describe certain behaviours: the postural unsteadiness and difficulty coordinating movement, with other possible signs such as tibulation (rhythmic head movements) or nystagmus (rapid involuntary movement of the eyes in the horizontal, vertical or rotary planes). However, it is not always possible to associate the disordered motor control seen in individuals with lesions of the cerebellum and its connections with specific cerebellar mechanisms.

The characteristics of movement disorders resulting from cerebellar dysfunction have been described since early in the twentieth century by Gordon Holmes (1917, 1922a,b, 1939). In the past seven decades, evidence from studies in neuroscience, neuroimaging and particularly in biomechanics has shed further light on both the

©2010 Elsevier Ltd
DOI: 10.1016/B978-0-7020-4051-1.00018-7

performance deficits associated with cerebellar lesions and the underlying impairments.

FUNCTIONAL ROLE OF THE CEREBELLUM

Although the cerebellum constitutes about 10% of the brain's total volume, it contains more than half the total number of neurons in the brain (Ghez 1991). The cerebellum regulates vestibular, spinal and cortical mechanisms by means of reciprocal neuronal connections. Structurally the cerebellum is composed of two main parts: the cerebellar cortex and the deep cerebellar nuclei (see below for further details). These parts receive afferent pathways from other parts of the brain regions, mainly the cerebral cortex. The efferent pathways that leave the cerebellum mainly arise from the deep nuclei, after receiving the outputs from the cerebellar cortex, and project back to the cerebral cortex and other regions. The cerebellum sends no pathways directly to the spinal cord but participates in at least three systems: a vestibulo-cerebellar system which modulates vestibular influences on posture and eye movements; a spino-cerebellar system which regulates muscle tone, posture and locomotion; and a cerebro-cerebellar system thought to play a role in regulating skilled movements (Gordon 1990).

The role of the cerebellum is sometimes described as enriching the quality of movement, acting as a regulatory centre for the control of motor activity and participating in the construction of synergies. The cerebellum plays an important role in the timing and sequencing of muscle activation during movement (Eccles 1977; Gilman et al 1981). It also regulates movement and posture indirectly by adjusting the output of major descending motor systems – for example, scaling the size of muscle contraction. In this sense, the cerebellum acts as a comparator to detect the difference between an intended movement and the actual movement, and, through its projections to the upper motor neurons, to reduce the error. In this role it would compensate for errors in movement by comparing intention with performance (Ghez 1991).

The cerebellum has the connections to carry out this role, receiving inputs from the periphery and from all levels of the CNS. Inputs include internal feedback (also called corollary discharge) related to the planning and forthcoming execution of movement. The cerebellum also receives external feedback about performance from sensory receptors (visual, tactile, proprioceptive, auditory) during movement and compares intended movement with the actual movement as it unfolds. Movements can, therefore, be corrected when they deviate from the intended course and the neural signals modified so that subsequent movements can achieve their goal.

In the traditional view the cerebellum has been considered to participate only in motor functions. There is, however, growing evidence for a cerebellar involvement in some aspects of cognitive processing, perception and language (Leiner et al 1993; Molinari et al 2002). The cerebellum has also been linked to higher order cognitive control processes frequently referred to as executive processing such as working memory, multitasking or inhibition (Bellebaum & Daum 2007). This may not be surprising given that movement and perception–cognition are closely related. After all, we are active participants in our environment, actively seeking out information and utilizing it to optimize the effectiveness of our goal-directed movements and to ensure that we achieve what we have set out to do. However, cerebellar involvement in cognitive function is still a topic under debate. The empirical evidence available so far does not yet allow a convincing theory of the mechanisms of a cerebellar involvement in cognitive function (Timmann & Daum 2007; Glickstein & Doron 2008).

Although the cerebellum contains both motor and sensory representations of the body, lesions to the cerebellum do not produce either paralysis or significant muscle weakness (Gordon 1990). Rather, cerebellar lesions may result in perceptuo-cognitive deficits such as deficits in estimating and comparing weights held in the hand (Holmes 1917, 1939; Mai et al 1989). Investigations performed with child and adult patients with focal lesions of the cerebellum have revealed a characteristic constellation of cognitive deficits, affecting executive, visuospatial, linguistic and behavioural functions (Bugalho et al 2006 and citations therein). Impaired perception of time intervals and velocity of moving objects have also been reported (Leiner et al 1989, 1991; Schmahmann 1991). It was proposed that the cerebellum can be characterized as a tracking system, its role in coordinating movement arising from the need to track moving objects and the body's own movements, and to analyse the sensory consequences (Paulin 1993). Interestingly, a recent study revealed that anticipatory postural adjustments during a bimanual action were intact in patients with either bilateral cerebellar degeneration or focal unilateral lesions (Diedrichsen et al 2005). In this experiment, patients with cerebellar lesions were able to adjust and reduce the postural force used to hold an object in one hand while the object was lifted with the other hand. However, compared with healthy controls, the cerebellar patients showed poorer timing adjustment. Taking together the evidence from experimental data, it is apparent that lesions to the cerebellum disrupt the normally smooth execution and coordination of movement and affect the ability to carry out intentions in a manner that is appropriate to the spatial and temporal requirements of the task and environment. As a result, the ability to perform tasks such as reaching out to an object, manipulating objects, walking and balancing is impaired.

FUNCTIONAL REGIONS OF THE CEREBELLUM

The cerebellum is a distinct and homogeneous anatomic section of the brain, divided into three lobes: anterior, posterior and flocculonodular. Longitudinal furrows divide it into the midline vermis and two hemispheres (Fig. 9.1). However, under the current view the cerebellum is divided into three distinct functional zones based on its afferent and efferent connectivity: the most medial zone (or the vermis), the intermediate zone and the lateral zone. All regions of the cerebellum play an important role in control and adjustment of balance and locomotion, each in different ways (Morton & Bastian 2007). The flocculonodular lobe is often considered a separate functional region (Morton & Bastian 2007). It receives inputs from the vestibular afferents and vestibular nuclei, and reticular

nuclei and Purkinje cells in the flocculonodular lobe project out to directly influence the vestibular nuclei for the control of eye movements, balance and locomotion.

The most medial zone of the cerebellum, the vermis, receives input from the primary vestibular, reticular and pontine nuclei, and from the spinal cord. It plays a primary role in regulating extensor tone, sustaining upright stance and dynamic balance control, and modulating the rhythmic flexor and extensor muscle activity that makes up the locomotor pattern (Morton & Bastian 2007).

The intermediate zone of the cerebellar hemispheres receives inputs from both ventral and dorsal spinocerebellar tracts, reticular nuclei and cerebral cortical areas (Brodal & Bjaalie 1997). This zone sends outputs to the red nucleus and the cerebral cortex via the thalamus (e.g., Asanuma et al 1983). Studies have reported that lesions to this zone cause little or no impairment to upright posture and balance during standing and walking in cats and monkeys (e.g., Thach et al 1992). It is thought that

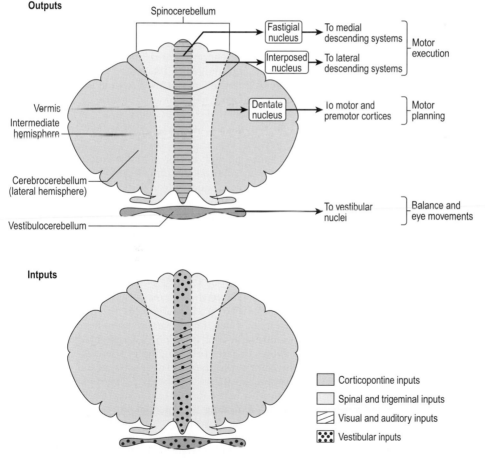

Figure 9.1 Three functional regions of the cerebellum showing outputs (*above*) and inputs (*below*). *(From Ghez 1991, with permission).*

the intermediate cerebellar region plays a fairly minimal role in controlling stance and posture and that it is more important for directing limb placement and regulating agonist–antagonist muscle pairs to control the relative timing, amplitude and trajectory of limb movements, especially in circumstances when more precision is required (Morton & Bastian 2007).

The lateral zone of the cerebellar hemisphere receives input primarily from primary motor, premotor, primary somatosensory and posterior parietal cortices, and also some from prefrontal and temporal cortical areas (e.g., Brodal & Bjaalie 1997; Glickstein 1997) and projects back to primary motor, premotor, parietal and prefrontal regions and other areas (e.g., Middleton & Strick 2001). Thus the lateral zone, through a 'feed-forward' mechanism, modulates cortical motor outputs to ensure precision in the control of the limbs, particularly during fast movement, by the precise timing of the sequence of agonist–antagonist interactions, enabling, for example, dexterity in manual tasks. It may play a significant role in making adjustments to the normal locomotor pattern in novel or complex circumstances or when strong visual guidance is required (Morton & Bastian 2007).

So, although the motor pattern may be determined by higher cortical centres, it appears that details of execution are left to subcortical, notably cerebellar, control mechanisms via specific functions of different anatomical regions of the cerebellum. The cerebellum may, therefore, spare us from having to think out every movement of a limb and enable us to act automatically in this regard (Eccles 1977).

ROLE OF THE CEREBELLUM IN ADAPTATION AND MOTOR LEARNING

Given its functional role in adjusting motor outputs, it is apparent that the cerebellum plays a major role in motor coordination to adapt to the requirements of the task as conditions change. It may, therefore, play a part in reorganizational and adaptive processes and in motor learning (Marr 1969; Glickstein 1992; Thach et al 1992; Halsband & Freund 1993). Motor learning is the means by which we acquire skilled movements and consign them to permanent memory (Saywell & Taylor 2008) with the involvement of multiple brain areas, including the cerebellum.

Thach (1980) proposed a link between adaptation of movement to unexpected circumstances and cerebellar olivary function. A classic experiment, in which able-bodied subjects standing on a movable platform responded to unexpected perturbations of the support surface, showed that, within a few trials, subjects had adapted their leg muscle activations to the novel conditions in order to

regain their balance (see Fig. 7.6) (Nashner & Cordo 1981). This adaptation involved a learning process in which a muscle's response to stretch was adjusted to restore balance. Individuals with cerebellar lesions, however, have difficulty adapting in such a way, with response to muscle stretch being neither functional nor adaptive (Nashner & Grimm 1978).

Motor learning requires a transition from non-specific responses to highly selective associations (Brooks 1986). A recent review by Saywell & Taylor (2008) suggests complex roles of the cerebellum in motor learning. According to the authors, these roles fall into two main categories: 1) skill acquisition and refinement encompassing a continuum from the cognitive through the associative stages of learning (Molinari et al 1997; Petrosini et al 2003; Boyd & Winstein 2004) and 2) skill automation and retrieval, which correlate with the autonomous stage of learning (Nicolson et al 1999; Nixon & Passingham 2001). There is evidence that motor skills learnt before a cerebellar lesion may remain intact and accessible by the patient (e.g., Petrosini et al 2003; Diedrichsen et al 2005) and that learning previously unknown skills, especially in a foreign environment, may be much harder to achieve (e.g., Diedrichsen et al 2005). This has an important implication for physiotherapists during assessment to explore specific information about tasks that were previously well learned and automatic. The motor sequences that have been well learned may be used to form the basis of treatment, reducing the amount of new motor learning required (Saywell & Taylor 2008).

To summarize, the present view is that the cerebellum is involved in:

- initiation and control of voluntary movement
- timing of movement/muscle action
- moment-to-moment correction of errors
- compensating for lesions of the cerebral cortex
- motor learning and adaptive adjustments.

AETIOLOGY

Lesions of the cerebellum may result from developmental abnormality (e.g., hydrocephalus or hypoxia at birth), traumatic brain injury, stroke, tumour or other space-occupying lesion, infection (e.g., encephalitis), demyelinating disease (e.g., multiple sclerosis), familial or hereditary disease (e.g., Friedreich's ataxia), degenerative disease, metabolic disease (e.g., myxoedema, Wilson's disease), vascular disease (e.g., vertebrobasilar artery insufficiency) or drug and alcohol intoxications. The most common causative factor is traumatic brain injury. It is not, therefore, common to see individuals demonstrating solely the signs of cerebellar dysfunction, since such signs are usually accompanied by signs of upper motor neuron dysfunction. This may be one reason for the relative lack of studies of individuals whose dysfunction results solely from cerebellar lesion.

CLINICAL SIGNS

Unilateral lesions of the cerebellum affect the ipsilateral side of the body. From knowledge of the specific afferent and efferent connections of the functional subdivisions, dysfunction characteristics appear to reflect the different functional compartments of the cerebellum (Diener & Dichgans 1992). For example, lesions of the lateral regions are accompanied by movement incoordination related to the intent of movement and reflect problems with preparation for movement. Other evident clinical signs of cerebellar dysfunction are delays in initiating and timing movement, terminal tremor, impaired temporal coordination of multijoint movement and spatial coordination.

Lesions of the vestibulo-cerebellum, with its connections to the vestibular system, are associated with disturbances of balance (increased postural sway with oscillations of head and trunk, staggering gait) and nystagmus. Since these disorders result from difficulty using vestibular information to coordinate movements of the body and eyes, no deficits are evident when the individual is totally supported, for example in supine.

Lesions of the central region result in problems reflecting the loss of 'updating' afferent information. Individuals find it difficult to adapt to changing circumstances. Amplitude of muscle force and timing muscle activation may, therefore, be inappropriate to the present reality as the action unfolds. Individuals with central lesions show abnormalities of balance with an absence of or diminished preparatory postural adjustments, poor timing of muscle onsets and poor recruitment of force. Actions which exemplify the impairments in force production include jumping and hopping, which may be impossible to perform, even by individuals who walk independently. The distinctive clinical signs used to categorize dysfunction, as described by Gordon Holmes, are:

- dysmetria
- dyssynergia
- dysdiadochokinesia
- rebound phenomenon
- tremor
- hypotonia
- dysarthria
- nystagmus.

Recent motion analysis studies of individuals with cerebellar lesions together with an accumulation of data related to how able-bodied individuals perform everyday actions and laboratory tasks are helping to clarify the picture of the motor impairments presented so long ago by Gordon Holmes.

In clinical practice the terms used by Holmes are still commonly used. However, more biomechanical descriptors are gradually appearing in the literature. These have the advantage to the physiotherapist of providing a means by which performance can be analysed, described and measured.

Ataxia

Ataxia is the general term used to describe abnormal coordination of movements. It is demonstrated by deficits in speed, amplitude of displacement, directional accuracy and force of movement (Brown et al 1990). Ataxia comprises the following movement disorders.

Dysmetria

Dysmetria (Fig. 9.2B) is demonstrated by inaccurate amplitude of movement and misplaced force and reflects the impairment in timing of muscle force typical of cerebellar ataxia. There is excessive extent of movement or overshooting (hypermetria) (Fig. 9.3) or deficient extent of movement or undershooting (hypometria). Hypermetric movements may be more marked in small, fast, aimed movements and postural adjustments, while hypometria is more evident in slow movements of small amplitude (Diener & Dichgans 1992). Cerebellar dysmetria occurs proximally and distally in the upper and lower limbs, affects both single-joint and multi-joint movements and is larger for movements performed as fast as possible (Manto 2009). The underlying impairment is thought to be in the agonist–antagonist relationship and in the duration of agonist contraction (Hallett et al 1975; Brooks & Thach 1981; Becker et al 1990).

Several studies of individuals with dysmetria point to difficulty in controlling the termination of movement (Fig. 9.4), specifically with braking or decelerating the movement. For example, when individuals with cerebellar lesions performed ballistic elbow flexion movements (Hallett et al 1975), they demonstrated co-contraction of both biceps and triceps brachii which was said to result in undershooting. It is, however, difficult to establish in such studies how much of the dyscontrol is primary, due to the lesion itself, and how much (or what part) to the individual's adaptive strategies developed in order to move effectively despite the underlying motor control deficit. Task-dependent changes in movement strategy (Brown et al 1990) used by individuals may explain the variability in some of the experimental studies. Dysmetria has also been proposed to result from perceptuo-motor deficits. Difficulty judging velocity and predicting movement outcome (errors in the estimation of movement, either of oneself or another body) would lead to errors in action (Leiner et al 1991; Paulin 1992, 1993).

Delayed movement initiation (see Fig. 9.2A) is demonstrated by increased reaction time (Marsden et al 1977;

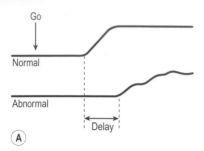

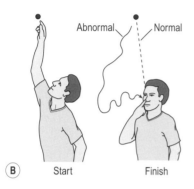

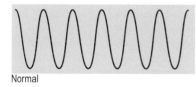

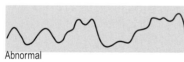

Figure 9.2 Typical clinical signs in cerebellar diseases. (A) A delay in the initiation of movement. When asked to flex both arms on a signal 'Go', subject moves L arm later than R. (B) Moving a hand from above the head to touch the tip of the nose exhibits dysmetria, with increased tremor as the hand nears the nose, (C) Dysdiadochokinesia seen on the lower trace. *(From Kandel et al 1991, after Thach and Montgomery 1990, by permission).*

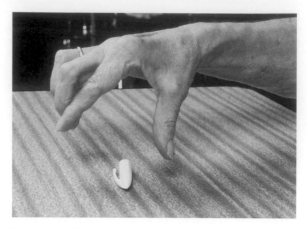

Figure 9.3 When reaching to pick up a pen top, dysmetria is illustrated by the over-wide grasp aperture.

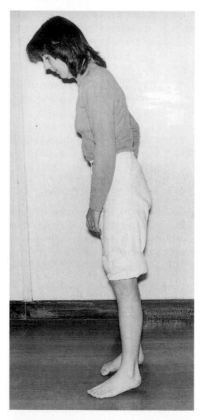

Figure 9.4 When asked to stop walking, there may be difficulty decelerating and halting the action.

Meyer-Lohmann et al 1977; Diener et al 1992) and is thought to be due to a delay in onset of movement-related discharge of neurons in the motor cortex (Diener et al 1993). This delay has been observed in several studies to occur at all joints involved in the action and in fast and slow movements (Beppu et al 1984). Results of studies in monkeys with lesions of the dentate nucleus (Spidalieri et al 1983; Beaubaton et al 1984) suggest that the cortico–ponto–neocerebellum loop, which has efferents to motor cortex through dentate and thalamus, is involved in movement initiation. Neurophysiological support comes from findings that neurons in the cerebellar cortex and the dentate nucleus change discharge frequency before cortical motor neurons (Vilis & Hore 1980; Hore & Flament 1988).

Rebound phenomenon

This phenomenon – lack of check – illustrates the dysfunction in the agonist–antagonist relationship, specifically the problem with braking of movement. It is demonstrated by asking the individual to flex the elbow isometrically against the examiner's resistance. When the resistance is suddenly released, the person is unable to stop the resultant movement, the limb overshoots and rebounds excessively. This is probably a form of hypermetria in that it illustrates the effects of a delay in the antagonistic response (Diener & Dichgans 1992).

Dysdiadochokinesia

This term denotes difficulty performing rapid alternating movements. It refers to the irregular pattern of movement seen when a person performs rapid alternating movements, such as pronating and supinating the forearm or repetitive tapping. The movements are performed clumsily and slowly. As the individual persists, the errors appear to increase, with amplitude of displacement becoming greater than necessary for the action (see Fig. 9.2C).

Tremor

Tremor is an oscillatory movement about a joint due to alternating contractions of agonists and antagonists. This tremor occurs during movement of the limb, not during rest, and is called intention, kinetic or goal-directed tremor. Intention tremor is tested mainly during the finger-to-nose test. It is different from parkinsonian tremor which is a resting tremor classically seen as a 'pill rolling' action of the hands. A classification system for tremor by Deuschl and colleagues (1998) may be a useful reference for the practicing clinicians. Cerebellar tremor is most marked at the end of the movement, for which reason it is frequently called a terminal tremor, or during the whole range of movement (Holmes 1939). Tremor may be greatest when visual cues are used (Sanes et al 1988). This sign may also be related to difficulty controlling the deceleration phase of the movement. A postural or truncal tremor (titubation) may be present when the person is attempting to stand or sit still. Brooks (1986) describes this as a decomposition of intended postural co-contraction of opposing muscles, consisting of inaccurate corrective movements of the whole body.

Dyssynergia

So-called 'decomposition of movement' demonstrates a lack of coordination between agonist, antagonist and other synergic muscles resulting in an absence of the normally smooth, sequential performance of various components of an action. Errors occur in the relative timing of segmental components of multijoint movements. These may be clearly seen in the heel-to-shin clinical test, in which the hip and knee of the moving limb normally flex then extend in one continuous and fluid movement. The individual with cerebellar dysfunction may perform the joint components independently of each other, producing a 'decomposed' movement. There may be a failure to brace joints against forces generated by movement more distally.

Hypotonia

Hypotonia is typically defined as diminished resistance to passive movement. It is said to be manifested in some people with cerebellar lesions as an unnatural increase in joint range on passive movement, called by André-Thomas and colleagues (1960) 'passivité' or 'extensibilité'. The wrist, for example, can be flexed or extended beyond what would be considered its typical range. The phasic reflexes are brisk and a pendular response is evoked if the limb is unsupported. Percussion to the patellar tendon is said to elicit a series of pendular oscillations.

Hypotonia could theoretically be explained by changes in tonic background activity of spinal interneurons, since cerebellar lesions lead to a decrease in phasic motor cortex neuronal discharge in some neurons (Hore & Flament 1988). It may be due to loss of the dynamic spindle response which would make the spindle less responsive to stretch. Patients seem to have difficulty increasing muscle 'stiffness'. According to some observers (e.g., Diener & Dichgans 1992), hypotonus is present only in the acute phase after a lesion. However, the mechanism remains elusive and it is not at all clear what hypotonus is or whether it is an independent entity at all. The typical method of testing, the pendular test, has been shown to be unable to differentiate between normal and cerebellar affected patients (van der Meche & van Gijn 1986).

Dysarthria

In this disorder of speech articulation symbols of speech are normal but mechanical aspects of speech are impaired. Speech is slurred and slow with prolonged syllables (scanning speech). There may also be a lack of coordination of oral musculature and breathing.

Nystagmus

Nystagmus denotes seesaw rhythmical movements of the eyes. This is a sign of vestibular dysfunction and may be present with a lesion involving the flocculonodular lobe of the cerebellum. When seen associated with a unilateral lesion, the oscillating eye may be deflected toward the side of the lesion.

All of the above characteristics of cerebellar dysfunction result in poor control when performing motor tasks, which can be summarized as: 1) errors of rate, amplitude, accuracy and force, evident during the ballistic phase of movements such as reaching and the swing phase of walking; 2) poor control over postural adjustments normally interrelated with voluntary movement; and 3) loss of fluidity of motion, that is poor timing and patterning of the synergic components. Patients attempt to accommodate their ataxia by a variety of different methods. Adaptive motor behaviours are described below.

Adaptive motor behaviour

As a result perhaps of the uncertainty and unpredictability of motor performance, individuals with cerebral dysfunction frequently appear to restrict their actions, and hold themselves stiffly with a wide base of support (Fig. 9.5) and arms outstretched. For example, they may shorten the range through which they move, or brace a segment or segments as a means of controlling dysmetria. In manipulating objects, rather than handling them at a distance from the body, the individual may confine the use of the hands to a position closer to the body or with forearms supported on a table (Fig. 9.6A). In reaching, a person may

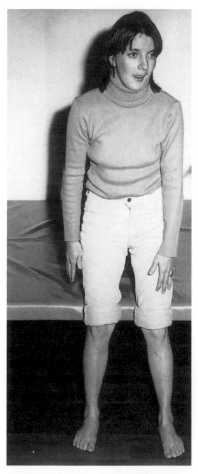

Figure 9.5 Balancing is usually difficult, particularly where a movement (in this case standing up from sitting) requires decelerating a considerable momentum. Note the wide base of support which is also typical of poor balance.

adapt to difficulty slowing the reach by using the support surface or object itself to brake the limb (Figs 9.7 and 9.8). These behaviours decrease the number of joints (and muscles) to be controlled.

In turning around, the person may take small steps instead of turning the body and pivoting on the feet. In individuals with relatively mild cerebellar signs, walking may be faster than appropriate, with large steps and a relatively wide base during double support. It is said that, at a certain level of disability, walking faster may be easier than walking slowly (Winter 1987). In this case, the ataxia and balance problems may be more clearly observed when the person is asked to walk slowly. However, walking may also be slower in some individuals, particularly in those who have very poor balance. Such an individual may take small steps to help restore balance, even when attempting to stand still. The major strategy for dealing with poor balance during standing or walking is to use the upper limbs (Balliet et al 1987) for support. In standing up, the hands may be used to assist at thighs-off (Fig. 9.9), perhaps adapting to a difficulty controlling the generation of extensor force required at this point in the action. Adaptive or compensatory phenomena are the person's natural response to the need to perform effective actions in the presence of incoordination.

Motor performance deficits

Much of what we know about cerebellar function has come from the study of monkeys and humans with cerebellar lesions. Since the availability of motion analysis methods, studies of biomechanical factors involved in actions performed by able-bodied individuals compared to those with cerebellar lesions are providing a clearer picture for the clinician of the nature of the movement deficits by providing information about performance which is of relevance to the clinic. Many studies have involved single-joint movements and the generalizability of their results to functional motor performance may be limited. Some of the apparent conflict in the literature may arise from the different types of action being performed by the subjects. Below is a review of some more functionally relevant studies.

Ataxic gait

One of the hallmarks of a cerebellar disorder is ataxic gait. Typical features of patients with ataxic gait are widened base, unsteadiness, irregularity of stepping both in direction and distance, and reduced stride length with a trend to reduced cadence (Palliyath et al 1998). When patients are asked to perform tandem gait walking, features of cerebellar ataxia such as dysmetria, hypometria, hypermetria and inappropriate timing of foot placement are often accentuated (Stolze et al 2002). Thus, in addition to other functional tests, tandem walking may be helpful in both training and testing progression.

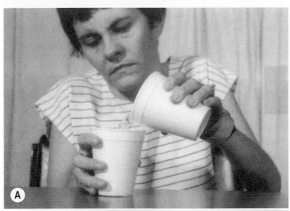

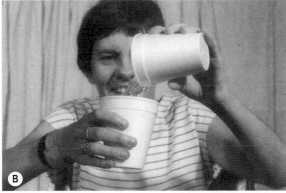

Figure 9.6 (A) This task makes little demand on coordination. (B) Practising pouring water from one cup to the other without arm support, however, increases the demands.

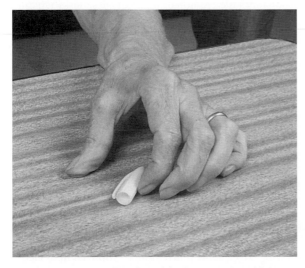

Figure 9.7 Dysmetria is adapted for by using the table to brake hand movement when reaching to pick up the pen top (see Fig. 9.3).

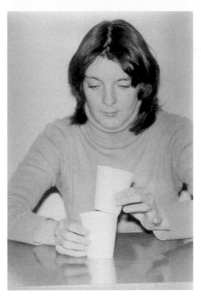

Figure 9.8 Putting one cup into the other is difficult so she uses the cups to brake the arm movement.

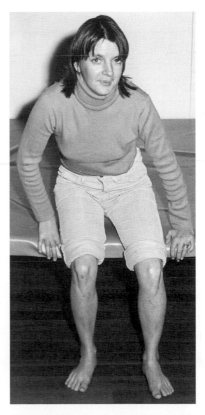

Figure 9.9 The hands are often used for support. Here they are also used to aid in propulsion of the body mass vertically.

Postural adjustments

Postural adjustments normally precede and accompany volitional body and limb movement (e.g., Belen'kii et al 1967; Bouisset & Zattara 1981; Cordo & Nashner 1982) and the muscle activation patterns which make up what are called postural adjustments appear to be specific to the task and the context in which the task is being performed (see Ch. 7). Postural adjustments (muscle activation patterns and segmental rotations), by appropriate shifts in the position of the body mass, ensure that the upcoming movement does not destabilize body equilibrium and cause either unnecessary sway or a fall.

Individuals with cerebellar lesions have difficulty maintaining a stationary position (particularly in standing) and problems with balance are evident whenever they perform any actions in which the centre of body mass moves beyond a certain limited perimeter. Individuals with cerebellar dysfunction demonstrate impaired performance on the rise-to-toes task as reflected in alterations of the magnitude and timing of their postural adjustments (Diener et al 1990, 1992). From the few biomechanical studies available, it appears that difficulties in balancing are due in part to an inability to time and grade muscle force appropriately, related to a deficit in information on status during ongoing movement (e.g., ongoing interactions between segments in multijoint actions). In addition, subjects may have vestibular dysfunction and a derangement of peripheral retinal information processing, which have been reported from studies of eye movements (Hood & Waniewski 1984). Both these impairments can affect balance control, as does the disruption of the coordination of limb and eye movements.

Rising on tiptoes in standing

This action normally comprises an initial shift forward of the body mass. Tibialis anterior, quadriceps and biceps femoris muscles (among others) have been shown to be active prior to heel raise, tibialis anterior to rotate the shank forward (and shift the body mass forward), quadriceps and biceps to stabilize the knee prior to the generation of extensor force at the ankle by the plantarflexor (triceps surae) muscles (Diener et al 1992). Timing of muscle activation and the pattern of force production is, therefore, critical to effective performance. In a study by Diener et al (1992), 18 men and women with cerebellar (vermis) lesions were asked to rise as fast as possible on tiptoes while standing on a forceplate. Their performance was compared with that of 10 able-bodied individuals. Subjects were videotaped and electromyographic (EMG) recordings were made of selected lower limb muscles. Two of the people with cerebellar signs were unable to perform the task. In one of these individuals, quadriceps activity built up slowly and was considerably delayed, its major burst occurring after triceps surae. Note that whereas, on average, the able-bodied subjects activated the synergic

quadriceps muscle some 11 ms after tibialis anterior, the subjects with cerebellar signs activated quadriceps on average 105 ms after tibialis anterior. As a result the knees flexed when the subject tried to rise on tiptoes and he had to drop back onto his heels. Among the other subjects, the deviations from normal varied. However, all groups showed relatively delayed latencies of muscle activation (See Holmes 1917; Hallett et al 1975 for arm and hand movements). These results clarify the nature of the deficits underlying the clinical sign of dyssynergia, with a failure of temporal coupling within synergic muscle groups that normally produces the smoothness of movement. The impairments described may underlie the difficulty commonly experienced in jumping and running.

Postural sway

In several studies, *postural sway in standing* has been found to be increased in individuals with cerebellar signs (see Mauritz et al 1981; Diener et al 1984; Dichgans & Diener 1987; Bronstein et al 1990), although decreased sway has been reported in patients with degenerative vermal lesions (Dichgans & Mauritz 1983). A recent magnetic resonance imaging study on alcoholics provides evidence of impaired postural balance in individuals with pathology of the anterior superior vermis of the cerebellum (Sullivan et al 2006). It should be noted that the relevance of postural sway in quiet standing as a test of balance is uncertain since postural sway seems variable even among able-bodied subjects.

Upper limb actions

There have been several studies of arm movements involving goal-directed reaching, pointing and specially designed laboratory tasks. Although many of these tasks typically involve the subjects moving as fast as possible, the results help clarify the mechanisms underlying dysfunction. Incoordination is particularly evident when individuals try to perform upper limb actions fast, although it can also be evident during slower movements. It is known that, in general, unskilled movements performed by able-bodied subjects involve a greater degree of muscle co-contraction than is evident when skill is attained. During learning to reach for an object, a limb is normally steadied (i.e., the path/trajectory is smoothed) by means of peripheral and visual feedback. As ability improves, co-contraction of muscles is decreased. The propulsive initial burst of agonist activity is increased and the braking opposition by antagonists is reduced until optimal control is reached (Brooks 1986).

Individuals with cerebellar disorders, however, in tasks which involve moving the forearm to follow a slowly moving target, show much more co-contraction of elbow muscles than able-bodied subjects (Beppu et al 1984). Even in studies of rapid single joint movements of the elbow, wrist or finger, patients with cerebellar dysfunction demonstrate an excessive extent of movement (hypermetria) at the joints being examined. One study showed that hypermetria was most marked in aimed movements with small 5° amplitudes (Hore et al 1991). Also characteristic of fast arm movements is a picture of decreased amplitude of peak acceleration and increased amplitude of deceleration (Hallett et al 1991; Hore et al 1991). It seems to be typical of cerebellar disorder that acceleration of a segment is brought about by agonist muscle activation that is less vigorous and more prolonged. In addition, deceleration is associated with delay in the onset of antagonist muscle activation in slow as well as fast movements, in single-joint and in multijoint movements (Hallett et al 1975; Marsden et al 1977; Becker et al 1990; Hallett et al 1991; Hore et al 1991). Both increased duration of agonist activation and delay in antagonist activation appear to contribute to dysmetria.

In one of the few investigations of a 'natural' multijoint movement, individuals with cerebellar signs were studied as they attempted to throw a ball at a target (Becker et al 1990). In performing this action, although subjects demonstrated normal sequencing of agonist arm muscles (elbow extensors, wrist flexors and hand opening), onset of antagonist biceps activation was premature. Subjects had difficulty consistently reproducing the same hand direction in a succession of movements and were, therefore, less accurate than able-bodied subjects. A later study of the dynamics of reaching found that the individuals with cerebellar dysfunction were unable to produce muscle torques that took into account interaction torques occurring in the limb during movement (Bastian et al 1996).

CLINICAL ASSESSMENT, MEASUREMENT AND EVALUATION

Clinical neurological tests

A series of tests are used which seem to reflect the underlying incoordination of movement. These tests were originally designed to test the major clinical signs according to Holmes. They remain useful in enabling the clinician to gain a descriptive picture of the movement deficits.

Finger-to-finger and finger-to-nose tests

The individual attempts to touch the index finger of the examiner with an outstretched arm. A fast response is encouraged as the examiner's arm is moved horizontally, the person attempting to follow. Alternatively, the individual attempts to touch in rapid succession the tip of his/her nose and the finger of the examiner. Any delay in movement initiation will be evident in this test, also terminal tremor and dysmetria. The test is done in standing if possible, and will therefore reveal any difficulty with

postural stabilization during the arm movement. The tester usually notes characteristics such as time taken and presence or absence of dysmetria and tremor. The reliability of a scaled version of this test has been examined in individuals with traumatic head injury and found to be poor when applied by physiotherapists, although it has been reported that the time taken could reliably be evaluated (Swaine & Sullivan 1993). Interestingly, it was found that cerebellar ataxia individuals showed no significant difference between eyes open and eyes closed on the finger-to-nose test (Notermans et al 1994). The apparent lack of reliability should not, however, detract from the test as a means of gaining a clear picture of terminal tremor.

Heel-to-shin test

In supine, the individual attempts to place the heel of one leg onto the shin of the other, near the knee, then to slide the heel down the shin towards the foot. Difficulty placing the heel illustrates the dysmetric component of dysfunction. The method of getting the heel onto the knee may illustrate the dyssynergic element, the individual flexing the hip and knee one after the other rather than flexing the limb in one synergic movement.

Rebound test

A strong isometric contraction of the elbow flexor muscles with the elbow flexed about 90° is resisted by the examiner, who suddenly releases the opposing force. Normally, release is followed by a small-amplitude movement of the forearm, which returns to its initial position after it stops. In an individual with cerebellar dysfunction, the movement of the forearm continues unchecked and the person can hit themselves quite forcefully with the hand if not prevented by the examiner. EMG activity in biceps brachii has been shown to persist after release of the opposing force, with delayed activation of the triceps. This is in contrast to the normal silent period in biceps together with activation of triceps, both occurring approximately 50 ms after release (Terzuolo & Viviani 1973).

Test for rapid alternating movements

In order to detect the presence of dysdiadochokinesia, the individual is asked to pat on a firm surface with one hand, rapidly alternating between palm up and palm down; that is, the forearm is rapidly supinated and pronated. The person with cerebellar dysfunction may perform the action slowly and with exaggerated supination and pronation range, seeming to have difficulty making the alternation. This phenomenon can be explained by the typical difficulty with movement initiation and by the dysmetria at the end of the movement (Diener & Dichgans 1992).

Romberg test for postural sway

This test is performed in standing. Subjects are asked to stand still with arms stretched forward at shoulder height, with eyes open then closed. Patients with cerebellar ataxia will show an increase in the observable body sway under the eyes closed condition.

There have been several attempts at developing quantified and meaningful tests. A study has reported four quantified tests for measuring ataxia (a modified Romberg, a quantified finger-to-nose test, tapping tests for both arms and legs), all of which were found to be reliable and correlated well with two other scales (see Notermans et al 1994). The Romberg test can be quantified using a force-plate to measure the centre of foot pressure (Black et al 1982).

Tests of motor performance

A functional activities evaluation is necessary to give a clear picture of the problems the individual is having with daily life. Suitable tests are described in Chapter 3. In evaluating functional performance, it is necessary to distinguish an individual's voluntary restriction of activity as an adaptation to the motor control deficits rather than as a primary cause of dysfunction. The ataxic characteristics may only be evident if the person is asked to change speed, to stop when asked, or to change direction. Since lack of consistency in movement is common following cerebellar lesions, it may be useful to record the number of repetitions performed in a consistent manner as a test of progress, or the number of successful repetitions in a given time. Two quantitative tests of hand coordination, the spiral test and nail test, have been developed and tested (Verkerk et al 1990). (The spiral test is described in Ch. 3.)

There have been other tests developed to assist clinicians to evaluate their health impact and treatment. For example, in 1997, an ad hoc committee of the World Federation of Neurology developed the International Cooperative Ataxia Rating Scale (ICARS) (Trouillas et al 1997), which involved a compartmentalized quantification of postural and stance disorders, limb ataxia, dysarthria and oculomotor disorders. However, the scale was criticized for lack of objectivity (Ferrarin et al 2005). Other tests include the BRAIN test, an acronym for bradykinesia akinesia incoordination. It assesses speed, accuracy and rhythmicity of upper limb movements, regardless of their physiological basis, during performance of alternating finger tapping on a computerized keyboard (Giovannoni et al 1999). The results of the test were found to correlate well with clinical rating scales in Parkinson's disease and cerebellar dysfunction. Alusi et al (2003) proposed a target board test for quantifying ataxia and dysmetria in the presence of tremor, while Ferrarin et al (2005) suggested that four tests, including walking, knee–tibia test, finger-to-nose and finger-to-finger test, would allow a better insight into motor disturbances in ataxic patients and this is a useful tool for the definition and follow-up of rehabilitation programmes.

Other commonly used functional tests. such as the 6-minute walk test, time-up-and go, nine-hole peg test (see Ch. 3), are also useful and appropriate for monitoring progression of patients with cerebellar dysfunction.

TRAINING

In general, the major objective of physiotherapy remains as it is for any individual with a lesion that affects the neuromuscular system; that is, to train optimal and effective performance of any actions with which the individual is having difficulty (see Ch. 2). It is likely that an organized training programme which ensures the opportunity for practice and which addresses the specific impairments interfering with controlled movement and effective goal achievement may be effective in either acute or chronic ataxia. For example, Balliet and colleagues (1987) reported positive results from a programme planned to improve independent walking in individuals with chronic cerebellar ataxia. Using body weight support for walking training on a treadmill and overground can improve ambulatory function (Cernak et al 2008).

Few studies have looked at the effectiveness of different physiotherapy interventions on reducing ataxia and tremor, as well as improving functional activities. As a consequence, the scientific evidence used to support clinical practice in physiotherapy is still at a low level. A recent systematic review by Martin and colleagues (2009) found only nine studies on the effects of training for cerebellar dysfunction. The majority of these studies are case studies or case series. In addition, translating research success into practice is limited by a lack of appropriate detail regarding these therapeutic interventions, and by an absence of motor performance measures examining specific actions (e.g., walking, balance and upper limb tests). It is apparent that there is a need for further high-quality research in this area.

Nonetheless, given what we currently understand about the motor control deficits and characteristics associated with cerebellar lesions, physiotherapists can train these patients in everyday skills by using declarative memory, that is a procedural memory formed during the learning process of a motor task, or premorbid skills (see Saywell & Taylor 2008 for further details). Environmental factors are also important factors for training success.

Specific objectives to be achieved within the context of individual actions are as follows:

- *To improve performance of functional movements and develop skill, specifically during actions such as standing up, sitting down, walking (including stairs and hills), reaching to take an object:*
  - Use external constraints to provide some steadiness, if this is necessary, to enable practice

of tasks that would otherwise be too difficult or require gross adaptations while moving the arm (pushing, pulling actions) and actions that involve the production of a rapid initial burst of agonist activity (e.g., jumping (Fig. 9.10), jogging (Fig. 9.11), throwing a ball).

- Train everyday actions in standing, with a narrow base of support and no arm support, in order to improve balance control.
- Organize practice of tasks that require predictive timing (e.g., bouncing a ball or hitting it with a bat; see Fig. 9.12).
- Train weightbearing exercises for lower limbs involving repetitive flexion–extension over fixed feet to improve intersegmental control/coordination, for example standing up and sitting down, squats, step-up and down, heels raise and lower (see Ch. 2). Emphasis is on smooth continuous performance, varied weight resistance-body weight, additional weights in vest.
- Provide exercises for the upper limbs in sitting and standing, involving picking up and placing games, with arms close to the body if control is difficult, increasing reaching distance; weightbearing exercises such as push-ups against the wall in standing, pulling games with weighted objects or resistance.
- Train dynamic stability of the trunk and limbs by practising tasks that rely on adapting or developing strategies to cope with increasingly demanding conditions. For example, tandem walking, walking in narrow spaces, on different surfaces and under bars or ropes, walking with eyes open and closed, and starting movements slowly with increases in movement complexity, balance demands, or speed (e.g., Gill-Body et al 1997).
- In practice of the activities and exercises above:
  – encourage performance of smooth movements of various amplitudes and speeds, including stopping and starting at different points in the range, in order to provide practice of controlling agonist/antagonist muscle activity.
  – train muscle control in parts of the range with maximum instability.

- *To set up a practice environment which enables the person to develop more control (accuracy) during practice by varying, for example:*
  - support conditions
  - timing constraints
  - environmental context.

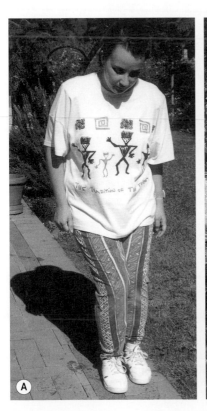
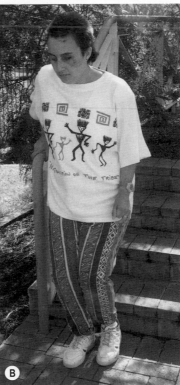

Figure 9.10 Jumping (A) from side to side keeping the legs together and (B) jumping off a step. Both of these actions involve the production of a rapid burst of agonist extensor activity to propel the body upward from the flexion counter-movement without a pause.

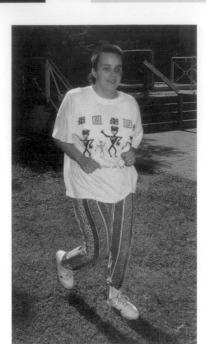

Figure 9.11 Jogging involves rapid bursts of muscle activity in a cyclical fashion. Stopping and starting in response to a command or as part of a game are also practised.

As the person gains more control of a particular action, there are several ways in which the therapist can increase complexity so as to push the individual to the limits of their effective performance.

- To provide challenge:
  - discourage/prevent use of the upper limbs for support
  - reduce the *possibilities* for support through the upper limbs
  - encourage increased amplitude of movement
  - add tasks that require speed alterations and changes in amplitude, direction and force
  - increase balance requirements
  - require that a complex movement (e.g., sit-to-stand, walking) stop immediately on request
  - reduce attentional demands of the action (e.g., by speaking during performance) to encourage automaticity.

Emphasis is placed on interesting, challenging actions, for example dart throwing (if necessary to a modified target), throwing a ball into a hoop, defending a wicket using a cricket bat (the bat can be used as an intermittent prop for balance), walking on a treadmill, throwing a ball through a basketball hoop, etc. (Fig. 9.13). Each of these actions makes certain demands on the individual that help the re-establishing of control if there is plenty of opportunity for practice. Treadmill walking enforces a constant and therefore predictable external timing, a suspended

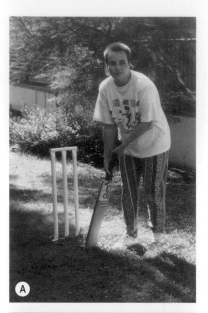

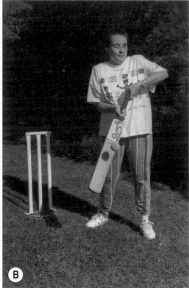

Figure 9.12 Playing cricket enables her to improve balance and coordination along with eye-hand coordination and predictive time-to-contact from a relatively stable position (A) with the ball on the ground and (B) raising the bat to hit the ball.

harness reduces the need for postural adjustment and prevents a fall – the amount of weightbearing through the legs can be controlled without having to use the arms for support (see Ch. 4). Jumping actions, such as jumping over a line on the floor or jumping down from a low step (see Fig. 9.10), provide the opportunity for practice of rapid generation of force (particularly in the calf muscles),

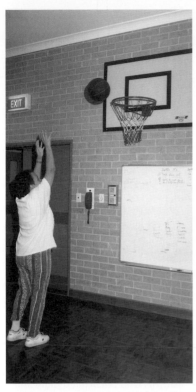

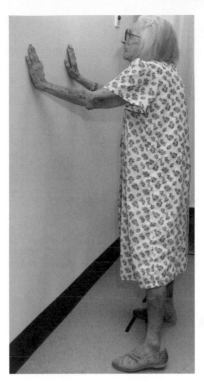

Figure 9.13 Goal throwing. Note that she has not been able to generate a sufficiently rapid and powerful burst of muscle activity to propel her on to her toes. Heel-raising exercises may increase strength and control in calf muscles.

Figure 9.14 Walking sideways with some support, keeping her body mass forward.

with associated intersegmental movements, and for switching between concentric and eccentric muscle action. As in any exercise and training programme designed to promote learning and motor control, it is important to focus on repetition and on varying task and environmental constraints.

Various forms of augmented feedback (see Ch. 2), particularly visual feedback, may assist the person to gain control over an action. For example, visual feedback about force production can assist patients with chronic cerebellar disease to sustain low isometric finger forces (Mai et al 1989). The use of weights can decrease movement errors (Sanes et al 1988) and a weighted belt may provide a means by which walking can be practised without using the hands for support. Many decades ago, Frenkel recommended exercises for individuals with sensory ataxia associated with spinal cord disease. Several of these involved augmented visual input and feedback, with patients walking along a line drawn on the floor, walking between two parallel lines and walking in footsteps drawn on the floor (Krusen et al 1971).

For patients who cannot maintain sitting or standing independently, actions can be practised with

modifications. For example, sitting with the arms supported on a table; walking sideways along a wall with the arms outstretched and hands on the wall (Fig. 9.14); standing up and sitting down with the hands on a table in front; use of a harness suspended from the ceiling to enable safe practice of actions in standing, and of walking.

In conclusion, there has been little interest in developing methods of treatment beyond helping the individual compensate for activity limitations with gait aids and limb weights (Martin et al 2009). However, there is now growing evidence that motor learning is possible with cerebellar damage (Boyd & Winstein 2004; Lacourse et al 2004; Ioffe et al 2006), and it is very likely that individuals with either acute or chronic ataxia are able to benefit from task-oriented training and exercises that encourage practice and challenge the person to the full extent of their capacity, with repetitive practice and discouraging the use of the arms for support. Detailed programmes with appropriate progression are essential for success in training cerebellar ataxia as in any exercise programme. There is as yet a paucity of good-quality clinical trials to demonstrate the effects of physiotherapy in cerebellar ataxia training. Indeed, there is a noticeable lack of documentation on therapy that addresses the specific motor control impairments and secondary adaptations.

REFERENCES

Alusi SH, Glickman S, Patel N et al 2003 Target board test for the quantification of ataxia in tremulous patients. Clin Rehabil 17:140–149.

André-Thomas A, Chesni Y, Saint-Anne Dargassies S 1960 The neurological examination of the infant, Heinemann, London.

Asanuma C, Thach WT, Jones EG 1983 Anatomical evidence for segregated focal groupings of efferent ramifications in the cerebellothalamic pathway of the monkey. Brain Res Rev 5:267–297

Balliet R, Harbst KB, Kim D et al 1987 Retraining of functional gait through the reduction of upper extremity weight-bearing in chronic cerebellar ataxia. Int Rehabil Med 8:148–153.

Bastian AJ, Martin TA, Keating JG et al 1996 Cerebellar ataxia: abnormal control of interaction torques across multiple joints. J Neurophysiol 76:492–509.

Beaubaton D, Trouche, E, Legallet E 1984 Neocerebellum and motor programming: evidence from reaction-time studies in monkeys with dentate nucleus lesions. In: Kornblum S, Requin J (eds) Preparatory states and processes. Erlbaum, London:303–320.

Becker WJ, Kunesch E, Freund H-J 1990 Coordination of a multijoint movement in normal humans and patients with cerebellar dysfunction. Can J Neurol Sci 17:264–274.

Belen'kii VY, Gurfinkel VS, Palt'sev YI 1967 Elements of control of voluntary movements. Biofitzika 12:134–141.

Bellebaum C, Daum I 2007 Cerebellar involvement in executive control. Cerebellum 6:184–192.

Beppu H, Suda M, Tanaka R 1984 Analysis of cerebellar motor disorders by visually guided elbow tracking movement. Brain 107:787–809.

Black FO, Wall C, Rockette HE et al 1982 Normal subject postural sway during the Romberg test. Am J Otolaryngol 3:309–318.

Bouisset S, Zattara M 1981 A sequence of postural movements precedes voluntary movement. Neurosci Lett 22:263–270.

Boyd LA, Winstein C J 2004 Cerebellar stroke impairs temporal but not spatial accuracy during implicit motor learning. Neurorehabil Neural Repair 18:134–143.

Brodal P, Bjaalie JG 1997 Salient anatomic features of the corticoponto-cerebellar pathway. Prog Brain Res 114:227–249.

Bronstein AM, Hood JD, Gresty MA et al 1990 Visual control of balance in cerebellar and Parkinsonian syndrome. Brain 113:767–779.

Brooks V B 1986 How does the limbic system assist motor learning? A limbic comparator hypothesis. Brain Behav Evol 29:29–53.

Brooks VB, Thach WT 1981 Cerebellar control of posture and movement. In: Brookhart JM, Mountcastle VB (eds) Handbook of physiology. American Physiological Society, Bethesda:877–946.

Brown SH, Hefter H, Mertens M et al 1990 Disturbance in human arm movement trajectory due to mild cerebellar dysfunction. J Neurol Neurosurg Psychiatry 53:306–313.

Bugalho P, Correa B, Viana-Baptista M 2006 Role of the cerebellum in cognitive and behavioural control: scientific basis and investigation models. Acta Med Port 19:257–267.

Cernak K, Stevens V, Price R et al 2008 Locomotor training using body-weight support on a treadmill in conjunction with ongoing physical therapy in a child with severe cerebellar ataxia. Phys Ther 88:88–97.

Cordo PJ, Nashner LM 1982 Properties of postural adjustments associated with rapid arm movement. J Neurophysiol 47:287–302.

Deuschl G, Bain P, Brin M 1998 Consensus statement of the Movement Disorder Society on Tremor. Ad Hoc Scientific Committee. Mov Disord 13(Suppl 3):2–23.

Dichgans J, Diener HC 1987 The use of short and long latency reflex testing in leg muscles of neurological patients. In: Struppler A, Weindl A (eds) Clinical aspects of sensory motor integration. Springer, Berlin:165–175.

Dichgans J, Mauritz K-H 1983 Patterns and mechanisms of postural instability in patients with cerebellar lesions. In: Desmedt JE (ed.) Motor control mechanisms in health and disease. Raven Press, New York.

Diedrichsen J, Verstynen T, Lehman SL et al 2005 Cerebellar involvement in anticipating the consequences of self-produced actions during bimanual movements. J Neurophysiol 93:801–812.

Diener HC, Dichgans J 1992 Review: pathophysiology of cerebellar ataxia. Mov Dis 7:95–109.

Diener HC, Dichgans J, Bootz F et al 1984 Early stabilization of human posture after sudden disturbances: influences of rate and amplitude of displacement. Exp Brain Res 56:126–134.

Diener HC, Dichgans J, Guschlbauer B et al 1990 Associated postural adjustments with body movement in normal subjects and patients with parkinsonism and cerebellar disease. Rev Neurol (Paris) 146:555–563.

Diener HC, Dichgans J, Guschlbauer B et al 1992 The coordination of posture and voluntary movement in patients with cerebellar dysfunction. Mov Dis 7:14–22.

Diener HC, Hore J, Ivry R et al 1993 Cerebellar dysfunction of movement and perception. Can J Neurol Sci 20(Suppl 3):S62–S69.

Eccles J 1977 Cerebellar function in the control of movement. In: Rose FC (ed.) Physiological aspects of clinical neurology. Blackwell, Oxford:157–178.

Ferrarin M, Gironi M, Mendozzi L et al 2005 Procedure for the quantitative evaluation of motor disturbances in cerebellar ataxia patients. Med Biol Eng Comput 43:349–356.

Ghez C 1991 The cerebellum. In: Kandel ER, Schwartz JH, Jessell TM (eds) Principles of neural science. Appleton and Lange, Norwalk:626–646.

Gill-Body KM, Popat RA, Parker SW et al 1997 Rehabilitation of balance in two patients with cerebellar dysfunction. Phys Ther 77:534–552.

Gilman S, Bloedel J, Lechtenberg R 1981 Disorders of the cerebellum, Davis, Philadelphia.

Giovannoni G, van Schalkwyk J, Fritz V et al 1999 Bradykinesia akinesia incoordination test (BRAIN test): an objective computerised assessment of upper limb motor function. J

Neurol Neurosurg Psychiatry 67:624–629.

Glickstein M 1992 The cerebellum and motor learning. Curr Opin Neurobiol 2:802–806.

Glickstein M 1997 Mossy-fibre sensory input to the cerebellum. Prog Brain Res 114:251–259.

Glickstein M, Doron K 2008 Cerebellum: connections and functions. Cerebellum 7:589–594.

Gordon J 1990 Disorders of motor control. In: Ada L, Canning C (eds) Key issues in neurological physiotherapy. Butterworth Heinemann, Oxford.25–50.

Guberman A 1994 Ataxia and cerebellar disorders. An introduction to clinical neurology – pathology, diagnosis and treatment, 1st edn. Little, Brown, New York:291.

Hallett M, Shahani BT, Young RR 1975 EMG analysis of patients with cerebellar deficits. J Neurol Neurosurg Psychiatry 38:1163–1169.

Hallett M, Berardelli A, Matheson J et al 1991 Physiological analysis of simple rapid movements in patients with cerebellar deficits. J Neurol Neurosurg Psychiatry 53:124–133.

Halsband U, Freund H-J 1993 Motor learning. Curr Opin Neurobiol 3:940–949.

Holmes G 1917 The symptoms of acute cerebellar injuries due to gunshot injuries. Brain 40:461–535.

Holmes G 1922a Clinical symptoms of cerebellar disease and their interpretation. The Croonian lectures 3. Lancet ii:59–65:111–115.

Holmes G 1922b Clinical symptoms of cerebellar disease and their interpretation. The Croonian lectures 1, 2. Lancet i:1177–1182, 1231–1237.

Holmes G 1939 The cerebellum of man. Brain 62:1–30.

Hood JD, Waniewski E 1984 Influence of peripheral vision upon vestibulo-ocular reflex suppression. J Neurol Sci 63:27–44.

Hore J, Flament D 1988 Changes in motor cortex neural discharge associated with the development of cerebellar limb ataxia. J Neurophysiol 60:1285–1302.

Hore J, Wild B, Diener HC 1991 Cerebellar dysmetria at the elbow, wrist and fingers. J Neurophysiol 65:563–571.

Ioffe ME, Ustinova KI, Chernikova LA et al 2006 Supervised learning of postural tasks in patients with poststroke hemiparesis, Parkinson's disease or cerebellar ataxia. Exp Brain Res 168:384–394.

Kandel ER, Schwartz JH, Jessell TM 1991 Principles of Neural Science. Appleton & Lange, Stamford, CT.

Krusen FH, Kottke FJ, Elwood PM 1971 Handbook of physical medicine and rehabilitation, 2nd edn. WB Saunders, Philadelphia.

Lacourse MG, Turner JA, Randolph-Orr E et al 2004 Cerebral and cerebellar sensorimotor plasticity following motor imagery-based mental practice of a sequential movement. J Rehabil Res Dev 41:505–524.

Leiner HC, Leiner AL, Dow RS 1989 Reappraising the cerebellum: what does the hindbrain contribute to the forebrain? Behav Neurosci 103:998–1008.

Leiner HC, Leiner AL, Dow RS 1991 The human cerebrocerebellar system: its computing, cognitive and language skills. Behav Brain Res 44:113–128.

Leiner HC, Leiner AL, Dow RS 1993 Cognitive and language functions of the human cerebellum. Trends Neurosci 16:444–447.

Mai N, Diener HC, Dichgans J 1989 On the role of feedback in maintaining constant grip force in patients with cerebellar disease. Neurosc Lett 99:340–344.

Manto M 2009 Mechanisms of human cerebellar dysmetria: experimental evidence and current conceptual bases. J Neuroeng Rehabil 6:10.

Marr D 1969 A theory of the cerebellar cortex. J Physiol 202:437–470.

Marsden CD, Morton PA, Morton HB et al 1977 Disorders of movement in cerebellar disease in man. In: Rose FC (ed.) Physiological aspects of clinical neurology. Blackwell, Oxford:197–199.

Martin CL, Tan D, Bragge P et al 2009 Effectiveness of physiotherapy for adults with cerebellar dysfunction: a systematic review. Clin Rehabil 23:15–26.

Mauritz KH, Schmitt C, Dichgans J 1981 Delayed and enhanced long-latency reflexes as the possible cause of postural tremor in late cerebellar atrophy. Brain 104:97–116.

Meyer-Lohmann J, Hore J, Brooks VB 1977 Cerebellar participation in generation of prompt arm movements. J Neurophysiol 40:1038–1050.

Middleton FA, Strick PL 2001 Cerebellar projections to the prefrontal cortex of the primate. J Neurosci 21:700–712.

Molinari M, Leggio MG, Solida A et al 1997 Cerebellum and procedural learning: evidence from focal cerebellar lesions. Brain 120:1753–1762.

Molinari M, Filippini V, Leggio MG 2002 Neuronal plasticity of interrelated cerebellar and cortical networks. Neuroscience 111:863–870.

Morton SM, Bastian AJ 2007 Mechanisms of cerebellar gait ataxia. Cerebellum 6:79–86.

Nashner LM, Cordo PJ 1981 Relation of automatic postural responses and reaction-time voluntary movements of human leg muscles. Exp Brain Res 43:395–405.

Nashner LM, Grimm RG 1978 Analysis of multiloop dyscontrols in standing cerebellar patients. Prog Clin Neurophysiol 5:300–319.

Nicolson RI, Fawcett AJ, Berry EL et al 1999 Association of abnormal cerebellar activation with motor learning difficulties in dyslexic adults. Lancet 353:1662–1667.

Nixon PD, Passingham RE 2001 Predicting sensory events. The role of the cerebellum in motor learning. Exp Brain Res 138:251–257.

Notermans NC, van Dijk GW, van der Graaf Y et al 1994 Measuring ataxia: quantification based on the standard neurological examination. J Neurol Neurosurg Psychiatry 57:22–26.

Palliyath S, Hallett M, Thomas SL et al 1998 Gait in patients with cerebellar ataxia. Mov Disord 13:958–964.

Paulin MG 1992 The role of the cerebellum in motor control and perception. Brain Behav Evol 41:39–50.

Paulin MG 1993 A model of the role of the cerebellum in tracking and controlling movements. Hum Mov Sci 12:5–16.

Petrosini L, Graziano A, Mandolesi L 2003 Watch how to do it! New advances in learning by observation. Brain Res Rev 42:252–264.

Sanes JN, LeWitt PA, Mauritz KH 1988 Visual and mechanical control of postural and kinetic tremor in cerebellar system disorders. J Neurol Neurosurg Psychiatry 51:934–943.

Saywell N, Taylor D 2008 The role of the cerebellum in procedural learning – are there implications for physiotherapists' clinical practice? Physiother Theory Pract 24:321–328.

Schmahmann JD 1991 An emerging concept: the cerebellar contribution to high function. Arch Neurol 48:1178–1187.

Spidalieri G, Busby L, Lamarre Y 1983 Fast ballistic arm movements triggered by visual, auditory and somaesthetic stimuli in the monkey. II. Effects of unilateral dentate lesion on discharge of precentral cortical neurons and reaction time. J Neurophysiol 50:1359–1379.

Stolze H, Klebe S, Petersen G et al 2002 Typical features of cerebellar ataxic gait. J Neurol Neurosurg Psychiatry 73:310–312.

Sullivan EV, Rose J, Pfefferbaum A 2006 Effect of vision, touch and stance on cerebellar vermian-related sway and tremor: a quantitative physiological and MRI study. Cereb Cortex 16:1077–1086.

Swaine BR, Sullivan SJ 1993 Reliability of the scores for the finger-to-nose test in adults with traumatic brain injury. Phys Ther 73:71–79.

Terzuolo CA, Viviani P 1973 Parameters of motion and EMG activities during some simple motor tasks in normal subjects and cerebellar patients. In: Cooper JS, Riklan M, Snider RS (eds) The cerebellum, epilepsy and behavior. Plenum Press, New York:173–215.

Thach WT 1980 The cerebellum. In: Mountcastle VB (ed.) Medical physiology. CV Mosby, St Louis:837–858.

Thach WT, Goodkin HG, Keating JG 1992 The cerebellum and the adaptive coordination of movement. Ann Rev Neurosci 15:403–442.

Thach WT, Montgomery EB 1990 Motor system. In: Pearlman AL, Collins RC (eds) Neurological pathophysiology, 3rd ed. Oxford University Press, New York:168–196.

Timmann D, Daum I 2007 Cerebellar contributions to cognitive functions: a progress report after two decades of research. Cerebellum 6:159–162.

Trouillas P, Takayanagi T, Hallett M et al 1997 International Cooperative Ataxia Rating Scale for pharmacological assessment of the cerebellar syndrome. The Ataxia Neuropharmacology Committee of the World Federation of Neurology. J Neurol Sci 145:205–211.

van der Meche FGA, van Gijn J 1986 Hypotonia: an erroneous clinical concept? Brain 109:1169–1178.

Verkerk PH, Schouten JP, Oosterhuis HJGH 1990 Measurement of the hand. Clin Neurol Neurosurg 92:105–109.

Vilis T, Hore J 1980 Central neural mechanisms contributing to cerebellar tremor produced by limb perturbations. J Neurophysiol 43:279–291.

Winter DA 1987 Biomechanics and motor control of human gait. University of Waterloo Press, Waterloo.

Chapter | 10 |

Somatosensory and perceptual–cognitive impairments

INTRODUCTION

Knowledge of the world comes through our senses (Kandel 2000). Information from the environment and from our own body is processed, stored and accessed in the central nervous system by a complex interaction of neuronal networks. This cortical integration to a sensory stimulus is influenced by the recent history of sensory experience (Merzenich et al 1988) and this may underlie the plasticity associated with the learning of tasks. Cortical integration of sensory information is also known to change dramatically with the individual's state of alertness.

Somatosensory, cognitive and perceptual impairments are found in many individuals with brain lesion (Wade et al 1985). These impairments contribute to poor motor control and have an impact on the individual's ability to participate in rehabilitation. Partial or complete loss of discrete sensations (tactile, proprioceptive) and disorders of cognition and perception (neglect, inattention) may be evident on testing and reflected in the individual's behaviour. Sensory impairment occurs most commonly following stroke and traumatic brain injury but is also associated with other brain lesions.

Sensory loss tends to involve discriminative and proprioceptive modalities more than others. Pain and temperature may be altered but are usually not lost. Cognitive and perceptual impairments commonly affect attention, memory, orientation, language and executive functions (National Stroke Foundation 2007). A critical domain of cognition is so-called executive function that controls, integrates, organizes and maintains other cognitive functions.

In a small number of patients a purely sensory stroke may be the only impairment and has a favourable prognosis (Fisher 1982). Lesions of the brainstem may result in hemianaesthesia and/or hemianalgesia on the contralateral or ipsilateral side, depending on the lesion site. Subthalamic lesions may result in spontaneous pain down the opposite side of the body and can result in considerable discomfort from touch stimuli to the skin and usually causes some degree of depression.

SOMATOSENSORY IMPAIRMENT

Loss of tactile and proprioceptive sensation following brain lesion is relatively common. Discrimination and

©2010 Elsevier Ltd
DOI: 10.1016/B978-0-7020-4051-1.00019-9

interpretation of information regarding movement, including perception of muscle force, texture and stereognosis, may be a major cause of functional disability, particularly in hand use. Although an individual may recover the ability to activate muscles and control the affected/paretic limb, and be able to demonstrate effective motor performance in the limited environment of the clinic, in the more natural environment of home the limb may not be used. Poor feedback from the glass in one's hand, the fork slipping out of the hand while eating, not knowing whether or not a leg will collapse when stepping off the kerb all contribute to lack of confidence.

It is very likely that tactile and proprioceptive sensation is critical for the regaining of effective motor function, particularly in hand and arm use, and for the learning of new skills (Kusoffsky et al 1982; Carr & Shepherd 1987, 1998). Monkeys with a deafferented limb have been shown to be capable of improving the use of the limb if they had training and if motivation was increased (Merzenich et al 1983). When both limbs were deafferentated, however, the monkeys were able to use the limbs in activities such as feeding early after the lesions (Knapp et al 1963). A recent brain imaging study showed that abolishing sensation by a pharmological blockade of the radial and median nerve in healthy human subjects caused an 'invasion' of the deafferented region of the brain by intact areas of the brain adjacent to it (Weiss et al 2004). It has been noted that when a limb is rarely used, is used only for the simplest of tasks, or where limb use is not trained, there is no stimulus for recovery to take place. Sensory impairments have tended to be neglected (Carey 1995) – we do not understand the problems, or what to do about them, or whether or not improvement on testing has generalized into, and can be taken to reflect, improved motor function.

Sensation usually functions in both regulatory and adaptive modes (Gordon 1987), guiding movements during their execution and correcting movements in order to improve the next attempt. The significance of the relationship between sensory and motor function is therefore a continuing subject of interest. More recently, however, experimentation has been directed increasingly to the relationship between motor and sensory function during the performance of real-life tasks. As a consequence, there is now an emerging body of knowledge of relevance to physiotherapists in developing strategies for testing and training sensory discrimination and motor performance in the clinic.

Patients with well-preserved sensation are generally believed by clinicians to achieve greater improvements in rehabilitation than those without. In the 1950s, this led to the design of several physiotherapy methods based on the belief that sensory inputs were likely to initiate muscle activity and improve motor control: for example, generalized sensory stimulation including ice and vibration (de Jersey 1979), fast brushing to specific dermatomes

(Stockmeyer 1967), rapid stretch to enhance muscle activity (Knott & Voss 1968) and the 'sensation' of more normal movements induced by the therapist's handling of the patient (Bobath 1990). It was hoped that improving sensory function would carry over to, and have a positive effect on, movement and function. However, the nervous system is selective in its use of sensory inputs, and non-specific sensory stimulation techniques have not been shown to be effective in improving either the perception of sensation or motor control. Research from neuroscience and cognitive science provides evidence that relatively arbitrary or non-specific stimulation of a passive recipient is unlikely to affect the awareness of specific sensation in people with discriminitive sensory dysfunction or motor performance.

A more modern understanding of the relationship between sensory information and motor output, the capacity of the brain to adapt and to selectively 'attend' to those inputs that contain the most relevant information to the task at hand (i.e., a more cognitively directed approach to motor training) has developed over the last few decades. In rehabilitation, challenging and meaningful problems posed to the hand as a sense organ (Yekutiel & Guttman 1993), for example, may be solved more by the patient attending to sensory inputs and their relationship to the task being attempted than by external and artificial stimulation.

Joint position and movement sense

Proprioception is made up of a range of sensations, including recognition of movement and heaviness and an awareness of its direction, position in space, sense of force and timing of muscular contraction (Gandevia 1996). Proprioceptive inputs are particularly critical to motor control in tasks involving multisegmental movement, such as manipulative actions, walking, standing up and sitting down, and balancing the body mass; that is, movements that require a fine degree of control (Jeannerod et al 1984). Preserving an upright posture requires a delicate interplay among sensory, motor and cognitive systems. Loss of proprioception, poor motor function and a low degree of independence in self-care have been reported. Sensory loss can be very specific. For example, a person with proprioceptive loss may recognize limb movement but not recognize the position of the limb or the direction of the movement.

A recent study of individuals post-stroke who could walk independently used a rigorous movement detection test at the ankle and reported a significant relationship between proprioceptive acuity and walking distance on the 6-minute walk test (Lee et al 2005). The authors suggested that reduced proprioception at the paretic ankle may contribute to a person's ability to position and load the foot during walking and that this would interfere with speed and attempts to move faster.

Tactile impairments

Sensory functions that involve localization and discrimination of stimuli such as stereognosis, two-point discrimination and the ability to recognize bilateral simultaneous stimuli are essential to effective use of the upper limbs in particular. Cutaneous afferent inputs are critical for the control of hand movements. Difficulty sustaining constant levels of muscle contraction without feedback results in slowness and clumsiness in many manual tasks (e.g., doing up buttons, writing). Grip force varies according to the friction properties of the object being handled – the more slippery the object the more force is normally generated by the finger flexor muscles (Johansson & Westling 1984). Several reports suggest that sensory impairments are linked to poor spontaneous use of a limb, particularly of the hand (Jeannerod et al 1984; Dannenbaum & Dykes 1988).

Stereognosis is the tactile identification of common objects and its absence is called astereognosis. It involves the recognition of physical properties including texture as well as the nature of the object. Normally touch and vision both provide this information. Stereognosis requires a normal threshold for touch in the palm of the hand. It is not an innate ability but grows and develops through appropriate experience and can develop to great heights of sensitivity in musicians and the visually impaired or can be almost absent in the hand of the person with congenital hemiplegia. The recognition of common objects is normally almost spontaneous in the adult.

Two-point discrimination is the ability to recognize two points when simultaneously applied with vision occluded. When the two points are at a particular distance from each other, and this depends on the part of the body touched, the two points are felt as one. The most sensitive areas are the lips, tongue, fingers and thumb.

Pain

Pain following stroke may originate centrally, when it is referred to as central post-stroke pain (CPSP). CPSP occurs in 2–8% of stroke patients (Andersen et al 1995). The pathophysiology of CPSP is unknown. Pain is often described as a burning or lacerating sensation with unpleasant tingling, pins and needles or numbness, and is often made worse by movement, touch and water. Several forms of pain relief have been suggested but evidence for efficacy is limited (National Stroke Foundation 2005).

Assessment

Evaluation of sensation includes tests of light touch, pin-prick, heat and cold, sense of passive movement and position, and stereognosis. Methods of testing are, however, largely subjective, with reliability and validity unconfirmed (Lincoln et al 1991). Winward and colleagues (1999) summarize the major problems that have contributed to subjective and unreliable sensory testing: lack of standardization of testing equipment and examiner protocols, heterogeneous nature of the lesion, absence of age-matched controls, and failure to consider or control for cognitive deficits. Quantifiable and reliable tests are required to identify signs of sensory loss in order to evaluate clinical effectiveness of intervention and its relationship to improving function.

A few years ago Lincoln and colleagues (1998) addressed some of the shortcomings of common sensory tests (see Ch. 3) This goes some way to increasingly standardize procedures. Carey and colleagues (1993) discuss in detail the assessment of somatosensory functions, stressing the importance of the use of quantified tests if they are to act as accurate guides to therapeutic intervention and provide meaningful information about outcome. More functionally-oriented and standardized tests have been designed and reported. Validity is a particular issue as the commonly used sensory tests were developed for testing peripheral nerve lesions, whereas in cerebral lesions emphasis needs to be on how the stimulus is perceived and interpreted and not only on conduction of specific peripheral nerves (Carey 1995).

Somatosensory-evoked potentials (SEP) are used to study the afferent projections from the limbs to the cerebral cortex (Kusoffsky et al 1982; Burke and Gandevia 1988; Watanabe et al 1989). SEP may also contribute toward providing a prognosis for motor recovery, especially in the upper limb (Kusoffsky et al 1982; Jacobs et al 1988; Zeman & Yiannikas 1989).

A thorough investigation of sensory loss after a brain lesion, its natural history, recovery, prognostic importance and treatment have been hampered by the use of unreliable and poorly standardized tests, in particular how sensory impairments relate to performance of functional activities and participation (Winward et al 1999).

Training

Task-oriented training is directed toward enabling the individual to perform critical everyday actions more effectively and efficiently in the relevant environment and involves practice of the actions themselves with the action and/or environment being modified if necessary to enable practice to take place. Motor impairments, muscle weakness and poor coordination are addressed by task-specific training and strengthening exercises with similar action patterns. Training is based on the knowledge that muscle activation, strength, coordination and proprioceptive and tactile feedback are specific to the task and the environment in which it is being performed.

A similar assumption is made about sensory functions since the system is selective in the inputs utilized for specific functional actions. Practice of meaningful tasks gives the neural system the opportunity to select and use those sensory inputs that are relevant to the action being performed. For example, practice of standing up and sitting down provides the opportunity to be aware of inputs from tactile and pressure receptors in the soles of the feet and kinaesthetic input from muscle and joint receptors, and may help the person to position and load the paretic foot (Dietz et al 1992).

Training task-specific hand functions involving a variety of common objects enables sensory training to be incorporated into motor training. It is probably critical to encourage, early after an acute lesion, simple exercises and activities using one or both hands as a means of 'driving' the reorganization of the brain and to prevent the phenomenon of 'learned non-use'. Examples of exercises and activities are given in Chapter 6. Training of bimanual activities such as unscrewing the lid from a jar and picking up a glass of water (Carr & Shepherd 2003) provide the opportunity for the individual to regain the ability to attend both to the motor act itself and the information being received from tactile receptors. When there is reduced sensory awareness, training includes cueing the individual into the sensory information required for the task. The hypothesis that sensory training may be more effective if incorporated into task training has not been tested in neurological rehabilitation. However, it is possible that practising real-life tasks may itself improve sensation if attention is directed to the goal of the task and how an object feels (i.e., its qualities), not to details of movement.

Where a person has a specific sensory impairment, such as astereognosis, specific training can be provided to assist the person to regain sensitivity. Such training does not need to be modality specific which may result in poor generalizability (Wynn-Parry & Salter 1975), but rather require the solving of meaningful sensory-identification problems. Several studies illustrate the potential for effective sensory retraining directed toward the cognitive manipulation of sensory information. A controlled trial of training sensory function demonstrated that somatosensory impairments could be improved even years after stroke (Yekutiel & Guttman 1993). The nature and extent of sensory loss were explored with the individual people. Emphasis was on sensory tasks the person could do and each session started and ended with these. Use was made of vision and the non-paretic hand to teach tactics of perception, and frequent rests and change of task were used to maximize concentration. Tasks included identification of number of touches or lines; identification of numbers and letters drawn on the arm and hand; 'find your thumb' when blindfolded; discrimination of shape, weight and texture of objects or materials placed in the hand; and passive drawing. Subjects were tested on location of touch, sense of elbow position, two-point discrimination and stereognosis. Only people in the treatment group made large gains on the sensory tests. However,

those with left hemiplegia improved less than those with right hemiplegia, suggesting that these patients needed additional training directed at other problems such as neglect or agnosia.

Carey and colleagues (1993) investigated the effects of a programme of task-specific training with two groups of four subjects 5–26 weeks following stroke, using an A (no intervention) B (training) quasi-experimental design. Training included attentive exploration and quantitative feedback. The results showed that marked improvement took place in the tactile and proprioceptive discrimination tasks tested, and that this improvement was maintained in most subjects for several weeks. Whether or not improved performance on sensory tests generalizes to improved motor performance and more use of the affected limb use needs to be investigated. Carey and others have more recently described generalized training effects (transfer of learning) within a sensory dimension post-stroke. These training programmes included attention to sensory stimuli, challenging and motivating tasks, graded exercises and feedback on accuracy and execution (for review see Carey 2006).

Despite evidence that sensory training may assist in improving hand function and despite reports of at least 60% of persons presenting with sensory dysfunction, retraining sensory function post-stroke is often overlooked (Schabrun & Hillier 2009).

VISUAL IMPAIRMENTS

Vision is our major source of information about the environment and our place in it. Hence, it has been called 'exproprioceptive' (Gibson 1966). Eye–head coordination is particularly critical for manipulating and negotiating the environment. We need the ability to locate and maintain a stable gaze on a fixed target, and to move our eyes while keeping the head still in order to locate objects in the peripheral field. In reaching out to pick up an object, there is a complex interaction between head, eye and hand movements. Movement is guided by visual information about location of the object and arm, and about the relationship between wrist, finger and hand movements just prior to and during the action of grasping (Jeannerod 1988).

Following stroke or traumatic brain injury, individuals may demonstrate visual impairments that have a negative impact upon their ability to engage actively in the rehabilitation process as well as throughout their daily lives. Visual impairments may result from oculomotor dysfunction (double vision, impaired saccadic movement), dry eyes and pre-existing retinal dysfunction (cataract or macular degeneration), or the cognitive and perceptual manipulations of those inputs (e.g., visual field loss and visuospatial agnosia).

The therapist needs to be informed about the state of the person's visual system, given its critical role in movement control. Individuals should have pre-existing visual impairments corrected by eye-glasses. An understanding of visual impairment enables the therapist to give consideration to environmental features such as glare and lighting during motor training.

Visual field loss

Not uncommon after stroke is loss of visual information from half the visual field. The term homonymous hemianopia is used when there is loss of half the visual field on the same side of each eye, cutting objects vertically and making it difficult or impossible to see objects within this part of the visual field (Fig. 10.1). Visual impairments can cause significant functional difficulties. The person may bump into objects on that side, miss utensils on the dinner tray or have difficulty reading. The person may not appreciate this loss of vision and may not compensate by moving the head unless advised to do so. Distinguishing a field loss from unilateral neglect can be difficult and requires specific testing. Compensation training is usually necessary. This includes the use of margin markers to aid reading and using eye and head movement to bring objects into view. The area of the blind field may decrease by learning to pay attention in detection tasks.

PERCEPTUAL–COGNITIVE IMPAIRMENTS

Stroke can affect cognitive as well as physical and sensory abilities (Wade et al 1985). Perceptual and cognitive impairments reflect the interactive links between perceptual and cognitive processes and commonly involve attention, memory, orientation, language and executive functions. Perceptual–cognitive disabilities include neglect, apraxia and agnosia. While cognition can be considered as the ability to process, sort, retrieve and interpret information, perception reflects the ability to process and interpret sensory information. Both are critical to successful functioning and interactions with the environment. Perceptual–cognitive impairments and dementia are common after stroke and there is usually some overlap, making problems difficult to diagnose (National Stroke Foundation 2005). These impairments have important implications for participation in rehabilitation and in the community and can compromise safety, particularly by provoking a fall.

Cognitive and perceptual impairments may include disorders of right–left discrimination, inattention, disorders of body image and unawareness of one (usually the left) side of space. The impairments are not clearly circumscribed but fuse into one another, and are taken to reflect

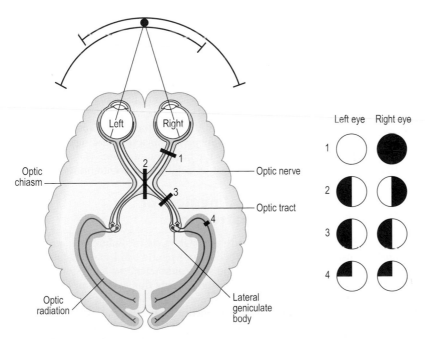

Figure 10.1 Visual field deficits produced by lesions at various points in the visual pathway. 1: Lesion of R optic nerve causes loss of vision in R eye. 2: Lesion of optic chiasm causes loss of vision in the temporal halves of both visual fields (bitemporal hemianopia). 3: Lesion of optic tract causes complete loss of vision in opposite half of visual field (contralateral hemianopia). 4: Lesion of optic radiation fibres causes loss of vision in upper quadrant of opposite half of visual field of both eyes. Partial lesions of visual cortex lead to partial field deficits on opposite side.

not only a failure of sensory awareness but more importantly of cognitive awareness of the problem (Critchley 1953). The impairments and the associated puzzling behavioural manifestations illustrate the close links between sensorimotor processes, and perceptual–cognitive processes. Their integration is critical for our existence in the environment. Perceptual–cognitive impairments are complex, not well understood and sometimes demonstrated by bizarre behaviours and responses and by striking manifestations of denial.

It is understood that lesions of the parietal lobes lead to abnormalities of body image and perception of spatial relations. Although it has been usual to consider that these deficits occur only after a lesion of the right (usually non-dominant) lobe, lesions of the left brain can also be followed by similar but less severe impairments.

Lesions of the left parietal lobe may be associated with *aphasia*, a disorder of language, and *agnosia*, an inability to perceive or know objects in the presence of normally functioning sensory pathways. For example, there may be an inability to recognize the form of an object by touch and therefore to recognize the object itself, or astereognosis may be present. Lesions of the right parietal lobe are typically associated with a lack of appreciation of the spatial aspects of sensory input from the left side of the body and the left extrapersonal space. Affected individuals are said to suffer neglect of the left side of space or visuospatial agnosia.

Apraxia

Apraxia is difficulty performing everyday activities not accounted for by weakness, sensory loss, incoordination, inattention or lack of comprehension. Apraxia may involve any movement. It is seen to affect even lip and tongue movement. For example, a person may be unable to lick the lips when asked to do so but will be observed to do so spontaneously when eating.

Apraxia is difficult to diagnose. Available assessments seem to test different aspects. It is sometimes described in functional terms such as dressing apraxia and walking apraxia but presently clinicians and researchers support the classical view of two forms: ideational and ideomotor (Leipmann 1920).

Ideational apraxia is characterized by absentmindedness and lack of purpose in performing various actions. For example, the person may pick up a matchbox, take out a match and strike it, but when asked to light a candle will instead do something inappropriate such as striking the candle on the matchbox.

Ideomotor apraxia hinders the individual's ability to select, sequence and use objects. The person may understand the purpose of the object but be unable to use it. For example, attempting to dress may result in putting the arm through the trouser leg. Attempting to walk after a stroke, the person seems to have no idea about the

movements required and may act impulsively, attempting to lift one foot without shifting weight onto the other, and can have difficulty following instructions or responding to feedback. Their behaviour may be thought to reflect intellectual deterioration rather than a lack of awareness of the appropriate movement at that time.

Several interventions have been tried including cueing, verbal or physical prompts at each stage of a task. A recent systematic review suggests that more quality research is needed in order to identify optimal intervention for apraxia (West et al 2009). It is also suggested that future researchers consider evaluating their treatment in terms of the patient's experience and outcome. Studies reviewed did not report quality of life issues or effects on family or carers.

Visual perceptual impairments

These may include distortion of the perception of verticality. Some stroke patients have impaired subjective visual vertical perception compared with able-bodied subjects (Snowdon & Scott 2005). A relationship between distorted perception of verticality and falling has been reported in elderly individuals, including those who have had a stroke. This can have a significant effect on preserving balance (Bonan et al 2006).

Other problems include difficulty appreciating the three-dimensional nature of objects, difficulty finding the way from place to place, discriminating numerical symbols, telling the time, visualizing a mental picture of familiar people and things and understanding the meaning of up–down, in–out, front–back. Some individuals have difficulty with figure–ground perception and are unable to distinguish an object from its background. Impairment in figure–ground perception has a particular effect on hand function and upon visual discrimination in general. A similar problem of discrimination may occur in auditory perception with the person unable to distinguish particular sounds from the background noise. The person may appear to be deaf or lacking in concentration.

Unilateral neglect or hemi-inattention

Unilateral neglect (ULN) is a failure to attend or respond to, identify or orient toward meaningful stimuli presented to the side contralateral to the lesioned hemisphere, typically the left side due to a lesion of the right parietal lobe. However, it is evident that some degree of visuospatial malfunction may also exist with left hemisphere lesions (Wilson et al 1987). Unilateral neglect is a perceptual–cognitive disability affecting the ability to carry out many everyday tasks and restricts a person's independence. There appears to be decreased ability to integrate visual and tactile sensory information leading to difficulty orientating the body in space. Although these impairments are most typically seen associated with stroke, they may also be present following traumatic brain injury or associated with a cerebral tumour.

Reported incidence of neglect varies considerably from as low as 29% to 85% of patients (Wilson et al 1987). However, the incidence reported probably depends on the methods of assessment, the tasks tested and on the definition of neglect. There have been few systematic investigations and there is no clear consensus on evaluating neglect. It is possible that neglect persists in some individuals despite lack of obvious behavioural indications.

Cognitive disorders such as ULN have serious effects on the outcome of rehabilitation, discharge destination, length of stay and independence (Barer 1990; National Stroke Foundation 2005). Impairments can involve perception, attention, memory and executive function (Calvanio et al 1993).

ULN is multidimensional and patients can display a combination of behaviours (Pierce & Buxbaum 2002). Heilman and colleagues (1993) described ULN according to the distribution (personal or spatial) or the modality (sensory or motor). *Personal neglect* is a failure to acknowledge stimuli on the contralateral side of the body; *spatial neglect* refers to failure to acknowledge stimuli in the contralateral side of space; *sensory neglect* is a deficit in awareness of contralateral stimuli (visual, auditory, somatosensory); and *motor neglect* is a failure to respond to a stimulus when the person is aware of it; that is, not due to weakness or spasticity.

The individual with neglect may fail to dress or wash the left side of the body or shave on the left (*autotopagnosia*) or may brush the teeth on one side only. The left side of space appears not to be 'seen' and a person may eat food only on one side of the plate (Fig. 10.2), start reading a sentence from the middle of the page, or fail to attend to objects and people on the left side. Difficulties with writing, reading and drawing also come under this general heading, together with impairments of line orientation and verticality perception. Walking through a doorway, the individual may veer to one side or bump into the door frame. The person may deny ownership of the left arm or leg, or deny the existence of hemiplegia (*anosognosia*). Riddoch & Humphreys (1994) point out the heterogeneity of the anatomical regions implicated in neglect in individuals following lesions to several different areas of the brain.

Lack of awareness of impairment or denial of impairment (agnosia – loss of knowledge) is sometimes seen following a brain lesion. Reasons for denial may range from a desire to avoid unpleasant problems or maintain positive self-regard, to a lack of awareness associated with unilateral neglect. The individual may appear indifferent or perplexed on confrontation or accept the problem on a broad level but fail to come to grips with the specific ways in which the problems are played out (Diller & Weinberg 1993). These authors suggest that the task for remediation is basically to facilitate the patient's discovery of their own impairment when they cannot achieve this on their own. Understanding the nature of the person's denial can help the therapist work out solutions with the patient.

The clinical signs of ULN are described both in the literature and in the clinic by different terms such as hemispatial neglect, hemispatial agnosia and hemi-inattention. The terminology may be unnecessarily misleading, the term 'neglect' suggesting some degree of carelessness or irresponsibility. The term 'inattention' infers that the person's behaviour is under volitional control. Perhaps the Greek word 'agnosia', a lack of knowledge or awareness, best reflects the person's dilemma as it describes a *selective* perceptual–cognitive disorder. The variability in terminology reflects the multicomponent nature of agnosia and it is likely that lack of knowledge about the underlying mechanisms is a contributing factor. It seems accepted that these phenomena cannot be explained in terms of a single underlying mechanism (Riddoch & Humphreys 1994).

Attention to the right side to the exclusion of the left seems very compelling to the affected individual. Stimuli in the right visual field seem to provide a strong magnet, making it difficult to disengage attention once it has been captured. For patients to be able to shift visual attention, they need to be able to disengage their attention from one target, shift it to another then focus on this new target (Herman 1992).

Recovery and trainability of everyday actions are likely to be affected in the presence of the barriers to functional effectiveness. Figure 10.3A shows that all patients started out at 1 week post-stroke at a similar level but varied widely by 7 weeks. The lower part shows the major source of this variability. The seven individuals had large right hemisphere lesions but the results show that the degree of recovery is inversely related to the amount of pre-stroke cortical atrophy (Calvanio et al 1993).

Typical strategies to draw attention to the affected side have included adapting the environment so that visual, auditory and tactile stimuli were presented to the neglected side. These strategies do not, however, address the range of different presentations of ULN following stroke and

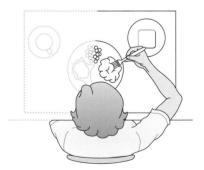

Figure 10.2 An individual with hemi-inattention may only eat food on one side of the plate.

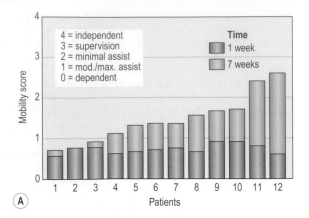

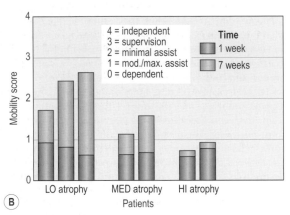

Figure 10.3 (A) Variation in recovery of mobility in 12 patients with R hemisphere stroke. All were severely impaired 1 week after admission to rehabilitation; at 7 weeks, they showed varied degrees of recovery. Mobility measures were performance on getting in and out of wheelchair, wheelchair driving, ambulation and stair climbing. (B) Variation in mobility of 7 of the above patients as a function of low, medium and high cortical atrophy by CT scan. *(From Calvanio et al (1993)).*

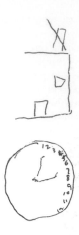

Figure 10.4 The type of drawing made by individuals with R hemisphere parietal lobe lesion.

have not provided scientific evidence of efficacy. They are of limited value, being dependent on the therapist to remind the individual. The difficulty remains that ULN patients tend not to direct their attention to the affected side unless specifically asked to do so (Riddoch & Humphreys 1987).

Assessment

Appropriate assessment of perceptual–cognitive impairment by trained staff (neuropsychologist or occupational therapist) is necessary to identify the type of impairment and guide the team in providing appropriate rehabilitation interventions and clues to assist in determining an individual's capacity to participate in rehabilitation. Careful observation by the physiotherapist of the person's

behaviour may provide useful clues to explain poor performance in motor training and identify points to be addressed.

There is no single test that can identify the syndrome in all patients nor will neglect behaviours manifest themselves in all tasks (Halligan et al 1991; Kinsella et al 1995). Neuropsychological assessment of visuospatial neglect may include various simple perceptual motor tasks involving, for example, line crossing (Albert 1973), cancellation tasks (Diller & Weinberg 1977), and drawing and copying tasks (Fig. 10.4). Other tests include drawing from memory, copying complex figures and performing visual matching tasks. Wilson and colleagues (1987) argue that such tests are not relevant to the problems encountered in everyday life. Just as tests of motor performance in everyday actions, reaching, walking and standing up give an indication of what to train so, Wilson and colleagues argue, behavioural tests of a selection of everyday skills provide the grounding for specific rehabilitation strategies, despite the absence of clearly defined underlying mechanisms.

The *behavioural inattention test* (see Ch. 3) was developed to provide such information (Wilson et al 1987; Stone et al 1991). It consists of items such as using a telephone, picture scanning, reading a menu, copying an address and sentence, and map navigation. It has been shown to be a valid and reliable test. An advantage of testing these tasks is that they suggest tasks that should be retrained.

A simple subjective *verticality test* involves holding an object such as a ruler in front of the person at different orientations, including the vertical, and asking the person to say which orientation is vertical. Alternatively, the individual is asked to match a ruler to the orientation of the examiner's ruler (Efferson 1995).

The *auditory perception test* involves, for example, snapping the fingers by the person's ear. This simple test enables the physiotherapist to gain some indication of hearing capacity.

Individuals who disregard one stimulus over another if applied bilaterally and simultaneously demonstrate *tactile inattention or extinction*. The person is unaware of stimulation on the affected side when this stimulus has to compete with a stimulus to the sound side. The ability to recognize both stimuli requires normal tactile localization which should be tested first.

Although there is some evidence of improvement in, for example, line crossing tests, there is no evidence of generalizability. A number of these studies appear potentially successful although generalization of training to untrained situations is rarely examined, nor is the retention of immediate benefit (Bowen & Lincoln 2007). Sample numbers are frequently small or only single case studies are studied and there are few controlled studies. The summary provided in a recent systematic review suggests that rehabilitation targeted at neglect appeared to improve an individual's ability to complete tests that included finding visual targets or marking the mid-point of a line. However, carryover into improved performance in a meaningful task, or ability to live independently, was not clear (Bowen & Lincoln 2007).

Training

Physiotherapy for individuals with ULN needs to address the attentional deficit in addition to contributing factors including coexisting sensorimotor impairments. It is likely that specific training to improve a person's performance on functionally relevant and concrete tasks, with emphasis on the individual paying attention to, concentrating on and orienting toward the relevant objects and their position in space, are critical along with strategies tailored to the contributing factors of neglect. Identification of the contributing factors enables treatment to be tailored to the individual's specific deficit.

Motion is powerful in capturing attention and directing it and our vision to a specific location in space (Dunai et al 1999). A moving stimulus may capture attention automatically. It is suggested that the general alerting characteristics of moving stimuli may activate the brainstem component of the attentional system, thereby reducing neglect (Butter et al 1990). Several clinical studies have provided evidence that moving visual cues are more compelling for reducing ULN than stationary cues (Mattingley et al 1994).

Given the importance of the visual system in our interactions with the external world, emphasis on attending to visual stimuli is a critical part of motor training. The individual is encouraged to search visually for particular objects in a complex environment, to identify objects they need to attend to in order to negotiate a complex environment and to pay attention to the therapist during a demonstration.

One implication from research in the area of unilateral attentional disorders is that training should involve specific cues found in everyday life. Cueing the patient to attend to the affected side has been shown to be beneficial but not necessarily transferable. Conversely, neglect can be exacerbated by presenting stimuli on both sides of the body simultaneously (Riddoch & Humphreys 1994).

In a single case study, after practice in negotiating an obstacle course, the subject showed improvement with cueing by the therapist but no generalization to other settings, at home or outside (Lennon 1994). However, the subject's spouse was able to use cueing to help the person negotiate other environments that led to fewer collisions and falls.

Improvements in neglect have been found with active intentional movements when movements are performed with the affected limb in the neglected part of extrapersonal space (Robertson & North 1993; Plummer et al 2001). Robertson and Noth (1993) also showed that active movement could reduce neglect but not sensory extinction, supporting the generally held view that different mechanisms subserve sensory extinction from those underlying neglect. A later report (Robertson & North 1994) suggests that improvements seen in neglect may disappear during bilateral active hand use (see Ch. 6). Computerized scanning and attentional training programmes have not been successful at generalizing into other tasks nor are they maintained once training has ceased (Robertson et al 1990).

Treatment regimes for cognitive and perceptual impairments are difficult to develop due to the lack of a clear understanding of the underlying mechanisms. Various rehabilitation strategies have been described but evidence of their benefit in reducing disability and improving independence is lacking. Some studies show promising results but fail to show generalizability of training to untrained situations.

Overall, rehabilitation aims to address specific deficits by increasing the person's awareness of the nature of their problem and by training them to reorient their attention to particular situations while practising motor tasks, such as walking, standing up and sitting down, reaching and manipulating objects. Specific training is also provided to address task-related perceptual–cognitive impairments with reinforcement provided during motor training sessions with the physiotherapist.

Given our lack of understanding, it is only possible to suggest ways to engage the person in their rehabilitation.

Some guidelines

- Emphasize visual scanning to search for targets or a particular object.
- Encourage the person to deal with what seems 'odd' and to use head and eye movement to locate apparently 'missing' objects.
- Use markers to help the person anchor their vision: for example, scan to the marker on the left of the page before starting to read.

- If attention is lost during training, assist the person to reorient before going on.
- Avoid using words with negative connotations and be sure not to nag.
- Do not use the term 'neglect' as it sounds like criticism.

In the acute phase following stroke, the manifestations of perceptual–cognitive impairments may be very pronounced, and early efforts to increase the person's awareness and understanding of the deficits may be critical to their general wellbeing and confidence. It is also important to help the person and relatives cope with the confusion they experience and the depression that may result from a feeling that they are mentally incompetent. Early and appropriate intervention can help the patient, relatives and therapist better understand the situation. Helping the person use intellectual knowledge both as a substitute for their lack of direct information and as a means of regaining direct knowledge may be helpful.

Some examples of early training include the following:

Impaired verticality

- Explain with a rod that the eyes and brain are providing incorrect information (playing tricks) and suggest the person focuses on an object known to be upright (such as the legs of the bed) and try to 'see' them as upright.

Not noticing food on the left of the plate

- Encourage the person to find the food on the left by exploring the plate with the fork or with fingers.
- When food is located on the left, the person is encouraged to identify what type of food it is and to concentrate on picking it up and eating it.

Avoiding attention to the left side during training

- Keep the right space free of distracting stimuli such as radio, TV, other people; suggest the person does not talk while paying attention; forewarn of a coming change in activity.
- Moving visual targets are more compelling than a stationary target.
- Start getting the individual's attention centrally, or even to the right, then move their attention toward the left.
- Use eye contact as a magnet to draw the person's attention to the left. Reward eye contact on the left with a smile.
- Challenge the individual by increasing complexity of the environment and task.

Training attention and concentration are critical parts of motor training that sets out to enable the individual to regain effective performance. It has been suggested that tasks that make demands on the depleted attentional resources of the lesioned hemisphere may increase arousal and consequently increase attention and decrease neglect (Riddoch & Humphreys 1994).

Memory deficits are a common complaint following stroke, traumatic brain injury, in multiple sclerosis and other neurological conditions. Individuals with memory impairments require a neuropsychological assessment to identify strengths and weaknesses combined with direct assessment of specific problems. Wilson (1995) lists eight points to encourage individuals with memory problems to encode, store and recall information (see Ch. 11). Memory training has typically focused on teaching the individual to use internal aids such as mnemonics, rehearsal and mental imagery and external memory aids such as notice boards, lists and microcassettes to improve the individual's independence and quality of life. These memory aids seem to be better than 'drill and practice' strategies. Technological advances have enabled the use of mobile phones, pagers and virtual environments. Many of these are strategies we all use, however memory impaired people may need encouragement to use them (Wilson 1995). A recent systematic review suggests that memory training plays a significant role in the individual's potential to adapt and compensate for the deficits (das Nair & Lincoln 2009).

Executive functions are those capacities that include several integrative cognitive processes by which people monitor, manage and negotiate the orderly execution of goal-directed activities of daily living (Cicerone et al 2005). They enable a person to engage successfully in independent performance and self-serving behaviours. If these executive functions are intact, a person can sustain considerable cognitive loss and still continue to be independent and productive (Lezak et al 2004). External cues such as a pager may be used to initiate everyday activities in people with impaired executive function (Wilson et al 2001).

In conclusion, despite the fact that somatosensory loss is relatively common following brain lesion, and stroke in particular, it remains a somewhat neglected problem as it was a decade ago (Carey 1995). The same can be said about visual and perceptual–cognitive impairments. Such impairments cause considerable difficulty for the individual through their impact on activities that require information about the environment. Rehabilitation methods directed at training specific functional actions involve learning by the patient. Such methods are likely to assist the person with somatosensory, visual and perceptual–cognitive impairments since they involve active participation of the individual, use of the environment to facilitate interaction, an emphasis on the need to pay attention to the task and the practice of concrete tasks. However, specific retraining of sensory awareness, with emphasis on paying attention to relevant sensory inputs, may be helpful for some individuals. In addition, people with severe cognitive deficits will need training of, for example, cognitive processes such as memory and attention.

REFERENCES

Albert ML 1973 A simple test of neglect. Neurology 23:658–664.

Andersen G, Vestergaard K, Ingeman-Nielsen M et al 1995 Incidence of central post-stroke pain. Pain 61:187–193.

Barer D 1990 The influence of visual and tactile inattention on predictions for recovery from acute stroke. Q J Med 74:21–32.

Bobath B 1990 Adult hemiplegia: evaluation and treatment, 3rd edn. Butterworth Heinemann, Oxford.

Bonan IV, Guettard E, Leman MC et al 2006 Subjective visual vertical perception relates to balance in acute stroke. Arch Phys Med Rehabil 87:642–646.

Bowen A, Lincoln N 2007 Cognitive rehabilitation for spatial neglect following stroke. Cochrane Database Syst Rev Issue 2. Art. No.: CD003586. DOI: 10.1002/14651858.CD003586.pub2.

Burke D, Gandevia SC 1988 Interfering cutaneous stimulation and the muscle afferent contribution to cortical potentials. Encephalog Clin Neurophysiol 70:118–125.

Butter CM, Kirsch NL, Reeves G 1990 The effect of lateralized dynamic stimuli on unilateral spatial neglect following right hemisphere lesions. Res Neurol Neurosci 2:39–46.

Calvanio R, Levine D, Petrone P 1993 Elements of cognitive rehabilitation after right hemisphere stroke. Behav Neurol 11:25–57.

Carey LM 1995 Somatosensory loss after stroke. Crit Rev Phys Rehabil Med 7:51–91.

Carey LM 2006 Loss of somatic sensation. In: Selzer M, Clarke S, Cohen L, et al (eds) Textbook of neural repair and rehabilitation. Vol II. Cambridge University Press, Cambridge:231–247.

Carey LM, Matyas TA, Oke LE 1993 Sensory loss in stroke patients: effective training of tactile and proprioceptive discrimination. Arch Phys Med Rehabil 74:602–611.

Carr JH, Shepherd RB 1987 A motor relearning programme for stroke, 2nd edn. Butterworth Heinemann, Oxford.

Carr JH, Shepherd RB 1998 Neurological rehabilitation: optimizing motor performance. Butterworth Heinemann, Oxford.

Carr JH, Shepherd RB 2003 Stroke rehabilitation: guidelines for exercise and training to optimize motor skill. Butterworth Heinemann, Oxford.

Cicerone KD, Dahlberg C, Malec JF et al 2005 Evidence-based cognitive rehabilitation: updated review of the literature from 1998 through 2002. Arch Phys Med Rehabil 86:1681–1692.

Critchley M 1953 The parietal lobes. Hafner, New York.

Dannenbaum RM, Dykes RW 1988 Sensory loss in the hand after sensory stroke: therapeutic rationale. Arch Phys Med Rehabil 69:833–839.

das Nair R, Lincoln N 2009 Cognitive rehabilitation for memory deficits following stroke. Cochrane Database Syst Rev Issue 3. Art. No.: CD002293. DOI: 10.1002/14651858.CD002293.pub2.

de Jersey M 1979 Report on a sensory programme for patients with sensory deficits. Aust J Physiother 25:165.

Dietz V, Gollhofer A, Kleiber M et al 1992 Regulation of bipedal stance: dependency on 'load' receptors. Exp Brain Res 89:229–231.

Diller L, Weinberg J 1977 Hemi-inattention and rehabilitation. The evolution of a rational treatment program. In: Weinstein EA, Friedland RP (eds) Advances in neurology. Raven Press, New York.

Diller L, Weinberg J 1993 Response styles in perceptual retraining. In: Gordon WA (ed.) Advances in stroke rehabilitation. Andover Medical Publishers, Boston:162–182.

Dunai J, Bennett K, Fotiades A et al 1999 Modulation of unilateral neglect as a function of direction of object motion. Neuroreport 10:1041–1047.

Efferson L 1995 Disorders of vision and visual perceptual dysfunction. In: Umphred DA (ed.) Neurological rehabilitation, 3rd edn. Mosby, St Louis:769–801.

Fisher CM 1982 Pure sensory stroke and allied conditions. Stroke 13:434–447.

Gandevia SC 1996 Kinesthesia: roles for afferent signals and motor commands. In: Rowell L, Shepherd JT (eds) Integration of motor, circulatory, respiratory and metabolic control during exercise. Oxford University Press, New York:128–172.

Gibson JJ 1966 The senses considered as perceptual systems. Houghton Mifflin, Boston.

Gordon J 1987 Assumptions underlying physical therapy intervention: theoretical and historical perspectives. In: Carr JH, Shepherd RB (eds) Movement science. Foundations for physical therapy in rehabilitation. Butterworth Heinemann, Oxford:1–30.

Halligan PW, Robertson IH, Pizzamiglio L et al 1991 The laterality of visual neglect after right hemisphere damage. Neuropsychol Rehabil 1:281–301.

Heilman KM, Watson RT, Valenstein E 1993 Neglect and related disorders. In: Heilman KM, Valenstein E (eds) Clinical neuropsychology, 3rd edn. Oxford University Press, Oxford:279–336.

Herman EWM 1992 Spatial neglect: new issues and their implications for occupational therapy practice. Am J Occup Ther 46:207–216.

Jacobs H, Vanderstaeten G, van Laere M et al 1988 SEPs and central somatosensory conduction time in hemiplegics. Electromyogr Clin Neurophysiol 28:355–360.

Jeannerod M 1988 Neural and behavioural organization of goal-directed movements. Oxford University Press, Oxford.

Jeannerod M, Michel F, Prablanc C 1984 The control of hand movements in a case of hemianaesthesia following a parietal lesion. Brain 107:899–920.

Johansson RS, Westling G 1984 Roles of glabrous skin receptors and sensorimotor memory in automatic control of precision grip when lifting rougher or more slippery objects. Exp Brain Res 56:550–564.

Kandel ER 2000 From nerve cell to cognition. In: Kandel ER, Schwartz JH, Jessel TM (eds) Principles of neural science, 4th edn. McGraw-Hill, New York:381–403.

Kinsella G, Packer S, Ng K et al 1995 Continuing issues in the assessment of neglect. Neuropsychol Rehabil 5:239–258.

Knapp HD, Taub F, Berman AJ 1963 Movements in monkeys with deafferented forelimbs. Exp Neurol 7:305–315.

Knott M, Voss DE 1968 Proprioceptive neuromuscular facilitation. Harper & Row, New York.

Kusoffsky A, Wadell I, Nilsson BY 1982 The relationship between sensory impairment and motor recovery in patients with hemiplegia. Scand J Rehabil Med 14:27–32.

Lee M-J, Kilbreath SL, Refshauge KM 2005 Movement detection at the ankle following stroke is poor. Aust J Physiother 51:19–24.

Leipmann H 1920 Apraxia. Ergebnisse der Gesamten Medizin 1:516–543.

Lennon S 1994 Task specific effects in the rehabilitation of unilateral neglect. In: Riddoch MJ, Humphreys GW (eds) Cognitive neuropsychology and cognitive rehabilitation. Erlbaum, London:187–203.

Lezak MD, Howieson DB, Loving DW 2004 Neuropsychological assessment, 4th edn. Oxford University Press, Oxford.

Lincoln NB, Crow JL, Jackson JM et al 1991 The unreliability of sensory assessments. Clin Rehabil 5:273–282.

Lincoln NB, Jackson JM, Adams SA 1998 Reliability and revision of the Nottingham Sensory Assessment for stroke patients. Physiotherapy 84:358–365.

Mattingley JB, Bradshaw JL, Bradshaw JA et al 1994 Horizontal visual motion modulates focal attention in left unilateral spatial neglect. J Neurol Neurosurg Psychiatry 57:1228–1235.

Merzenich MM, Kaas JH, Wall J et al 1983 Topographic reorganization of somatosensory cortical areas 3b and 1 in adult monkeys following restricted deafferentation. Neuroscience 8:33.

Merzenich MM, Recanzone G, Jenkins WM et al 1988 Cortical representational plasticity. In: Rakie P, Singer W (eds) Neurobiology of the neocortex. Wiley, New York:41–67.

National Stroke Foundation 2005 Clinical guidelines for stroke rehabilitation and recovery. National Stroke Foundation, Melbourne.

National Stroke Foundation 2007 Clinical guidelines for acute stroke management. National Stroke Foundation, Melbourne.

Pierce SR, Buxbaum LJ 2002 Treatments of unilateral neglect: a review. Arch Phys Med Rehabil 83:256–268.

Plummer P, Morris M, Dunai J 2001 Physical therapy for stroke patients with unilateral neglect: the role of visual cues and limb activation strategies. Phys Ther Rev 6:175–188.

Riddoch MJ, Humphreys GW 1987 Perceptual and action systems in unilateral visual neglect. In: Jeannerod M (ed.) Neurophysiological and neuropsychological aspects of spatial neglect. Elsevier, Amsterdam:151–181.

Riddoch MJ, Humphreys GW 1994 Towards an understanding of neglect. In: Riddoch MJ, Humphreys GW (eds) Cognitive neuropsychology and cognitive rehabilitation. Erlbaum, London:125–149.

Robertson IH, North N 1993 Active and passive activation of left limbs: influence on visual and sensory neglect. Neuropsychology 31:293–300.

Robertson IH, North NT 1994 One hand is better than two: motor extinction of left hand advantage in unilateral neglect. Neuropsychology 32:1–11.

Robertson IH, Gray JM, Pentland B et al 1990 Microcomputer-based rehabilitation for unilateral left visual neglect: a randomised controlled trial. Arch Phys Med Rehabil 62:476–483.

Schabrun SM, Hillier S 2009 Evidence for the retraining of sensation after stroke: a systematic review. Clin Rehabil 23:27–39.

Snowdon N, Scott O 2005 Perception of vertical and postural control following stroke: a clinical study. Physiotherapy 91:165–170.

Stockmeyer SA 1967 An interpretation of the approach of Rood to the treatment of neuromuscular dysfunction. Am J Phys Med 46:900–956.

Stone SP, Wilson B, Wroot A et al 1991 The assessment of visuo-spatial neglect after acute stroke. J Neurol Neurosurg Psychiatry 54:345–350.

Wade D, Skilbeck C, David R et al 1985 Stroke: a critical approach to diagnosis, treatment and management. Chapman and Hall, London.

Watanabe Y, Shikano M, Ohba M et al 1989 Correlation between somatosensory evoked potentials and sensory disturbance in stroke patients. Clin Electroencephalogr 20:156–161.

Weiss T, Miltner WHR, Liepert J et al 2004 Rapid functional plasticity in the primary somatomotor cortex and perceptual changes after nerve block. Eur J Neurosci 20:3413–3423.

West C, Bowen A, Hesketh A et al 2009 Interventions for motor apraxia following stroke. Cochrane Database Syst Rev Issue 1. Art. No.: CD004132. DOI: 10.1002/14651858.CD004132.pub2.

Wilson BA 1995 Management and remediation in brain-injured adults. In: Baddeley AD, Wilson BA, Watts FN (eds) Handbook of memory disorders. John Wiley, Chichester:451–479.

Wilson B, Cockburn J, Halligan P 1987 Development of a behavioral test of visuospatial neglect. Arch Phys Med Rehabil 68:98–102.

Wilson BA, Emslie HC, Quirk K et al 2001 Reducing everyday memory and planning problems by means of a paging system: a randomised control crossover study. J Neurol Neurosurg Psychiatry 70:477–482.

Winward CE, Halligan PW, Wade DT 1999 Somatosensory assessment after central nerve damage: the need for standardized clinical measures. Phys Ther Rev 4:21–28.

Wynn-Parry CB, Salter M 1975 Sensory reeducation after median nerve lesions. Hand 8:250–257.

Yekutiel M, Guttman E 1993 A controlled trial of the retraining of the sensory function of the hand in stroke patients. J Neurol Neurosurg Psychiatry 56:241–244.

Zeman BD, Yiannikas C 1989 Functional prognosis in stroke: use of somatosensory evoked potentials. J Neurol Neurosurg Psychiatry 52:242.

Stroke

Written with Julie Bernhardt

INTRODUCTION

Stroke refers to neurological signs and symptoms, usually focal and acute, that result from disease involving cerebral blood vessels. The brain is highly susceptible to disturbance of its blood supply. Anoxia and ischaemia lasting only seconds can cause neurological signs, and within minutes, irreversible neural damage. Although the cerebrovasculature has specific anatomical and physiological features that are designed to protect the brain from circulatory compromise, when these protective mechanisms fail, the result is a stroke.

Aetiology and pathology

Disorders of the cerebral circulation include any disease of the vascular system that causes ischaemia (insufficiency of blood supply depriving tissue of both oxygen and glucose) or infarction (tissue death) of the brain or spontaneous haemorrhage into the brain or subarachnoid space. Strokes are either occlusive (due to closure of a blood vessel) or haemorrhagic (due to bleeding from a vessel). Both types of stroke may occur at any age, including infancy, from many causes including cardiac disease,

©2010 Elsevier Ltd
DOI: 10.1016/B978-0-7020-4051-1.00020-5

infection, trauma, neoplasm, vascular malformation and immunological disorders. The three most commonly recognized risk factors include hypertension, diabetes mellitus and heart disease, with hypertension the most important of these factors.

Most occlusive strokes are due to atherosclerosis and thrombosis or embolus and most haemorrhagic strokes are associated with hypertension or aneurysm. Haemorrhage may occur at the brain's surface (extraparenchymal), for example from rupture of a congenital aneurysm at the circle of Willis, causing a subarachnoid haemorrhage. This type of stroke is the least common of all stroke types. More commonly, haemorrhage may be intraparenchymal, occurring from rupture of vessels damaged by longstanding hypertension which may cause a blood clot or haematoma within the cerebral hemispheres, in the brainstem or the cerebellum. Rapid intracerebral accumulation of blood under arterial pressure may act as an expanding lesion, displacing or compressing adjacent brain tissue, limiting the blood supply. If ischaemia is temporary, there may be little or no pathological evidence of tissue damage. When ischaemia is sufficiently severe and prolonged, neurons and other cellular elements die (infarction).

The most commonly seen stroke syndrome is caused by infarction in the territory of the middle cerebral artery with contralateral weakness, sensory loss, homonymous hemianopia (visual field impairment) and, depending on which hemisphere is involved, either language disturbance (in general, a left hemisphere lesion) or impaired spatial perception (in general, a right hemisphere lesion). A history of abrupt loss of focal cerebral function of some kind constitutes the fundamental basis of the stroke diagnosis.

Cerebral infarction is responsible for between 67% and 80% of all first strokes, primary intracranial haemorrhage for between 7% and 20% and subarachnoid haemorrhage for about 1–7% (Feigin et al 2003).

Incidence

After coronary heart disease and cancer, stroke is the third most common cause of death in western countries and is the most important single cause of severe disability in people living in their own homes. In addition to the personal and family burden of stroke, costs of care also place a considerable burden on the community. Lifetime costs per patient have been estimated as between AU$45 000 (Dewey et al 2001) and US$60 000–US$230 000 (Feigin et al 2003), with the costs of informal caregiving (provided by family/friends to help patients live at home after stroke) a considerable hidden cost to society. In Australia, lifetime caregiver costs are estimated at AU$332 million (Dewey et al 2002).

The number of deaths due to stroke has been estimated as 5.5 million worldwide, with two-thirds of deaths occurring in less-developed countries (World Health Organization 2008). It is not clear whether this is due to racial, environmental (including health services) or social factors. Mortality appears to be declining however, most notably in developed countries such as Japan, North America and western Europe (Feigin et al 2003), although reliable data from less-developed countries are often difficult to obtain.

Stroke incidence has been estimated to be 1.5–2 per 1000 population (Lindley 2008). Incidence varies between countries, but not markedly so. Men tend to be younger (70 years) than women (75 years) when they first experience a stroke. The age-specific incidence of stroke progressively increases with every decade of life, estimated as 0.1–0.3 cases per 1000 per year for those aged <45 years, rising to 12.0–20.0 cases per 1000 per year for those aged 75–84 years (Feigin et al 2003), with the highest age-specific rates occurring in Japan, Russia and the Ukraine. What these figures mean is that, on average, there is a 10-fold increase in stroke incidence from childhood to early adulthood, another 10-fold increase from early adulthood to middle age, and a further increase of the same magnitude from middle age to old age (Lindley 2008). Almost 20% of strokes in Australia occur in people under the age of 55 (Australian Institute of Health and Welfare 2004).

Stroke prevalence is extremely difficult to measure since some patients die early after onset and many of the patients are not disabled. Overall prevalence rates are around 10 per 1000 population, which would equate to around 50 per 1000 for those over 65 years (Lindley 2008). Prevalence data, despite the difficulties associated with obtaining an accurate estimate, are useful for the planning of medical and support services required to properly care for people with stroke.

Blood supply to the brain

Efficient blood flow to the central nervous system delivers oxygen, glucose and other nutrients and removes carbon dioxide, lactic acid and other metabolic products. At rest, the brain, which is only 2% of total body weight, receives 15% of the cardiac output of blood and consumes about 25% of the total inspired oxygen. The brain receives this rich supply of blood through four major arteries, two vertebral arteries and two internal carotid arteries (Fig. 11.1A) which anastomose at the base of the brain to form the circle of Willis. The protective importance of the circle of Willis is illustrated by the fact that minor deviations from the classic structure are common. The four major arteries branch intracranially to form the main arterial branches of the brain (Fig 11.1B). Extensive anastamatic connections between blood vessels can protect the brain when part of its vascular supply is blocked.

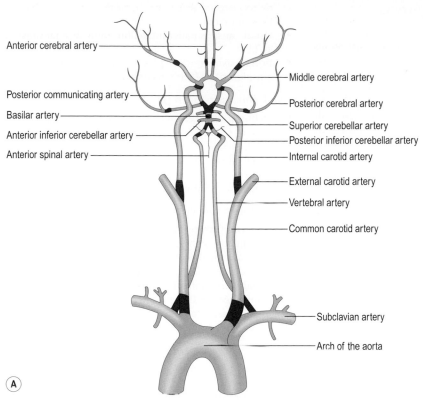

Figure 11.1A Blood vessels of the brain. Dark areas indicate common sites of atherosclerosis and occlusion. *(From Kandel ER, Schwartz JH, Jessell TM eds (1991) Principles of Neural Science, 3rd ed. pp 1042. Appleton and Lange, Norwalk, CT, by permission).*

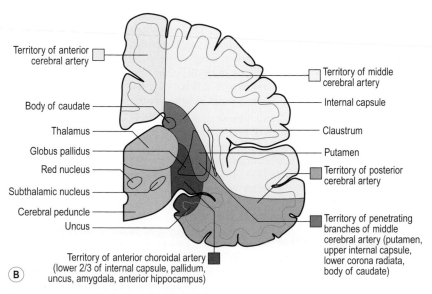

Figure 11.1B Cerebral arterial areas. *(From Kandel ER, Schwartz JH, Jessell TM (eds) (1991) Principles of Neural Science, 3rd ed 1042. Appleton and Lange, Norwalk, CT, by permission).*

Classification and prognosis

The key clinical features of stroke are its sudden onset and the presence of focal neurological signs and symptoms. Typically, patients with stroke have been well prior to the event. Isolated vertigo and loss of consciousness without focal neurological signs are rarely due to stroke.

The similarities between minor ischemic stroke and *transient ischaemic attack* (TIA) are strong. TIA has traditionally been defined as rapidly developing clinical signs of focal or global disturbance of cerebral function lasting fewer than 24 hours, with no apparent non-vascular cause. However, recently there has been considerable support to change this definition and shorten the duration of TIA to 1 hour as TIAs rarely last longer than this (Albers et al 2002). Furthermore, new evidence has confirmed that TIA is associated with a much higher risk of subsequent stroke than was previously believed, with half of the risk seen within the first 48 hours of symptom onset. Consequently, the principles of assessment and management of TIA should now follow those outlined for ischaemic stroke and treatments to prevent stroke need to be established early. Five factors that increase the risk of subsequent stroke are: diabetes mellitus; age >60 years; symptom duration >10 minutes; motor or speech impairments; and high blood pressure (>140/90 mmHg) (National Stroke Foundation 2007a). Risk stratification tools have been validated (e.g., the ABCD^2 tool) and are now recommended to help clinicians target those patients most at risk of subsequent stroke.

The classic *stroke* definition comprises rapidly developing clinical symptoms and/or signs of focal and at times global loss of cerebral function, with symptoms lasting more than 24 hours with no apparent cause other than that of vascular origin (Hatano 1976). There is a wide range of severity, from recovery in a few days through to persistent disability and death. The Oxfordshire Community Stroke Project (OCSP) classification (Bamford et al 1991) has become a common method of classifying stroke subtype and it can assist with prognostication. Below are listed the defining features of the classification, together with the usual cause and a comment on prognosis for each subtype (Dewey & Bernhardt 2007).

TACI (total anterior circulation infarct)

- **Defining features:** ipsilateral motor and/or sensory deficit *and* higher cortical dysfunction, e.g., dysphasia, neglect *and* homonymous hemianopia.
- **Usual cause:** large middle cerebral artery infarct due to embolism from the heart or proximal arterial source.
- **Prognosis:** high likelihood of death and long-term dependency.

PACI (partial anterior circulation infarct)

- **Defining features:** two of three deficits present in TACI *or* higher cortical dysfunction alone *or* restricted motor/sensory deficit, e.g., confined to one limb or face and hand.
- **Usual cause:** smaller infarct but same arterial causes as TACI.
- **Prognosis:** better prognosis for recovery than TACI but high risk of early recurrence.

LACI (lacunar infarct)

- **Defining features:** pure motor hemiparesis, pure sensory stroke, sensorimotor stroke, ataxic hemiparesis.
- **Usual cause:** small, deep infarct due to small vessel disease.
- **Prognosis:** relatively good.

POCI (posterior circulation infarct)

- **Defining features**: brainstem signs, cerebellar dysfunction without ipsilateral long-tract signs (i.e., not ataxic hemiparesis) *or* isolated homonymous hemianopia.
- **Usual cause**: infarct in the posterior cerebral hemisphere, brainstem or cerebellum, due to large or small vessel disease or cardiac embolism.
- **Prognosis**: variable.

ICH (intracerebral haemorrhage)

- **Defining features:** signs depend on site and size of haemorrhage.
- **Usual cause:** multiple.
  - *Deep location:* usually due to rupture of small, deep perforating artery; often associated with hypertension.
  - *Superficial/lobar location:* cerebral amyloid angiopathy often the cause; older patients.
  - *Other common causes:* arteriovenous malformation/cavernoma; ruptured saccular aneurysm; coagulopathy.
- **Prognosis:** often worse than ischaemic stroke, with high risk of death in the hours to days after stroke. Survivors of ICH have similar functional, quality of life outcomes as other stroke survivors.

Immediately after stroke it is difficult to predict the extent of eventual recovery. Some strokes are rapidly fatal, particularly very large ischemic (TACI) or haemorrhagic strokes, contributing to a mortality of 10% within the first week of stroke. Models developed to help predict devastating (dead, very disabled) or good outcome (alive, little disability) after stroke have been found to discriminate outcome in 80% of cases (Johnston et al 2003). However, these models are not intended to influence management, but rather to help researchers adjust outcome data from clinical trials or epidemiological studies (Counsell et al 2002) and it is well known that there are patients who improve unexpectedly and others who do poorly despite having a good predicted prognosis (Bonita & Beaglehole 1988; Barer & Mitchell 1989; Lincoln et al 1990; Jørgensen et al 1995). Nevertheless, older age and worse stroke severity (often measured using the National Institutes of Health Stroke Scale (NIHSS) appear to strongly influence outcome after stroke. In addition to these factors, premorbid heart disease and dementia impact on mortality and stroke recurrence (Appelros et al 2003), plasma glucose >8 mmol/L predicts poor prognosis independent of age, stroke severity or stroke subtype (Weir et al 1997) while functional independence and living alone pre-stroke, early consciousness and the ability to walk post-stroke predict survival in a non-disabled state at 6 months (Counsell et al 2002). As you can see, there is no single model that can help us predict long-term outcome soon after stroke. After about 2 weeks post-stroke, good prognostic signs include urinary continence, young age, mild stroke, rapid improvement, good perceptual abilities and no cognitive disorders. However, patients who do not demonstrate these signs may still do well in the long term.

In fact, the great majority of patients who survive the first month after a stroke will improve and many return to pre-stroke levels of function. Approximately 50–60% of stroke survivors become functionally independent, with little difference between those whose stroke was due to cerebral infarction or primary intracerebral haemorrhage. In the Copenhagen study, a study of a large, unselected group of stroke patients, 81% of those who survived their stroke went home (Jørgensen et al 1995). An Australian incidence study of all first-ever strokes found that among 3-month stroke survivors, 74% required assistance with activities of daily living and received informal care from family or friends, two-thirds of whom were women who provided care during family or leisure time (Dewey et al 2002). Patients with pure motor stroke appear more likely to be independent at 6 months (93%) compared with those experiencing motor, somatosensory and visual (hemianopia) disturbances (50%) (Patel et al 2000). However, functional outcome does not necessarily predict placement after discharge from hospital. Some families take home individuals who require considerable care.

The extent to which recovery depends on what the patient does in rehabilitation, what the person actually experiences, is not known, but it is likely that both rehabilitation methods and the environment itself play a significant part in recovery processes. Early active mobilization (Johansson 2000; Calautti & Baron 2003) and a focus on tasks that are challenging and meaningful (Nudo 2003) seem to be effective in optimizing neural plasticity and functional recovery.

Survival after stroke

About 20% of first-ever stroke patients die within a month, the prognosis being much better for cerebral infarction than for intracerebral haemorrhage (about 10% vs 50% dead) (Bamford et al 1990). Mortality in the first few days is almost always due to the brain lesion itself, intracerebral haemorrhage or large cerebral infarcts with associated oedema causing brain shift and herniation or direct disruption of vital brainstem centres by the lesion. Sudden death only occurs as a consequence of intracranial haemorrhage (Bamford et al 1990). Deaths after the first week are more likely to be due to indirect consequences of the brain lesion (e.g., bronchopneumonia and pulmonary embolism) or concurrent cardiac disease.

After the first month, the risk of death declines (about 6% per annum) but it is still about twice that in the general population because stroke patients are particularly likely to die of a further stroke and even more likely to die of the consequences of other vascular disease (Lindley 2008).

Management of modifiable risk factors for stroke can reduce likelihood of further stroke (and prevent stroke occurring in the first place). High blood pressure, high blood cholesterol, diabetes, smoking, atrial fibrillation and excessive alcohol are the most important modifiable risk factors. Although not considered 'independent' risk factors for stroke, obesity and lack of exercise contribute to hypertension, high cholesterol and diabetes, and therapists have a key role to play in preventing future stroke through management of obesity and exercise. Medical management of the key modifiable risk factors is briefly outlined below.

ACUTE STROKE

Admission to hospital

Unlike 10–15 years ago, stroke is now considered a medical emergency, requiring the same urgent attention as a heart attack. 'Time is brain' is the new catch cry with an estimated 1.9 million neurons and 14 billion synapses lost every minute following a stroke (Saver 2006). Rapid transfer to a hospital with a specialist stroke service represents best practice and public health campaigns in many countries focus on educating the public about signs of stroke and promote an 'act fast' message. This major shift in stroke management has primarily been driven by the emergence of two proven treatments for acute stroke: 1) intravenous thrombolysis or tissue plasminogen activator and 2) stroke units. Thrombolysis involves the administration of a clot-dissolving drug (alteplase) which, if administered within 3–4.5 hours of stroke onset, can completely reverse the damaging effects of an occluded vessel. However, it must be delivered early and can only occur after a rapid computerized tomography (CT) scan has excluded haemorrhage as the cause of symptoms.

Treatment within a stroke unit (a geographically located ward, manned by a multidisciplinary team) is the other evidence-based acute stroke intervention. Risk of recurrent events for those with stroke and TIA are highest in the first days after stroke, and stroke units have been proven to reduce death and long-term disability when compared to treatment in general medical wards (Langhorne 2000). There are a range of care models included in the meta-analysis demonstrating the benefits of organized stroke units. These include: *acute stroke units* (short stay, diagnostic wards); *comprehensive stroke units* (acute plus rehabilitation provided, longer stay); and *rehabilitation stroke units* (delayed onset of care, rehabilitation only, mixed or stroke alone). Evidence for stroke units is strongest for those that incorporate rehabilitation. Important aspects of effective stroke unit care are thought to include: 1) accurate and rapid stroke diagnosis, likely causation and associated risk factors; 2) evidence-based treatments; 3) close monitoring of neurological status and physiological parameters; 4) prevention of the complications of stroke and recurrent stroke; and 5) early institution of rehabilitation focused on achieving functional goals and early development of an individualized discharge plan (Dewey & Bernhardt 2007). Surprisingly, full implementation of these proven and cost-effective interventions has been difficult to achieve and access to stroke unit care and/or thrombolysis varies within a country and from one country to the next.

Medical management of all strokes

Early diagnosis and management

Accurate diagnosis of the cause of stroke dictates many acute management decisions, so diagnostic testing often dominates the early phase of care for people with both TIA and stroke. Brain imaging, CT or magnetic resonance imaging (MRI) is urgently requested since stroke can be mimicked by other serious pathology (e.g., subdural haematoma) and making a distinction between ischaemic and haemorrhagic stroke is not possible on clinical grounds alone. Brain imaging also confirms eligibility for thrombolysis. Early CT imaging is frequently normal in ischaemic stroke or changes may be subtle, but haemorrhage is generally visible. If the initial scan is normal and there is any doubt about the diagnosis, CT imaging is often repeated after 3–7 days or a more sensitive MRI is performed.

An electrocardiogram is commonly requested (to exclude atrial fibrillation, acute coronary syndrome and evidence of structural or ischaemic heart disease), as are studies of electrolytes and renal function, blood sugar level, full blood examination and erythrocyte sedimentation rate (Dewey & Bernhardt 2007). Other investigations are tailored to the individual patient and their stroke syndrome taking into account the severity of the stroke and comorbidities.

Carotid ultrasound and/or imaging may be urgently requested for patients with stroke or TIA who may be candidates for carotid artery surgery which can prevent further stroke, particularly if performed early after first symptoms. Echocardiography may be indicated in some patients to search for a cardiac or aortic source of embolism.

Patients with ischemic stroke or TIA will usually be started on daily aspirin within 48 hours of stroke onset. Antiplatelet therapy with aspirin significantly reduces risk of further stroke and those unable to tolerate aspirin can be treated with alternative drugs (Dewey & Bernhardt 2007). Intravenous heparin is no longer recommended because it is associated with an increased risk for intracerebral haemorrhage (ICH).

Major brain swelling can be a complication of large hemispheric infarcts and hemicraniectomy within 48 hours has been shown to substantially improve outcome from this complication.

Patients with haemorrhagic stroke (ICH) due to anticoagulation have the anticoagulation urgently reversed to prevent further expansion of the stroke lesion. Surgical evacuation of the haemorrhage may be considered in a few select patients (e.g., cerebellar hemisphere haemorrhage >3 cm), but is no longer routinely practised.

General care

It remains uncertain whether elevated blood pressure should be lowered acutely after ischaemic stroke with some guidelines recommending toleration of blood pressures up to 220/120 mmHg without treatment in the first hours to days of stroke unless a concomitant disease dictates otherwise. In patients treated with thrombolysis, blood pressure is more tightly controlled to ≤185/110 mmHg as higher blood pressures are associated with an increased risk of ICH. It is generally accepted that blood pressure lowering in ICH patients is indicated to reduce further risk of bleeding. Hyperglycaemia and hypoglycaemia are avoided and oxygen supplementation is provided when patients are hypoxic.

Expert nursing care is a key aspect of effective stroke unit care. Although management of impairments from stroke must be individualized, good general care that ensures the patient is comfortable, properly hydrated, fed and toileted, monitored reliably, turned regularly and suitably positioned, that the airway is kept clear and swallowing is safe is vital. Frequent monitoring of neurological status and physiological variables (e.g., heart rate, oxygen saturation, blood pressure, blood sugar) aids early detection and treatment of complications.

Complications after stroke are common, with 62–85% of patients experiencing at least one complication within the first few months after stroke (Langhorne 2000). Neurological worsening is common early after stroke, with stroke progression reported in up to 40% of cases. Secondary complications such as urinary tract and chest infections, pressure sores, falls, deep vein thrombosis, pulmonary embolism and musculoskeletal pain occur more frequently. Disorders of mood, such as depression and anxiety, are likely to be under reported (Dewey & Bernhardt 2007). Intrinsic factors (e.g., age, comorbidities, stroke severity) are also associated with increased complication risk post-stroke. Good nursing care, combined with *early active rehabilitation*, is believed to play an important role in reducing complications and improving the outcomes seen for patients treated in organized stroke units. Specific recommendations for management of common complications can be found in a number of stroke clinical guidelines (Adams et al 2003; National Stroke Foundation 2007a).

Modifiable risk factor management

Hypertension. Hypertension is the most important modifiable risk factor for recurrent stroke. Most patients with stroke or TIA, even those with 'normal' blood pressure, should be commenced on antihypertensive medication while still in the acute hospital.

Atrial fibrillation. In patients with TIA/ischaemic stroke and atrial fibrillation, valvular disease or recent myocardial infarction, warfarin (international normalized ratio (INR) 2–3) is appropriate secondary prevention, unless there is a clear contraindication. The benefits for stroke prevention clearly outweigh the risks of serious haemorrhage in this population. The most appropriate timing for starting warfarin for secondary prevention is uncertain and stroke physicians vary in their practice, although commencing as soon as possible after TIA, once CT scanning has excluded ICH, and delaying warfarin commencement for 1–2 weeks for stroke patients is considered reasonable (National Stroke Foundation 2007a). Before warfarin is begun, aspirin should be used.

Diabetes. Elevated blood sugar level is common in patients presenting with stroke or TIA and good glycaemic control is essential for prevention of the long-term microvascular and non-vascular complications of this disease. Standard methods for controlling blood sugar level within normal ranges should be used for those with stroke.

Hypercholesterolaemia. Lowering lipids with statin therapy in patients with TIA and stroke significantly reduces stroke risk with no significant increase in haemorrhagic stroke and this treatment should be commenced while the patient is still in hospital.

Smoking and alcohol use. Cigarette smoking and excessive use of alcohol are potent risk factors for stroke. Individually tailored programmes to help change behaviour are available and should be encouraged in those at risk (National Stroke Foundation 2007a).

RECOVERY AFTER STROKE

Around 10% of stroke patients may experience a period of marked impairment of consciousness following stroke. They are generally those patients who have experienced large middle cerebral artery infarcts (TACI) or intracerebral haemorrhage. In some cases, a decision will be made to provide palliative care (treatment to relieve symptoms of life-threatening stroke) rather than active care. Those who receive palliative care will often die of their stroke and therapist involvement in palliative care will vary according to the needs of the patient and their family. Decompressive surgery (removal of part of the skull to relieve pressure) will be performed in some patients with cerebral oedema, however these patients will generally be managed in intensive care following surgery. Once back on the stroke ward they can be treated the same as other patients with stroke, with the exception of the need for extra care of the now vulnerable brain.

Patients who experience a *prolonged period of unconsciousness* may require intubation if their respiratory function is compromised. Physiotherapy is required to prevent retention and pooling of secretions, atelectasis and bronchopneumonia, and may include the following interventions.

Respiratory function

- Regular and frequent turning.
- Sitting out of bed in a supportive chair and mobilization as possible.
- Mechanical suction, postural drainage, manual hyperinflation if unconscious and continuous positive airway pressure (CPAP) once conscious.

Musculoskeletal integrity

- *Range of motion exercises* are probably not helpful beyond aiding a person's comfort. When passively moving the glenohumeral joint, particular care should be taken to avoid damage to the soft tissues and impingement at the glenohumeral joint which is likely to occur when passively moving the arm into abduction without external rotation. Early active exercises (including standing) are likely to be more beneficial as a means of preventing secondary changes associated with disuse.
- *Positioning* to maintain at-risk muscles and soft tissue in a lengthened position and to prevent muscle shortening and increased stiffness (e.g., at-risk muscles in the upper limb include internal rotators and adductors of the shoulder and long finger and thumb flexors; at-risk muscles in the lower limb include the plantarflexors, hip and knee flexors) may be helpful.
- *Active exercises* should be instituted as soon as possible and need not wait until the patient regains full consciousness. Early active exercise (in sitting and standing) can increase consciousness level and reduce the likelihood of medical complications associated with bed rest, for example pneumonia and deep vein thrombosis, which are common after stroke.

Early mobilization

In general, active rehabilitation can commence if there is no progression of neurological deficits within 24–48 hours (Indredavik et al 1991). Early onset of rehabilitation would be expected to influence not just the rate and extent of physical recovery by preventing disuse related to long periods of rest (see Ch. 8) and maintaining cardiorespiratory fitness, but also to have a role in minimizing cognitive deterioration, depression and anxiety after stroke. Physiotherapists obviously have a key role to play here. Early mobilization (helping patients to get out of bed, sitting, standing or walking as appropriate) is now recommended in a number of clinical guidelines for acute stroke care (Adams et al 2003; National Stroke Foundation 2007a; Lindsay et al 2008). However, guideline recommendations typically state that mobilization should begin as soon as possible after stroke. These somewhat vague directives reflect the absence of a strong evidence base. If mobilization of stroke patients within hours of stroke was straightforward, then we could expect it to be standard practice throughout the world, but it is not. Instead, the practice remains controversial (Diserens et al 2006; Bernhardt 2008) and existing studies provide promising but limited evidence of the benefits of early exercise on functional recovery (Indredavik et al 1999), early depression (Cumming et al 2008), complications (Bernhardt et al 2009) and healthcare costs (Tay-Teo et al 2008). A recent Cochrane review concludes that although further research is needed in the field, there is no evidence that countries that practise early mobilization as part of standard care should stop (Bernhardt et al 2009).

In Trondheim, Norway, one comprehensive stroke unit has been practising early mobilization for nearly 20 years with impressive patient results. On average, first out-of-bed activity commences within 17 hours of stroke onset. A physiotherapist and nurse take a staged approach to the first mobilization, first sitting the patient up in bed, then over the edge of the bed (Fig. 11.2A), then into a chair (or standing (Fig 11.2B) as appropriate), carefully monitoring oxygen saturation, blood pressure, consciousness and heart rate throughout the procedure. Patients are not left

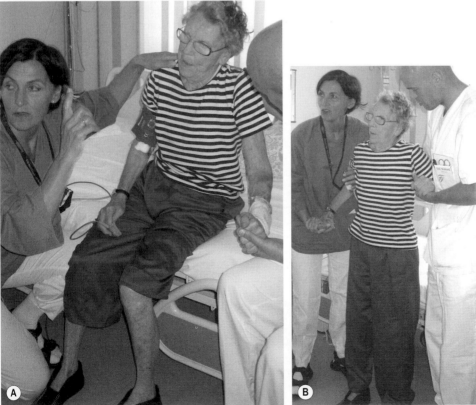
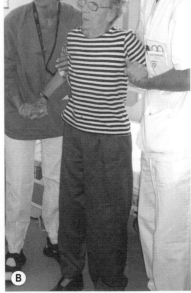

Figure 11.2 (A) Early mobilization: When she first sat up she was very dizzy, so she is monitored carefully before progressing into standing. (B) Her first experience of standing upright after her stroke. Her condition is monitored before she progresses on to more active practice. *(Courtesy of Anne Løge & colleagues, St Olavs Hospital, Trondheim, Norway).*

to sit in a chair longer than 50 minutes following the first mobilization. Tilt-in-space wheelchairs that allow rapid lowering of the back of the chair are often used, and these are helpful in cases of large blood pressure drops that can occur in the first day(s) after stroke.

Once this first mobilization has been successfully completed, the patient is then assisted frequently throughout the day to repeat out-of-bed activity, progressively increasing activity as able (Bakke 1995). Early *and frequent* mobilization does influence patient activity. One study which compared patient activity within this early mobilization centre in Norway to well-established acute stroke units in Melbourne, Australia found that Trondheim patients spent twice as long standing and walking and less time lying in bed (Bernhardt et al 2008). They also found that patients changed position (from lying to sitting to standing) throughout the day twice as often as patients in Melbourne. This approach contrasts with hospitals in which a rest in bed (often flat) policy is maintained for up to 3 days after stroke (Diserens et al 2006). Physicians who order rest in bed do so because of concern that getting patients up out of bed may lead to loss of blood flow to an already compromised cerebral circulation.

Due to the controversy surrounding the practice, and the need for clearer guidelines, a large, international, multicentre randomized controlled trial (AVERT) is currently underway (Bernhardt et al 2006). The primary purpose of the trial is to test whether early and frequent mobilization results in fewer deaths and less disability at 3 months after stroke compared to current stroke practices. A cost-effectiveness substudy is also underway. Results are expected in 2012.

Although commencing rehabilitation within hours of stroke is somewhat controversial, it is well accepted that rehabilitation should begin as soon as possible after stroke. The number of studies comparing interventions commenced at different time points after stroke are few, however they do support earlier onset of training. In one study, a comparison of two groups of patients, one that began rehabilitation within 3 days after acute hospital admission and another that commenced rehabilitation after 4–15 days, indicated that the early intervention group was discharged earlier, was more likely to walk independently and to go home (e.g., Hayes & Carroll 1986). In a comprehensive review of the literature on outcome following stroke, delay in onset of rehabilitation correlated with poor outcome in a number of studies (Cifu & Stewart 1996). Rehabilitation early after stroke has also been suggested to improve long-term social and economic costs (Dombovy et al 1986).

The traditional view of neurological rehabilitation is that it reduces impairment and minimizes disability. Intensive rehabilitation is expensive and there are, in most countries, limited and diminishing resources. In attempts to address the role of rehabilitation in reducing disability and improving quality of life, there is an ongoing debate in the literature on major issues. What type of rehabilitation for stroke is most effective (Langhorne et al 2009)? Where should rehabilitation take place? When should it start? Who are most likely to benefit from intensive rehabilitation? Are group intervention programmes as effective as one-to-one therapy (Wevers et al 2009)? Although significant inroads have been made in answering some of these questions, major methodological problems of studies include the following:

- The variety of measurement tools used and failure to measure outcomes of importance to the patient (e.g., function, participation, quality of life).
- Studies are often small and underpowered (therefore unable to find a result either way).
- Huge variation in treatment methods provided, location, timing post-stroke make pooling of results across studies (e.g., for meta-analysis) difficult.
- Heterogeneity of patients studied and lack of repeated measures.
- Most importantly, the failure of authors to describe or define accurately the interventions used and the intensity.

Another important question is: what type of movement rehabilitation is most effective at improving functional outcome? It is argued in this book that newer, more scientifically-based and active task-related training of motor performance and fitness together with a deeper understanding of the need to prevent deleterious musculoskeletal changes may result in a better outcome than the commonly used 'approaches'. This is particularly so given that there is only equivocal support for the effectiveness of these (e.g., Bobath/neurodevelopmental treatment, Brunnstrom) (Kollen et al 2009). What patients *do* following stroke, the *use* to which they put their affected limbs and their *experiences* appear to affect brain reorganization (see Ch. 1). It is becoming clear that the amount and type of physical and mental activity, attitudes of staff and the attitude and motivation of the patient will impact upon brain reorganization post-stroke.

PROBLEMS IN BODY STRUCTURE AND FUNCTION

In the initial stage following stroke, the system is in a state of cerebral shock, but as a result of reparative processes that occur following the lesion, such as resolution of cerebral oedema, absorption of damaged tissue and improved local vascular flow, functionality of neural tissue is restored and the patient starts to improve. Tissue recovery seems to be a relatively fast process. All recovery beyond the immediate reparative stage probably reflects use and experience, the learning process and the brain's ability to reorganize. It is necessary to accept that there is a link between brain plasticity (i.e., anatomical, physiological and functional reorganization) and the methods used in rehabilitation. It is clear that neural elements are inherently flexible, responding to use and experience (see Ch. 1).

The sensorimotor, cognitive, psychological and behavioural impairments that may be seen in patients following stroke vary from patient to patient. The most typical are discussed below.

Sensorimotor impairments and secondary adaptive changes

The site and size of the cerebrovascular lesion and the amount of collateral blood flow initially determine the degree of motor deficit, which may range from slight incoordination to complete paralysis of the upper and lower limbs and face on one side of the body (hemiplegia or hemiparesis). Deficits in motor control have also been reported on the other side of the body (Newham 2005), and may be related to the bilateral activation of some skeletal muscles. Coexistence of sensory deficits adds to the overall motor deficits, the two systems being functionally interrelated. Sensory loss tends to involve discriminative and proprioceptive modalities more than affective modalities (Carey 2006). Pain, touch and temperature sensitivity may be impaired but are usually not lost unless the lesion is peripheral to the thalamus when they may be associated with anaesthesia. Joint position sense may be severely impaired. There may be loss of two-point discrimination and stereognosis, and failure to recognize a touch stimulus if another is simultaneously delivered to the intact side of the body. Disorders of perception and cognition, such as visuomotor agnosia, are described in Chapter 10. Strokes can affect other areas of the brain, including the cerebellum and its projections, and clinical signs reflect these sites.

Lesions affecting the cortical motor areas and their projections cause characteristic clinical signs. Some reflect the loss of particular functions controlled by the damaged system, for example, impaired innervation of spinal motor neurons results in disabled muscle activation, with *weakness and loss of or disordered motor control*; others, such as *reflex hyperactivity or spasticity*, may emerge after the lesion. Secondary features, particularly evident where there is moderate to severe weakness and loss of motor control, include adaptive changes in muscles and other soft tissues.

Most critical for their effects on functional performance are decreased muscle activation and weakness, and loss of motor control due to impaired central innervation (e.g., Burke 1988; Landau 1988; Gracies 2005a,b). Normally, muscle activation results in force generation that produces muscle forces whose magnitudes and timing characteristics are specific for the task being performed. Poorly innervated muscles may not generate sufficient force for effective task performance. The effects of impaired innervation include:

- reduced muscle activation and difficulty sustaining muscle activity
- reduced muscle force generation and poor timing of peak forces leading to slowness of movement
- poor control of synergistic muscle activity
- lack of skill (dexterity) due to loss of fine motor control/impaired coordination.

These impairments are initially the result of the neural lesion. They may be augmented as time passes by secondary neural and soft tissue changes due to changes in motor performance. Individuals with impaired activation have difficulty supporting, propelling and balancing the body mass over the feet in actions such as standing up and sitting down and walking, and difficulty controlling the joints of the upper limb in actions involving the hand. They lack skill in these taken-for-granted activities that enable us to function in our daily lives.

Motor and sensory loss has the greatest effect on the limbs. Proximal limb and trunk muscles tend to have greater representation in both hemispheres (Brust 1991), for example paraspinal muscles are relatively unaffected in unilateral cerebral lesions. Similarly, the facial muscles of the forehead and muscles of the pharynx and jaw are represented in both hemispheres and are usually spared.

Muscle weakness, including slowness to reach peak force and loss of motor control, causes limitations to functional movement and results in inactivity. Muscle weakness and inactivity lead to secondary adaptation of soft tissue, particularly muscle. Adaptive changes may emerge quite early after stroke and include increased muscle stiffness, muscle contracture, stretch reflex hypersensitivity and other changes within soft tissues. Over time, decreased physical activity leads to a decline in physical fitness. These adaptive musculoskeletal changes contribute to functional disability and their significance is increasingly being understood. Chapter 8 provides a detailed review.

A major feature of the neuromotor system is its *adaptability*. Throughout our lives we learn to adapt our motor performance in order to learn new skills that require changed neuromuscular configurations, and to adapt to different circumstances such as injury. Adaptations to the way we move in response to weakness and loss of motor control are evident after stroke from the person's initial attempts at a purposeful action and throughout the process of recovery. The movement that emerges reflects the person's 'best' attempts, the most biomechanically advantageous movement given the effects of the lesion, the dynamic possibilities in the musculoskeletal linkage and the environment in which the action is performed (see Fig. 6.8).

Adaptive movements that emerge during rehabilitation represent both the initial attempts of the individual to move, using muscles that can be most easily activated, as well as the restraining effects of adaptive length-associated changes in muscles and other soft tissue. That is, the way in which the patient attempts to achieve a goal reflects the degree and distribution of muscle weakness, motor incoordination and the loss of soft tissue extensibility that impose mechanical restraints on movement. Exaggerated force may be generated by stronger and more easily activated muscles as the individual struggles to perform the action required to carry out a task.

REHABILITATION

Stroke manifests itself in many different ways. For this reason, there is considerable variability in sensorimotor, perceptuo-cognitive and behavioural impairments. The role of rehabilitation is to provide a coordinated programme consisting of a multidisciplinary team of health professionals, doctors, nurses, physiotherapists, occupational therapists, speech pathologists and dietitians. The team may be expanded to include other disciplines, for example psychologists and neuropsychologists. The person with a stroke and their family members should be acknowledged as important members of the team.

As soon as possible after a stroke, the focus changes from a medical and sickness orientation to emphasis on exercise and training planned to regain effective functioning in daily life. The rehabilitation environment can be a direct facilitator of rehabilitation goals if it is an environment organized toward health, fitness, mental and physical stimulation, and learning. The patient should be dressed in clothes suitable for exercising, including appropriate shoes. Motor training should start as soon as vital signs are stable. The person is assisted into sitting and standing immediately in order to begin the process of coping with gravity: learning again how to move about in a gravitational environment without using the arms for support and without falling.

The patient is encouraged to be an active participant in a rehabilitation and recovery process designed to optimize functional performance of motor actions, exercising the musculoskeletal system to increase force production and motor control, and to preserve muscle contractility and extensibility. Training of critical actions, standing up and sitting down (Fig. 11.3), walking, reaching and

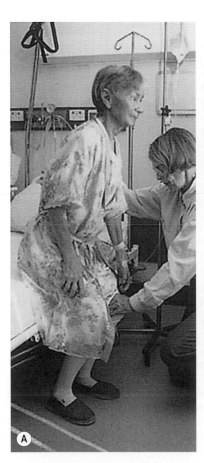
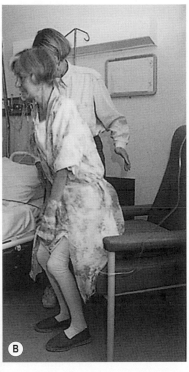

Figure 11.3 Both bed and chair are adjusted to a suitable height to enable practice of STS and SIT with (A) manual guidance to stabilize the foot and (B) stand-by assistance.

manipulation, and balancing (controlling the centre of body mass over the base of support) is based on an understanding of the dynamics of these actions and of how people acquire skill.

A typical physiotherapy session includes balancing activities in sitting and standing, for example reaching beyond arm's length, standing up and sitting down, walking and manipulation, as described in Chapters 4–7. Achieving sitting balance without using the arms for support early after stroke impacts positively on many critical functions – eye contact, communication, visual scanning of the environment, body orientation in space and attentional capacity.

Training methods take account of movement biomechanics, exercise science, muscle characteristics, environmental context and the nature of impairments. The methods used in training are similar to those already shown to be effective in promoting motor learning and in optimizing muscle strength, endurance, fitness and skill in sports and other training programmes for healthy and disabled subjects. The techniques used for encouraging learning include goal identification, instruction, feedback as methods of focusing attention, technological and mechanical aids, and practice (see Chs 2 and 4–7; Carr & Shepherd 2003).

These rehabilitation methods are not yet in common use in stroke, their use held back by continuing reliance on the old 'approaches' view of therapy (e.g., the Bobath approach) despite the lack of evidentiary support. Focus on an 'approach' rather than the specific content of therapy delivery has held back the investigation and practice of science- and evidence-based methods in the clinic, methods that are clearly described and more congruent with current scientific understanding and that have increasing evidentiary support.

However, it is encouraging to see that stroke foundations in several countries, including Australia, Canada, the UK, the USA and The Netherlands, are endeavouring to provide stroke rehabilitation recommendations based on best evidence. The *Clinical Guidelines for Stroke Rehabilitation and Recovery* developed by the Australian National Stroke Foundation (2005) take up current scientific views, and refreshingly make no mention of physiotherapy 'approaches', instead providing guidelines (including levels of evidence) for clinical practice that include early mobilization, task training, physical activity and interventions to improve fitness and mobility. A recent systematic review of motor recovery after stroke recommends that motor training should focus on high-intensity, repetitive, task-specific practice and feedback (Langhorne et al 2009).

Task-oriented training

The major focus of physiotherapy is the optimization of functional motor actions. Optimizing motor performance in this context refers to training a person's performance to

be as effective and as efficient as possible in achieving a functional goal: 'effective' means goal achieved, 'efficient' means the least physiological cost (e.g., ability to walk at a pace that allows a person to carry out daily tasks).

Methods of intervention designed to increase strength and skill, endurance, fitness and wellbeing are included briefly below and the reader should refer to Chapters 2–7 for more detail. General principles of task-specific training following stroke include the following:

- Encouraging muscle activation and movement utilizing kinesiological principles such as elimination of gravity to reduce magnitude of forces required, switching between eccentric, concentric and isometric contractions. Where muscles are very weak, such techniques as functional electrical stimulation (FES) may preserve the integrity of muscle and enable an increase in strength.
- Increasing muscle strength and control using task- and context-specific repetitive exercise so that training increases strength that is relevant to the task and context (i.e., relative, not absolute strength). An added benefit of enhanced physical activity is in preventing or minimizing unwanted soft tissue changes, since active exercise increases blood flow to soft tissues and preserves tissue extensibility.
- Prevention of muscle stiffness and soft tissue contracture by active stretching during training. Muscles and muscle groups most at risk of shortening include ankle plantarflexors (particularly soleus), internal rotators and adductors of the shoulder joint, elbow flexors, forearm pronators, wrist, finger, thumb flexors and adductors. People at particular risk of developing contracture require prolonged positioning of muscles in a lengthened position to maintain range of motion.
- Increasing endurance and physical conditioning/fitness.
- Providing concrete, rather than abstract, goals to train motor control.
- Modifying the action or environment to achieve a more effective outcome if an action can only be performed with ineffective movements.

Treadmill training with and without body weight support (by suspension harness)

This is increasingly shown to be associated with positive outcomes (see Langhorne et al 2009 for review). It is an effective way to augment time spent in gait practice (Moseley et al 2005). Treadmill training with body weight support is well tolerated and effective in the early phase of recovery and may be the only means of practising gait for more severely affected and dependent walkers (Barbeau & Visintin 2003). If performed with sufficient intensity and with an increasing incline, treadmill walking can increase endurance (Moseley et al 2005) and physical fitness. A movable suspension harness attached to an overhead track, or a Lite-Gait® trainer enables a patient to practise walking without fear of falling (see Ch. 5).

Constraint of non-paretic limb and task-oriented practice

This methodology is described in detail in Chapter 6. Randomized controlled trials have shown that, in the later stages of rehabilitation, a combination of meaningful task-oriented training and intensive practice plus a strategy to enforce movement of the paretic limb can be effective in individuals who have some ability to extend actively their wrist and fingers. There is limited evidence that this methodology can be effective in the early stages and with individuals with moderate to severe activity limitations.

Training balance

Balance is the ability to control the body's centre of mass over the base of support and respond to stumbles and slips quickly enough to prevent a fall. Balance is trained simultaneously as part of functional motor actions of which balance is an integral part. Although many different types of intervention are available, some are more likely to result in improvement in balance and prevent falls; for example, challenging and progressive balance exercises performed in weightbearing positions that minimize use of the upper limbs for support (see Ch. 9). These training methods have been shown to be effective in preventing falls and improving functional motor performance (Dean et al 2000; Eng et al 2003; Salbach et al 2004; Krebs et al 2007; Lord et al 2007; Olivetti et al 2007; Sherrington et al 2008a,b).

Functional strength training

Strength training is in large part a matter of neural adaptation, improving control over muscle activation, increasing efficiency of contraction, learning again how to move and coordinate force generation relative to the functional actions being relearned. Studies in healthy subjects indicate that a number of neural adaptations occur in the process of getting stronger in terms of the ability to:

- recruit more motor units
- increase the frequency of motor unit discharge
- increase the synchronization of motor unit activity (e.g., Hakkinen & Komi 1983; Rutherford & Jones 1986; Rutherford 1988).

Lower limb strength training

Training to increase strength, endurance and motor control consists of exercises selected according to an individual's needs at a specific time. In general, the major muscle groups on which to concentrate in the lower limb are the extensors of the hips, knees and ankles, ankle dorsiflexors and hip abductors, for support, balance and propulsion. Functional weightbearing exercises are methods of choice for lower limb tasks. Exercises include repetitive practice of standing up and sitting down, step-ups and step-downs, semi-squats to reach for an object, walking overground, up and down ramps, stair climbing and descent, treadmill walking with or without body-weight support. These activities are graded to the individual's level of performance while the individual is being encouraged to increase load, increase speed and number of repetitions. The ability to balance is also being trained as an integral part of these actions. Generally speaking, progression includes increasing load to increase strength, increasing repetitions for increasing muscle endurance, and increasing speed which may increase muscle power.

The environment can be modified to enable practice; for example, a critical factor enabling a weak person to load the paretic leg to stand up and sit down is the provision of a chair that is optimal for an individual's height and strength (see Fig. 11.3). Some exercises are directly task specific, others can be expected to generalize into improved performance of similar actions. Number of repetitions should take the person to the point of muscle fatigue; without this amount of effort, progress may not be made.

Upper limb strength training

In the upper limb, strength must be sufficient for reaching, carrying, picking up and manipulating objects. Task-related upper limb strength training is necessary for dealing successfully with load: for example, carrying and manipulating objects requires variable amounts of strength depending on the weight of the object; unscrewing a jar needs a strong grasp and sufficient stabilizing muscle strength at other joints to get the job done. Strengthening exercises include lifting and lowering actions, grasping (grasp and turn, grasp and squeeze) and pushing actions. Exercises with hand weights or elastic bands can involve lifting and lowering, pulling, pushing and grasping.

Sensorimotor and perceptual–cognitive training

In general, patients with well-preserved sensation are likely to have better outcomes in rehabilitation than those who do not. More cognitively directed training developed over the last decades engages the individual in practice of meaningful everyday actions, with the environment and/or the action modified to enable participation. In this way, the neural system can select those sensory inputs relevant to the action being performed.

Specific sensory training, however, may assist the individual to regain sensitivity by attending to sensory inputs and their relation to the task being practised. For example, specific training of stereognosis may improve hand function; attending to sense of pressure and load through the feet while practising standing up and sitting down, reaching out in standing or standing up from a small squat may help the person to be more aware of loading the paretic limb.

Visuospatial perception is critical for successful interaction with the environment and the people and objects within it. Perceptual–cognitive deficits are complex and are a factor in lack of progress in many patients following stroke. Current interventions do not have high-level evidentiary support – some specific methods show promising results, however generalizability of training to untrained situations is more problematic. Chapter 10 includes some practical ways of engaging the patient by, for example, focusing attention on appropriate cues or scanning the environment.

Physical conditioning (aerobic fitness)

Emphasis in stroke rehabilitation has been primarily placed on the neurological impairments with little attention to cardiorespiratory adaptation to physical inactivity. Reduction in levels of physical activity as a consequence of stroke leads to a deterioration in both exercise capacity and physical conditioning and is a significant determinant of poor health in individuals with chronic stroke (Pang et al 2005). Added to this, many individuals following stroke are elderly and may have been deconditioned before their stroke.

Adaptation to physical inactivity after stroke further threatens the individual's ability to meet the energy demands of everyday life, particularly the elevated energy demands of gait abnormalities and activities of daily living. Low physical endurance limits the individual's ability to perform household tasks and to maintain their preferred walking pace as a result of exercise intolerance (Ryan et al 2000). Among stroke survivors investigated 1 year post-stroke, the most striking area of difficulty was low endurance as measured by the 6-minute walk test (Mayo et al 2005). Exercise training to enhance exercise capacity should be initiated early in the rehabilitation process and continue after discharge.

There are several reports of improved aerobic capacity in chronic stroke with appropriate training including bicycle ergometry (Potempa et al 1995), graded treadmill walking (Macko et al 1997, 2005; Pohl et al 2002) and a combination of aerobic and strengthening exercises (Teixeira-Salmela et al 1999). In graded treadmill training it appears that increasing speed rather than duration best optimizes the gains in aerobic fitness.

Exercise and physical activity are known to have positive effects on the able-bodied young and elderly, and in disabled individuals. The results of studies highlighting the benefits of aerobic exercise to improve both the physical and mental wellbeing of individuals following stroke suggest that all patients should participate in aerobic training unless there are contraindications such as a history of serious cardiac disease, for example myocardial infarction, or uncontrolled blood pressure (Pang et al 2005).

Intensity of training, increasing practice and dosage

It is clear from several studies of time-use during rehabilitation that only a small part of the patient's day is typically spent in exercise and training (see Ch. 1). There is evidence that rehabilitation programmes may not be sufficiently vigorous to prevent physical deconditioning (MacKay-Lyons & Makrides 2002; Kelley et al 2003). Time-use, intensity of exercise and delivery of physiotherapy during rehabilitation are currently receiving more attention. A number of reviews have shown that intensity of training, time spent in therapy as well as task specificity are the main determinants of functional improvement in stroke (Richards et al 1993; Kwakkel et al 2004; van Peppen et al 2004).

It is therefore important that physiotherapists move away from reliance on hands on, one-to-one therapy, given for a short period in the day, to a more efficient use of time, one in which patients practise in small groups in, for example, a circuit training class. One or two therapists or an aide can supervise several individuals in a group. An interesting paper gives details of the methods used to increase practice, providing evidence that this leads to improved outcomes that are retained over time (Ada et al 2006).

Results of a recent meta-analysis support the use of task-oriented circuit class training to improve walking competence and gait-related activities in chronic stroke (Wevers et al 2009). Other benefits summarized by the authors include the potential for a reduction in staff-to-patient ratios. From the individual's perspective, classes encourage group dynamics. Circuit training can start early after stroke and should not be left to the chronic stage; for example, one study in the review recruited subjects with a mean time of 43 days from stroke (Blennerhassett & Dite 2004). Classes can be customized to an individual's ability in terms of intensity, frequency and duration.

Technological developments

New technologies such as electromechanical-assisted gait trainers and arm trainers (see Mehrholz et al 2007, 2009 for systematic reviews), ceiling suspension systems with a harness for walking practice without fear of falling, computer games, virtual reality training systems (see Fig. 12.10) and non-robotic trainers have the potential to enhance motivation and increase the time spent practising. These systems are being designed as a means of overcoming the waste of rehabilitation time that typically occurs when patients spend large parts of the day inactive. For the patient who enters the rehabilitation gymnasium, these machines provide symbols of exercise and activity, exciting and challenging, suggesting activity and participation are expected.

Aids

Ankle–foot orthoses. The impact of ankle–foot orthoses on gait following stroke is equivocal. There is some evidence of immediate improvements in selected patients but there has been little long-term follow-up (Leung & Moseley 2003; Tyson & Kent 2009). The significance of kinematic and temporal changes on daily functioning, implications for the general population and the issue of compliance are largely unresearched (Leung & Moseley 2003). If a device is being considered for a particular individual, it is recommended that walking speed is measured while using the orthosis as the individual's chosen walking speed will give an indication of the relative merits or otherwise of the device (Olney 2005).

Orthoses can be designed to optimize muscle activity at a joint. For example, a small splint or strapping to hold the thumb abducted at the carpometacarpal joint enables practice of grasp and release and may optimize thumb muscle activity. Taping over the gluteus maximus on the paretic side can lead to an immediate improvement in hip extension (Kilbreath et al 2006), and may help the individual get the idea of hip extension at the end of stance phase of gait.

One-arm drive wheelchairs. The propulsion of a wheelchair with the non-paretic arm and leg is inconsistent with the aim of directing the person's attention to the paretic limbs since only the non-paretic arm and leg are being exercised. Learning to depend on a limb to substitute for an impaired limb not only reduces the use of the impaired limb but also increases the likelihood of losing any residual capacity (Kolb 1995).

Walking aids. All walking aids (parallel bars, walking frame, quadripod/four-point cane) impose some mechanical constraint. A simple *walking stick* interferes least with balance and walking and may provide some assistance.

LANGUAGE, COGNITIVE AND AFFECTIVE IMPAIRMENTS

Modern cognitive psychology and brain science have led us to appreciate that all mental processes consist of perceiving, thinking, learning and remembering, and even the simplest task requires the coordination of several regions of the brain. Impairments following stroke can be categorized as disorders of language that also interfere with cognitive function (dysphasia/aphasia); disorders of perception–cognition (i.e., of perception, orientation,

memory, executive functioning); and depression and other emotional and behavioural disturbances. All these impairments affect the individual's mental state and have the potential to affect significantly the individual's ability to participate in and benefit from rehabilitation. Perceptual–cognitive impairments, such as unilateral neglect or agnosia, are described in Chapter 10.

Aphasia

The aphasias (usually dysphasia, since there is rarely a total loss of language) are disturbances of language caused by an insult to specific regions of the brain (usually regions of the left cerebral cortex), with lesions in different parts of the cortex causing selective disturbances. The problem of understanding language is called *receptive* aphasia, and that of producing the correct word or sequence of words, *expressive* aphasia. Since language is distinguished from other kinds of human communication by its creativity, form, content and use, and since, in both its written and spoken forms, it represents social and interactive activities (Mayeux & Kandel 1991), loss or impairment has a profound effect on the individual.

The aphasias are often distinct from disorders of speech which result from weakness and incoordination of muscles controlling the vocal apparatus, which are classified as: *dysarthria*, a disturbance of articulation; *dysphonia*, a disturbance in vocalization; and *dyspraxia*, impaired planning and sequencing of muscles used for speech.

There is no universally accepted classification for the aphasias. However, several types can be distinguished (Mayeux & Kandel 1991). Wernicke's aphasia is characterized by a deficit in comprehension and severe difficulty in reading and writing. Lesions causing this problem are usually in the dominant temporal lobe. In Broca's aphasia, comprehension is usually preserved but language expression is affected. Lesions are usually in the dominant frontal lobe. Broca's aphasia, also called 'expressive' or 'non-fluent aphasia', may result in almost complete loss of language expression to a slowed, deliberate speech utilizing only key words and simple grammatical structure. Comprehension of both spoken and written language is less disturbed than in Wernicke's aphasia. Other types of aphasia include nominal aphasia, a difficulty in naming objects or people, and global aphasia, an inability to speak or comprehend language, read or write, repeat or name objects.

The stroke patient with aphasia suddenly finds he/she is unable to understand spoken language, read, speak or write and to communicate the simplest needs. These deficits isolate the individual and may, not surprisingly, lead to anger and frustration as attempts to communicate fail. Early diagnosis of language impairment by a speech pathologist is essential to identify the person's specific problems so that the family and rehabilitation team can understand the nature and extent of the communication deficits and the best ways of communicating.

Most people with aphasia experience spontaneous improvement within weeks or months of stroke (Pedersen et al 1995). However, recovery can be prolonged and persistent problems may have profound and pervading consequences for the individual's quality of life and employment opportunities, and lead to a feeling of social isolation.

Intervention varies with the type and severity of aphasia and may include: constraint-induced therapy (forced use of language); massed practice; therapies directed at optimizing preserved abilities; group training; use of communication partners; and/or computer-based therapies. At present, however, many interventions are not underpinned by high-level evidence. Earlier commencement of therapy does appear to be more effective than delaying intervention (National Stroke Foundation 2007a).

Below are some suggestions to assist physiotherapists to communicate with aphasic patients before they have the benefit of an assessment and plan of management by the speech pathologist:

- Do not exclude the individual from the conversation, or answer for him/her.
- Keep sentences short and simple without too much information.
- Provide time for the person to respond and to switch from one topic to another.
- Phrase questions so that they can be answered with yes/no or some other form of response where there is expressive aphasia.
- Use gestures, situational cues, visual prompts, facial expression to enhance communication and comprehension.
- Engage in eye contact since eye contact facilitates communication and more positive attitudes (Mehrabian 1969).
- Be honest in establishing communication and a relationship with the individual. For example, if the therapist does not understand a response, it is better to say so and ask the individual to try again. Prompts such as 'Is it about your appointment time?' may help, as may diverting behaviour if the individual becomes very frustrated.
- Discourage perseveration on words and phrases as it interferes with real communication.

Disorders of speech execution, *dysarthria*, due to facial muscle paresis and/or sensory loss, may lead to problems eating and dribbling, which can be of great concern to the person and their families. Some clinicians report success with facial muscle re-education using exercise with visual feedback. Often muscle weakness improves over time.

Cognitive function

Approximately two-thirds of stroke survivors experience difficulties with carrying out mental tasks that require processes such as attention, memory, orientation, language and executive function. This impaired cognitive function is associated with poorer recovery from stroke, higher rates of institutionalization, poorer quality of life and higher healthcare costs (Claesson et al 2005; Pasquini et al 2007). Early screening by a trained clinician is essential. More detailed assessment should help clinicians and families understand how best to manage the person with cognitive impairment.

It should be noted that neuropsychological tests of cognition may demonstrate a variety of impairments in elderly stroke patients, not all of which would have a marked effect on everyday life. Some impairments may have been present before stroke with no apparent effect upon ability to function in their own environment. It is likely that these individuals may have coped quite well with everyday levels of stress despite certain cognitive impairments. Clearly, however, some patients with pre-existing impairments in cognitive function are unable to cope with the demands placed on them by the new sensorimotor and/or language impairments following stroke and the stress imposed by the unfamiliar environment in which they find themselves. All patients with apparent cognitive problems require evaluation and the development of treatment plans to help them participate actively in the rehabilitation process.

There is an ongoing debate concerning the effectiveness of cognitive retraining. For example, a systematic review found that interventions directed at improving attention improved attention but had no functional overflow (Lincoln et al 2000). External cues (e.g., pager) for memory deficits may help prompt memory, and may also be used to help patients plan, solve problems and self-monitor (executive function), but studies are inconclusive. Interestingly, physical activity has now been shown to have a positive effect on cognitive function in a range of populations (Heyn et al 2004). At present, however, there is no clear evidence of benefit in people with stroke. Meanwhile the physiotherapist and other clinicians have to deal daily with patients with perceptual–cognitive impairments (see Ch. 10). As a good rule of thumb, therapists should consider the following when working with such a person:

- Keep information simple.
- Reduce the amount of information given at any one time.
- Ensure there is minimal distraction.
- Make sure information is understood; for example, ask the person to repeat the information in his or her own words.
- Encourage the person to link or associate information with material already known.
- Encourage the person to ask questions.
- Use the 'little and often' rule (Baddeley 1992).
- Make sure learning occurs in different contexts to promote generalization.

Other strategies include rearranging the environment; for example, having rooms clearly labelled or direction markers on the floor, so that the individual has to rely less on memory. Use of external aids such as notebooks, diaries, microcassettes and personal digital assistants (PDAs), mobile phones and other electronic recording devices should also be encouraged. These are strategies we all use. Wilson (1995) reports how a woman who could not find her way around a rehabilitation centre dictated the directions onto a microcassette that she listened to when she needed to find a particular department.

Dementia

Dementia is a serious and progressive decline in mental function, in memory and in acquired intellectual skills (Srikanth et al 2003). Stroke can contribute to progressive mental decline, but rarely is the sole cause of dementia.

Normal ageing is associated with characteristic changes in the brain and behaviour that vary widely among individuals but in most cases do not seriously compromise the quality of life. Although dementia is age related, it is not an inevitable consequence of ageing and many individuals age without substantial loss of intellect. The neurobiological processes of age-related mental changes are poorly understood (Goldman & Côté 1991).

Depression

Sudden stroke comes as a huge shock to most people and it is normal for a patient's mood to be affected. However, in one-fifth to one-third of patients, more severe and prolonged symptoms of depression appear within the first year of stroke. Diagnosing depression is difficult, particularly early following stroke, when symptoms of stroke (e.g., aphasia, flat affect or monotonous voice, emotional lability) and/or changes in sleep patterns or fatigue can mask or mimic symptoms of depression (Lindley 2008).

Nevertheless, it is well recognized that this common complication following stroke often goes undiagnosed and untreated. Therapists and nurses are often the ones who notice symptoms first (Lindley 2008) and family may also help diagnose changes in mood. Stroke-associated depression can impede rehabilitation and place stress on carers, and has been associated with increased risk of death, including death from suicide (Hackett et al 2008).

While spontaneous recovery from depression is possible, depression persists in about one-third of cases. Pharmacological treatments have shown benefits in people with stroke, however they are also associated with increased harm (Hackett et al 2008) and need to be carefully prescribed after accurate diagnosis. Counselling and problem-solving interventions can also be tried (National Stroke Foundation 2007a), but evidence is limited.

There appears to be a strong association between self-efficacy (the degree to which a patient feels in control of their own management), self-care and depression in stroke patients undergoing rehabilitation (Robinson-Smith et al 2000). Identifying strategies to improve patient confidence and expectations of self care should be an important goal of the rehabilitation team and here too exercise may play an important role.

Other emotional and behavioural disturbances

Anxiety, emotionalism (frequent crying), outbursts of uncontrolled behaviour and hostility can also occur following stroke but are much less common than depression (Agency for Health Care Policy and Research 1995). Apathy and 'undue cheerfulness' have also been described, particularly in individuals with right hemisphere stroke (Price 1990). There are no proven treatments for these mood disorders, but spontaneous recovery does occur in some cases. Positive attitudes towards the individual by all members of staff often help patients and families cope with these changes. Having the patient dress as soon as possible in day clothes and encouraging both men and women to take an interest in their appearance all help to improve an individual's self-image and have a positive effect on all those with whom the person comes in contact.

If a patient appears unmotivated, the cause should be investigated. There is consensus among rehabilitation professionals that a patient's level of motivation will influence outcome. Motivation, however, is not easy to measure, and personal (e.g., gender, personality, education coping capacity, etc.) as well as environmental factors (being in hospital, staff expectations, degree of autonomy) interact in complex ways. It is difficult, if not impossible, to separate the effect of damage to the brain following stroke from personal and environmental factors when considering a patient's level of motivation. Decades ago Seligman described a phenomenon he called learned helplessness, or passivity. A recent study has shown that patients undergoing rehabilitation reported being strongly influenced by a range of environmental factors such as the unstimulating hospital environment, overprotective family and nurses, the way in which information is communicated by health professionals and the making of comparisons with other patients' performance (Holmqvist 2001). Involving patients in goal setting and planning of their rehabilitation program has been shown to improve motivation. As therapists, we need to find ways to overcome the barriers to patient involvement that are often inherent in the physical structure and/or the established processes and policies of rehabilitation environments.

Dysphagia

Dysphagia, or difficulty swallowing, affects up to half of all people affected by stroke and may lead to aspiration of saliva, food or liquids. As a consequence, immediately after a stroke, eating and drinking are not allowed until swallowing ability has been carefully checked. Medical complications associated with dysphagia include aspiration pneumonia, malnutrition and dehydration. 'Silent' aspiration is common and early detection and treatment are important in preventing both aspiration and dehydration from inadequate oral intake. People with dysphagia often require additional fluids via intravenous, subcutaneous or enteral (using a nasogastric tube or percutaneous endoscopic gastrostomy (PEG)) routes. Strategies to prevent complications include: fluid and diet modification to make food and drink thicker and safer to swallow; sitting a person upright in a chair during meals, with the head tilted slightly down; and use of safe swallowing strategies (National Stroke Foundation 2007a). These include: taking small mouthfuls of food and small sips of fluids; alternate mouthfuls of food and drink; closing the jaw; allow a number of swallows after each mouthful; using a cup with a spout for fluids; taking time during meals and stopping if the voice sounds 'wet' or if there is coughing, choking or pooling of food in the mouth.

In many individuals, swallowing function returns within the first few weeks of stroke. Videofluoroscopy using a modified barium swallow may be used to evaluate the pharyngeal phase of swallowing and the mechanism of aspiration in patients whose problem persists beyond the early stage of recovery. The testing of therapies for dysphagia is relatively new, however resisted exercises, specialized electrical simulation and thermal tactile simulation show promise (National Stroke Foundation 2007a). Those with severe dysphagia who do not respond to training may require nasogastric tube feeding.

Bladder and bowel function

Urinary incontinence is common but usually transient following stroke. Clearly, some of the problems are related to motor and sensory impairments, difficulty communicating (which interferes with making the need known to others), enforced immobility, as well as cognitive and perceptual deficits and inability to recognize the need to void. There is, however, some evidence of neurological deficits leading to either retention or overflow or both (e.g., Gelber et al 1993). Gelber and colleagues summarize the major mechanisms for post-stroke incontinence as: disruption of the neuromicturition pathways resulting in bladder hyporeflexia and urge incontinence; functional incontinence associated with cognitive and language deficits, with normal bladder function; and bladder hyporeflexia and overflow incontinence associated with concurrent neuropathy or medication. Each type of dysfunction requires targeted management. Careful assessment of continence status and medication use, and a clear diagnosis are important to continence management. Post-void bladder scanning is becoming more common as a technique to guide assessment and management following stroke. In cases where incontinence persists, urodynamic studies may also be useful in diagnosing the cause of incontinence and a urologist referral should be requested.

Early assumption of the standing position and early ambulation can help individuals overcome incontinence.

Use of a commode or toilet should be encouraged rather than a bed pan or bottle. Men should be encouraged to stand to void.

For people with urge incontinence, a prompted voiding schedule (where staff prompt an individual to go to the toilet at regular intervals) combined with anticholinergic drugs and bladder retraining can help. A bladder retraining programme may use a range of techniques including timed voiding (development of a schedule that fits with a person's habits and aims to reduce 'accidents'), pelvic floor exercises and use of distraction and relaxation techniques to extend time between toilet stops. For people with urinary retention, intermittent catheterization for those with severe retention is favoured over routine use of indwelling catheters. For those people with functional incontinence, the whole team need to be aware of the cues provided by the person indicating a need to toilet and respond quickly and appropriately. Clothing that accommodates the person's dexterity should be provided and toilet signage may need to be more clearly marked.

Therapists should always be aware of continence problems and communicate clearly with the nursing staff about any programmes underway in order to reinforce voiding cues, ensure access to toilet facilities and avoid embarrassing accidents during treatment which add to the individual's loss of self-esteem and interfere with time spent in active rehabilitation. Containment aids (pads) can help reduce the incidence of obvious accidents but should not be the only form of management for those affected by incontinence.

Alteration in bowel function, either diarrhoea or constipation, may be associated with immobility. Constipation is by far the more common and is assessed and treated by paying attention to pre- and post-stroke bowel habits, diet, fluid intake, laxative use and activity.

PATIENT AND FAMILY EDUCATION

The provision of education to both patients and families is considered a key feature of organized stroke care and stroke survivors and families express a strong need for information (National Stroke Foundation 2007a). Many models of education exist, however education programmes typically include lectures and/or group discussions on the pathophysiology of stroke, the adaptability of the brain, the physical and emotional affects of stroke, ways of communicating, coping strategies and how to prevent further strokes.

Education is probably a very helpful part of the recovery process, yet little is know about the best time to engage patients and their families in education or the most effective method of providing the information they seek. It is likely that education needs to be offered at multiple time points in the recovery process and there is some evidence to suggest that allowing patients and carers a number of opportunities to ask questions and seek clarification can reduce stress and depression (Smith et al 2007). In the early stages after stroke, patients and their families may feel overwhelmed. Nevertheless, as many patients are discharged directly home after a period of acute care, education provision needs to occur here. Education programmes offered in rehabilitation are often more comprehensive and may also address the challenges of transition to home after long periods in hospital, and carer and patient support in the home environment. Today, many stroke support agencies provide access to education materials for survivors, often in a range of languages, and these can be a good resource for clinicians.

THE ROLE OF THE FAMILY IN STROKE RECOVERY

The effects of stroke and stroke rehabilitation are mostly described in terms of functional gains. The consequences of stroke on everyday life of the patient and family are typically inadequately described and poorly understood. Patients are seldom asked to evaluate their experiences during rehabilitation although there are several insightful publications written by individuals who have survived a stroke and rehabilitation (e.g., Griffiths 1970; Brodal 1973; Smits & Smits-Boon 2000; O'Kelly 2005; Bolte Taylor 2008).

Major challenges for the individual after a stroke are coming to terms with the losses associated with disability or handicap, coping with a changed identity as a disabled person and with the way this affects self-image and social relationships. The process of adjustment may take considerable time and go through several phases (Lewinter & Mikkelsen 1995).

There is some evidence that family interactions can affect eventual outcome either positively or negatively (Evans et al 1987). This probably depends on the strength of the relationship prior to stroke. Family members often help to reinforce therapeutic objectives, however Evans and colleagues (1992) caution that expecting families to assist with treatment when they are not coping well themselves can be counterproductive. Family members contribute to patient recovery through provision of emotional and practical support and the level of support provided by family can influence the rate and extent of recovery (Tsouna-Hadjis et al 2000).

The majority of individuals who survive a stroke return to live at home and the alteration in family lifestyle can be considerable. In a review of the literature, Evans and colleagues (1992) identified the need for family education, advocacy and supportive counselling to foster cooperation and social support after stroke.

There are several clinical studies that indicate that the level of functioning at discharge from rehabilitation decreases after that discharge (e.g., Paolucci et al 2001). A survey in the UK showed a paucity of follow-up services beyond the most basic of community therapy or support. This was compounded by poor communication between professionals and between patients, carers and professionals, and high levels of patient dissatisfaction and low expectations by professionals of patients' abilities (Tyson & Turner 2000). Both inadequate family education and preparation for the patient's return home may be reasons for these findings. Another reason may be a lack of emphasis on the need for continuing exercise and training after discharge.

Sexual concerns are rarely addressed by the patient, spouse or professional team, yet sexual dysfunction has been found to be common after stroke (Monga et al 1986) and a source of disharmony in a relationship. In a semi-structured interview in which individuals were asked to report on their experiences in rehabilitation, those interviewed expressed a need for more sexual counselling (Lewinter & Mikkelsen 1995). One subject reported that sexual concerns were a taboo subject and that some staff members 'fled' when it was introduced, highlighting the need for sexual issues to be addressed during rehabilitation. The first national rehabilitation audit in Australia found that only 13% of patients were offered advice about sexual issues after stroke (National Stroke Foundation 2008). Many post-stroke sexual problems are related to emotional causes such as fear, dependency in self-care, anxiety and changes in body image.

DISCHARGE PLANNING AND RETURN TO THE COMMUNITY

One of the most poorly managed areas of the stroke recovery pathway is return to the community. Patients who return home directly after even a short period of acute hospital care are often extremely anxious and at a loss about how to go on with their lives. Those patients who return home after longer periods of hospitalization can have great difficulty (as can their families) in adjusting to life back in the community. Many patients express a feeling of being 'abandoned' by their treating teams (National Stroke Foundation 2007a). Major oversights in post-discharge stroke management include lack of community exercise facilities for the disabled, lack of carer support and poor access to transport. There has been little emphasis on the obvious need for individuals with disability to continue exercise and training post-discharge, not only to maintain but also to progress their functional abilities and levels of physical fitness.

In some hospitals, supported discharge programmes have been used with good effect to ease transition of patients from acute services back into the community (Early Supported Discharge Trialists 2004). However, supported discharge programmes vary widely and many services are focused on reducing hospital length of stay rather than improving the experience of transition for the stroke survivor. One model in Norway (Indredavik et al 2000) is focused on helping patients make the transition to home-based care through the use of a dedicated coordinator. This individual liaises between family and support services and provides a stable point of contact for the patient and their family as they negotiate their way through the first months of transition to home. Patients managed under this model have shown excellent long-term outcomes (Fjaertoft et al 2003).

In the long term, stroke survivors and their families often move from reliance on hospital-based support services to community-based supports. In a follow-up study carried out in Sweden 5–6 years after stroke, patients who experienced a good quality of life were all married, lived at home, participated in active leisure activities and were continuing to train/exercise on their own (Wadell et al 1987). Locally run stroke support groups can link individuals with other stroke survivors in their community, and this social support may be of great benefit to some survivors and their families.

Ongoing participation in exercise is important for all stroke survivors. Exercise helps maintain fitness and participation, but also has a very real protective function, helping to prevent recurrent stroke and further cardiovascular disease, reducing the risk of falls, increasing physical independence and improving quality of life (Gordon et al 2004). Exercises directed at maintaining or improving aerobic function, strength, flexibility and neuromuscular control are all strongly recommended for stroke survivors (Gordon et al 2004). The challenge for many survivors is finding a person with the right expertise to assist with the prescription and supervision of their programme and finding a suitable community-based venue. As with healthy individuals, exercise prescription needs to consider personal preferences and it is unlikely that there will ever be a 'one size fits all' programme. Nevertheless, physiotherapists are well placed to have a major role in this area and further development of post-stroke exercise programmes is urgently needed.

In conclusion, there have been considerable advances in the early recognition, faster assessment and early thrombolytic treatment of acute stroke in the 10 years since the first edition of this book was published. Major advances in knowledge have also increased our understanding of the impairments resulting from an acute stroke, the nature of adaptive changes in muscle and their effects on function. Advances in physiotherapy practice based on scientific findings in motor learning, exercise science and biomechanics and research into the effects of new rehabilitation methods are contributing to the development of an increasingly sound evidence base. There are encouraging findings that many methods used by physiotherapists have the potential to improve outcome. Research using advanced imaging techniques shows that the brain can reorganize after damage as individuals relearn functional tasks, with many repetitions and a great deal of exercise and practice. The National Stroke Foundation in Australia pointed out recently, referring to acute care, that 'organized stroke care remains the cornerstone of effective stroke care and must remain the priority …' (2007b). The next step in stroke rehabilitation must be a move to science- and evidence-based practice, and to an organized programme of intensive task-oriented rehabilitation.

REFERENCES

Ada L, Dean CM, Mackey FH 2006 Increasing the amount of physical activity undertaken after stroke. Phys Ther Rev 11:91–100.

Adams HJ, Adams R, Brott T et al 2003 Guidelines for the early management of patients with ischemic stroke: a scientific statement from the Stroke Council of the American Stroke Association. Stroke 34:1056–1083.

Agency for Health Care Policy and Research (AHCPR) 1995 Clinical practice guidelines, 16. Poststroke rehabilitation. US Department of Health and Human Services, Rockville, MD.

Albers GW, Caplan LR, Easton JD et al 2002 Transient ischemic attack – proposal for a new definition. New Engl J Med 347:1713–1716.

Appelros P, Nydevik I, Viitanen M 2003 Poor outcome after first-ever stroke: predictors of death, dependency, and recurrent stroke within the first year. Stroke 34:122–126.

Australian Institute of Health and Welfare (AIH) 2004 Heart, stroke and vascular diseases – Australian facts 2004. Australian Institute of Health and Welfare, National Heart Foundation, National Stroke Foundation of Australia:528.

Baddeley AD 1992 Memory theory and memory therapy. In: Wilson BA, Moffat N (eds) Clinical management of memory problems, 2nd edn. Chapman and Hall, London:1–31.

Bakke F 1995 The acute treatment of stroke. In: Harrison MA, Rustad RA (eds) Physiotherapy in stroke management. Edinburgh, Churchill Livingstone:215–222.

Bamford J, Dennis M, Sandercock P et al 1990 The frequency, causes and timing of death within 30 days of a first stroke: the Oxfordshire Community Stroke Project. J Neurol Neurosurg Psychiatry 53:824–829.

Bamford J, Sandercock P, Dennis M et al 1991 Classification and natural history of clinically identifiable subtypes of cerebral infarction. Lancet 337:1521–1526.

Barbeau H, Visintin M 2003 Optimal outcomes obtained with body-weight support combined with treadmill training in stroke subjects. Arch Phys Med Rehabil 84:1458–1465.

Barer DH, Mitchell JRA 1989 Predicting the outcome of acute stroke: do multivariate models help? Q J Med 74:27–39.

Bernhardt J 2008 Very early mobilization following acute stroke: controversies, the unknowns and a way forward. Ann Indian Acad Neurol 11:S88–S98.

Bernhardt J, Dewey H, Collier J et al 2006 A Very Early Rehabilitation Trial (AVERT). Int J Stroke 1:169–171.

Bernhardt J, Chitravas N, Lidarende MI et al 2008 Not all stroke units are the same: a comparison of physical activity patterns in Melbourne, Australia and Trondheim, Norway. Stroke 39:2059–2065

Bernhardt J, Thuy MNT, Collier J et al 2009 Very early versus delayed mobilisation after stroke. Cochrane Database Syst Rev Issue 1: Art.No.: CD006187.DOI:10.1002114651858. CD006187.pub2.

Blennerhassett J, Dite W 2004 Additional task-related practice improves mobility and upper limb function early after stroke: a randomized controlled trial. Aust J Physiother 50:219–224.

Bolte Taylor J 2008 My stroke of insight. Hodder and Stoughton, London.

Bonita R, Beaglehole R 1988 Recovery of motor function after stroke. Stroke 19:1497–1500.

Brodal A 1973 Self-observation and neuroanatomical considerations after a stroke. Brain 96:675–694.

Brust JCM 1991 Cerebral circulation: stroke. In: Kandel ER, Schwartz JH, Jessell TM (eds) Principles of Neural Science, 3rd edn. Appleton and Lange, Norwalk, CT:1041–1049.

Burke D 1988 Spasticity as an adaptation to pyramidal tract injury. In: Waxman SG (ed.) Advances in neurology, 47. Functional recovery in neurological disease. Raven Press, New York:401–423.

Calautti C, Baron J 2003 Functional neuroimaging studies of motor recovery after stroke in adults: a review. Stroke 34:1553–1566.

Carey LM 2006 Loss of somatic sensation. In: Selzer M, Clarke S, Cohen L et al (eds) Textbook of neural repair and rehabilitation. CUP, Cambridge:231–247.

Carr JH, Shepherd RB 2003 Stroke rehabilitation. Guidelines for exercise and training to optimize motor skill. Butterworth Heinemann, Oxford.

Cifu DX, Stewart DG 1996 A comprehensive, annotated reference guide to outcome after stroke. Crit Rev Phys Rehabil Med 8:39–86.

Claesson L, Linden T, Skoog I et al 2005 Cognitive impairment after stroke – impact on activities of daily living and costs of care for elderly people. The Goteborg 70+ Stroke Study. Cerebrovasc Dis 19:102–109.

Counsell C, Dennis M, McDowall M et al 2002 Predicting outcome after acute and subacute stroke: development and validation of new prognostic models. Stroke 33:1041–1047.

Cumming TB, Collier J, Thrift AG et al 2008 The effect of very early mobilisation after stroke on psychological well-being. J Rehabil Med 40:609–614.

Dean CM, Richards CL, Malouin F 2000 Task-related circuit training improves performance of locomotor tasks in chronic stroke: a randomized controlled pilot trial. Arch Phys Med Rehabil 81:409–417.

Dewey H, Bernhardt J 2007 Acute stroke patients. Early hospital management. Aust Fam Physician 36:904–912.

Dewey H, Thrift A, Mihalopoulos C et al 2001 The cost of stroke in Australia from a societal perspective: results from the North East Melbourne Stroke Incidence Study (NEMESIS). Stroke 32:2409–2416.

Dewey HM, Thrift AG, Mihalopoulos C et al 2002 Informal care for stroke survivors: results from the North East Melbourne Stroke Incidence Study (NEMESIS). Stroke 33:1028–1033.

Diserens K, Michel P, Bogousslavsky J 2006 Early mobilisation after stroke: review of the literature. Cerebrovasc Dis 22:183–190.

Dombovy ML, Sandok BA, Basford JR 1986 Rehabilitation for stroke: a review. Stroke 17:363–369.

Early Supported Discharge Trialists 2004 Services for reducing duration of hospital care for acute stroke patients. Cochrane Database Syst Rev Issue 4: Art.No.: CD000443. DOI:10.1002/14651858.CD000443. pub2.

Eng JJ, Chu KS, Kin CM 2003 A community-based group exercise program for persons with chronic stroke. Med Sci Sports Exerc 35:1271–1278.

Evans RL, Bishop DS, Matlock AL et al 1987 Family interaction and treatment adherence after stroke. Arch Phys Med Rehabil 68:513–517.

Evans RL, Hendricks RD, Haselkorn JK et al 1992 The family's role in stroke rehabilitation. A review of the literature. Am J Phys Med Rehabil 71:135–139.

Feigin VL, Lawes CMM, Bennettt DA et al 2003 Stroke epidemiology: a review of population-based studies of incidence, prevalence, and case-fatality in the late 20th century. Lancet Neurol 2:43–53.

Fjaertoft H, Indredavik B, Lydersen S 2003 Stroke unit care combined with early supported discharge: long-term follow-up of a randomized controlled trial. Stroke 34:2687–2962.

Gelber DA, Good DC, Laven LJ et al 1993 Causes of urinary incontinence after acute stroke. Stroke 24:378–382.

Goldman J, Côté L 1991 Aging of the brain: dementia of the Alzheimer's type. In: Kandel ER, Schwartz JH, Jessell TM (eds) Principles of neural science. Appleton and Lange, Norwalk, CT:974–983.

Gordon N, Gulanick M, Costa F et al 2004 Physical activity and exercise recommendations for stroke survivors. Circulation 109:2031–2041.

Gracies J 2005a Pathophysiology of spastic paresis. I: paresis and soft tissue changes. Muscle Nerve 31:535–551.

Gracies JM 2005b Pathophysiology of spastic paresis. II: emergence of muscle overactivity. Muscle Nerve 31:552–571.

Griffiths V 1970 A stroke in the family. Pitman, London.

Hackett ML, Anderson CS, House A et al 2008 Interventions for treating depression after stroke. Cochrane Database Syst Rev Issue 4: Art. No.: CD003437. DOI 10.1002/14651858. CD003437.pub3.

Hakkinen K, Komi PV 1983 Electromyographic changes during strength training and detraining. Med Sci Sports Exerc 15:455–460.

Hatano S 1976 Experience from a multicentre stroke register: a preliminary report. Bull World Health Organ 54:541–553.

Hayes SH, Carroll SR 1986 Early intervention care in the acute stroke patient. Arch Phys Med Rehabil 67:319–321.

Heyn P, Abreu BC, Ottenbacher KJ 2004 The effects of exercise training on elderly persons with cognitive impairment and dementia: a meta-analysis. Arch Phys Med Rehabil 85:1694–1704.

Holmqvist LW 2001 Environmental factors in stroke rehabilitation: being in hospital itself demotivates patients. BMJ 322:1501–1502.

Indredavik B, Bakke F, Slordahl S et al 1991 Benefits of a stroke unit: a randomized controlled trial. Stroke 22:1026–1031.

Indredavik B, Bakke RPT, Slordahl SA et al 1999 Treatment in a combined acute and rehabilitation stroke unit: which aspects are most important? Stroke 30:917–923.

Indredavik B, Fjaertoft H, Ekeberg G et al 2000 Benefit of an extended stroke unit service with early supported discharge: a randomized controlled trial. Stroke 31:2989–2994.

Johansson B 2000 Brain plasticity and stroke rehabilitation. The Willis lecture. Stroke 31:223–230.

Johnston KC, Connors AF, Wagner DP et al 2003 Predicting outcome in ischemic stroke: external validation of predictive risk models. Stroke 34:200–202.

Jørgensen HS, Nakayama H, Raaschou HO et al 1995 Outcome and time course of recovery in stroke. Part 1: outcome. The Copenhagen stroke study. Arch Phys Med Rehabil 76:399–405.

Kandel ER, Schwartz JH, Jessell TM 1991 Principles of neural science. Appleton and Lange, Norwalk, CT.

Kelley JO, Kilbreath SL, Davis GM et al 2003 Cardiorespiratory fitness and walking ability in subacute stroke patients. Arch Phys Med Rehabil 84:1780–1785.

Kilbreath S, Perkins S, Crosbie J et al 2006 Gluteal taping improves hip extension during stance phase of walking following stroke. Aust J Physiother 52:53–56.

Kolb B 1995 Brain, plasticity and behavior. Lawrence Erlbaum Associates, Mahwah, NJ.

Kollen BJ, Lennon S, Lyons B et al 2009 The effectiveness of the Bobath

concept in stroke rehabilitation: what is the evidence? Stroke 40:e89–97.

Krebs DE, Scarborough DM, McGibbon CA 2007 Functional vs strength training in disabled elderly outpatients. Am J Phys Med Rehabil 86:93–103.

Kwakkel G, van Peppen R, Wagenaar RC et al 2004 Effects of augmented exercise therapy time after stroke: a meta analysis. Stroke 35:2529–2536.

Landau WM 1988 Parables of palsy, pills and PT pedagogy: a spastic dialectic. Neurology 38:1496–1499.

Langhorne P 2000 Organisation of acute stroke care. Br Med Bull 56:436–443.

Langhorne P, Coupar F, Pollack A 2009 Motor recovery after stroke: a systematic review. Lancet Neurol 8:741–754.

Leung J, Moseley A 2003 Impact of ankle–foot orthoses on gait and leg muscle activity in adults with hemiplegia. Physiotherapy 89:39–55.

Lewinter M, Mikkelsen S 1995 Patients' experience of rehabilitation after stroke. Disabil Rehabil 17:3–9.

Lincoln NB, Jackson JM, Edmans JA et al 1990 The accuracy of predictions about progress of patients on a stroke unit. J Neurol Neurosurg Psychiatry 53:972–975.

Lincoln NB, Majid MJ, Weyman N 2000 Cognitive rehabilitaiton for attention deficits following stroke. Cochrane Database Syst Rev Issue 4, Art.No.: CD002842.D01:10.1002/14651858. ID002842.

Lindley RI 2008 Stroke. Oxford University Press, Oxford.

Lindsay P, Bayley M, Hellings C et al 2008 Canadian best practice recommendations for stroke care (updated 2008). CMAJ, 179:e-supplement. Online. Available: http://www.cmaj.ca/content/vol179/issue12/#supplement.

Lord S, Sherrington C, Menz H et al 2007 Falls in older people. Cambridge University Press, Cambridge.

MacKay-Lyons MJ, Makrides L 2002 Cardiovascular stress during a contemporary stroke rehabilitation program: is the intensity adequate to induce a training effect? Arch Phys Med Rehabil 83:1378–1383.

Macko RF, DeSouza CA, Tretter LD et al 1997 Treadmill aerobic training reduces the energy expenditure and

cardiovascular demands of hemiparetic gait in chronics stroke patients: a preliminary report. Stroke 28:326–330

Macko RF, Ivey FM, Forrester LW et al 2005 Treadmill exercise rehabilitation improves ambulatory function and cardiovascular fitness in patients with chronic stroke. Stroke 36:2206–2211.

Mayeux R, Kandel R 1991 Disorders of language: the aphasias. In: Kandel ER, Schwartz JH, Jessell TM (eds) Principles of neural science. Appleton and Lange, Norwalk, CT:834–851.

Mayo NE, Wood-Dauphine S, Ahmed S et al 2005 Disablement following stroke. Disabil Rehabil 27:258–268.

Mehrabian A 1969 Significance of posture and position in the communication of attitude and status relationships. Psychol Bull 71:359–372.

Mehrholz J, Weiner C, Kugler J et al 2007 Electromechanical-assisted gait training for walking after stroke. Cochrane Database Syst Rev Issue 4. Art. No.: CD006185. DOI: 10.1002/14651858.CD006185.pub2.

Mehrholz J, Platz T, Kugler J et al 2009 Electromechanical and robot-assisted arm training for improving arm function and activities of daily living after stroke. Cochrane Database Syst Rev Issue 4. Art. No.: CD006876. DOI: 10.1002/14651858.CD006876. pub2.

Monga TN, Lawson JS, Inglis J 1986 Sexual adjustment in stroke patients. Arch Phys Med Rehabil 67:19–22.

Moseley A, Stark A, Cameron ID et al 2005 Treadmill training and body weight support for walking after stroke. Cochrane Database Syst Rev Issue 4. Art. No.: CD002840. DOI: 10.1002/14651858. CD002840.pub2.

National Stroke Foundation 2005 Clinical guidelines for stroke rehabilitation and recovery. National Stroke Foundation, Melbourne.

National Stroke Foundation 2007a Clinical guidelines for acute stroke management. National Stroke Foundation, Melbourne.

National Stroke Foundation 2007b Walk in our shoes: stroke survivors and carers report on support after stroke. National Stroke Foundation, Melbourne.

National Stroke Foundation 2008 National stroke audit post acute services. National Stroke Foundation, Melbourne.

Newham DJ 2005 Muscle performance after stroke. In: Refshauge K, Ada L, Ellis E (eds) Science-based rehabilitation: theories into practice. Elsevier, Oxford:67–86.

Nudo RJ 2003 Functional and structural plasticity in motor cortex: implications for stroke recovery. Phys Med Rehabil Clin N Am 14:S57–S76.

O'Kelly D 2005 A patient's perspective. In: Barnes M, Dobkin B, Bogousslavsky J (eds) Recovery after stroke. Cambridge University Press, Cambridge:637–645.

Olivetti L, Schurr K, Sherrington C et al 2007 A novel weight-bearing strengthening program during rehabilitation of older people is feasible and improves standing up more than a non-weight-bearing strengthening program: a randomized trial. Aust J Physiother 53:147–153.

Olney SJ 2005 Training gait after stroke: a biomechanical perspective. In: Refshauge K, Ada L, Ellis E (eds) Science-based rehabilitation: theories into practice. Elsevier, Oxford:159–184.

Pang MYC, Eng JJ, Dawson AS et al 2005 A community-based fitness and mobility exercise program for older adults with chronic stroke: a randomized, controlled trial. J Am Geriatr Soc 53:1667–1674.

Paolucci S, Grasso MG, Antonucci G et al 2001 Mobility status after inpatient stroke rehabilitation: 1 year follow-up and prognostic factors. Arch Phys Med Rehabil 82:2–8.

Pasquini M, Leys D, Rousseaux M et al 2007 Influence of cognitive impairment on the institutionalisation rate 3 years after a stroke. J Neurol Neurosurg Psychiatry 78:56–59.

Patel AT, Duncan P, Lai SM et al 2000 The relation between impairments and functional outcomes poststroke. Arch Phys Med Rehabil 81:1357–1363.

Pedersen PM, Jorgensen HS, Nakayama H et al 1995 Aphasia in acute stroke: incidence, determinants and recovery. Ann Neurol 38:659–666.

Pohl M, Mehrholz J, Ritschel C et al 2002 Speed-dependent treadmill training in ambulatory hemiparetic stroke patients: a randomized controlled trial. Stroke 33:553–558.

Potempa K, Lopez M, Braun LT et al 1995 Physiological outcomes of aerobic exercise training in hemiparetic stroke patients. Stroke 26:101–105.

Price TR 1990 Affective disorders after stroke. Stroke 21(Suppl 11):12–13.

Richards CL, Malouin, F, Wood-Dauphinee S et al 1993 Task-specific physical therapy for optimization of gait recovery in acute stroke patients. Arch Phys Med Rehabil 74:612–620.

Robinson-Smith G, Johnston MV, Allen J 2000 Self-care self-efficacy, quality of life and depression after stroke. Arch Phys Med Rehabil 81:460–464.

Rutherford OM 1988 Muscular coordination and strength training implications for injury rehabilitation. Sports Med 5:196–202.

Rutherford OM, Jones DA 1986 The role of learning and coordination in strength training. Eur J Appl Physiol 55:100–105.

Ryan AS, Dobrovolny L, Silver KH et al 2000 Cardiovascular fitness after stroke: role of muscle mass and deficit severity. J Stroke Cerebrovasc Disord 9:1–8.

Salbach NM, Mayo NE, Wood-Dauphinee S et al 2004 A task-orientated intervention enhances walking distance and speed in the first year post stroke: a randomized controlled trial. Clin Rehabil 18:509–519.

Saver JL 2006 Time is brain – quantified. Stroke 37:263–266.

Sherrington C, Pamphlett PI, Jacka J et al 2008a Group exercise can improve participants' mobility in an outpatient rehabilitation setting: a randomized controlled trial. Clin Rehabil 22:493–502.

Sherrington C, Whitney JC, Lord SR et al 2008b Effective exercise for the prevention of falls: a systematic review and meta-analysis. J Am Geriatr Soc 56:2234–2243.

Smith J, Forster A, House A et al 2007 Information provision for stroke patients and their caregivers. Cochrane Database Syst Rev Issue 3 Art.No.: CD001919. DOI10.1002/14651858. CD001918.pub2.

Smits JG, Smits-Boone EC 2000 Hand recovery after stroke: exercise and results measurements. Butterworth Heinemann, Oxford.

Srikanth VK, Thrift AG, Saling MM et al 2003 Increased risk of cognitive impairment 3 months after mild to moderate first-ever stroke: a community-based prospective study of nonaphasic English-speaking survivors. Stroke 34:1136–1143.

Tay-Teo K, Moodie M, Bernhardt J et al 2008 Economic evaluation alongside a phase II, multi-centre, randomised controlled trial of very early rehabilitation after stroke (AVERT). Cerebrovasc Dis 26:475–481.

Teixeira-Salmela L, Olney SJ, Nadeau S et al 1999 Muscle strength and physical conditioning to reduce impairment and disability in chronic stroke survivors. Arch Phys Med Rehabil 80:1211–1218.

Tsouna-Hadjis E, Vemmos KN, Zakopoulos N et al 2000 First-stroke recovery process: the role of family social support. Arch Phys Med Rehabil 81:881–887.

Tyson SF, Kent RM 2009 Orthotic devices after stroke and other non-progressive brain lesions. Cochrane Database Syst Rev. Article withdrawn.

Tyson S, Turner G 2000 Discharge and follow-up for people with stroke: what happens and why. Clin Rehabil 14:381–392.

van Peppen RP, Kwakkel G, Wood-Dauphinee S 2004 The impact of physical therapy on functional outcomes after stroke: what's the evidence? Clin Rehabil 18:833–862.

Weir CJ, Murray GD, Dyker AG et al 1997 Is hyperglycaemia an independent predictor of poor outcome after acute stroke? Results of a long term follow up study. BMJ 314:1303.

Wevers L, van de Port I, Vermue M et al 2009 Effects of task-oriented circuit class training on walking competency after stroke: a systematic review. Stroke 40:2450–2459.

Wilson BA 1995 Management and remediation in brain-injured adults. In: Baddeley AD, Wilson BA, Watts FN (eds) Handbook of memory disorders. John Wiley, Chichester:451–479.

World Health Organization 2008 The world health report 2008. Geneva, Switzerland.

Appendix: The shoulder

The hand is the focal point for movement of the upper limb. Moving and placing the hand is brought about by the functional apparatus of the upper limb, which comprises the controlled and complex activation of many muscles, plus mechanical interactions between the glenohumeral (GH) joint, the scapula moving on the thoracic wall and at the clavicle. Muscle attachments between the spine, pelvis, thoracic cage, scapula and humerus add to the complexity. After a stroke that results in severely reduced muscle activation, loss of motor control and subsequent immobilization of the limb, the potential for development of pain in the shoulder area and wrist, swelling of the hand and subluxation of the GH joint is considerable in those people whose activity limitations are the most severe. Early rehabilitation should focus primarily on task-oriented training, targeting controlled movement of the GH joint, and using electrical stimulation and mechanical arm trainers when muscles are very weak. These may be the best methods for facilitating optimal recovery of upper limb function and preventing secondary complications (see Kumar & Swinkels 2009).

GLENOHUMERAL JOINT SUBLUXATION

Adaptive changes to the soft tissues around the GH joint may occur in individuals with severe muscle weakness and an immobilized arm, particularly if the arm is dependent or in the same position for long periods (see Fig. 6.8B). The weight of the limb appears to cause an overstretching of paretic muscles and other soft tissues that normally would stabilize the GH joint when the arm is dependent (Fig. 11.4) and displacement of the head of the humerus may occur. Moderate to severe weakness of muscles of the rotator cuff leaves joint integrity dependent on passive structures – joint capsule, ligaments and inactive muscles. Early lengthening of the joint capsule was shown in an arthrographic study reported many decades ago (Miglietta et al 1959).

Downward rotation of the scapula caused by the weight of the paretic limb has been considered a contributing mechanical cause of subluxation by repositioning the glenoid fossa more vertically (Cailliet 1991). However, a radiological report of a group of people after stroke found no relationship between scapulohumeral orientation and subluxation (Culham et al 1995), and it has been shown in a recent study of healthy individuals, using a new measuring device, that the scapula is normally tilted downward (Price et al 2001). There is really no evidence that altered scapulohumeral position plays a role in subluxation, and extreme muscle weakness or paralysis, adaptive soft tissue

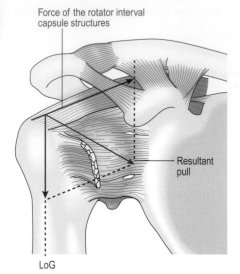

Force of the rotator interval capsule structures

Resultant pull

LoG

Figure 11.4 Mechanism for stabilization of the dependent arm. With the arm relaxed by the side, the downward pull of gravity is opposed by passive tension in the rotator interval capsule (superior capsule and GH ligament, coracohumeral ligament). The resultant of these opposing forces stabilizes the humeral head on the glenoid fossa. *(From Levangie PK & Norkin CC (2005)* Joint Structure & Function. A Comprehensive Analysis, *4th ed. pp 255. FA Davis, Philadelphia, by permission).*

changes, flexed thoracic spine plus absence of active arm movement remain the probable major contributors to GH malalignment (Linn et al 1999). Indeed, there is a tendency for subluxation to decrease as range of active shoulder abduction increases and as significant motor recovery occurs (Zorowitz 2001).

Whether GH subluxation is a contributing factor in the development of pain in the shoulder region is not clear and remains controversial (Joynt 1992; Lo et al 2003). Some studies have reported a statistical relationship between subluxation and pain (van Ouwenwaller et al 1986; Roy et al 1995), however several studies report patients with subluxation and no pain, even when subluxation was moderate to severe (Ikai et al 1998; Zorowitz 2001). Subluxation is frequently present in patients with pain, severe muscle weakness and activity limitations – but causation cannot be assumed.

One possible cause of brief episodes of pain at the subluxed joint during movement is pinching of soft tissue (stretched capsular and rotator cuff tissue) during active (or passive) movement. Sharp pain on movement at a particular point during movement (often between 60° and 120° of abduction), which may be due to impingement of the humerus on acromion, can be relieved by gentle distraction at the joint during training. When GH abductor and flexor muscles are very weak, reaching actions in flexion and abduction should be practised with the limb supported on a table so that movement of the shoulder can be achieved without impingement (see Fig. 6.13). An elevated position changes the angle/line of pull of abductor and flexor muscles and simplifies the mechanics of the movement, enabling pain-free limb movement even when muscles are very weak. Active retraining of muscles around the shoulder, with small-range reaching movements into abduction, external rotation and flexion, with a major focus on controlling muscle activity around the joint, may help in avoiding the negative effects of disuse and misuse, and enable the individual to develop better control of the limbs (Figs 6.13 & 6.14). There is no evidence that supportive devices developed so far are effective in preventing subluxation (Ada et al 2005b, 2008).

PAIN

Some patients develop pain in the shoulder following stroke, reporting pain either over a specific site or an ache radiating down the arm. The major causes appear related to weakness/paralysis of muscles around the joint, poor coordination of shoulder movement and immobility of the limb for long periods of the day with resultant adaptive changes in soft tissues. Causative factors include pre-existing degenerative or trauma-induced changes in the GH joint area, and trauma occurring to the unprotected shoulder post-stroke caused when the person is assisted to sit up and stand.

Some patients develop pain as part of *complex regional pain syndrome* (CRPS), reflex sympathetic dystrophy (RSD) or shoulder–hand syndrome. This condition is characterized by pain, stiffness, swelling and discolouration of the involved limb. Reports citing frequency of this syndrome are variable and its cause is unknown, although immobility and GH joint inflammation appear to contribute.

Shoulder pain is most evident in those whose motor impairment and activity limitations are severe (Chae et al 2007; Sackley et al 2008). Recent studies have found that shoulder pain may occur in about 30–40% of survivors, with the likelihood of increasing over time in the 6 months following stroke (Gamble et al 2000; Ratnasabapathy et al 2003; Lindgren et al 2007; Rajaratnam et al 2007).

Pain can be a factor in poor recovery of upper limb function following stroke – a significant degree of pain can cause inhibition of muscle action at the shoulder and discourage participation in upper limb training. Broader effects of pain include diminished quality of life, depression and poor sleep (Chae et al 2007). Localized tenderness over supraspinatus or biceps brachii may be present. Pain may be present at rest or only when the arm is moved passively or during attempts at active movement.

Wide variations in reports of pain incidence may reflect the nature of the investigations carried out (e.g.,

methodology, heterogeneity of the populations studied). They may also reflect multifactorial causations, diversity in rehabilitation methods and whether or not early and active motor training is provided with a mandated care-of-shoulder programme. When there is muscle weakness and imbalance around the shoulder, early training should emphasize active shoulder movement. Therapy methods should place emphasis on encouraging controlled contractions of GH external rotator, abductor and flexor muscles and associated shoulder girdle movements within a task-specific exercise and training programme. Surprisingly, focus may still be on the effects of spasticity and its reduction (Turner-Stokes & Jackson 2002; Ryerson 2007) instead of on muscle weakness and imbalance, preventing/minimizing soft tissue stiffness and contracture, training limb movement and, where possible, promoting or 'driving' active functional use of the limb.

Complexity of shoulder movement. Normally, when the upper limb is in active use, effective function is brought about by complex mechanical interactions between structures that comprise the shoulder complex – humerus, acromion, clavicle, thoracic wall and sternum. In order to understand the potential for injury after stroke it is useful to reflect on the complex nature of the shoulder region. *Anatomy and biomechanics* reflect the complex mobility of the limb. Ginn and colleagues (1997) have pointed out that the mobile base of the GH joint, the scapula, is suspended from the skeleton via the acromioclavicular joint and coracoclavicular ligament. At the GH joint, the passive structures that provide stability at other joints are designed also to facilitate mobility. The articular surfaces of the humeral head and the glenoid fossa of the scapula lack congruity, and the joint capsule itself is thin and lax, allowing 2–3 cm of distraction between the articular surfaces. The ligaments are few and provide stability only in limited ranges of motion. The shoulder region depends on muscles and their synchronized activity to provide stability.

Raising the arm may seem a simple action but it is not. For example, during abduction of the arm between 0° and 30°, most of the movement takes place at the GH joint. After 30° the ratio of GH-to-scapulothoracic movement is about 5:4, meaning that the humerus moves 5° on the glenoid fossa while the scapula moves 4° on the thorax (Poppen & Walker 1976; Donatelli 2004; Greenfield et al 2004). Even a simple movement at the shoulder is brought about by the controlled action of many muscles that link humerus to scapula, and humerus and scapula to thorax and pelvis (Fig. 11.5). Some muscles are stabilizers, others prime movers. Deltoid (middle fibres) and supraspinatus are major abductors of the GH joint (Fig. 11.6) but many muscles contribute to this action by ensuring the joint movement is controlled appropriately for the task being carried out. Since deltoid is attached to the scapula, muscles linking the scapula to the spine (such as trapezius,

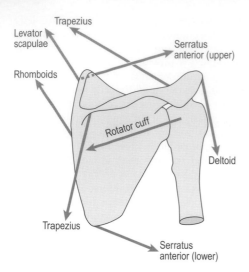

Figure 11.5 Muscles of the shoulder girdle and major forces acting on the shoulder girdle. *(From Peat 1986, with permission).*

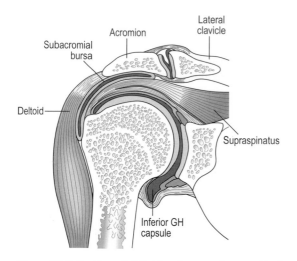

Figure 11.6 Position of deltoid and supraspinatus with the arm at rest by the side. In this position the superior capsule is taut and the inferior capsule is slack. *(From Levangie PK & Norkin CC (2005) Joint Structure & Function. A Comprehensive Analysis, 4th ed. pp 249. FA Davis, Philadelphia, by permission).*

serratus anterior) act to stabilize and control scapular movement. The pull of the deltoid muscle to abduct the arm tends to displace the humeral head upwards in the glenoid fossa and it is counteracted normally by the musculotendinous (rotator) cuff, formed by the blending of four muscles with the capsule (teres minor, infraspinatus, supraspinatus and subscapularis) (Levangie & Norkin 2005). The rotator cuff stabilizes the humeral head into the fossa. Attachment of these muscles and of biceps brachii close to the GH joint enhances their role as

stabilizers. Other muscles around the GH joint also contribute to stability of the joint. The application of these combined stabilizing muscle forces at the GH joint, together with the action of deltoid on the humeral head, provides the counterforce necessary to abduct the humerus.

Effects of weakness, loss of coordination and adaptive soft tissue changes. The brain lesion impacts the mechanism of the shoulder complex when there is a reduction in descending inputs to spinal motor neurons and disturbance of motor control mechanisms. When the resulting muscle weakness is severe and the limb is not used, this provokes adaptive changes in soft tissues, including increased passive intrinsic muscle stiffness and contracture of the muscles that are held at a shortened length (see Fig. 6.8B).

The mechanisms of scapulohumeral coordination and control of the limb are grossly disturbed by muscle weakness and length-associated muscle and capsular changes. If muscles have variable levels of innervation or if there is pain due to impingement or inflammatory processes, an imbalance of muscle forces is evident on any attempt at active movement (Bohannon & Smith 1987). Poor motor control of muscles of the shoulder complex results in altered joint mechanics when the patient attempts to move the limb. Changed intersegmental mechanics may be a major cause of impingement trauma, and training needs to be carefully carried out to avoid repetitive injury. Mechanical derangements can lead to inflammation of the supraspinatus where it crosses the head of the humerus below the acromion, of the tendon of biceps brachii in the humeral groove, and bursitis.

Inability to externally rotate the GH joint actively through range and to abduct the arm seem particularly critical factors in the development of a stiff shoulder and pain. Several studies point to significant relationships between weakness of GH external rotators and abductors, diminished range of external rotation (due to increased stiffness or contracture of internal rotators and adductors) and pain (Bohannon et al 1986; Bohannon 1988; Zorowitz et al 1995; Wanklyn et al 1996; Rajaratnam et al 2007). An objective in early rehabilitation is the preservation of musculoskeletal integrity as a means of helping the individual regain optimal functional hand recovery (Shepherd & Carr 1998). A major focus of early motor training should be on encouraging activation of these muscles, with specific exercises involving external rotation with the arm by the side and elbow flexed and with the arm straight and resting on a table (see Fig. 6.15). (See Ch. 6 for details.)

Changes in response to muscle weakness, immobility and disuse are becoming better understood and are described in detail in Chapters 6 and 8. Changes in muscles immobilized in a shortened position include connective tissue remodelling and reduction in sarcomere number, and, if positioning persists and there is minimal regaining of active movement, contracture becomes established. Changes in muscle morphology and mechanics lead to a marked increase in muscle stiffness and changes in muscle spindle sensitivity can occur.

Spasticity has been considered a cause of pain, with the assumption that spastic muscles hold the limb immobilized by 'spastic contracture' of muscles such as scapula retractors and GH joint adductors and internal rotators (Bobath 1990; Turner-Stokes & Jackson 2002). There is no evidentiary support for this assumption and a more likely explanation is that resistance to passive movement is the result of adaptive viscoelastic changes in muscles held short in response to prolonged immobility (see Fig. 6.9 and Ch. 8). Muscles that become shorter and stiffer restrict both passive and active joint movement. For example, contracture of GH adductor and internal rotator muscles anchors the humerus to the scapula and prevents the coordinated scapulohumeral movement that normally occurs during movements of the arm. Muscle contracture, reduced range of motion and repeated trauma including impingement have been shown to be associated with joint changes typical of adhesive capsulitis in the able-bodied population as well as after stroke (Bruckner & Nye 1981; Rizk et al 1984; Lo et al 2003; Ludewig & Reynolds 2009). A recent study using MRI scans of 89 individuals with post-stroke shoulder pain and paresis found that partial rotator cuff tears (particularly age-dependent tears of supraspinatus) and tendinopathies (mostly of supraspinatus, infraspinatus and subscapularis) were highly prevalent (Shah et al 2008). These findings point to the need for a focus on training of rotator cuff muscles, with exercises to improve shoulder dynamics and reduce the potential for wear and tear (Blennerhassett 2009).

Pre-existing degenerative changes. Older people may have sustained injuries to the shoulder at some time or may have developed arthritic and general 'wear-and-tear' changes to the GH joint (Ratnasabapathy et al 2003). Degenerative changes in periarticular soft tissues occurring with increasing age include thickening and shredding of biceps brachii tendon; calcific deposits in rotator cuff tendons; and thinning and fraying of supraspinatus muscle (Hakuno et al 1984; Shah et al 2008). Any increase in the angle of thoracic kyphosis with decreased thoracic extension is associated with decreased range of unilateral, but particularly of bilateral, arm elevation (Crawford & Jull 1993). In people with severe thoracic kyphosis, decreased capacity to lift the arms high above the head can influence the performance of both unimanual and bimanual actions. These findings point to the need to take particular care with the shoulder from the time a person, particularly an elderly individual, is admitted to acute care following stroke. A gentle stretch of the thoracic spine into extension can be applied by a rolled-up towel along the spine (see Fig. 13.5) and may be helpful where the spine is stiff.

Trauma to the unprotected arm. The shoulder without muscle control is virtually defenseless. Trauma to the unprotected limb has been implicated in the cause of shoulder pain (Cailliet 1980; Wanklyn et al 1996; Turner-Stokes & Jackson 2002) and capsulitis is known to follow on from even relatively minor trauma in the non-stroke population. In the presence of extreme weakness following stroke, when the limb is moved passively by its own weight as in turning over in bed, or when moved by another person, there is potential for injury due to the absence of normally occurring protective mechanisms. The altered mechanics caused in part by the limitations on movement imposed by the altered length of tissue, together with thoracic stiffness, can also subject bone and soft tissue to stresses that cause inflammation, soft tissue damage and pain. Pre-existing tendinopathies or inflammatory states such as capsulitis, tendinitis and bursitis may be aggravated. Potential causes of injury in the hospital environment include:

- assisting the person to shift position by pulling on or holding the arm
- poor self-care, for example in a person with inattention, so-called 'neglect'
- passive range of movement and pulley exercises.

There have been few investigations of the environmental factors leading to injury. In one study, the authors reported that lifting patients by pulling on the arm was a rather common occurrence, even when staff had been advised not to (Wanklyn et al 1996). They found that those who most needed help with getting in and out of bed, standing up and sitting down on a chair were most likely to suffer shoulder pain, suggesting that assisting by holding the arm can be a causative factor.

Passive range of motion exercises to a paralysed arm, including overhead pulley exercises, were implicated in injury or reactivation of previous inflammatory states in several early studies (Cailliet 1980; Griffin 1986; Kumar et al 1990). Passive movements can cause impingement-related pain or repeated minor trauma to muscle fibres or capsule. Impingement of the head of the humerus against the acromion occurs if the shoulder is passively or actively abducted without external humeral rotation (Hawkins & Murnaghan 1984) (Fig. 11.7). This can cause inflammation and can put stress on ischaemic or damaged soft tissues. Poor control of muscles that link the scapula to the thorax and spine affect scapula movement, interfering with rotation and protraction when the arm is moved into elevation. This effect is magnified if muscles linking scapula to humerus are short and stiff (particularly adductor and internal rotator muscles).

Difficulties with diagnosis. Despite the fact that shoulder pain can be a common complication reported after stroke, the cause may not be subject to a careful diagnostic evaluation (e.g., X-ray, ultrasound, clinical evaluation) as it would be in a non-stroke population. Similarly, the site and type of pain are rarely presented in published studies, although this may be critical information. Although the causes of shoulder pain are multifactorial and, in individual patients, may not be at all clear, evaluation is required to enable training to be planned.

A preliminary study attempting to identify pain-producing structures found that those in the subacromial area appeared to be common sites of pain, perhaps related to inflammation or trauma, or impingement of the head of the humerus against the acromion process due to disturbed shoulder mechanics (Joynt 1992) (Fig. 11.8). Recent studies have reported adhesive capsulitis as a potential cause of pain (Ikai et al 1998; Lo et al 2003). Patients with capsulitis had restricted passive shoulder external rotation and abduction, and a higher incidence of shoulder–hand syndrome. A study of 67 individuals found that the amount of shoulder pain was related most to loss of movement at the shoulder. Amount of pain was unrelated to subluxation, spasticity, muscle strength or sensation (Joynt 1992). Causes of pain have been summarized as rotator cuff tears, adhesive capsulitis, osteoarthritis, bicipital or supraspinatus tendinitis, bursitis, and as part of complex regional pain syndrome (Zorowitz 2001; Ratnasabapathy et al 2003).

Since there are few studies that have examined the cause of shoulder pain in individual subjects post-stroke, the best methods of prevention and intervention remain unclear (National Stroke Foundation 2005). Nevertheless, specific subgroups of patients probably require specific interventions (Price et al 2001) and a clinical evaluation is necessary to develop a plan for intervention. It is likely that developments in imaging techniques and future investigations will enable a better understanding of shoulder dysfunction.

In summary, the factors predisposing to the development of a painful stiff shoulder are as follows:

- Paralysis or severe weakness of muscles around the GH joint that results in persistent immobility of the limb.
- Positioning for lengthy periods of the day with the GH joint in internal rotation and adduction.
- Adaptive changes to soft tissues, for example increased muscle stiffness, and changed muscle fibre length and morphology in response to paresis and inactivity, gravitational effects and limb position.
- Muscle imbalance causing mechanical derangement during movement and resulting in impingement of the humerus on the scapula.
- Compounding effects of:
  - pre-stroke degeneration of cartilage, bone and soft tissues around the GH joint
  - post-stroke injury to the unprotected shoulder region of the paretic limb, exacerbating pre-existing degenerative changes and causing inflammation of soft tissues.

These factors can be responsive to intervention; some could probably be prevented by the newer training

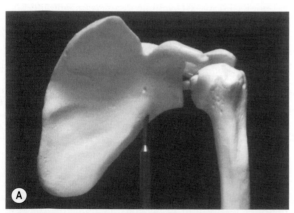

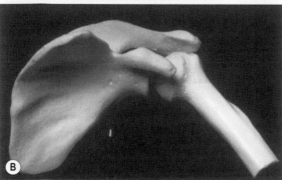

Figure 11.7 Scapular-humeral anatomical relationships: External rotation of the humerus during abduction ensures that the greater tuberosity of the humerus rotates out of the way of the acromion process.

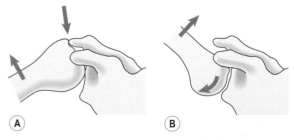

Figure 11.8 (A) Without downward sliding of the humeral head's articular surface as the arm abducts, the head will roll up the glenoid fossa and impinge on the coracoacromial arch. (B) With downward sliding of humeral head as the humerus abducts, a full range of motion can occur without impingement. *(From Levangie PK & Norkin CC (2005) Joint Structure & Function. A Comprehensive Analysis, 4th ed. pp 253. FA Davis, Philadelphia, by permission).*

methods that are now increasingly in use as clinical practice evolves.

Pain prevention

Research has not yet identified the most effective methods of prevention of pain and its treatment. In clinical practice, avoidance of a stiff painful shoulder after stroke depends on awareness of the negative sequelae of muscle weakness, inactivity and disuse, and of the susceptibility of the unprotected shoulder to injury. We know that a stiff painful shoulder can occur in those whose stroke has resulted in moderate to severe muscle weakness; we understand that causative mechanisms are multifactorial and that some could be prevented. The next steps are to investigate methods of eliciting potential muscle activity in the

moderately and severely compromised shoulder region, test the effects of an early start to task-specific training in unimanual and bimanual tasks, and test the effects of a programme of care aimed at preventing avoidable injury, pain caused by trauma and immobility. Outcome studies should include data on type of pain and severity, site of pain, what triggers it, any pre-existing episodes of pain, details of intervention and follow-up.

The following box shows an example of a preventive programme with guidelines for shoulder care and early active exercise that should involve all staff and start in the acute care facility. This programme is developed out of current knowledge and, where it is available, from evidence.

The National Stroke Foundation's clinical guidelines for acute stroke management (2007) and for

---

Shoulder pain prevention programme

- Early task-oriented training of reaching in all directions (modified and assisted if necessary) – regaining active coordinated movement at the shoulder is a major deterrent to the development of a stiff shoulder. Careful attention is paid to GH alignment and to external rotation of the humerus during abduction.
- Emphasis on active pain-free exercise for GH external rotation, abduction, flexion and elevation (Figs 6.13 & 6.14). Avoid impingement of the head of the humerus on the scapula.
- Positioning for at least 30 minutes each day sitting at a table, with the GH joint in external rotation and abduction (Fig. 11.9) (Ada et al 2005a) plus task-related exercises in this position. Pay attention to thoracic spine posture.
- Arm positioning in a wheelchair on an arm trough, lap board or other arm support (Turton & Britton

- 2005) in mid-pronation/supination and GH rotation.
- Avoid prolonged GH internal rotation/adduction, for example in a sling. There is no reliable evidence that a sling prevents subluxation (Turton et al 2004); wearing a sling is associated with decreased GH external rotation range (Ada et al 2008). If a sling is used it should be worn for very short periods at a time, and staff must be aware of negative consequences.
- Functional electrical stimulation to deltoid and supraspinatus muscles (Ada & Foomchomcheay 2002) to prevent/minimize subluxation.
- Avoid damaging events – passive range of motion and self-assisted pulley exercises (Kumar et al 1990), pulling on the arm when helping sit-to-stand (Wanklyn et al 1996), lying on the affected limb.

---

stroke rehabilitation and recovery (2005) include these interventions, providing the levels of available evidence. They stress that particular emphasis should be placed during the acute phase on prevention of shoulder pain and prevention of subluxation, as no clear evidence exists for effective treatments once they occur.

There is some evidence that positioning during the day can be effective at preventing contracture of internal rotator and adductor muscles, but to be effective the patient also needs active exercise and training. For example, a recent study showed that including 30 minutes with the limb positioned in maximum GH external rotation on a table plus 10 minutes of task-oriented shoulder exercises significantly reduced development of internal rotator contractures in a small group of people within 3 weeks of their stroke compared to a control group (Ada et al 2005a).

Major aspects of training and exercise

These are as follows:

- Therapists need skill in using methods of eliciting and training muscle activity in muscles such as upper trapezius, serratus anterior, deltoid, supraspinatus, biceps and triceps brachii, and external rotators of the GH joint. Exercise should start early, with active concentric and eccentric exercises, and involve simple modified reaching and manipulation tasks (Fig. 11.10; Figs 6.13–6.15). When muscles are active, intensive training is likely to increase contractile strength, the timing and speed of force production, and coordinated action between

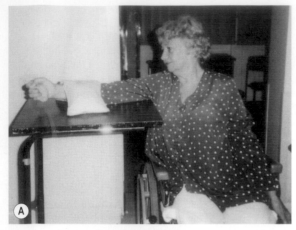

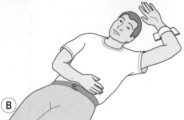

Figure 11.9 Examples of positioning to preserve length in shoulder muscles, (A) sitting at a table, (B) lying down. A sandbag can be used to keep the arm in position. (a) In this position, exercises to improve grip strength (particularly of 4th and 5th fingers which are weak), finger extension and pronation/supination can be practised.

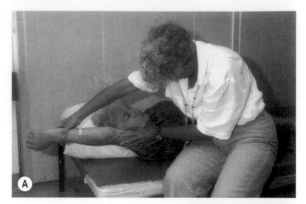

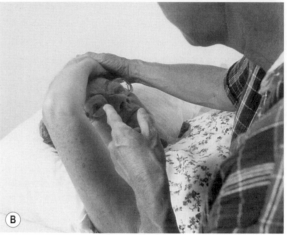

Figure 11.10 (A) Post-stroke: Practice of raising the arm and lowering it in an elevated position. The therapist guides the path of the limb and encourages her to keep the arm close by her head as she moves the arm off the pillow and down again. The distance moved is increased as her muscle control improves. (B) Practice of eccentric and concentric activity of shoulder muscles (principally pectorals) as she tries to move the elbow to touch the therapist's finger and to control an eccentric contraction as she moves the elbow back to the pillow.

the muscles involved. Exercises are task related for maximum transfer to daily life.

- Task practice is modified to take account of muscle weakness (Fig. 11.10). Pain from impingement may be avoided by controlling the limb through small pain-free arcs, gradually increasing this range. The patient is encouraged to practise shoulder shrugging during the day to overcome the dragging effect of a heavy weak limb.

- Conditions are set up to enable the patient to practise frequently throughout the day. Motivating strategies help the person focus attention, concentrating on the task of eliciting and sustaining muscle force while practising tasks. Strapping applied to the shoulder (Fig. 11.11) may help focus the person's attention on contracting the muscles around the shoulder, and the support it gives may increase comfort. Strapping has been shown to limit the development of pain and to decrease pain in the shoulder (Hanger et al 2000; Griffin & Bernhardt 2006).

- Constraint of the non-paretic limb plus intensive exercise (several hours per day) for the affected limb

has been tested extensively as part of the EXCITE trial (Wolf et al 2006, 2007, 2008) in which inclusion criteria required that participants could extend the wrist (10°) and fingers (20°). There have been some tests with individuals with moderately severe weakness but some ability to move the limb. Positive results were reported (see Bonifer et al 2005; Ploughman et al 2008) and also in early rehabilitation after stroke (Dromerick et al 2000).

- Bilateral actions are also a focus of training (see Ch. 6 for discussion).

- Neuromuscular stimulation, used with and without EMG triggering early in rehabilitation, has the aim of

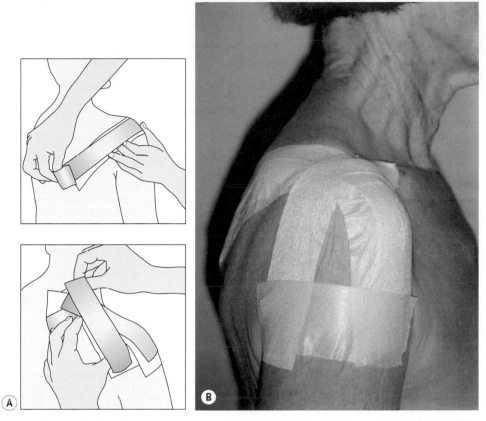

Figure 11.11 (A,B) Strapping to provide some support for the upper limb. Fixomull stretch tape (BSNmedical) is used under the Sports Tape or Leukoplast (BSNmedical) to protect the skin. (A) Upper: The first piece passes over the front of the shoulder to a short distance down the scapula. Lower: 2 pieces are pulled upward over the shoulder and held in place by a lower cross-piece. *(Courtesy of J. McConnell)*

preserving muscle fibre contractility and stimulating functional recovery of critical muscles such as supraspinatus and deltoid. Functional electrical stimulation (FES) to shoulder muscles may prevent the development of subluxation (Faghri et al 1994; Linn et al 1999) and may reduce existing subluxation (Baker & Parker 1986; Chantraine et al 1999; Kobayashi et al 1999), although evidence is weak so far. FES to posterior deltoid and supraspinatus significantly increased arm function, muscle activity and joint range in one study when compared to a control group (Faghri et al 1994). Patients in the experimental group received FES for 6 hours a day for 6 weeks. A systematic review (Price & Pandyan 2001) found evidence of a positive effect in reducing severity of subluxation and in improving pain-free range of passive external rotation but no significant effect on motor recovery of the upper limb. A meta-analysis reported that early application of electrical stimulation that evoked a motor response in deltoid and supraspinatus was effective in preventing shoulder subluxation (Ada & Foongchomcheay 2002).

- Robotic and non-robotic training devices to drive or enable active movement in people with severe paresis are being developed (see Ch. 6). If successful, such devices could increase independent practice time. The first study to examine the effects of a simple EMG-triggered non-robotic device in training reaching in patients with severe muscle weakness has shown significant improvements in all impairment and activity measures tested (Barker et al 2008) (see Fig. 6.21).

In conclusion, there is evidence that motor training, with an emphasis on motor learning, training that includes the use of imagery, electrical stimulation with and without biofeedback and practice of repetitive tasks can be effective in decreasing motor impairment after stroke. In addition, care with handling, training movements in elevation, the use of strapping and avoidance of overhead pulley exercises can decrease or prevent pain in the paretic limb (see Barreca et al 2003 for systematic review).

REFERENCES

Ada L, Foomchomcheay A 2002 Efficacy of electrical stimulation in preventing or reducing subluxation of the shoulder after stroke: a meta-analysis. Aust J Physiother 48:257–267.

Ada L, Goddard E, McCully J et al 2005a Thirty minutes of positioning reduces the development of shoulder external rotation contracture after stroke: a randomized controlled trial. Arch Phys Med Rehabil 86:230–234.

Ada L, Foongchomcheay A, Canning C 2005b Supportive devices for preventing and treating subluxation of the shoulder after stroke. Stroke 36:1818–1819.

Ada L, Foongchomcheay A, Canning C 2008 Supportive devices for preventing and treating subluxation of the shoulder after stroke. Cochrane Database Syst Rev Issue 1. Art. No.: CD003863. DOI: 10.1002/14651858.CD003863.pub2.

Baker LL, Parker K 1986 Neuromuscular electrical stimulation of the muscles surrounding the shoulder. Phys Ther 66:1930–1937.

Barker R, Bauer S, Carson RG 2008 Training of reaching in stroke survivors with severe and chronic upper limb paresis using a novel nonrobotic device: a randomized controlled clinical trial. Stroke 39:1800–1807.

Barreca S, Wolf SL, Fasoli S et al 2003 Treatment interventions for the paretic upper limb of stroke survivors: a critical review. Neurorehabil Neural Repair 17:220–226.

Blennerhassett J 2009 Personal communication.

Bobath B 1990 Adult hemiplegia: evaluation and treatment, 3rd edn. Heinemann, London.

Bohannon RW 1988 Relationship between shoulder pain and selected variables in patients with hemiplegia. Clin Rehabil 2:111–117.

Bohannon RW, Smith MB 1987 Assessment of strength deficits in eight paretic upper extremity muscle groups of stroke patients with hemiplegia. Phys Ther 67:522–525.

Bohannon RW, Larkin PA, Smith MB et al 1986 Shoulder pain in hemiplegia: statistical relationship with five variables. Arch Phys Med Rehabil 67:514–516.

Bonifer NM, Anderson KM, Arciniegas DB et al 2005 Constraint-induced movement therapy after stroke: efficacy for patients with minimal upper-extremity motor ability. Arch Phys Med Rehabil 86:1867–1873.

Bruckner FE, Nye CJS 1981 A prospective study of adhesive capsulitis of the shoulder ('frozen shoulder') in a high risk population. Q J Med 198:191–204.

Cailliet R 1980 The shoulder in hemiplegia. FA Davis, Philadelphia.

Cailliet R 1991 Shoulder pain. FA Davis, Philadelphia.

Chae J, Mascarenhas D, Yu DT et al 2007 Poststroke shoulder pain: its relationship to motor impairment, activity limitation and quality of life. Arch Phys Med Rehabil 88:298–301.

Chantraine A, Baribeault A, Uebelhart D et al 1999 Shoulder pain and dysfunction in hemiplegia: effects of functional electrical stimulation. Arch Phys Med Rehabil 80:328–331.

Crawford HJ, Jull GA 1993 The influence of thoracic posture and movement on range of arm elevation. Physiother Theory Pract 9:143–148.

Culham EG, Noce RR, Bagg SD 1995 Shoulder complex position and glenohumeral subluxation in hemiplegia. Arch Phys Med Rehabil 76:857–864.

Donatelli R 2004 Functional anatomy and mechanics. In: Donatelli R (ed.) Physical therapy of the shoulder, 4th edn. Churchill Livingstone, St Louis:11–28.

Dromerick AW, Edwards D, Hahn M 2000 Does the application of constraint-induced movement therapy during acute rehabilitation reduce arm impairment after ischaemic stroke? Stroke 31:2984–2988.

Faghri PD, Rodgers MM, Glaser RM et al 1994 The effects of functional electrical stimulation on shoulder subluxation, arm function recovery, and shoulder pain in hemiplegic stroke patients. Arch Phys Med Rehabil 75:73–79.

Gamble GE, Barberan E, Bowsher D et al 2000 Post stroke shoulder pain: more common than previously realized. Eur J Pain 4:313–315.

Ginn KA, Herbert RD, Khouw W et al 1997 A randomized, controlled clinical trial of a treatment for shoulder pain. Phys Ther 77:802–811.

Greenfield BR, Donatelli R 2004 Impingement syndrome and impingement-related instability. In: Donatelli R (ed.) Physical therapy of the shoulder, 4th edn. Churchill Livingstone, St Louis, MI, pp291–317.

Griffin JW 1986 Hemiplegic shoulder pain. Phys Ther 66:1884–1893.

Griffin A, Bernhardt J 2006 Strapping the hemiplegic shoulder prevents development of pain during rehabilitation: a randomized controlled trial. Clin Rehabil 20:287–295.

Hakuno A, Sashika H, Ohkawa T et al 1984 Arthrographic findings in hemiplegic shoulders. Arch Phys Med Rehabil 65:706–711.

Hanger HC, Whitewood P, Brown G et al 2000 A randomized controlled trial of strapping to prevent post-stroke shoulder pain. Clin Rehabil 14:370–380.

Hawkins RJ, Murnaghan JP 1984 The shoulder. In: Cruess RL, Rennee WR (eds) Adult orthopaedics, Vol. 2. Churchill Livingstone, New York.

Ikai T, Tei K, Yoshida K et al 1998 Evaluation and treatment of shoulder subluxation in hemiplegia: relationship between subluxation and pain. Am J Phys Med Rehabil 77:421–426.

Joynt RL 1992 The source of shoulder pain in hemiplegia. Arch Phys Med Rehabil 73:409–413.

Kobayashi H, Onishi H, Ihashi K et al 1999 Reduction in subluxation and improved muscle function of the hemiplegic shoulder joint after therapeutic electrical stimulation. J Electromyogr Kinesiol 9:327–336.

Kumar P, Swinkels A 2009 A critical review of shoulder subluxation and its association with other post-stroke complications. Phys Ther Rev 14:13–25.

Kumar R, Matter EJ, Mehta AJ et al 1990 Shoulder pain in hemiplegia. The role of exercise. Am J Phys Med Rehabil 69:205–208.

Levangie PK, Norkin CC 2005 Joint structure and function. A

comprehensive analysis 4th edn. FA Davis, Philadelphia.

Lindgren I, Jonsson A-C, Norrving B et al 2007 Shoulder pain after stroke. Stroke 38:343–348.

Linn SL, Granat MH, Lees KR 1999 Prevention of shoulder subluxation after stroke with electrical stimulation. Stroke 30:963–968.

Lo S-F, Chen SY, Lin HC et al 2003 Arthrographic and clinical findings in patients with hemiplegic shoulder pain. Arch Phys Med Rehabil 84:1786–1791.

Ludewig PM, Reynolds JF 2009 The association of scapular kinematics and gleno-humeral joint pathologies. J Orthop Sports Phys Ther 39:90–104.

Miglietta O, Lewitan A, Rogoff JB 1959 Subluxation of the shoulder in hemiplegic patients. N Y State J Med 59:457–460.

National Stroke Foundation 2005 Clinical guidelines for stroke rehabilitation and recovery. National Stroke Foundation, Melbourne.

National Stroke Foundation 2007 Clinical guidelines for acute stroke management. National Stroke Foundation, Melbourne.

Ploughman M, Shears J, Hutchings L et al 2008 Constraint-induced movement therapy for severe upper-extremity impairment after stroke in an outpatient rehabilitation setting: a case report. Physiother Can 60:161–170.

Poppen NK, Walker PS 1976 Normal and abnormal motion of the shoulder. J Bone Joint Surg 58A:195–200.

Price CIM, Pandyan AD 2001 Electrical stimulation for preventing and treating post-stroke shoulder pain: a systematic Cochrane review. Clin Rehabil 15:5–19.

Price CI, Rodgers H, Franklin P et al 2001 Glenohumeral subluxation, scapula resting position, and scapula rotation after stroke: a noninvasive evaluation. Arch Phys Med Rehabil 82:955–960.

Rajaratnam BS, Venketasubramanian N, Kumar PV et al 2007 Predictability of simple clinical tests to identify shoulder pain after stroke. Arch Phys Med Rehabil 88:1016–1021.

Ratnasabapathy Y, Broad J, Baskett J et al 2003 Shoulder pain in people with a stroke: a population-based study. Clin Rehabil 17:304–311.

Rizk TE, Christopher RP, Pinals RS et al 1984 Arthrographic studies in painful hemiplegic shoulders. Arch Phys Med Rehabil 65:254–256.

Roy CW, Sands MR, Hill LD et al 1995 The effect of shoulder pain on outcome of acute hemiplegia. Clin Rehabil 9:21–27.

Ryerson SD 2007 Hemiplegia. In: Umphred DA (ed.) Neurological rehabilitation, 5th edn. Mosby, St Louis:857–901.

Sackley C, Brittle N, Patel S et al 2008 The prevalence of joint contractures, pressure sores, painful shoulder, other pain, falls, and depression in the year after a severely disabling stroke. Stroke 39:3329–3334.

Shah RR, Haghpanah S, Elovic EP et al 2008 MRI findings in the painful poststroke shoulder. Stroke 39:1808–1813.

Shepherd RB, Carr JH 1998 The shoulder following stroke: preserving musculoskeletal integrity. Top Stroke Rehabil 4:35–53.

Turner-Stokes L, Jackson D 2002 Shoulder pain after stroke: a review of the evidence base to inform the development of an integrated care pathway. Clin Rehabil 16:276–298.

Turton AJ, Britton E 2005 A pilot randomized controlled trial of a daily muscle stretch regime to prevent contractures in the arm after stroke. Clin Rehabil 19:600–612.

van Ouwenwaller C, Laplace PM, Chantraine A 1986 Painful shoulder in hemiplegia. Arch Phys Med Rehabil 67:23–26.

van Peppen RPS, Kwakkel G, Wood-Dauphinee S et al 2004 The impact of physical therapy on functional outcomes after stroke: what's the evidence? Clin Rehabil 18:833–862.

Wanklyn P, Forster A, Young J 1996 Hemiplegic shoulder pain (HSP): natural history and investigation of associated features. Disabil Rehabil 18:497–501.

Wolf SL, Winstein CJ, Miller JP et al 2006 Effect of constraint-induced movement therapy on upper extremity function 3 to 9 months after stroke. JAMA 296:2095–2104.

Wolf SL, Newton H, Maddy D et al 2007 The EXCITE trial: relationship of intensity of constraint induced movement therapy to improvement in the Wolf Motor Function Test. Restor Neurol Neurosci 25:549–562.

Wolf SL, Winstein CJ, Miller JP et al 2008 Retention of upper limb function in stroke survivors who have received constraint-induced movement therapy: the EXCITE randomized trial. Lancet Neurol 7:33–40.

Zorowitz RD 2001 Recovery patterns of shoulder subluxation after stroke: a six-month follow-up study. Top Stroke Rehabil 8:1–9.

Zorowitz RD, Idank D, Ikai T et al 1995 Shoulder subluxation after stroke: a comparison of four supports. Arch Phys Med Rehabil 76:763–771.

Chapter | 12 |

Traumatic brain injury

Written with Anne Moseley and Leanne Hassett

INTRODUCTION

Trauma is the commonest cause of death under the age of 35 years in most developed countries and head injury is the commonest cause of accidental death. Head injury or traumatic brain injury (TBI) are terms used to describe a physical injury to the brain by an external mechanical force or projectile, that results in loss of consciousness, post-traumatic amnesia and neurological impairments. TBI is most commonly the result of road accidents, industrial and sporting accidents, attempted suicides and interpersonal violence. The sequelae can have a devastating effect on the individual's lifestyle and future aspirations, creating general health and social problems, causing disruption for family members and marital strain, affecting role-relationships and fostering economic hardship (McKinlay et al 1981).

The beginning of the systematic study of the effects of TBI can be traced to World War II. In this early work, much was learned about the deficits following penetrating injuries to the brain in servicemen with gunshot wounds. The majority of TBI individuals seen in hospitals these days are classified as closed TBI, i.e. the skull is not actually penetrated.

The type of trauma sustained in road accidents (e.g. blunt impact or acceleration-deceleration) usually results in diffuse brain damage with a variety of physical, cognitive and behavioural problems. As the younger age groups tend to be over-represented and because life expectancy is lowered by only an average of 7 years after TBI (Harrison-Felix et al 2004), the role of rehabilitation is critical in order to maximize quality of life by improving function and participation.

Following a period of unconsciousness, the majority of individuals are left with a combination of physical and cognitive impairments which vary as a consequence of the severity of the lesion, the nature of brain damage and medical complications. Changes in behaviour, mood and personality after TBI have been documented and are considered by many clinicians to be among the most difficult problems to manage effectively. Behaviour problems range from minor irritability and passivity to disinhibited and psychotic behaviour. Cognitive, behavioural and personality changes are far more frequently associated with long-term functional disability and family stress than are physical impairments (Marsh et al 2002, Morton & Wehman 1995).

©2010 Elsevier Ltd
DOI: 10.1016/B978-0-7020-4051-1.00021-7

EPIDEMIOLOGY

It has been suggested that TBI is one of the five most prevalent neurological conditions affecting the central nervous system, together with cerebrovascular disease, epilepsy, Parkinson's disease and migraine (Wade & Langton Hewer 1987). Estimates of prevalence and incidence vary depending on such factors as whether or not all grades of severity and all who are hospitalized are included, urban versus rural location, country and the research methodology used (Abelson-Mitchell 2008). The incidence per 100,000 population ranges from 108 to 392 (Abelson-Mitchell 2008). A well-designed study which followed a cohort of 1,265 New Zealanders from birth to 25 years reported an overall prevalence of TBI of 32% (McKinlay et al 2008). About ten per cent of these were classified as moderate to severe (McKinlay et al 2008).

In all studies, males outnumber females by at least 2 : 1 (Abelson-Mitchell 2008, McKinlay et al 2008), and the injuries in which males are involved tend to be more severe (Slewa-Younan et al 2004). Several risk factors have been suggested as predisposing individuals to the likelihood of sustaining a TBI. Consumption of alcohol increases the risk of head trauma (Puljula et al 2007), and about half of all injuries are transport related (Abelson-Mitchell 2008). Wearing seatbelts in cars and the use of helmets by both motor bike riders and cyclists reduces the risk of sustaining a severe TBI from a road traffic accident (Javouhey et al 2006).

The pattern and severity of injury as well as the resulting outcome are extremely variable and are dependent in part on the criteria used for classification. In the United States it has been estimated that 1.4 million people sustain a TBI each year, and of these 3.6% die, 79.6% attend the accident and emergency department only, and 16.8% are hospitalized (Langlois et al 2006). The overall mortality from TBI amongst those seen in accident and emergency departments is relatively small since most of these individuals have minor TBI. Mortality amongst those hospitalized, however, is high. Approximately 24% of these individuals die and 20% survive with persistent and severe disability (Myburgh et al 2008). Of those who survive, outcome is typically defined by global categories listed on the 5-point Glasgow Outcome Scale (GOS) [death; persistent vegetative state; severe disability; moderate disability; good recovery] (Jennett & Teasdale 1981) or the 8-point Glasgow Outcome Scale Extended (GOSE) [death; persistent vegetative state; lower severe disability; upper severe disability; lower moderate disability, upper moderate disability; lower good recovery; upper good recovery] (Wilson et al 1998) (Chapter 3). Even those who achieve a good recovery on the GOS may have significant psychological impairment that interferes with a return to premorbid levels of function (Whyte & Rosenthal 1993). The economic and social impact is enormous. While estimates of return to work vary considerably, only about 20% of people with moderate to severe TBI are employed 1-year post-injury (Arango-Lasprilla et al 2008).

Those patients who suffer a brief loss of consciousness (≤20 minutes) and post-traumatic amnesia (PTA) of less than 24 hours, encompass the vast majority of TBI individuals. A percentage of these individuals are likely to have persistent problems. In injuries commonly referred to as mild, the individual may not suffer any loss of consciousness, although there may be a period of brief altered consciousness, and the individual returns to normal activities after several days without any problems. In other 'mild' injuries, a post-concussional syndrome consisting of symptoms like headaches, irritability, anxiety, dizziness, fatigue, and impaired concentration may persist for months or even years (e.g. Jakola et al 2007).

PATHOPHYSIOLOGY

TBI may occur as a result of a direct blow to the head, or the head may be injured indirectly from an impact to other parts of the body. Direct injury may be blunt or penetrating. Blunt or acceleration-deceleration injuries commonly result in multiple injuries of the body as well as widespread brain damage. The impact to the head may cause scalp injuries, deformation of the skull with or without fractures, or depressed fractures which may lacerate and perforate the dura mater and brain.

Mechanism of brain damage

The mechanisms that produce brain damage in trauma are varied and complex and include both intracranial and extracranial factors (Table 12.1). Intracranial mechanisms of brain damage are typically divided into *primary damage*, in which the effects are largely immediate, and delayed or *secondary damage* that occurs some time after the injury. Both affect the eventual morbidity and mortality of the individual. In general, primary brain damage produces an immediate effect on level of consciousness while secondary brain damage produces a late deterioration in the level of consciousness and development of focal signs. Hypoxic and ischaemic brain damage can be minimized by effective and early resuscitation. It is chiefly in the treatment of secondary brain damage, which is potentially preventable or treatable, that medical and surgical intervention has advanced over the past decade or so.

The injuries associated with extracranial mechanisms are many and may include fractures to the extremities, spine (with or without spinal cord damage) and pelvis, damage to the rib cage and underlying organs, rupture of abdominal viscera, and facial injuries. These insults and the associated haemorrhage are often responsible for

Table 12.1 Classification of mechanisms of brain damage following trauma

Extracranial mechanisms

Hypoxia
Hypotension

Intracranial mechanisms

Primary brain damage
  diffuse axonal injury
  laceration
  contusion
  haemorrhage
    subdural
    epidural
    subarachnoid and intraventricular spaces
Secondary brain damage
  brain swelling
    vasogenic oedema
    cytotoxic oedema
  cerebral blood vessel constriction

Adapted from Mendelow (1993a) by permission.

ischaemic brain damage largely as a result of hypoxia and hypotension.

Primary brain damage

The primary neuropathology of TBI, which occurs at the time of injury, is classified as focal (contusion, laceration and haemorrhage due to contact) and diffuse (diffuse axonal injury due to acceleration/deceleration) (Werner & Engelhard 2007). Diffuse axonal injury, or microscopic damage to the neurofilament subunits within the axonal cytoskeleton, is a predominant feature of TBI due to motor vehicle and other high-speed causes of injury (Meythaler et al 2001). The main regions affected are the parasagittal white matter of the cerebral cortex, corpus callosum, and the pontine-mesencephalic junction adjacent to the superior cerebellar peduncles (Meythaler et al 2001). Diffuse axonal injury can occur in the absence of focal injuries (Topal et al 2008), occurs in mild, moderate and severe TBI, and is primarily responsible for the initial loss of consciousness (Meythaler et al 2001). The degree of diffuse axonal injury is associated with the severity of injury, long-term disability and cognitive impairment (Hou et al 2007, Meythaler et al 2001).

Cerebral laceration and contusion (or cortical bruising) occurs principally at the crests of the gyri and expands to variable depths depending on the severity of the injury. Contusion may occur where the brain strikes the skull at the site of the externally applied force (coup) or at a point 180 degrees from this site of impact, where the brain strikes the skull (contra coup) (Provenzale 2007). Contusions also occur on the under-surface of the frontal lobes and at the temporal tips due to translational movements of the brain on the bony contours of the floor of the anterior and middle cranial fossae (Provenzale 2007). In contrast to diffuse axonal injury, contusions may result from relatively low-velocity impact such as in blows to the head and falls. They may also cause multiple small intracerebral haemorrhages and occasionally more extensive bleeding. Cerebral contusions are not directly responsible for loss of consciousness but are risk factors for development of seizures, and may produce focal cognitive and sensorimotor impairments (Mendelow & Teasdale 1983).

Haemorrhage may occur in three areas of the brain (subdural haemorrhage, epidural haemorrhage, and haemorrhage into the subarachnoid and intraventricular spaces) (Provenzale 2007) due to shearing forces on blood vessels and laceration. Subdural haemorrhage occurs with forceful strikes to the skull and is commonly associated with skull fracture.

Another form of primary brain damage is laceration following penetration of the brain by a projectile or skull fragment. Associated with these, there is often a surrounding zone of damage caused by release of kinetic energy (Mendelow 1993a).

Secondary brain damage

The primary injury initiates a cascade of neuropathologic processes that result in more severe and widespread brain damage. The primary injury may cause a reduction of blood flow and oxygen supply to the brain, cerebral metabolic flow uncoupling, and impairment of cardiovascular autoregulation, leaving the brain vulnerable to secondary damage. The neuropathologic processes involved in secondary damage include release of excitotoxic levels of excitatory neurotransmitters (e.g. glutamate), impaired calcium homeostasis, generation of oxygen free radicals (e.g. superoxides), and inflammatory processes (Werner & Engelhard 2007). The consequences of these neuropathic processes include cerebral oedema, cerebral vasospasm (constriction of blood vessels), and hypoxia, which in turn lead to a critical reduction in cerebral blood flow, potentially leading to ischaemic neuronal death (Matthews et al 1995, Werner & Engelhard 2007).

Cerebral oedema is common after brain injury and is classified as vasogenic or cytotoxic. Vasogenic brain oedema is caused by cellular damage to the blood-brain barrier. The damaged barrier allows uncontrolled ion and protein transfer from the intravascular to the extracellular brain compartments leading to water accumulation in the extracellular space. Cytotoxic brain oedema is described as intracellular water accumulation in neurons, astrocytes, and microglia. It is caused by increased cell membrane permeability for ions, and ionic pump failure. Both types of cerebral oedema lead to increased intracranial pressure (ICP) and potentially ischaemic neuronal death (Vincent & Berre 2005, Werner & Engelhard 2007).

The space inside the cranium is occupied by the brain and its coverings, blood vessels, together with blood and cerebrospinal fluid. The sum of these three volumes is normally constant, so that an increase in any one occurs at the expense of the others. Since the skull is rigid, the space available is finite and an increase in intracranial mass associated with oedema, for example, causes an increase in ICP. As ICP rises, cerebral blood flow may fall. The relationship between ICP and cerebral blood flow can be described by the following equation:

Cerebral perfusion pressure =
  mean arterial blood pressure – intracranial pressure
e.g. Rowland et al 1991.

Therefore, any mechanism that leads to sufficient increase in ICP or low blood pressure, can decrease cerebral perfusion pressure and cause ischaemic damage (Deem 2006). This in turn increases cerebral oedema and the cycle continues (Mendelow 1993).

Treatment to lower ICP is recommended when it reaches a threshold of 20mmHg (Bratton et al 2007d). If ICP rises to approximately 40 to 45mmHg, the forces on the brain may cause the brain to shift from where pressure is rising to a compartment where it is lower, causing herniation of brain tissue through openings in the skull (e.g. foramen magnum herniation) or dura (e.g. tentorial herniation) (Deem 2006). Herniation ultimately results in brainstem compression with increase in systemic arterial blood pressure, bradycardia, and irregular breathing followed by apnoea. A poor outcome is likely with brain herniation, particularly if it is not corrected immediately (Deem 2006).

A reduction in mortality and severity of injury are seen when secondary brain damage is minimized (Carney & Ghajar 2007). For this reason, early intervention is focused on minimizing this damage. This is primarily achieved by optimizing cerebral perfusion and oxygenation, minimizing increases in ICP, and treatment of cerebral oedema (Ling & Marshall 2008). The Brain Trauma Foundation has developed evidence-based guidelines for the initial management of severe traumatic brain injury, with the third edition published in 2007 (Carney & Ghajar 2007). The majority of recommendations are based on level II (guideline) and level III (option) evidence and include the use of hyper-osmolar therapy (e.g. Mannitol) to reduce ICP (Bratton et al 2007b) and jugular venous saturation and brain tissue oxygen monitoring to ensure adequate oxygenation (Bratton et al 2007e).

Measures of severity

Depth of initial coma, duration of coma and length of post-traumatic amnesia (PTA) are considered to be indices of severity of TBI and predictors of outcome (Sherer et al 2008). More severe (deeper) coma and longer periods of coma and PTA are typically associated with poorer prognosis.

The Glasgow Coma Scale (GCS) (Teasdale & Jennett 1974) is the most widely used measure of the severity of coma and has provided clinicians with a relatively precise definition of coma (Chapter 3). The GCS was designed to provide a system of monitoring the comatose patient that is consistent when used by different observers, and the results of which are easily accessible to different members of the team. It consists of three features which are independently observed: eye opening, motor response and verbal response.

The initial GCS score is used to classify the injury severity as severe (GCS ≤ 8), moderate (GCS 9–12) or mild (GCS 13–15) (Jennett & Teasdale 1981). There is some disagreement about which GCS score to use, with some studies using the emergency department admission GCS and others using the lowest or highest GCS recorded in the first 24 hours (Sherer et al 2008). In early studies, the initial GCS was highly predictive of outcome at 6 months as measured by the Glasgow Outcome Scale (GOS) (Jennett & Teasdale 1981). Acute medical interventions for moderate to severe TBI in common usage today (e.g. sedation, intubation, ventilation, paralysis) may influence the GCS score and make measurement of severity less accurate (Stocchetti et al 2004).

The duration of coma and the length of PTA appear to be better preditors of functional outcome compared to the initial GCS (Sherer et al 2008). A number of different definitions of duration of coma have been used, including the interval from injury to spontaneous eye opening (Andrews et al 2002), the following of commands (Sherer et al 2008), and scoring ≥8 on the GCS (Wade 1992). The commonly accepted criteria for classifying severity of trauma using the duration of coma are: >6 hours for severe, 20 minutes to ≤6 hours for moderate, and ≤20 minutes for mild (Bond 1986).

PTA is the period of impaired consciousness that extends from the initial injury until continuous memory for ongoing events is restored (Levin et al 1982). This period is characterized by several cognitive and behavioural disturbances, including anterograde amnesia (i.e. the inability to lay down memories from after the injury from one day to the next), restlessness, agitation, fatigue and confabulation (Ahmed et al 2000). The duration of PTA can be measured by a number of scales, including the Modified Oxford PTA Scale (MOPTAS) (Fortuny et al 1980, Tate et al 2001), the Galveston Orientation and Amnesia Test (GOAT) (Levin et al 1979) and the Westmead PTA Scale (Shores et al 1986) (Chapter 3). The commonly accepted criteria for classifying severity using the duration of PTA are: >4 weeks for extremely severe, 1–4 weeks for very severe, 1–7 days for severe, 1–24 hours for moderate, and <1 hour for mild (Jennett & Teasdale 1981, Russell 1932).

Interestingly, the likely duration of PTA can be estimated reasonably accurately using the day post-injury that PTA testing commenced and the PTA scores from the first

5 days of testing (Tate et al 2001). Tate and colleagues (2001) argue that this prediction is very useful not only to plan the rehabilitation program but also to support the family of the person with TBI. A longer duration of PTA is a strong prognostic indicator for being non-productive (i.e. not returning to work or school, or being unemployed) 1-year post-injury (Willemse-van Son et al 2007).

MANAGEMENT OF ACUTE TRAUMATIC BRAIN INJURY

TBI presents a considerable problem of management. Preservation of life and prevention of secondary brain damage are the first priorities in the emergency treatment of the brain-injured and multi-injured individual, involving the expertise of a wide range of health professionals. Skilled and forward-looking management in the immediate stage can prevent many subsequent disabilities, a fact which must not be overlooked in the urgent concern to save life (Hitchcock 1971)

Improvements in acute care management over the past 30 years have contributed to a dramatic reduction in mortality from TBI (Lu et al 2005). These improvements include use of evidence-based guidelines in clinical practice, advances in neuromonitoring and neuroimaging, early aggressive neurosurgical interventions, and preventing and treating comorbid conditions such as infections (Ling & Marshall 2008)

There is no typical clinical picture following TBI. Nevertheless, the first priorities for pre-hospital staff are resuscitation, assessment of airways and prevention of aspiration. Hypotension (systolic blood pressure < 90mmHg) and hypoxaemia (PaO_2 < 60mmHg) must be avoided to minimize the risk of secondary brain damage (Bratton et al 2007a). An initial neurological evaluation using a scale such as the GCS is also conducted in the field to assist with categorizing the severity of injury and to triage the patient (Bazarian et al 2003).

When the patient arrives at the emergency department, a non-contrast enhanced CT scan should be performed as soon as possible (Ling & Marshall 2008). This enables the identification of any conditions appropriate for neurosurgical intervention (e.g. presence of expanding intracranial hematoma, or malignant cerebral oedema) (Ling & Marshall 2008). Haematomas may need evacuation. Decompressive craniectomy is an emerging clinical management approach to aggressively combat rising ICP, however, data is still conflicting and large randomized controlled trials are underway.

If neurosurgery is not required, the patient may be admitted to intensive care. TBI patients are preferably nursed in a neurosurgical or specialized brain-injury intensive care unit and there is some evidence to suggest that the provision of these facilities improves outcome (Patel et al 2002). Monitoring of vital signs and coma are routinely performed. It is recommended that ICP monitoring be conducted in all patients with severe TBI and abnormal CT scan (Bratton et al 2007c) as it enables early recognition of intracranial hypertension (e.g. Frost 1987) and prevention of secondary brain damage (Frost 1985, Shapiro 1975). Observation of progression of the clinical picture from the moment of injury is critical to management. Any patient whose level of consciousness deteriorates should be considered to have a haematoma (Mendelow 1993a) and requires immediate investigation.

Respiratory function

The management of the TBI individual varies depending on the severity of the problems. The management of respiratory function of the comatose TBI patient is complex. It requires an understanding of the relationship between pulmonary, cardiovascular and neurological function, and of the mechanical and physiological effects of respiratory techniques, since inappropriate intervention can exacerbate the problems of hypoxia and hypercapnia. Early control of the airway by endotracheal tube and controlled ventilation is paramount to reduce the likelihood of hypoxemia, hypocapnia, or hypercapnia, to protect the airway from aspiration (e.g. of vomitus) and reduce ICP (Helm et al 2002).

Control of breathing is normally a complex interaction of a number of mechanisms. Brain tissue requires adequate oxygenation in order to function and the respiratory system relies on drive from the brain to control ventilation. In the TBI patient, injury can cause abnormalities or dysfunction of any or all of the mechanisms that provide for adequate oxygenation and ventilation (Mackay et al 1997). For example, lung function may be compromised by damage to the lung or chest wall (e.g. pulmonary contusion, fractured ribs), or damage to the respiratory centres of the brain. Similarly, brain function may be compromised if the respiratory system is damaged by changing the arterial blood oxygen and carbon dioxide content delivered to the damaged brain tissue. This can affect cerebral autoregulation, alter cerebral perfusion pressure, and potentially cause ischaemia (Baigelman & O'Brien 1981).

Patients with mild or moderate brain injuries (GCS > 8) who have adequate arterial blood gases, no respiratory dysfunction or signs of deterioration, are usually not ventilated but their inspired oxygen concentration is increased since the oxygen requirements of the damaged brain are greater than those of the undamaged brain (Mackay et al 1997). In the severe brain injured patient (GCS ≤ 8), hypoventilation or apnoea may be present, reflected by hypercapnia ($PaCO_2$ > 45mmHg) and severe hypoxemia (PaO_2 < 60mmHg). This situation requires immediate intubation, oxygenation, and ventilatory support (Mackay et al 1997). Patients may also be paralysed and sedated. Ventilation and the associated paralysis and sedation decrease cerebral blood volume and prevent potentially noxious stimuli and inadequate respiration from causing further brain damage. Paralysis and sedation are usually discontinued after three days, and, when patients are able to maintain adequate blood gases, they are extubated. If prolonged mechanical ventilation is required, early tracheostomy is generally recommended (Rozet & Domino 2007).

Pulmonary complications (e.g. pneumonia, atelectasis, adult respiratory distress syndrome) are the most frequent medical complication associated with TBI, dramatically contributing to mortality (Rozet & Domino 2007). Therefore, respiratory treatment is an essential part of the care of the person with TBI. The major aims of physiotherapy intervention as part of the team involved in the initial management of the person with TBI are to:

- Improve respiratory function and
- Prevent respiratory complications and secondary brain damage

by ensuring adequate ventilation and clearing of excessive secretions. The major respiratory problems amenable to intervention are hypoventilation, impaired mucociliary clearance, hyperventilation and ventilation/perfusion mismatch (Cook 2003).

Physiotherapy interventions such as positioning, percussion, manual hyperinflation, and suctioning can affect intracranial variables (e.g. ICP and mean arterial blood pressure), with adverse events more likely to occur when these variables are outside normal levels prior to commencement of treatment (Zeppos et al 2007). The benefits and risks of intervention need to be carefully weighed, intracranial variables (ICP and cerebral perfusion pressure) closely monitored, and interventions modified or shortened according to need (Imle et al 1997). For example, postural drainage typically needs to be modified since the head-dependent position is contraindicated where there is a risk of increasing ICP.

The other major goal of physiotherapy during the acute phase when the patient is comatose and therefore immobilized, is the prevention of muscle and soft tissue contracture in order to maintain musculoskeletal integrity.

Musculoskeletal integrity

Impaired motor control and coma effectively immobilize the individual following TBI, who is then vulnerable to the musculoskeletal and cardiorespiratory adaptations associated with bed rest, reduced physical activity and disuse. Soft tissue changes and reduced cardiorespiratory fitness are likely to impede rehabilitation by interfering with active and intense training designed to improve motor performance.

Immobilization of skeletal muscle is known to induce both muscle atrophy and impairment of contraction. Muscle tissue responds selectively and differentially to the demands placed on it, altering its structure (length, volume, cross-sectional area) in response to changes in the operating conditions (Tabary et al 1981, Tabary et al 1976). Muscle force production and levels of physical activity have an important relationship with other components of the musculoskeletal system such as tendons, ligaments and bones. Deprivation of mechanical stresses normally imposed on the skeleton by the musculature can result in demineralization of the skeleton (McLellan 1993). Furthermore, loading of bones and joints is important in order to preserve bone mass and density and to maintain healthy articular cartilage (Akeson et al 1980).

Soft tissue contractures are reported to be common following TBI, with a prevalence of 11–81% (Fergusson et al 2007, Moseley et al 2008). Muscles at particular risk of shortening due to the effects of position (and immobilization) include hip and knee flexors, ankle plantarflexors and inverters, shoulder adductors and internal rotators, elbow flexors, forearm pronators, wrist and finger flexors, thumb flexors and adductors or any other muscle held persistently at a short length. Animal studies have shown that when muscle is subjected to imposed and maintained change in length, it undergoes anatomical, biochemical and physiological changes (Gossman et al 1982). These length-associated changes can be induced by many factors including immobilization, muscle imbalance, postural malalignment or, as is typical, a combination of these. Furthermore, these changes start to occur within a few hours of immobilization and can have a profound effect on motor performance.

A typical animal model used in studying the effect of imposed changes of length on muscle involves immobilizing a joint in a plaster cast (for an overview see Herbert 2005). When immobilized in a shortened position, muscle loses sarcomeres (while muscle immobilized in a lengthened position adds sarcomeres) (Coutinho et al 2004). Loss of sarcomeres results in the remaining sarcomeres being pulled out to a length which affects the ability of the muscle to generate tension, with maximum tension being developed at the immobilized length (Tabary et al 1972, Williams 1990, Williams & Goldspink 1973). Connective tissue in muscle immobilized in a shortened position changes in alignment (orientation and crimp pattern) and increases in concentration relative to the muscle tissue (Jarvinen et al 2002), which also contributes to the muscles becoming shorter and stiffer. In functional terms, an increase in stiffness of muscle has an adverse effect on motor function since it will take an increased amount of force to lengthen the muscle actively during movement. It is thought that connective tissue remodelling is associated with lack of movement (Akeson et al 1987) both in terms of lack of stretch applied and reduced muscle activity, whereas the stimulus for muscle fibre adaptation results from the imposed length (Tabary et al 1972). Range of joint motion is reduced, therefore, both by the shortening of muscle fibres and by loss of muscle compliance (increased stiffness). In addition to impaired muscle compliance, tendon (Herbert & Crosbie 1997) and ligament and joint capsule (Akeson et al 1987, Akeson et al 1980) also lose extensibility following immobilization.

Electrically induced constant contraction of the muscle when it is held at a shortened length appears to exaggerate the rate and quantity of sarcomere loss (Tabary et al 1981). Spasticity and dystonic posturing following severe TBI may, therefore, lead to more rapid development of contracture.

Muscle weakness and atrophy are well known adaptations associated with disuse. Interestingly the effect of disuse in non-trained healthy subjects has been found to be most obvious in highly active antigravity muscles, such as triceps surae (White & Davies 1984), particularly the slow-twitch soleus and quadriceps. For example, atrophy of quadriceps has been detected as early as 3 days after immobilization (Lindboe & Platou 1984). The decrease in muscle strength, found when a muscle is immobilized in the shortened position, appears to be greater than that attributable to decrease in size alone.

The major aim in preserving musculoskeletal integrity in people with TBI is to prevent or minimize adaptive changes in soft tissue, in particular to prevent muscle shortening and increased stiffness by:

- Applying passive stretch to the at-risk muscles and soft tissues.
- Loading bone and cartilage.
- Task-related training that involves active stretching during the lengthening phase of actions.

Passive stretch is used clinically to prevent (or treat) contracture. The duration of passive stretch recommended varies widely, from passive range of motion and other very brief stretch applied with the therapist's hands (Harvey et al 2009, Light et al 1984) to longer stretches by positioning using equipment, and continuous stretch applied using serial casting (Moseley 1997).

Although recommended in rehabilitation texts, it appears that passive range of motion (PROM) and brief stretch have little effect on preventing development of (or treating) contracture. In a recent clinical trial evaluating the effects of PROM exercises in people with spinal cord injury, 6 months of regular passive movements to the ankle joint had very small effects on ankle mobility compared to no intervention (mean between-group difference in passive ankle dorsiflexion was 4 degrees, 95% confidence interval 2–6 degrees) (Harvey et al 2009).

PROM may also have deleterious effects on soft tissue. A possible relationship between trauma produced by forceful passive movements and neurogenic heterotopic ossification was reported many years ago (Silver 1969) and immobilization with intermittent forceful manipulation can induce heterotopic ossification in experimental animals (Vanden Bossche et al 2008). Passive ranging performed too vigorously or in too large a range can cause

micro tears in muscle. Such tears cause bleeding into the muscle which leads to ossification, or myositis ossificans, a form of heterotopic ossification, and further loss of mobility. Early signs of myositis include decreased range of movement, increased pain and swelling. The most common sites are around the elbow, shoulder and hip (Horn & Garland 1990).

Since spasticity is velocity-dependent (see Chapter 8), PROM exercises performed too quickly may cause an increase in hyperreflexia. Conversely, in the presence of muscle weakness and paralysis, PROM exercises performed at the end of range may overstretch and damage periarticular connective tissue. This is especially likely in joints that rely on the braking activity of muscles for protection at end of range, such as the glenohumeral joint.

If passive exercises are the only way of moving joints in a person with TBI with severe weakness (or paralysis) or altered levels of consciousness, they should probably be performed slowly, with care taken at the end of range not to cause abnormal stress. In this case, passive movements of the limbs also provide an opportunity to make some contact with the individual, with the therapist (or relative) describing the movements being performed.

Passive stretch can be applied for longer periods of time by positioning and using equipment. For example, the calf muscles can be stretched for periods of 30–60 minutes by standing with the support of a tilt table with a wedge placed under the feet to maximize the stretch (e.g. Ben et al 2005) (Fig 12.1). This standing also loads the bones and cartilage of the lower limbs, providing a weight-bearing stimulus to maintain bone mineral density. Stretches of longer duration (e.g. 8 hours or overnight) can be applied using splints (e.g. see Harvey et al 2006). Clinical trials evaluating the effects of prolonged low load stretch have produced equivocal and conflicting results, while prolonged stretch appears to be superior to brief stretch (Light et al 1984) other trials report negligible difference between prolonged stretch and no stretch treatment conditions (Ben et al 2005, Harvey et al 2006).

In the first days post-injury, the comatose patient can be positioned in side lying or semi-prone to help prevent the development of contractures. A pillow placed between the slightly flexed legs prevents the hips from adducting. The upper limb may be positioned on a pillow with the shoulder girdle protracted and the elbow extended. Inflatable plastic blow-up splints or foam splints may be useful in maintaining position.

As soon as vital signs are stable, in particular blood pressure and ICP, periods of sitting (Fig 12.2) and standing, if necessary with external constraints, are instituted. The standing position loads bones, and applies stretch to soft tissue predisposed to developing contracture, e.g. lower limb flexors. Patients can be placed in the upright standing position on a tilt table (Fig 12.1). This procedure does not produce dynamically distributed compression forces through the bones as would occur in the natural

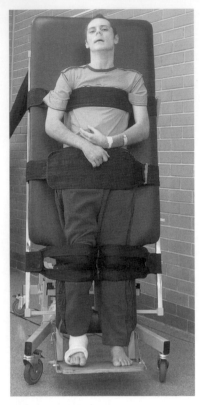

Figure 12.1 Standing on a tilt table. Note the footplate is angled upwards and there is a serial cast on the right ankle to apply stretch to the calf muscles. A high table may be placed in front of a tilt table to enable participation in cognitive, reaching and manipulative activities while adjusting to the vertical position.

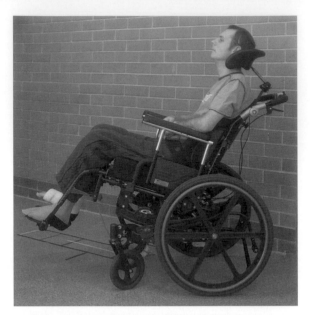

Figure 12.2 A tilt-in-space wheelchair (Quickie IRIS Tilt Wheelchair) allows a patient to be sat upright to engage in therapy and assist with postural control. The chair can be tilted back to change the distribution of pressure and allow rest. The headrest can be removed to encourage strengthening of neck extensor muscles. Footplates are adjusted to keep ankles in a plantargrade position.

process of standing up. However, if patients need to be stood up slowly to control blood pressure changes, a tilt table is essential. Furthermore, using a tilt table may be the only way to get a person into standing and to stay there for a sufficiently long period to stretch soft tissue at risk of shortening.

Since the upright position is vital for the proper functioning of many organs, other possible benefits of having the patient stand for periods during the day may include:

- Stimulation of internal functions such as bowel movements and bladder emptying.
- Improved ventilation (the abdominal contents move down giving more space for lung expansion, redistributing air flow to basal lobes, and changing perfusion/ventilation ratio).
- Decreased ICP as cerebral venous return is increased provided autoregulation is intact.
- Improved arousal, attention and interaction with other people and the environment.

Since the upright position can result in large drops in cerebral blood flow if autoregulation is compromised, blood pressure and ICP should be monitored during initial attempts to stand the patient.

The use of serial casting has been found to be effective in both preventing (Sullivan et al 1988) and correcting contracture (Moseley 1997, Moseley et al 2008) in people with TBI. Applying casts with muscle in a lengthened or neutral position stretches the connective tissue elements and may provide a stimulus for the muscle to add sarcomeres to the muscle fibre as reported in animal studies (Tabary et al 1972). Sullivan and colleagues (1988) comment that casting has been more successful when patients at risk of developing contracture are immediately placed in casts rather than waiting for contracture to occur.

The critical features in applying casts are described by Sullivan and colleagues (1988) and Moseley (1997). Casts are applied with minimum padding in order to prevent movement and ensure a sustained stretch (Fig 12.3a). When casting a two-joint muscle, a lengthened position is more easily achieved if the cast is applied while the muscle is not lengthened over the other joint (Fig 12.3b). Monitoring of circulation is initiated as soon as casts are applied and they need to be changed regularly to examine the condition of the skin. Another reason for changing casts

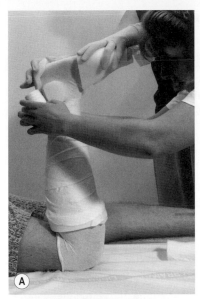

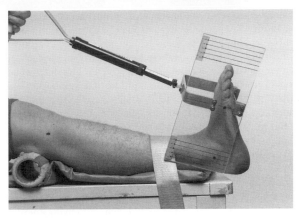

Figure 12.4 A torque-controlled measurement procedure. A known torque is applied to produce passive ankle dorsiflexion in a standardized testing position. Ankle angle is measured using skin surface markers and photography. *(From Moseley, A. (1997) The effect of casting combined with stretching on passive ankle dorsiflexion in adults with traumatic head injuries. Physical Therapy, 77, 240–259, by permission).*

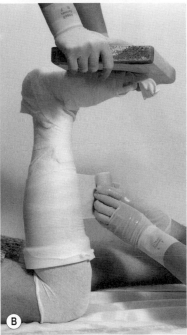

Figure 12.3 Application of cast, (A) Application of stockinette and padding over bony prominences prior to casting, (B) Soleus muscle is stretched into maximum obtainable dorsiflexion using a board placed on the plantar surface of the foot while the cast is applied. Note that with the knee in flexion, the gastrocnemius muscle is not lengthened over both joints. *(From Moseley. A. (1997) The effect of casting combined with stretching on passive ankle dorsiflexion in adults with traumatic head injuries. Physical Therapy, 77, 240–259, by permission).*

regularly is to measure joint range to ensure that muscle shortening is in fact being prevented/corrected (Fig 12.4). The therapist applying the cast needs to be technically skilled in order to prevent complications. Muscle relaxants and sedating drugs may be necessary to achieve a lengthened position in the awake individual. These drugs, however, tend to depress brain function and should be avoided if possible.

Maintaining functional muscle length is critical to the re-establishing of active self-initiated functional movement. For motor training to be effective, muscles must be of functional length not only so that movement of the necessary amplitude can be performed but also so that the muscles can generate tension over the necessary range of movement. Note that it is only by lengthening the muscle that the range, over which the muscle can actively generate tension, can be increased. Casting may be imperative if exercise and training are not sufficient to lengthen muscle actively.

Altered levels of consciousness

There are three main disorders of consciousness after TBI. Coma is a state of unconsciousness in which there is neither arousal nor awareness (Plum & Posner 1980). Eyes remain closed and there is an absence of sleep/wake cycles. As the definition implies, there is no motor response to command and no speech. Coma exists in the early period after injury and usually lasts no longer than 3–4 weeks. Individuals who remain unconscious for more than a few weeks can evolve into a vegetative state which is characterized by the presence of spontaneous sleep-wake cycles but absence of cortical activity (Jennett & Plum 1972). The vegetative state describes a condition in which the patient demonstrates no signs of cognition but may return to wakefulness with the eyes open in response to verbal stimuli. Although sleep/wake cycles, normal blood pressure and normal respiration are present, the patient is unable to engage in verbal interaction or produce organized, discrete motor responses (Garner & Valadka 1994). The patient appears to be 'awake but not aware'. Individuals who show inconsistent evidence of consciousness are classified as being in a minimally conscious state (Giacino et al 2002). A minimally conscious state has recently been defined as "a condition of severely altered consciousness in which minimal but definite behavioral evidence of self or environmental awareness is demonstrated" (Giacino et al 2002, pp 350–1).

There is a need to distinguish between the type of altered consciousness (and between altered consciousness and locked-in syndrome, for an overview see Giacino et al 2002) in order to plan the rehabilitation program and support the family of the person with TBI. New technologies are being developed to assist this process (e.g. magnetic resonance imaging and magnetic resonance spectroscopy), but these still lack sufficient accuracy to make a differential diagnosis (Weiss et al 2007). Until these diagnostic tools have been fully validated, classification needs to be based on careful and systematic clinical observation of the person with TBI. A number of clinical assessments have been developed to monitor the minimally conscious state (for an overview see Giacino & Whyte 2005). For example, the Western Neuro Sensory Stimulation Profile (Ansell & Keenan 1989) systematically assesses arousal/attention, auditory/visual/tactile response and expressive communication domains, and has been used to track emergence from the minimal conscious state in people with TBI (Taylor et al 2007).

The environment around the TBI individual with altered consciousness needs to be taken into account. If environmental effects are not considered, the unconscious person is not only deprived of normal sensory input but many of the necessary observations may produce stimulating and painful sensory input throughout 24 hours each day (e.g. turning, tracheal stimulation, attention to hygiene, feeding). The physiotherapist's contribution needs to take account of the timing of interventions.

Family involvement, education and counselling are important considerations. Both family and team members need to understand the importance of speaking to the patient, of the need to consider the patient's feelings during conversation around the bed, of the need to preserve a sense of dignity by ensuring that he or she is appropriately covered, and of providing specific input which encourages some active response from the patient. The family can provide important information about the patient's favourite name, interests, likes and dislikes.

Recovery from coma

Recovery from coma manifests itself with periods of opening of the eyes. This is evidence that the mechanisms concerned with wakefulness are recovering. The minimally conscious state may follow the period of coma. During this phase the person with TBI starts to inconsistently demonstrate conscious awareness of self or their environment. The Aspen Neurobehavioral Conference Workgroup outlined 4 criteria that characterize entry into the minimally conscious state (Giacino et al 2002). At least one of these criteria needed to be observed:

- Following simple instructions.
- Gestural or verbal yes/no responses
- Intelligible verbalizations
- Purposeful movements or affective behaviours that are contingent on relevant environmental stimuli (e.g. appropriate smiling or reaching to grasp an object).

Emergence from the minimally conscious state, as defined by the Aspen Group, is characterized by consistent and reliable functional communication and/or the functional use of 2 different objects (Giacino et al 2002). Functional communication was operationally defined as providing accurate yes/no responses 100% of the time to 6 situational orientation questions on 2 consecutive assessments. An example of a situational orientation question is: "Are you sitting down?". Functional object use was defined as the appropriate use of at least 2 different objects (e.g. bringing a comb to the head) on 2 consecutive assessments. Emergence from the minimal conscious state indicates a readiness to engage in more intensive rehabilitation.

Several interventions (including pharmacologic and sensory stimulation programs) to accelerate recovery of consciousness have been investigated, but none has proven effective (Giacino & Whyte 2005). Current best practice involves the prevention of complications (e.g. contracture, pressure areas, respiratory infection) and maintaining nutrition while the individual recovers consciousness. The establishment of regular testing to monitor emergence from coma, the vegetative state or the minimally conscious state is useful for the rehabilitation team and the family.

The re-establishment of swallowing, unassisted breathing, effective coughing and communication through facial expression, gesture and language is essential if the patient is to resume more normal function. At the stage when the patient is emerging from coma, the establishment of an unambiguous and easy way to produce a yes/no response is critical to re-establishing some form of communication. Options to augment communication include eye gaze, facial expression, gesture and communication boards with letters (Fig 12.5), symbols or pictures.

Once patients can breathe unaided for several minutes they are disconnected from the ventilator for short periods.

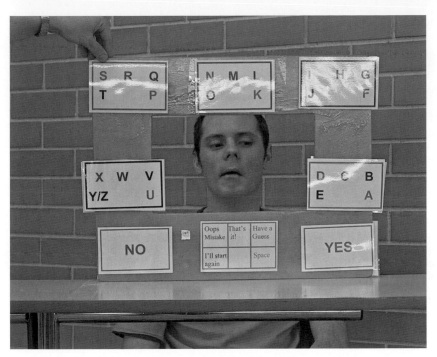

Figure 12.5 Critical to early rehabilitation is the need to establish meaningful communication with a patient. This young man is able to use eye gaze with this double-sided communication board to answer simple questions.

Tension and anxiety, which may precipitate respiratory distress, are to be avoided. Periods of unassisted breathing are increased in duration and frequency. Articulation, phonation and eating are dependent upon control of breathing. Patients who have both a nasogastric and tracheostomy tube need training to improve co-ordination of these functions once the tubes are removed. Sitting with erect trunk and head are critical pre-requisites for swallowing, improved lung expansion and coughing as well as fostering orientation, eye contact and communication. If the individual cannot sit unsupported or hold the head upright some form of external restraint may be necessary (Fig 12.2).

The reticular formation (neurons in the brain stem extending through the medulla, pons and midbrain) is considered to mediate aspects of arousal (Kelly & Dodd 1991). It is likely, therefore, that the erect position facilitates arousal by providing a change in the orientation of the head and neck. Standing is also critical for proper functioning of many organs, including regaining control over continence.

After emergence from unconsiousness, the individual with TBI is usually amnesic and exhibits disturbed behaviour (Jennett & Teasdale 1981). During this period of PTA there is severe anterograde memory disorder (amnesia for events occurring after the precipitating trauma) in association with other problems such as disorientation, restlessness, agitation, fatigue and confabulation (Ahmed et al

2000). The most common behaviours observed early in the PTA period (i.e. in more than 20% of cases) are poor concentration, no self monitoring, wandering, agitation, incoherent verbalization, and aggression (Weir et al 2006).

Since PTA involves anterograde amnesia, it is a common belief that new learning cannot take place during this phase. As a consequence, functional assessment and intensive rehabilitation are often delayed until after the individual has emerged from PTA (Tate et al 2000). However, procedural learning (i.e. the learning of skills) may be preserved during PTA (Ewert et al 1989, Weir et al 2006). Ewert and colleagues (1989) illustrated this in a small group of people in PTA after TBI. While these patients had a stable impairment for memory of declarative tasks (i.e. recognition of the words used in mirror reading, questionnaire concerning details of the previous testing session), their performance improved in a number of procedural tasks (i.e. mirror reading, mazes, pursuit tracking task). This suggests that people with TBI have the capacity to learn motor skills and may benefit from task-related training while in PTA.

Appropriate behavioural and environmental strategies are needed to facilitate active participation in task-related training by the patient in PTA. Approaches that may increase involvement include:

- Practice of whole tasks that are relevant to the patient (rather than parts of tasks).

- Structuring the environment to make the task easier to perform.
- The use of concrete goals.
- Using demonstration and performing the exercise with the patient.
- Minimizing the amount of manual guidance and instruction.
- Performing a large number of repetitions of practice.
- Providing short, frequent sessions.
- Removing distractions and triggers for outbursts of aggressive behaviour from the training environment.

The PTA phase can be difficult for both relatives and staff to deal with but it is important that the patient's natural recovery is not impeded by heavy sedation. Families require reassurance since, having ceased to fear for the survival of the individual, they may now be very concerned about the future. Families need early counselling to be able to cope with altered behaviour, to be prepared for difficulties likely to occur, and be given some short-term objectives as well as some hint of the ultimate degree of recovery that is expected. The establishment of daily testing to monitor emergence from PTA is useful for the rehabilitation team and the family, as the expected duration of PTA can now be estimated reasonably accurately (Tate et al 2001).

The end of PTA is a crucial stage in the recovery process and is associated with the restoration of other mental skills. Emergence from PTA is a gradual process with marked variability between patients. Amnesia appears to resolve before disorientation (Tate et al 2000). The most common pattern of resolution of disorientation is orientation to person, followed by orientation to place, followed by orientation to time (Tate et al 2000, Weir et al 2006). The typical PTA behaviours also gradually resolve, with incoherent verbalization and aggression resolving early, followed by wandering and agitation, and poor concentration and no self monitoring being the last to resolve (Weir et al 2006).

Bladder and bowel function

While urinary (Chua et al 2003, Leary et al 2006) and faecal (Leary et al 2006) incontinence are relatively common after TBI, bladder and bowel management is not routinely addressed in interdisciplinary management (Leary et al 2006). Factors that contribute to incontinence include muscle weakness, cognitive impairment and neurogenic bladder and bowel dysfunction. Slowed mobility, poor communication and impaired initiation also contribute to incontinence. Neurogenic bladder dysfunction is assessed by measuring urinary retention after an individual voids (Chua et al 2003). After a thorough evaluation, intervention could include an external collecting device, pelvic floor muscle training, mobility and communication training, or a bladder training program.

REHABILITATION: AN OVERALL VIEW

Rehabilitation of the TBI individual requires the provision of comprehensive interdisciplinary rehabilitation services including physiotherapist, occupational therapist, social worker, speech pathologist, neuropsychologist, clinical psychologist, doctor, nurse, recreation officer and vocational rehabilitation counsellor. Rehabilitation should begin in the acute surgical or intensive care unit and continue in a rehabilitation centre or the person may visit the rehabilitation centre from home or transitional living centre, an arrangement which helps the person bridge the gap between hospital-based facilities and re-entry into the community. At periodic intervals, the patient and family need assistance in coming to terms with the person's changing physical, mental and social capabilities. Rehabilitation of the severely brain-damaged individual may continue for many years and some patients will require long-term care.

The issue of predicting outcome, time course and degree of recovery is complex and may be affected by many factors. The study of outcome from rehabilitation of TBI has been hampered by lack of agreement on methods for monitoring the process of recovery, or the degree of recovery finally reached, as well as the diversity of populations studied. In a systematic review of prospective cohort studies, Willemse-van Son and colleagues (2007) concluded that the strong prognostic factors for long-term disability were older age, pre-injury unemployment, pre-injury substance abuse, and more disability at rehabilitation discharge, while the strong prognostic factors for being non-productive were pre-injury unemployment, longer PTA, more disability at rehabilitation admission, and pre-injury substance abuse.

TBI is by nature a diffuse and multifocal insult. For this reason there is great variability in sensorimotor, cognitive, behavioural and personality impairments depending on many factors including the pattern, extent and severity of the damage. The therapist is faced with understanding the complex interaction of the many physical, cognitive and behavioural impairments.

Cognitive and behavioural impairments

It has long been realized that it is the cognitive impairments and changes in personality and behaviour that have the most profound consequences in terms of rehabilitation and social reintegration (Jennett & Teasdale 1981, Marsh et al 2002, Wood & Rutterford 2006). Jennett and Teasdale (1981) describe the effect of these deficits on the family and the individual. As these authors point out, suffering a TBI, even brief concussion, is a significant experience for anyone. The severely injured person wakes up after days or sometimes weeks unable to recall anything that occurred in that time. Unbeknown to the individual, relatives have been fearing for his or her life but are now concerned about mental status. Insight into the situation and implications for the future, however, may take months to develop. It is often only when the individual with TBI goes home that the extent of the effects of the injury on the person and the family are fully realized.

Cognition

A wide variety of cognitive impairments have been reported, the most common being disorders of learning and memory, the rate of information processing and attention, and executive function (Draper & Ponsford 2008, Mathias & Wheaton 2007, Millis et al 2001, Tate et al 1991). These impairments are evident early after moderate to extremely severe TBI (Tate et al 1991) and are still present 5–10 years post-injury (Draper & Ponsford 2008, Millis et al 2001). While these cognitive impairments are relatively common after TBI, the combination of impairments exhibited by individuals is highly varied (Tate et al 1991). For a good overview of cognitive impairment after TBI readers are directed to Lezak (1995).

Impairment of memory and learning is frequently identified by patients and their relatives. Memory has several components, including working memory, immediate memory (both verbal and visual), learning rate, use of semantic knowledge, forgetting rate, sensitivity to interference, retrograde amnesia, and prospective memory (Vakil 2005). While the exact nature of memory and learning impairments is difficult to unravel using neuropsychological testing, it is likely that the relearning of motor tasks in the individual with memory impairment will require a larger number of repetitions of practice. Using worksheets, photographs and video footage to record the exercises to be performed and the goals of therapy may facilitate task-related training.

Memory aids and strategies can also be used by the individual with TBI to cope with everyday life. In a recent survey of 101 people with self-reported memory impairment after acquired brain injury (69 with TBI), the remembering strategies used successfully by more than 40% of the group were wall calendars or charts, notebooks, lists, appointment diaries, asking others to remind them, using mental retracing to find missing objects, and alarm clocks (Evans et al 2003). There was a significant relationship between being independent and using 6 or more memory aids or strategies. The successful use of memory aids could be predicted by four variables: (1) lower current age; (2) shorter time since injury; (3) use of more memory aids premorbidly; and, (4) less marked attentional impairment (Evans et al 2003). Electronic memory aids (e.g. a paging system, mobile phone reminders) have also been shown to increase the success of carrying out everyday activities such as self care tasks, taking medication and attending appointments (Culley & Evans 2009, Wilson et al 2001).

Impairment of attention can include difficulty in selectively directing attention to the task at hand, in dividing attention between tasks, in sustaining attention over time and in overall attention capacity (Mathias & Wheaton 2007). Information processing speed can have marked effects on cognitive function, particularly on attention (Mathias & Wheaton 2007). Task-related training is possible in the presence of attention deficits and slowed processing speeds. Strategies which can assist with directing and sustaining attention include training interesting tasks that are relevant to the individual, using clear visual or auditory cues and feedback, and modifying the environment in order to remove distractions. Providing feedback on the time taken to complete a number of repetitions of a task (e.g. the time taken to step up onto a block 10 times) may increase speed.

Dividing attention across two or more tasks is required for skilled performance of open tasks (e.g. using public transport or walking down a busy corridor) (Gentile 2000). However, people with acquired brain injury (including TBI) exhibit slowed performance or increased errors when they perform two tasks (i.e. dual task condition) compared to when they perform a single task in isolation, and this decrement in performance is not observed in healthy controls (Haggard et al 2000). A preliminary study suggests that practice under dual-task conditions improves performance in people with TBI (Evans et al 2009).

A neuropsychological assessment as described by Lezak (1995) provides a picture of the individual's cognitive strengths and weaknesses. Interventions to rehabilitate cognitive impairment after TBI can be broadly divided into interventions to remediate the specific cognitive function (e.g. drills and computer tasks) and interventions which focus on learning compensatory strategies in order to cope with chronic cognitive deficits. There have been three extensive systematic reviews which have evaluated the effectiveness of cognitive rehabilitation (Cicerone et al 2000, Cicerone et al 2005, Rohling et al 2009). The most recent concludes that there is strong evidence that rehabilitation of attention improves attention outcomes, while memory rehabilitation produced moderate size effects on measures of memory (Rohling et al 2009).

Executive dysfunction involves impairment of high-level organisation abilities that encompass planning, decision-making, self-monitoring, problem-solving, inhibition and attention. As described by Lezak (1995), these aspects allow individuals to engage in purposeful, self-focused activities. Impairments in this area have a broad impact on communication, social interactions and behaviour. Therapy for executive dysfunction focuses on training multiple steps, strategic thinking and multi-tasking in individual and group sessions, and can have immediate and lasting effects on measures of cognitive impairment, activity and participation (Kennedy et al 2008). Strategies that may facilitate task-related training in the presence of executive dysfunction include using worksheets, photographs and video footage to record the exercises to be performed, and providing clear cues, instructions, feedback, and goals.

Behaviour

Impaired regulation of mood and behaviour is evident after TBI, and it is increasingly understood that disorganized behaviour seen after frontal lobe damage is related to impairments in the cognitive domain (Lezak 1995, Ylvisaker et al 2003). Behaviours can be broadly classified as impaired drive or dyscontrol (Ylvisaker et al 2003). Behaviours allied with impaired drive or arousal include reduced initiation, apathy, loss of interest, lethargy, slowness, inattentiveness, reduced spontaneity, unconcern, lack of emotional reactivity, and dullness. Behaviours related to dyscontrol include disinhibition, impulsiveness, lability, reduced anger control, aggressiveness, sexual acting out, perseveration, and generally poor social judgment.

The prevalence and severity of these neurobehavioural sequelae are difficult to estimate. Neurobehavioural symptoms were present 1-year post-injury in about two-thirds of a cohort of 164 adults admitted to hospital with a diagnosis of TBI, and about 40% had 3 or more symptoms (Deb et al 1999). Behaviours reported as causing moderate to severe problems in more than 10% of the cohort were sleep problems (17%), impatience (15%), irritability (14%), mood swings (14%), socialization problems (13%), and fatigue (13%) (Deb et al 1999). In contrast, the caregivers of 62 people with moderate or severe TBI rated the following items from the Head Injury Behaviour Rating Scale as being problematic 1-year post-injury: impatience (73%), impulsivity (63%), overly sensitive (61%), childish (60%), argumentative (58%), anger (55%), difficulty in becoming interested in things (53%), lacks motivation (53%), depressed (52%), anxious (52%), and poor insight (50%) (Marsh & Kersel 2006). Of 79 people with TBI admitted to a specialist rehabilitation service because of their challenging behaviour, verbal aggression was assessed to be the most prevalent behaviour (89%), followed by inappropriate social behaviour (81%), physical aggression directed at other people (48%), and lack of initiation (41%) (Kelly et al 2008).

It has been emphasized by Ylvisaker and colleagues (2003, p. 16) that rehabilitation for people with TBI with challenging behaviours does not involve the "piecemeal reduction of behaviors considered unacceptable by others, but rather a comprehensive lifestyle change, including construction of a meaningful role of personal value". The framework for intervention is based on applied behaviour analysis, with therapy provided to develop behaviours required to construct meaningful roles (Ylvisaker et al 2003). Applied behaviour analysis involves investigation

of both the antecedents and consequences of the behaviour. Antecedents are the events and circumstances that occur before the behaviour and set the conditions that 'trigger' the behaviour to occur. For example, careful observations revealed that transition between activities, changes in routine, requests without choice, and the use of specific language (like saying 'no' or 'however' in response to a request from the patient) were triggers for physical aggression in a child with TBI (Pace et al 2005). Antecedent-focused strategies that have been used successfully in TBI rehabilitation include environmental simplification, consistency and modulation, carefully planned staff communication with patients, clearly specified and agreed upon treatment goals and schedules, and the use of signs, prompts and reminders (Ylvisaker et al 2003). The consequences of the behaviour component of applied behaviour analysis involves rewarding instances of appropriate behaviour and ignoring instances of inappropriate behaviour. Rewards that have been used in TBI rehabilitation include social (e.g. praise, interest and social interaction), food and the earning of money, points or tokens (Ylvisaker et al 2003).

A small proportion of people with TBI present with serious challenging behaviours that preclude the individual from rehabilitation and community reintegration. For this sub-group, behaviour modification in a highly structured environment (e.g. a behaviour unit) is required. The program is based on positive reinforcement (tokens, privileges, interest, attention and praise) of all appropriate behaviour and the strict avoidance of such reinforcement of inappropriate and socially unacceptable behaviours (Eames & Wood 1985, Wood 1987). The goals of treatment as summarized by Eames et al (1990) are:

- Reward all instances of appropriate behaviour.
- Withhold rewards that are currently maintaining maladaptive behaviour.
- Withhold all sources of positive reinforcement for a brief period after each instance of maladaptive behaviour (time-out from positive reinforcement).
- Apply a predeclared penalty following the maladaptive behaviour.
- Apply an aversive consequence following extremely severe or resistant maladaptive behaviour.

Communication

Sarno's detailed studies (Sarno 1980, 1984) have shown that *impaired communication* is a common consequence of TBI. Except in the case of focal left hemisphere damage, language dysfunction following TBI differs considerably from the aphasias seen following stroke. Adequate speech is often present (i.e. good results on conventional language tests) but language may be ineffective at a conversation level (Togher 2000). Whereas individuals with aphasia often communicate better than they talk, individuals with TBI frequently talk better than they communicate (Milton

& Wertz 1986). These cognitive-communication difficulties are a manifestation of the underlying cognitive and behavioural impairments experienced by the individual with TBI (e.g. memory, self-regulation, divided attention). New strategies for optimizing language and communication are being developed that involve training the communication partners of the person with TBI (Togher et al 2004) and social skills training for the individual (McDonald et al 2008).

In the period of recovery characterized by confusion and generally inappropriate behaviour, communication management includes tolerance for slow and cumbersome speech, use of orientational and pertinent cues, strategies to focus attention (addressing the individual by name, waiting for eye contact, and use of prompts), and positive interaction with the individual. Other ways of encouraging communication summarized by Ylvisaker and Urbanczyk (1994) and Togher and colleagues (2004) include:

- Simplifying language in both form and content.
- Modifying the environment so that communication is likely to be successful.
- Understanding the features of different types of communication interactions in order to improve communication success.
- Using cues relevant to the type of communication interaction.
- Communicating respect for the individual.
- Avoiding being patronizing.
- Redirecting agitated or perseverant behaviour.

Task-related training

Due to the diffuse nature of TBI, primary sensorimotor impairments are variable and complex and may include weakness, loss of co-ordination, hyperreflexia, rigidity, cerebellar ataxia, tremor, dyskinesia, sensory loss (impairments in basic sensation or of perceptual processing) and commonly a combination of these. Added to these neurological impairments, some individuals may have other associated physical injuries, including fractures, spinal cord injury and cranial nerve injury. Many individuals also enter rehabilitation with secondary musculoskeletal, cardiorespiratory and metabolic sequelae, and in some instances a combination of all of these, which interferes with performance of everyday activities and skills. Low aerobic capacity and increased fatiguability may limit the individual's ability to participate in motor training. The major objective of physiotherapy is to train effective and efficient performance of functional actions which the individual cannot perform or can only perform with difficulty.

The physiotherapist needs an understanding of the pathophysiology of the primary sensorimotor impairments (see Chapters 8–10) and the adaptations or compensations that emerge as the patient attempts to perform everyday actions. The major role of the physiotherapist is

to train the individual to perform everyday actions more effectively, including sitting and standing balance, reaching and manipulation tasks, walking, stairclimbing, and running. Motor training is described in Chapters 2 and 4–7. Some other important details of physiotherapy intervention particularly relevant to rehabilitation of the individual with TBI, however, are discussed below.

Physiotherapy evaluation primarily involves observation and analysis of the effects of sensorimotor impairments. Information is also gathered about the individual's communication, cognitive, and behavioural impairments, and any other relevant information (e.g. presence of double-vision, hearing impairments). All of these impairments affect the individual's ability to participate actively in motor training. Early assessment may be complicated because the patient is dysphasic, may have a short attention span, inappropriate or antisocial behaviours and impaired short-term memory. The physiotherapist needs to consider physical, cognitive and social demands of the task in order to clarify where task breakdown occurs. In other words, problems in functional performance may be due not only to primary sensorimotor impairments but also to distraction from performing the task because of other impairments such as irritability, short-term memory loss, short attention span, apathy or lack of motivation.

The focus of measurement (Chapter 3) should be on real world functional performance, i.e. performance of everyday actions as measured on a functional scale, e.g., the Motor Assessment Scale (MAS) (Carr et al 1985), the Rivermead Motor Assessment (Lincoln & Leadbitter 1979), or the High level Mobility Assessment Tool (HiMAT) (Williams et al 2005). Some special-purpose tests, e.g. sensory tests, walking and running velocity (Chapter 3), motor fitness tests (Hassett et al 2007, Rossi & Sullivan 1996, Vitale et al 1997) are also used to establish the major reason for impaired motor performance and/or to get a baseline measure. When muscle contracture is present, measurement of joint range using standardized procedures (Ada & Herbert 1988) is necessary in order to monitor effectiveness of intervention aimed at reducing stiffness and increasing muscle extensibility. Measurement of muscle strength may be helpful. However, measurement of isolated muscles does not indicate how that muscle works in a multijoint movement (e.g. the ability to sustain a contraction, to time a contraction within a synergy to achieve a specific goal).

Some critical factors in motor training for the TBI individual are to:

- Direct the individual's attention to the critical biomechanical features of the action.
- Modify the task to achieve success.
- Organize the environment to force use and participation.
- Practice routines using the same verbal or non-verbal cues.

- Provide concrete goals (rather than abstract ones).
- Decrease prompts as performance improves.
- Monitor performance throughout the day.
- Provide reinforcers.
- Establish goals for each session.
- Give feedback that is concrete and accurate.
- Graph progress for the individual.
- Provide pictorial (and/or written) instructions.
- Evaluate effects of training.

Physiotherapy should be biased toward functional performance of concrete tasks (Figs 12.6, 12.7, 12.8), with enjoyable activities (Figs 12.9, 12.10) and repetitive exercise (Figs 12.11, 12.12). The use of group exercise, such as a circuit class, can be an effective method to provide additional practice of motor tasks in a motivating environment (Fig 12.13).

To keep the patient focused on practising tasks, the physiotherapist needs to be inventive and creative to ensure that the activities practised in therapy are perceived as relevant to the individual's needs. It is only in a more natural and challenging environment, e.g. walking in a busy corridor, stepping onto and off an escalator, crossing a busy street, rather than the artificial setting of the therapy centre that the individual may gain insight into his or her disability and the need to train and practice.

Some TBI individuals simply fail to act without extensive cuing and imposed structure. Since the cognitive and behavioural impairments tend to predominate after TBI, a highly structured, consistent and reinforcing environment is required to ensure active participation in training as well as sufficient time-on-task to improve performance. Steps in structuring environmental settings to change behaviour during therapy sessions include systematic observation and assessment, and the provision of a comprehensive continuum of structure throughout the rehabilitation centre with reinforcement by all staff and relatives. Less restrictive options can be instituted as improvement occurs. For example:

- Observe patient's behaviour in different settings and with different people.
- Analyse environmental variables that affect the patient's behaviour either positively or negatively.
- Remove variables that trigger or reinforce unwanted/maladaptive behaviours and replace them with variables that reinforce desired behaviours.
- Evaluate effects of environmental modification.
- Progress and modify intervention to facilitate further improvement.

Cardiorespiratory conditioning

The aetiology of cardiorespiratory deconditioning after TBI is multi-factorial, with both central and peripheral adaptations occurring due to the initial brain damage, trauma, and prolonged and extreme physical inactivity. Not only are many patients very deconditioned at the start

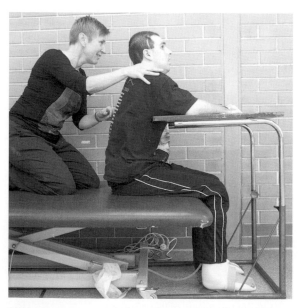

Figure 12.6 This young man requires full thigh support and a table to support his arms to enable him to stay balanced in sitting with minimal support. The therapist is encouraging him to look at some pictures placed directly in front of him.

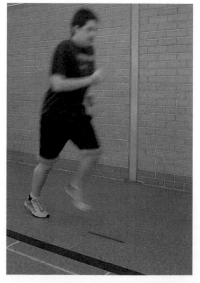

Figure 12.7 Jogging is an important motor task to train for many people to enable return to pre-injury work and leisure activities. Jogging involves large rapid bursts of muscle activity in a cyclical fashion. Stopping and starting in response to a command or as part of a game are also practiced.

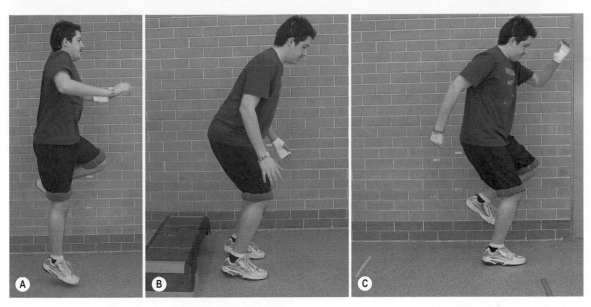

Figure 12.8 (A) Hopping, (B) jumping off a step and (C) leaping. All three of these actions involve the production of a rapid initial burst of agonist extensor activity to propel the body upward (A) (B) and forward (C) from the flexion counter-movement (without a pause between the two phases).

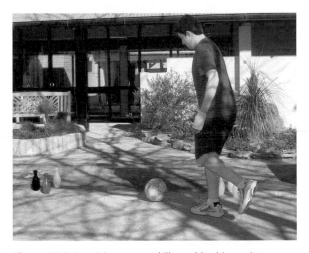

Figure 12.9 Practicing soccer skills enables him to improve balance and co-ordination along with eye-hand/foot co-ordination and predictive time-to-contact. In this task he has to dribble a ball around a figure-of-eight path. Other activities can include kicking a ball against a wall or between two people, and catching a ball to prevent a goal.

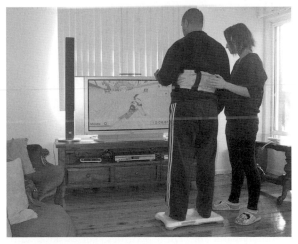

Figure 12.10 Using computer games. This patient is playing the ski slalom game on the Nintendo Wii Fit to improve balance and co-ordination.

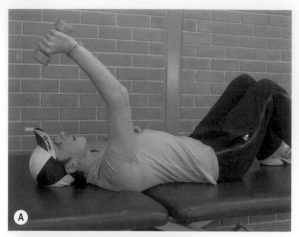

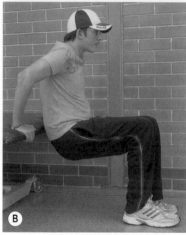

Figure 12.11 Progressive resistance strength training. The triceps can initially be strengthened (A) in supine with a weight added as the muscles become stronger, and (B) progressed to triceps dips.

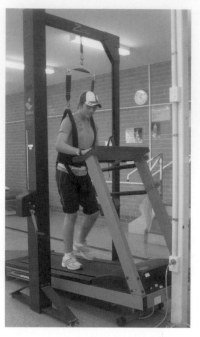

Figure 12.12 Walking on a treadmill with or without bodyweight support enables task specific practice of walking as well as providing a cardiorespiratory fitness training effect if the intensity (speed and incline) and duration are sufficient. A heart rate monitor can be used to ensure the patient's heartrate is within their training heart rate zone.

of active rehabilitation, but many may remain deconditioned for a number of years post injury. Aerobic capacities as low as 65% (Bhambhani et al 2003) to 74% (Hunter et al 1990) of age-predicted values have been measured in people with TBI greater than one year post injury. The consequences of deconditioning and physical inactivity may include increased physical fatigue (Jankowski & Sullivan 1990), participation restriction in pre-injury work and leisure activities (Jankowski & Sullivan 1990, Rossi & Sullivan 1996), changes in body composition (Bhambhani et al 2005), and an increase risk of comorbid conditions such as diabetes and heart disease (Booth et al 2000).

Conditioning programs are prescribed to increase physical activity and combat cardiorespiratory deconditioning (Sullivan et al 1990). The American College of Sports Medicine has developed specific guidelines for implementing a conditioning program for people with a brain injury, however these are yet to be validated (Palmer-McLean & Harbst 2003). The guidelines recommend aerobic exercise three to five times per week, at an intensity of 40 to 70% of $\dot{V}_{O_2\,peak}$ or 13/20 rating of perceived exertion (RPE), and a duration of 20 to 60 minutes using the appropriate mode (e.g. walking, swimming, cycling) depending on the individual's physical ability. Strength, flexibility, and neuromuscular training are also recommended as part of the conditioning program.

Types of conditioning programs that have been investigated in people with TBI include circuit training classes (Bhambhani et al 2005, Jankowski & Sullivan 1990, Sullivan et al 1990) (Fig 12.13), individual exercise utilizing gymnasium equipment (Bateman et al 2001, Hunter et al 1990, Mossberg et al 2002, Wolman et al 1994) (Fig 12.12), aquatic exercise classes (Driver et al 2004, Driver et al 2006), functional retraining (Canning et al 2003) (Fig 12.12), and home-based and fitness centre-based exercise programs (Hassett et al 2009). The environment in which the conditioning program is prescribed needs to be considered. For example, use of virtual reality technology (Grealy et al 1999) or exercise classes with an atmosphere akin to that found in a fitness centre (Sullivan et al 1990) may be beneficial for people with impairments of

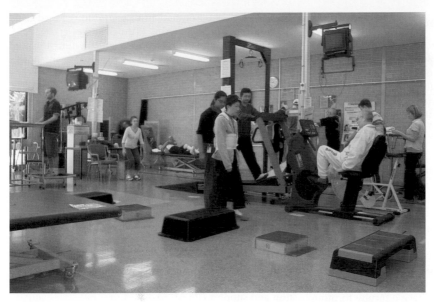

Figure 12.13 Circuit class. This circuit class includes a combination of task-related training and cardiorespiratory fitness stations.

attention or drive. Similarly, a quiet environment with one-to-one supervision may be more suited for an individual with behavioural disturbances. Potential benefits of a physical conditioning program include:

- Increased cardiorespiratory fitness (Hunter et al 1990).
- Prevention of comorbid diseases such as cardiovascular disease (Booth et al 2000).
- Decreased resistance to physical fatigue (Jankowski & Sullivan 1990).
- Enhanced ability to participate in other aspects of the rehabilitation program (Sullivan et al 1990).
- Improved psychological functioning (Moran 1976) and cognition (Grealy et al 1999).
- Establishing general healthy behaviour (Driver et al 2006).
- Assisting in gaining normal sleep patterns (Sullivan et al 1990).
- Improved community integration (Sullivan et al 1990).

In a recent Cochrane systematic review the efficacy of fitness training in people with TBI was investigated (Hassett et al 2008). This review was unable to confirm that fitness training reverses cardiorespiratory deconditioning or has any other health benefits (e.g. improved psychological functioning) in people with TBI. It was, however, able to confirm that fitness training was a safe and well accepted intervention to implement in this group.

It has been reported (Jankowski & Sullivan 1990, Wolman et al 1994) that people with TBI took a long time within an exercise session to reach their training heart rate, and that some individuals were unable to reach the prescribed training heart rate at all within an exercise session. Therefore a longer duration exercise session may be required to allow more time for the individual to reach their training heart rate or to compensate if they are only able to exercise at a lower intensity. This suggests that clinicians should carefully prescribe the duration and intensity of conditioning programs in order to optimize the relative exercise dosage. Additionally, monitoring of the exercise dosage using heart rate monitors would enable confirmation of the actual training dose achieved.

The reliability and/or validity of a number of fitness tests for adults with TBI have now been established. These include a symptom-limited cycle ergometer test (Bhambhani et al 2003), a graded treadmill test (Mossberg & Greene 2005), a timed walking test (Mossberg 2003), and the modified 20-metre shuttle test (Hassett et al 2007, Vitale et al 1997). An attempt has been made to establish reliability in a battery of motor performance and fitness tests in children and adolescents (age range 8–17) (Rossi & Sullivan 1996). The components tested were based on criteria which included flexibility, muscle strength, cardiorespiratory endurance, agility, power, balance, speed and co-ordination. Specific items tested included: agility run, standing broad jump, hand grip strength, vertical jump, 50 yard dash, soft ball throw, soccer dribble test and chin-up hang. Successful reintegration into sports and physical activities, whether for health, leisure or competition, provides children and adolescents following TBI with a sense of accomplishment (Haley et al 1990). It is probably similar for adults.

Community reintegration

Community reintegration refers to effective role performance in the community setting (Burleigh et al 1998) and is seen to encompass reintegration in the three areas of social network, home, and productive activities (Willer et al 1993). In a study of people with TBI two to five years post discharge from rehabilitation, 40% still performed poorly in all three areas of community reintegration (Doig et al 2001).

Cognitive impairments such as memory problems, reduced speed of processing, problem-solving and organizational skills are the problems most often complained of by the patient and relatives. These impairments may prevent the individual from re-entering the work force and educational and vocational systems. They also present difficulties for the individual in maintaining an independent lifestyle and often require financial assistance for basic living requirements. Poor social skills are another common problem experienced by people with TBI that leads them to lose pre-injury friendships and have difficulty forming new friendships. Poor social skills can impact on employment opportunities, reduce quality of life, and lead to social isolation (McDonald et al 2008). Post-traumatic epilepsy can also be an important factor in terms of family and social acceptance and employment opportunities.

Return to work is a key component of rehabilitation and is increasingly being seen as a therapeutic, social as well as economic need for the person with TBI (Wehman et al 2005). In the literature, return to work rates after TBI range from 12 to 70% (Shames et al 2007). A number of interacting factors have been found to influence successful return to work including pre-morbid characteristics, injury factors, post-injury impairments, and personal and environmental factors. It is becoming accepted that a significant proportion of people with TBI, including those with severe injuries, are able to return to some form of employment if sufficient and appropriate effort is invested (Shames et al 2007). For those who are unable to return to work, many will face years of social isolation and hardship.

Some form of continuing assistance is needed for many individuals and their families. Education, support, self-help and sports for the disabled groups assist in fulfilling some of these needs. For those individuals who have ongoing rehabilitation needs and goals, they should have access to follow-up outpatient or community-based rehabilitation to suit their needs (Turner-Stokes et al 2005). Improvements in language and cognitive function and ongoing medical and behavioural assistance to ameliorate mood swings and frustration are some of the ongoing needs identified by TBI individuals and their families. Community mobility may be limited for a variety of reasons ranging from physical to the purely cognitive or behavioural. Lack of adequate recreational facilities whether for health, leisure or competition is viewed as a major barrier to successful reintegration (Rimmer et al 2004).

There are relatively few published studies on sexuality following TBI, despite the fact that sexual problems can cause significant distress (Ponsford 2003). Disturbances in sexual function, either organic or behavioural, may include hypersexuality, hyposexuality, impotence, loss of feeling of attractiveness and an inability to engage in intimate interpersonal relationships (Griffith et al 1990). It is important that rehabilitation professionals do not ignore sexual problems and provide assessment, guidance, education and support (Ponsford 2003).

In conclusion, improved emergency care, quicker and safer transportation to specialized hospitals, and advances in acute medical management are saving the lives of many TBI victims who, 20–30 years ago, would have succumbed to the metabolic, haemodynamic and other complications that follow brain trauma (National Institute of Health (USA) 1998). As a result, there are an ever-increasing number of survivors of severe injury, mostly children and young adults, who are rapidly familiarizing us with the tragic phenomenon of physically fit young people whose brains have been damaged significantly (Lezak 1995). The occurrence of some of the once commonly seen physical sequelae, such as contracture and heterotopic ossification, has been lessened, but cognitive and behavioural impairments in many individuals still represent the most significant obstacles to reintegration in the community. There are a variety of financial and medicolegal issues which can also complicate the rehabilitation process, and complex ethical issues related to the treatment of patients in minimally conscious state or persistent vegetative state. For those who emerge from coma, the goal of successful community reintegration should guide all rehabilitation intervention.

REFERENCES

Abelson-Mitchell N 2008 Epidemiology and prevention of head injuries: literature review. J Clin Nurs 17:46–57.

Ada L, Herbert R 1988 Measurement of joint range of motion. Aust J Physiother 34:260–262.

Ahmed S, Bierley R, Sheikh JI et al 2000 Post-traumatic amnesia after closed head injury: a review of the literature and some suggestions for further research. Brain Inj 14:765–780.

Akeson WH, Amiel D, Abel MF et al 1987 Effects of immobilization on joints. Clin Orthop Relat Res 219:28–37.

Akeson WH, Amiel D, Woo SL-Y 1980 Immobility effects on synovial joints. The patho-mechanics of joint contracture. Biorheology 17:95–110.

Andrews PJ, Sleeman DH, Statham PF et al 2002 Predicting recovery in patients suffering from traumatic brain injury by using admission variables and physiological data: a comparison between decision tree analysis and logistic regression. J Neurosurg 97:326–336.

Ansell BJ, Keenan JE 1989 The Western Neuro Sensory Stimulation Profile: a tool for assessing slow-to-recover head-injured patients. Arch Phys Med Rehabil 70:104–108.

Arango-Lasprilla JC, Ketchum JM, Williams K et al 2008 Racial differences in employment outcomes after traumatic brain injury. Arch Phys Med Rehabil 89:988–995.

Baigelman W, O'Brien JC 1981 Pulmonary effects of head trauma. Neurosurgery 9:729–740.

Bateman A, Culpan FJ, Pickering AD et al 2001 The effect of aerobic training on rehabilitation outcomes after recent severe brain injury: a randomized controlled evaluation. Arch Phys Med Rehabil 82:174–182.

Bazarian JJ, Eirich MA, Salhanick SD 2003 The relationship between pre-hospital and emergency department Glasgow coma scale scores. Brain Inj 17:553–560.

Ben M, Harvey L, Denis S et al 2005 Does 12 weeks of regular standing prevent loss of ankle mobility and bone mineral density in people with recent spinal cord injuries? Aust J Physiother 51:251–256.

Bhambhani Y, Rowland G, Farag M 2003 Reliability of peak cardiorespiratory responses in patients with moderate to severe traumatic brain injury. Arch Phys Med Rehabil 84:1629–1636.

Bhambhani Y, Rowland G, Farag M 2005 Effects of circuit training on body composition and peak cardiorespiratory responses in patients with moderate to severe traumatic brain injury. Arch Phys Med Rehabil 86:268–276.

Bond MR 1986 Neurobehavioural sequelae of closed head injury. In: Grant I, Adams KM (eds) Neuropsychological Assessment of Neuropsychiatric Disorders. Oxford University Press, New York:347–373.

Booth FW, Gordon SE, Carlson CJ et al 2000 Waging war on modern chronic diseases: primary prevention through exercise biology. J Appl Physiol 88:774–787.

Bratton SL, Chestnut RM, Ghajar J et al 2007a Guidelines for the management of severe traumatic brain injury. I. Blood pressure and oxygenation. J Neurotrauma 24:S7–S13.

Bratton SL, Chestnut RM, Ghajar J et al 2007b Guidelines for the management of severe traumatic brain injury. II. Hyperosmolar therapy. J Neurotrauma 24:S14–S20.

Bratton SL, Chestnut RM, Ghajar J et al 2007c Guidelines for the management of severe traumatic brain injury. VI. Indications for intracranial pressure monitoring. J Neurotrauma 24:S37–S44.

Bratton SL, Chestnut RM, Ghajar J et al 2007d Guidelines for the management of severe traumatic brain injury. VIII. Intracranial pressure thresholds. J Neurotrauma 24:S55–S58.

Bratton SL, Chestnut RM, Ghajar J et al 2007e Guidelines for the management of severe traumatic brain injury. X. Brain oxygen monitoring and thresholds. J Neurotrauma 24:S65–S70.

Burleigh SA, Farber RS, Gillard M 1998 Community integration and life satisfaction after traumatic brain injury: long-term findings. Am J Occup Ther 52:45–52.

Canning CG, Shepherd RB, Carr JH et al 2003 A randomized controlled trial of the effects of intensive sit-to-stand training after recent traumatic brain injury on sit-to-stand performance. Clin Rehabil 17:355–362.

Carney NA, Ghajar J 2007 Guidelines for the management of severe traumatic brain injury. Introduction. J Neurotrauma 24:S1–S2.

Carr JH, Shepherd RB, Nordholm L et al 1985 Investigation of a New Motor Assessment Scale for stroke patients. Phys Ther 68:175–180.

Chua K, Chuo A, Kong KH 2003 Urinary incontinence after traumatic brain injury: incidence, outcomes and correlates. Brain Inj 17:469–478.

Cicerone KD, Dahlberg C, Kalmar K et al 2000 Evidence-based cognitive rehabilitation: recommendations for clinical practice. Arch Phys Med Rehabil 81:1596–1615.

Cicerone KD, Dahlberg C, Malec JF et al 2005 Evidence-based cognitive rehabilitation: updated review of the literature from 1998 through 2002. Arch Phys Med Rehabil 86:1681–1692.

Cook N 2003 Respiratory care in spinal cord injury with associated traumatic brain injury: bridging the gap in critical care nursing interventions. Intensive Crit Care Nurs, 19:143–153.

Coutinho EL, Gomes AR, Franca CN et al 2004 Effect of passive stretching on the immobilized soleus muscle fiber morphology. Braz J Med Biol Res 37:1853–1861.

Culley C, Evans JJ 2009 SMS text messaging as a means of increasing recall of therapy goals in brain injury rehabilitation: A single-blind within-subjects trial. Neuropsychol Rehabil, 1–17.

Deb S, Lyons I, Koutzoukis C 1999 Neurobehavioural symptoms one year after a head injury. British Journal of Psychiatry 174:360–365.

Deem S 2006 Management of acute brain injury and associated respiratory issues. Respir Care 51:357–367.

Doig E, Fleming J, Tooth L 2001 Patterns of community integration 2–5 years post-discharge from brain injury rehabilitation. Brain Inj 15:747–762.

Draper K, Ponsford J 2008 Cognitive functioning ten years following traumatic brain injury and rehabilitation. Neuropsychology 22:618–625.

Driver S, O'Connor J, Lox C et al 2004 Evaluation of an aquatics programme on fitness parameters of individuals with a brain injury. Brain Inj 18:847–859.

Driver S, Rees K, O'Connor J et al 2006 Aquatics, health-promoting self-care behaviours and adults with brain injuries. Brain Inj 20:133–141.

Eames P, Haffey WJ, Cope N 1990 Treatment of behavioural disorders. In: Rosenthal M, Bond MR, Griffith ER et al (eds) Rehabilitation of the Adult and Child with Traumatic Brain Injury, 2nd edn. F.A. Davis, Philadelphia:410–432.

Eames P, Wood RL 1985 Rehabilitation after severe brain injury: a follow-up study of a behaviour modification approach. J Neurol Neurosurg Psychiatry 48:613–619.

Evans JJ, Greenfield E, Wilson BA et al 2009 Walking and talking therapy: improving cognitive-motor dual-tasking in neurological illness. J Int Neuropsychol Soc 15:112–120.

Evans JJ, Wilson BA, Needham P et al 2003 Who makes good use of memory aids? Results of a survey of people with acquired brain injury. J Int Neuropsychol Soc 9:925–935.

Ewert J, Levin HS, Watson MG et al 1989 Procedural memory during posttraumatic amnesia in survivors of severe closed head injury. Implications for rehabilitation. Arch Neurol 46:911–916.

Fergusson D, Hutton B, Drodge A 2007 The epidemiology of major joint contractures: a systematic review of the literature. Clin Orthop Relat Res 456:22–29.

Fortuny LA, Briggs M, Newcombe F et al 1980 Measuring the duration of post traumatic amnesia. J Neurol Neurosurg Psychiatry 43:377–379.

Frost EAM 1985 Management of head injury. Can Anaesth Soc J 32:S32–SS9.

Frost EAM 1987 Central nervous system trauma. Anesthesiol Clin North America 5:565–585.

Garner SH, Valadka AB 1994 Medical management and principles of head injury rehabilitation. In: Finlayson MAJ, Garner SH (eds) Brain Injury Rehabilitation: Clinical Considerations. Williams and Wilkins, Baltimore, MD:83–101.

Gentile AM 2000 Skill acquisition: action, movement, and neuromotor processes. In: Carr JH, Shepherd RB (eds) Movement Science: Foundations for Physical Therapy in Rehabilitation, 2nd. Aspen Publishers, Rockville, MD:111–187.

Giacino J, Whyte J 2005 The vegetative and minimally conscious states: current knowledge and remaining questions. J Head Trauma Rehabil 20:30–50.

Giacino JT, Ashwal S, Childs N et al 2002 The minimally conscious state: definition and diagnostic criteria. Neurology 58:349–353.

Gossman MR, Sahrmann SA, Rose SJ 1982 Review of length-associated changes in muscle. Phys Ther 62:1799–1808.

Grealy MA, Johnson DA, Rushton SK 1999 Improving cognitive function after brain injury: the use of exercise and virtual reality. Arch Phys Med Rehabil 80:661–667.

Griffith ER, Cole S, Cole TM 1990 Sexuality and sexual dysfunction. In: Rosenthal M, Bond MR, Griffith ER et al (eds) Rehabilitation of the Adult and Child with Traumatic Brain Injury, 2nd edn. F.A. Davis, Philadelphia:206–224.

Haggard P, Cockburn J, Cock J et al 2000 Interference between gait and cognitive tasks in a rehabilitating neurological population. J Neurol Neurosurg Psychiatry 69:479–486.

Haley SM, Cioffi MI, Lewin JE et al 1990 Motor dysfunction in children and adolescents after traumatic brain injury. J Head Trauma Rehabil 5:77–90.

Harrison-Felix C, Whiteneck G, DeVivo M et al 2004 Mortality following rehabilitation in the Traumatic Brain Injury Model Systems of Care. NeuroRehabilitation 19:45–54.

Harvey L, de Jong I, Goehl G et al 2006 Twelve weeks of nightly stretch does not reduce thumb web-space contractures in people with a neurological condition: a randomised controlled trial. Aust J Physiother 52:251–258.

Harvey LA, Herbert RD, Glinsky J et al 2009 Effects of 6 months of regular passive movements on ankle joint mobility in people with spinal cord injury: a randomized controlled trial. Spinal Cord 47:62–66.

Hassett LM, Harmer AR, Moseley AM et al 2007 Validity of the modified 20-metre shuttle test: assessment of cardiorespiratory fitness in people who have sustained a traumatic brain injury. Brain Inj 21:1069–1077.

Hassett LM, Moseley AM, Tate R et al 2008 Fitness training for cardiorespiratory conditioning after traumatic brain injury. Cochrane Database Syst Rev, (2), CD006123.

Hassett LM, Moseley AM, Tate RL et al 2009 Efficacy of a fitness centre-based exercise programme compared with a home-based exercise programme in traumatic brain injury: a randomized controlled trial. J Rehabil Med 41:247–255.

Helm M, Hauke J, Lampl L 2002 A prospective study of the quality of pre-hospital emergency ventilation in patients with severe head injury. Br J Anaesth 88:345–349.

Herbert R 2005 How muscles respond to stretch. In: Refshauge K, Ada L, Ellis E (eds) Science-based Rehabilitation: Theories into Practice. Butterworth Heinemann, London:107–130.

Herbert RD, Crosbie J 1997 Rest length and compliance of non-immobilised and immobilised rabbit soleus muscle and tendon. Eur J Appl Physiol Occup Physiol 76:472–479.

Hitchcock ER 1971 Summary of emergency care of head and multiple injury. In Head Injuries. Proceedings of an International Symposium, Churchill Livingstone, Edinburgh and London:201–203.

Horn LJ, Garland DE 1990 Medical and orthopaedic complications associated with traumatic brain injury. In: Rosenthal M, Bond MR, Griffith ER et al (eds) Rehabilitation of the Adult and Child with Traumatic Brain Injury, 2nd edn. F.A. Davis, Philadelphia:107–126.

Hou DJ, Tong KA, Ashwal S et al 2007 Diffusion-weighted magnetic resonance imaging improves outcome prediction in adult traumatic brain injury. J Neurotrauma 24:1558–1569.

Hunter M, Tomberlin JA, Kirkikis C et al 1990 Progressive exercise testing in closed head-injury subjects: comparison of exercise apparatus in assessment of a physical conditioning program. Phys Ther 70:363–371.

Imle P, Mars M, Ciesla N et al 1997 The effect of chest physical therapy on intracranial pressure and cerebral perfusion pressure. Physiother Can 49:48–55.

Jakola AS, Muller K, Larsen M et al 2007 Five-year outcome after mild head injury: a prospective controlled study. Acta Neurol Scand 115:398–402.

Jankowski LW, Sullivan SJ 1990 Aerobic and neuromuscular training: effect on the capacity, efficiency and fatiguability of patients with traumatic brain injuries. Arch Phys Med Rehabil 71:500–504.

Jarvinen TA, Jozsa L, Kannus P et al 2002 Organization and distribution of intramuscular connective tissue in normal and immobilized skeletal muscles. An immunohistochemical, polarization and scanning electron microscopic study. J Muscle Res Cell Motil 23:245–254.

Javouhey E, Guerin A-C, Chiron M 2006 Incidence and risk factors of severe traumatic brain injury resulting from road accidents: a population-based study. Accid Anal Prev 38:225–233.

Jennett B, Plum F 1972 Persistent vegetative state after brain damage: a syndrome in search of a name. Lancet 299:734–747.

Jennett B, Teasdale G 1981 Management of Head Injuries. F.A. Davis, Philadelphia.

Kelly G, Brown S, Todd J et al 2008 Challenging behaviour profiles of people with acquired brain injury living in community settings. Brain Inj 22:457–470.

Kelly JP, Dodd J 1991 Anatomical organization of the nervous system. In: Kandel ER, Schwartz JH, Jessell TM (eds) Principles of Neuroscience, 3rd edn. Appleton and Lange, Norwalk, CT:273–282.

Kennedy MR, Coelho C, Turkstra L et al 2008 Intervention for executive functions after traumatic brain injury: a systematic review, meta-analysis and clinical recommendations. Neuropsychol Rehabil 18:257–299.

Langlois JA, Rutland Brown W, Thomas KE 2006 Traumatic Brain Injury in the United States: Emergency Department Visits, Hospitalizations, and Deaths. Centers for Disease Control and Prevention, National Center for Injury Prevention and Control, Atlanta (GA).

Leary SM, Liu C, Cheesman AL et al 2006 Incontinence after brain injury: prevalence, outcome and multidisciplinary management on a neurological rehabilitation unit. Clin Rehabil 20:1094–1099.

Levin HS, Benton AL, Grossman RG 1982 Neurobehavioural Consequences of Closed Head Injury Oxford University Press, New York.

Levin HS, O'Donnell VM, Grossman RG 1979 The Galveston Orientation and Amnesia Test. A practical scale to assess cognition after head injury. J Nerv Ment Dis 167:675–684.

Lezak MD 1995 Neurophysiological Assessment 3rd edn. Oxford University Press, New York.

Light KE, Nuzik S, Personius W et al 1984 Low-load prolonged stretch vs. high-load brief stretch in treating knee contractures. Phys Ther 64:330–333.

Lincoln N, Leadbitter D 1979 Assessment of motor function in stroke patients. Physiotherapy 65:48–51.

Lindboe CF, Platou CS 1984 Effect of immobilization of short duration on the muscle fibre size. Clin Physiol 4:183–188.

Ling GS, Marshall SA 2008 Management of traumatic brain injury in the intensive care unit. Neurol Clin 26:409–426.

Lu J, Marmarou A, Choi S et al 2005 Mortality from traumatic brain injury. Acta Neurochir (Wien), 95:281–285.

Mackay LE, Chapman PE, Morgan AS 1997 Respiratory management of the brain-injured patient. In: Aspen (eds) Maximising Brain Injury Recovery: Integrating Critical Care and Early Rehabilitation Publishers, Gaithersburg:331–395.

Marsh NV, Kersel DA 2006 Frequency of behavioural problems at one year following traumatic brain injury: correspondence between patient and caregiver reports. Neuropsychol Rehabil 16:684–694.

Marsh NV, Kersel DA, Havill JA et al 2002 Caregiver burden during the year following severe traumatic brain injury. J Clin Exp Neuropsychol 24:434–447.

Mathias JL, Wheaton P 2007 Changes in attention and information-processing speed following severe traumatic brain injury: a meta-analytic review. Neuropsychology 21:212–223.

Matthews DS, Matthews JN, Aynsley-Green A et al 1995 Changes in cerebral oxygen consumption are independent of changes in body oxygen consumption after severe head injury in childhood. J Neurol Neurosurg Psychiatry 59:359–367.

McDonald S, Tate R, Togher L et al 2008 Social skills treatment for people with severe, chronic acquired brain injuries: a multicenter trial. Arch Phys Med Rehabil 89:1648–1659.

McKinlay A, Grace RC, Horwood LJ et al 2008 Prevalence of traumatic brain injury among children, adolescents and young adults: prospective evidence from a birth cohort. Brain Inj 22:175–181.

McKinlay WW, Brooks DN, Bond MR et al 1981 The short-term outcome of severe blunt head injury as reported by relatives of the injured persons. J Neurol Neurosurg Psychiatry 44:527–533.

McLellan DL 1993 Rehabilitation in neurology. In: Walton J (eds) Brain's Diseases of the Nervous System, 10th edn. Oxford University Press, Oxford:768–783.

Mendelow AD 1993a Head injury. In: Walton J (eds) Brain's Diseases of the Nervous System, 10th edn. Oxford University Press, Oxford:184–196.

Mendelow AD 1993b Raised intracranial pressure, cerebral oedema, hydrocephalus, and intracranial tumours. In: Walton J (eds) Brain's Diseases of the Nervous System, 10th edn. Oxford University Press, Oxford:144–183.

Mendelow AD, Teasdale GM 1983 Pathophysiology of head injuries. Br J Surg 70:641–650.

Meythaler JM, Peduzzi JD, Eleftheriou E et al 2001 Current concepts: diffuse axonal injury-associated traumatic brain injury. Arch Phys Med Rehabil 82:1461–1471.

Millis SR, Rosenthal M, Novack TA et al 2001 Long-term neuropsychological outcome after traumatic brain injury. J Head Trauma Rehabil 16:343–355.

Milton SB, Wertz RT 1986 Management of persistent communication deficits in patients with traumatic brain injury. In: Uzzell BB, Gross Y (eds) Clinical Neuropsychology of Intervention. Martinus Nijhoff Publishing, Boston:223–256.

Moran AJ 1976 Six cases of severe head injury treated by exercise in addition to other therapies. Med J Aust, 396–397.

Morton MV, Wehman P 1995 Psychosocial and emotional sequelae of individuals with traumatic brain injury: a literature review and recommendations. Brain Inj 9:81–92.

Moseley AM 1997 The effect of casting combined with stretching on passive ankle dorsiflexion in adults with traumatic head injury. Phys Ther 77:240–247.

Moseley AM, Hassett LM, Leung J et al 2008 Serial casting versus positioning for the treatment of elbow contractures in adults with traumatic brain injury: a randomized controlled trial. Clin Rehabil 22:406–417.

Mossberg KA 2003 Reliability of a timed walk test in persons with acquired brain injury. Am J Phys Med Rehabil 82:385–390.

Mossberg KA, Greene BP 2005 Reliability of graded exercise testing after traumatic brain injury: submaximal and peak responses. Am J Phys Med Rehabil 84:492–500.

Mossberg KA, Kuna S, Masel B 2002 Ambulatory efficiency in persons with acquired brain injury after a rehabilitation intervention. Brain Inj 16:789–797.

Myburgh JA, Cooper DJ, Finfer SR et al 2008 Epidemiology and 12-month outcomes from traumatic brain injury in Australia and New Zealand. J Trauma 64:854–862.

National Institute of Health (USA) 1998 Rehabilitation of persons with traumatic brain injury. NIH Consens Statement 16:47–57.

Pace GM, Dunn EK, Luiselli JK et al 2005 Antecedent interventions in the management of maladaptive behaviours in a child with brain injury. Brain Inj 19:365–369.

Palmer-McLean K, Harbst K 2003 Stroke and brain injury. In: Durstine JL, Moore GE (eds) ACSM's Exercise Management for Persons with Chronic Diseases and Disabilities, 2nd edn. Human Kinetics, Champaign, IL:238–246.

Patel HC, Menon DK, Tebbs S et al 2002 Specialist neurocritical care and outcome from head injury. Intensive Care Med 28:547–553.

Plum F, Posner JB 1980 The Diagnosis of Stupor and Coma, 3rd edn. Blackwell, Oxford.

Ponsford J 2003 Sexual changes associated with traumatic brain injury. Neuropsychol Rehabil 13:275–289.

Provenzale J 2007 CT and MR imaging of acute cranial trauma. Emerg Radiol 14:1–12.

Puljula J, Savola O, Tuomivaara V et al 2007 Weekday distribution of head traumas in patients admitted to the emergency department of a city hospital: effects of age, gender and drinking pattern. Alcohol Alcohol 42:474–479.

Rimmer JH, Riley B, Wang E et al 2004 Physical activity participation among persons with disabilities: barriers and facilitators. Am J Prev Med 26:419–425.

Rohling ML, Faust ME, Beverly B et al 2009 Effectiveness of cognitive rehabilitation following acquired brain injury: a meta-analytic re-examination of Cicerone et al.'s (2000, 2005) systematic reviews. Neuropsychology 23:20–39.

Rossi C, Sullivan SJ 1996 Motor fitness in children and adolescents with traumatic brain injury. Arch Phys Med Rehabil 77:1062–1065.

Rowland LP, Fink ME, Rubin L 1991 Cerebrospinal fluid: blood-brain edema and hydrocephalus. In: Kandell JH, Schwartz JH, Jessell TM (eds) Principles of Neuroscience. Appleton and Lange, Norwalk, CT:1050–1060.

Rozet I, Domino KB 2007 Respiratory care. Best Pract Res Clin Anaesthesiol 21:465–482.

Russell WR 1932 Cerebral involvement in head injury. Brain 35:549–603.

Sarno MT 1980 The nature of verbal impairment after closed head injury. J Nerv Ment Dis 168:685–692.

Sarno MT 1984 Verbal impairment after closed head injury: report of a replication study. J Nerv Ment Dis 172:475–479.

Shames J, Treger I, Ring H et al 2007 Return to work following traumatic brain injury: trends and challenges. Disabil Rehabil 29:1387–1395.

Shapiro HM 1975 Intracranial hypertension: therapeutic and anesthetic considerations. Anesthesiology 43:445–471.

Sherer M, Struchen MA, Yablon SA et al 2008 Comparison of indices of traumatic brain injury severity: Glasgow Coma Scale, length of coma and post-traumatic amnesia. J Neurol Neurosurg Psychiatry 79:678–685.

Shores EA, Marosszeky JE, Sandanam J et al 1986 Preliminary validation of a clinical scale for measuring the duration of post-traumatic amnesia. Med J Aust 144:569–572.

Silver JR 1969 Heterotopic ossification: a clinical study of its possible relationship to trauma. Paraplegia 7:220.

Slewa-Younan S, Green AM, Baguley IJ et al 2004 Sex differences in injury severity and outcome measures after traumatic brain injury. Arch Phys Med Rehabil 85:376–379.

Stocchetti N, Pagan F, Calappi E, et al 2004 Inaccurate early assessment of neurological severity in head injury. J Neurotrauma 21:1131–1140.

Sullivan SJ, Richer E, Laurents F 1990 The role of and possibilities for physical conditioning programmes in the rehabilitation of traumatically brain-injured persons. Brain Inj 4:407–414.

Sullivan T, Conine TA, Goodman M, et al 1988 Serial casting to prevent equinis in acute traumatic head injury. Physiother Can 40:346–350.

Tabary J, Tardieu C, Tardieu G et al 1981 Experimental rapid sarcomere loss with concomitant hypoextensibility. Muscle Nerve 4:198–203.

Tabary JC, Tabary C, Tardieu C et al 1972 Physiological and structural changes in the cat's soleus muscle due to immobilization at different lengths by plaster cast. J Physiol 224:231–244.

Tabary JC, Tardieu C, Tardieu G et al 1976 Functional adaptation of sarcomere number of normal cat muscle. J Physiol (Paris) 72:277–291.

Tate RL, Fenelon B, Manning ML et al 1991 Patterns of neuropsychological impairment after severe blunt head injury. J Nerv Ment Dis 179:117–126.

Tate RL, Perdices M, Pfaff A et al 2001 Predicting duration of posttraumatic amnesia (PTA) from early PTA measurements. J Head Trauma Rehabil 16:525–542.

Tate RL, Pfaff A, Jurjevic L 2000 Resolution of disorientation and amnesia during post-traumatic amnesia. J Neurol Neurosurg Psychiatry 68:178–185.

Taylor CM, Aird VH, Tate RL et al 2007 Sequence of recovery during the course of emergence from the minimally conscious state. Arch Phys Med Rehabil 88:521–525.

Teasdale G, Jennett B 1974 Assessment of coma and impaired consciousness. Lancet 304:81–84.

Togher L 2000 Giving information: the importance of context on communicative opportunity for people with traumatic brain injury. Aphasiology 14:365–390.

Togher L, McDonald S, Code C et al 2004 Training communication partners of people with traumatic brain injury: a randomised controlled trial. Aphasiology 18:313–335.

Topal NB, Hakyemez B, Erdogan C et al 2008 MR imaging in the detection of diffuse axonal injury with mild traumatic brain injury. Neurol Res 30:974–978.

Turner-Stokes L, Disler PB, Nair A et al 2005 Multi-disciplinary rehabilitation for acquired brain injury in adults of working age. Cochrane Database Syst Rev 3:CD004170.

Vakil E 2005 The effect of moderate to severe traumatic brain injury (TBI) on different aspects of memory: a selective review. J Clin Exp Neuropsychol 27:977–1021.

Vanden Bossche L, Van Maele G, Rimbaut S et al 2008 Free radical scavengers have a preventive effect on heterotopic bone formation following manipulation of immobilized rabbit legs. Eur J Phys Rehabil Med 44:423–428.

Vincent JL, Berre J 2005 Primer on medical management of severe brain injury. Crit Care Med 33:1392–1399.

Vitale AE, Jankowski LW, Sullivan SJ 1997 Reliability of a walk/run test to estimate aerobic capacity in a brain-injured population. Brain Inj 11:67–76.

Wade DT 1992 Measurement in Neurological Rehabilitation Oxford University Press, Oxford.

Wade DT, Langton Hewer R 1987 Epidemiology of some neurological diseases with special reference to work load on the NHS. Int Rehabil Med 8:129–137.

Wehman P, Targett P, West M et al 2005 Productive work and employment for persons with traumatic brain injury: what have we learned after 20 years? J Head Trauma Rehabil 20:115–127.

Weir N, Doig EJ, Fleming JM et al 2006 Objective and behavioural assessment of the emergence from post-traumatic amnesia (PTA). Brain Inj 20:927–935.

Weiss N, Galanaud D, Carpentier A et al 2007 Clinical review: Prognostic value of magnetic resonance imaging in acute brain injury and coma. Crit Care 11:230.

Werner C, Engelhard K 2007 Pathophysiology of traumatic brain injury. Br J Anaesth 99:4–9.

White MJ, Davies TM 1984 The effects of immobilization after lower leg fractures on the contractile properties of human triceps surae. Clin Sci 66:277–282.

Whyte J, Rosenthal M 1993 Rehabilitation of the patient with traumatic brain injury. In: DeLisa JA (eds) Rehabilitation Medicine: Principles and Practice, 2nd edn. J.B. Lippincott Company, Philadelphia:825–860.

Willemse-van Son AH, Ribbers GM, Verhagen AP et al 2007 Prognostic factors of long-term functioning and productivity after traumatic brain injury: a systematic review of prospective cohort studies. Clin Rehabil 21:1024–1037.

Willer B, Rosenthal M, Kreutzer J et al 1993 Assessment of community integration following rehabilitation for traumatic brain injury. J Head Trauma Rehabil 8:75–87.

Williams G, Robertson V, Greenwood K et al 2005 The high-level mobility assessment tool (HiMAT) for traumatic brain injury. Part 1: item generation. Brain Inj 19:925–932.

Williams PE 1990 Use of intermittent stretch in the prevention of serial sarcomere loss in immobilized muscles. Ann Rheum Dis 47:316–317.

Williams PE, Goldspink G 1973 The effect of immobilization on the longitudinal growth of striated muscle fibres. J Anat 116:45–55.

Wilson BA, Emslie HC, Quirk K et al 2001 Reducing everyday memory and planning problems by means of a paging system: a randomised control crossover study. J Neurol Neurosurg Psychiatry 70:477–482.

Wilson JT, Pettigrew LE, Teasdale GM 1998 Structured interviews for the Glasgow Outcome Scale and the extended Glasgow Outcome Scale: guidelines for their use. J Neurotrauma 15:573–585.

Wolman RL, Cornall C, Fulcher K et al 1994 Aerobic training in brain-injured patients. Clin Rehabil 8:253–257.

Wood RL 1987 Brain Injury Rehabilitation: A Neurobehavioural Approach. Croom Helm, London.

Wood RL, Rutterford NA 2006 Demographic and cognitive predictors of long-term psychosocial outcome following traumatic brain injury. J Int Neuropsychol Soc 12:350–358.

Ylvisaker M, Jacobs HE, Feeney T 2003 Positive supports for people who experience behavioral and cognitive disability after brain injury: a review. J Head Trauma Rehabil 18:7–32.

Ylvisaker M, Urbanczyk B 1994 Assessment and treatment of speech, swallowing and communication disorders following traumatic brain injury. In: Finlayson MAJ, Garner SH (eds) Brain Injury Rehabilitation: Clinical Considerations. Williams and Wilkins, Baltimore, MD:157–186.

Zeppos L, Patman S, Berney S et al 2007 Physiotherapy in intensive care is safe: an observational study. Aust J Physiother 53:279–283.

Chapter | 13 |

Parkinson's disease

Written with Colleen Canning

INTRODUCTION

The basal ganglia are made up of four nuclei (the striatum, consisting of the caudate, putamen and ventral striatum; the globus pallidus; the substantia nigra, consisting of pars reticulata and pars compacta; and the subthalamic nucleus) which participate in the control of movement and other functions. These nuclei do not make direct output to or receive input from the spinal cord. Their primary input is from the cerebral cortex and thalamus and their output is directed to the brainstem via the thalamus, back to the prefrontal, premotor and motor cortices. Diseases which affect the basal ganglia produce characteristic types of movement disorders: tremor and other involuntary movements; poverty and slowness of movement without paralysis; and changes in muscle tone and posture. In addition to movement disorders, diseases of the basal ganglia have non-motor effects on behaviour, cognition and emotion.

Inputs from the cerebral cortex, thalamus and brainstem are directed to the striatum. The striatum projects to the globus pallidus and substantia nigra, giving rise to the major outputs from the basal ganglia (DeLong 2000). The basal ganglia incorporate a number of circuits linking the thalamus and the cerebral cortex, engaging different portions of the basal ganglia and thalamus and mediating different functions. These circuits include the skeletomotor circuit, the oculomotor circuit, the prefrontal circuits and the limbic circuit. These circuits are relatively inde-

©2010 Elsevier Ltd
DOI: 10.1016/B978-0-7020-4051-1.00022-9

pendent, although anatomical evidence shows some convergence in the substantia nigra (DeLong 2000).

The role of the basal ganglia in movement control remains unclear despite anatomical studies (e.g., Parent 1990), cerebral blood flow studies (e.g., Seitz & Roland 1992), single cell recordings in conscious animals (e.g., Brotchie et al 1991a,b) and numerous clinical studies (e.g., Schwab et al 1954; Talland & Schwab 1964). It is now clear from anatomical studies that the motor component of the basal ganglia is incorporated in a loop originating in the motor sensory cortex and terminating in the supplementary motor area (SMA) and premotor area. The basal ganglia are considered to be involved in higher-order aspects of motor control; i.e., the planning and execution of complex motor performance. It appears that the SMA and the basal ganglia may work together to run well-learned and predictable movement sequences. Based on the numerous inputs from virtually all areas of the cerebral cortex to the basal ganglia, it has been speculated that the basal ganglia may also be involved in many functions besides motor control.

Motor disturbances in diseases of the basal ganglia characteristically produce either excessive movements or diminished movement (Wichmann & DeLong 1993). A major breakthrough in understanding how basal ganglia dysfunction may lead to either excessive movements as in Huntington's disease or to reduced movement (akinesia) in Parkinson's disease (PD) has come from the finding that there are two pathways that mediate striatal influences over activity of the thalamocortical neurons: a direct pathway that tends to facilitate ongoing motor behaviour and an indirect pathway that dampens motor activity (Goldman-Rakic & Selemon 1990). Excessive involuntary movements are characterized by: tremor (rhythmic, oscillatory), athetosis (writhing movements), chorea (abrupt movements of the limbs and facial muscles) and ballismus (wild swinging movements of the limbs). Diminished movement is characterized by: poverty and slowness of movement without paralysis and dystonia (a persistent posture of the body which can result in distorted alignment of the body).

PD (paralysis agitans) is the most common disease affecting the basal ganglia and is the major subject of this chapter. The clinical features of other diseases of the basal ganglia, for example Huntington's disease and Wilson's disease, can be found in general neurology texts (e.g., Goetz 2007).

Parkinsonism is a clinical syndrome characterized by a disorder of movement consisting of tremor, rigidity, elements of bradykinesia (slowness of movement), hypokinesia (reduced excursion of movement) and akinesia (slowness in initiating movement and loss of spontaneous movement), and postural abnormalities (e.g., Marsden 1994). PD consists of the clinical syndrome of parkinsonism associated with a distinctive pathology. It was James Parkinson (1817) who first described the 'shaking palsy'

which now bears his name. Since then the site of neurologic degeneration that results in PD has been identified but the aetiology of the disease is still unknown (idiopathic PD). There are many other diseases that present with clinical features of parkinsonism. These include parkinsonism-plus syndromes, such as progressive supranuclear palsy and multiple system atrophy, drug-induced parkinsonism and vascular parkinsonism (Goetz 2007).

PD is a slowly progressive degenerative disease that affects some 3 in 1000 of the general population, and 1 in 100 people over 60 (Rajput 1992; De Rijk et al 2000). The mean age of onset is early to mid-60s, men are slightly more commonly affected than women and people of all ethnic backgrounds are affected. Five to 10% of cases are classified as young-onset PD, with initial symptoms evident as early as age 20. Juvenile-onset PD is rare with symptoms arising before the age of 20 (Samii et al 2004).

PD was the first disease to be identified as a molecular disease (DeLong 2000). In the late 1950s, Carlsson (1959) observed that 80% of the dopamine in the brain is localized in the basal ganglia, an area that contributes less than 0.5% of the total brain weight. Not long after this, Hornykiewicz (1966), on post mortem examination, found that dopamine was drastically reduced in patients with PD and that a specific defect in transmitter metabolism was shown to have a causal role in the disease. These findings led to the development of levodopa therapy. Prior to these advances, PD progressed relentlessly and was a cause of miserable disability (Hoehn & Yahr 1967).

PATHOPHYSIOLOGY

Neurochemically, PD is characterized by a disturbance of the central dopaminergic pathway from the substantia nigra to the striatum (Agid et al 1990). In addition to a reduction of dopamine, pathological findings include depigmentation and neuronal loss in the substantia nigra and the presence of Lewy bodies (eosinophilic inclusions) and pale bodies (neurofilament interspersed with vacuolar granules) with consequent changes to neural conduction in the nigrostriatal pathway. Lewy body pathology is found in the brainstem, spinal cord and cortex as well as the basal ganglia and is not specifically indicative of PD (Goetz 2007). Approximately 80% of nigrostriatal dopaminergic neurons are lost before symptoms become noticeable (Korman & James 1993). Recent work by Braak and colleagues (2004) has challenged the traditional view that the pathological process in PD begins in the substantia nigra. A 6-stage pathological process based on Lewy body distribution is proposed. Stages 1 and 2 are considered pre-clinical stages with olfactory bulb and anterior olfactory nucleus degeneration occurring in stage

1, followed by lower brainstem degeneration in stage 2. Stages 3 and 4 involve the basal ganglia and forebrain and stages 5 and 6 extend involvement to the cortex. Although the loss of striatal dopamine is considered to account for most of the cardinal signs of PD (i.e., tremor, bradykinesia, rigidity and postural instability), other motor and non-motor impairments which respond poorly to levodopa are likely to be mediated through other deficit transmitter systems (norepinephrine, serotonin, cholinergic) due to degeneration of lower brainstem nuclei, locus caeruleus and dorsal raphe (Goetz 2007).

AETIOLOGY

The cause of PD is unknown in the majority of cases. Known autosomal dominant and recessive forms of PD account for 5% of cases, usually causing young-onset parkinsonism. For the remaining 95% of cases, the cause is unknown. PD is likely to be caused by a complex interaction of genetic and environmental factors, with risk factors for PD including a positive family history, male gender, head injury, exposure to pesticides, consumption of well water and rural living (DeLong & Juncos 2008).

Diagnosis is primarily clinical and is based on medical history and physical examination and improvement of symptoms and signs with dopaminergic treatment (Samii et al 2004). It is thought that patients with PD may have a long pre clinical period (Korman & James 1993).

Clinical signs

Tremor at rest, rigidity, bradykinesia (or akinesia) and postural instability are considered to be the four cardinal features of PD (Jankovic 2008).

Tremor is defined as approximately rhythmic, involuntary and roughly sinusoidal movement of a body part (Sethi 2003). By convention, tremor is classified by the behavioural situation in which it occurs, regardless of the underlying mechanism (Findley 1988). Tremor at rest is a cardinal sign of PD and is often the first sign of the disease (Marsden 1994). It typically occurs unilaterally at a frequency of 4–6 Hz and is more prominent distally. Body parts commonly affected by resting tremor are the hands, feet, lips, chin and jaw. Resting tremor is usually suppressed by voluntary activity, sleep and complete relaxation. Postural tremor of similar frequency to resting tremor (observed while voluntarily maintaining a position against gravity) and/or kinetic tremor at 8–12 Hz (occurring during any voluntary movement) may also be present (Jankovic 2008).

Although the origin of the resting tremor is still disputed, it appears that it results from oscillations in a hyperactive long loop reflex pathway, triggered by an endogenous mechanism at the thalamic level which is influenced by peripheral afferents, chiefly the 1A afferents (Delwaide & Gonce 1988). Recent work shows that the frequency of tremor in different extremities is not consistent, suggesting that different oscillators underlie parkinsonism tremor in different extremities (Bergman & Deuschl 2002).

Rigidity is characterized by increased stiffness throughout range of passive movement at a joint. This stiffness has the same intensity in both extensor and flexor muscles and may be regularly interrupted at a 4–6 Hz frequency by the cogwheel phenomenon, a result of rigidity superimposed on, or interrupted by, tremor. The degree of rigidity is relatively independent of stretch speed. In some instances, however, the resistance to stretch is inversely proportional to speed, being greatest when movement is slow. The degree of rigidity is not necessarily constant, stiffness being reinforced by stress, anxiety and movement of a contralateral limb or in a standing rather than a seated individual. The major cause of rigidity in PD is thought to be hyperactivity in the long loop reflex pathways, probably in the cortex (Delwaide et al 1991).

Mechanical changes in the muscles have also been shown to contribute to resistance to passive movement, particularly in more severe cases (Dietz et al 1981, 1988; Watts et al 1986). It has also been proposed that rigidity may be partly due to adaptive behaviour in response to postural instability (Horak et al 1992; Broussolle et al 2007). Abnormal axial rigidity has recently been measured in the trunk and hips during slow trunk and hip rotation movements in standing and this rigidity was unresponsive to levodopa (Wright et al 2007). However, rigidity is not considered to contribute to reduced mobility and quality of life to the same extent as bradykinesia (e.g., Dural et al 2003).

Bradykinesia, used as an umbrella term to describe slowness of or absence of movement (Berardelli et al 2001), is the most disabling manifestation of PD. Bradykinesia is often used synonymously with two related terms: akinesia and hypokinesia. Strictly speaking, bradykinesia refers to slowness of movement, while hypokinesia refers to reduced amplitude of movement. Akinesia refers to reduced spontaneous movement (such as facial expression) or associated movements (such as arm swing while walking). Akinesia also includes slowness to initiate movement and freezing while moving. The bradykinesia which is evident during single joint movements (Hallett & Khoshbin 1980) is exaggerated during the performance of simultaneous tasks (Talland & Schwab 1964) or sequential movements. For example, when sequential movements are performed such as walking, progressive reductions in speed of walking and amplitude of step length are observed, which may lead to freezing and an inability to proceed. Although the various manifestations of bradykinesia are related, they may evolve independently and are not necessarily correlated with each other (Evarts et al 1981). Bradykinesia affects the performance of all motor actions and their associated postural adjustments (e.g., reaching and manipulation, sit to stand), and articulation and phonation.

The mechanisms underlying bradykinesia are still not well understood. Current theories suggest that bradykinesia is due to a failure of the basal ganglia to reinforce the cortical mechanisms that prepare and execute motor commands (Berardelli et al 2001). Even when electromyograph (EMG) onset is within normal limits, the magnitude of EMG is reduced, resulting in delayed movement onset and reduced size and speed of movement (e.g., Berardelli et al 2001). When movements are cued, or attention is directed towards the size and/or speed of the movement, many movements can be normalized (e.g., Berardelli et al 2001; Morris et al 2006). It is hypothesized that this reflects the brain's ability to compensate for the basal ganglia deficit, utilizing alternate structures such as lateral premotor areas. Compensation, however, does not appear to be limitless and this is evident when bradykinesia re-emerges when more than one task is performed at the same time.

Freezing, that is, difficulty in starting or continuing rhythmic repetitive movements such as speech, handwriting and gait, is a well-known and incapacitating problem in PD. The neural mechanism responsible for freezing remains unclear, however freezing should be considered a distinct clinical sign of PD with some independence from bradykinesia and hypokinesia. Freezing of gait (FOG) is an episodic gait disturbance, typically experienced when walking through an enclosed space or when turning (Bloem et al 2004). Festination (i.e., progressive shortening of stride length and increasing cadence) often occurs prior to freezing. During freezing, the feet appear to stick to the floor while momentum carries the centre of body mass forward. Patients feel as though their feet are 'glued to the ground' and the likelihood of falls is increased. While FOG occurs more frequently in cluttered environments, in stressful circumstances or when the patient is distracted, it can be improved when focused attention or cues are used (Giladi & Nieuwboer 2008).

Classification

It is difficult to get a clear and consistent picture of the nature of the motor and non-motor deficits in PD for several reasons. First, a number of subtypes have been identified suggestive of different pathologies or, in fact, a number of Parkinson's *diseases* (Lewis et al 2005; Halliday et al 2008; Weiner 2008). Second, marked differences can be observed in the same participant when tested at different times of the day or when participants are asked to withhold their drugs for a period of time prior to testing (e.g., Evarts et al 1981). Despite the variability within and between patients, it is helpful to classify the degree and extent of clinical disability in PD. The most commonly utilized scales are the Hoehn and Yahr scale (Hoehn & Yahr 1967) and the Unified Parkinson's Disease Rating Scale (UPDRS) (Fahn et al 1987) (see Ch. 3).

MOTOR CONTROL AND MOTOR PERFORMANCE DEFICITS

A decline in function may occur even before a diagnosis of PD is established. Early symptoms may be vague and non-specific, such as inexplicable tiredness, unwarranted fatigability and mild muscular aches and cramps, all potentially contributing to increasing incapacity (Stern & Lees 1991). Cognitive impairment, particularly affecting executive function and memory, is also evident in more than 25% of newly-diagnosed patients (Muslimovic et al 2005). Excessive levels of physical and mental fatigue are common and independently contribute to poor quality of life (Havlikova et al 2008). Depression may compound the situation and may influence the individual's participation in activities. As the disease progresses, clinical signs and symptoms, including tremor which may result in spills of drinks and food, speech difficulties, diminished facial expression and the possibility of drooling, may lead to embarrassing and upsetting incidents causing the individual to feel socially unacceptable and isolated. Difficulty in initiating movement such as in gait and 'freezing' on a social outing may compromise independence and confidence.

Individuals with PD have been studied performing meaningful tasks in an attempt to add insight into the role of the basal ganglia in motor control. Since these studies illustrate the motor control deficits as well as motor performance deficits, the findings should assist the physiotherapy clinician to understand these and to develop and test scientifically-based intervention strategies. Studies typically involve the investigation of reaction time (RT), movement time (MT) and the ability to perform simultaneous or sequential movements.

Reaction time and movement time

Patients with PD undoubtedly have difficulty initiating movement. In 1925, Wilson reported delayed RT in a patient with unilateral parkinsonism when asked to sit up from a supine position by using dynamometers to record contraction of the rectus femoris. Evarts and colleagues (1981) reported a high degree of variability in RT between patients and within the same individual at different times in a simple pronation/supination arm movement. The authors reported that although, in general, RT and MT were prolonged in PD, overall MT was more severely affected than RT. The degree of slowing in simple movements, however, is often not correlated with the degree of clinical bradykinesia (Benecke et al 1986; Berardelli et al 1986).

Execution of sequential movements

The generalized movement slowing seen in PD is characterized clinically by slowness of both simple single joint ballistic movements which usually undershoot (Hallett & Khoshbin 1980) and movement sequences (Benecke et al 1987). It has been suggested that slowness of movement may be more marked for movement sequences performed automatically (Schwab et al 1954).

Many of the critical everyday actions that individuals with PD have difficulty in performing, such as sit-to-stand (Fig. 13.1) and walking, are made up of sequential movements. In a series of studies, Benecke and colleagues (1987) demonstrated that movement sequences are slower in patients with PD compared with normal participants. When patients performed sequential movements, not only were the individual movements slower than normal but the interval when switching between the two sequences

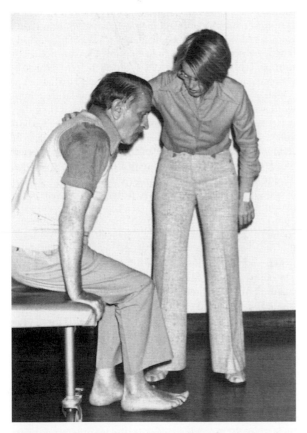

Figure 13.1 An attempt to stand up illustrates decreased amplitude of trunk flexion at the hips and dorsiflexion at the ankles. He has difficulty initiating horizontal momentum and changing from the horizontal to vertical sequence of the action. Note he has not moved his right foot back.

was also prolonged. Georgiou and colleagues (1993) suggest that the greater severity of deficit with movement sequences compared with individual movements may arise from the decrease in amplitude and speed of each component the further down the sequence it is produced.

Execution of simultaneous tasks

Patients with PD not only have difficulty in executing a motor task involving sequential movements but also in carrying out simultaneous tasks. A striking clinical feature of PD is the difficulty experienced when attempting to perform two motor tasks at the same time. Schwab and colleagues (1954) had patients with PD draw lines perpendicular to the mid-point of each side of a triangle with the dominant hand while squeezing the bulb of an ergometer with the other hand. Able-bodied participants were able to perform these two acts simultaneously with ease whereas this ability was lost or impaired in the PD participants who tended to make sequential movements by performing first one task then the other.

In an attempt to elucidate further the deficit in performing simultaneous movements, Benecke and colleagues (1986) had PD participants perform several simple movements as rapidly as possible and then combine these; for example, squeeze an isometric force transducer and flex the elbow. Movement times for each simple movement were slower than able-bodied participants. When two movements were combined, there was a further slowing of the movement seen in an increase in MT. The extra slowness found in both sequential and simultaneous movements has been reported to be closely related to the degree of clinically evaluated bradykinesia and conventional neurological examination (Benecke et al 1986). Bradykinesia was evaluated on time taken to complete a pegboard task and the number of touches between thumb and finger in a specified time.

The underlying mechanisms responsible for the motor deficits in performing learned automatic movement sequences in PD remain unclear. These mechanisms appear to fall into two categories: deficits in the motor plan or motor set, that is, a failure in the ability to match and maintain the amplitude of a cortically selected movement plan; and defective internal cue production causing progressive slowing of sequences of movement. When both deficits occur concurrently or when one is severe, festination and freezing may result (Iansek et al 2006). One function of the basal ganglia may be the provision of internal cues for the performance of well-learned activities or movement sequences (Phillips et al 1993; Morris et al 1995).

The *performance deficits* in PD have been studied in several actions critical to independence – gait, postural adjustments and reach-to-grasp as well as respiratory and oromotor function.

Gait

The most frequently observed gait disorders are slowness of movement and difficulty in initiation. The individual with PD is observed to walk with short, shuffling steps (marche à petit pas), uneven step lengths, a typical flexed posture (Fig. 13.2), reduced movement of the arms and decreased angular displacement of the lower limb joints (e.g., Murray et al 1978; Blin et al 1990). These problems tend to become more severe as the disease progresses and are associated with a loss of independence and an increased incidence of falls. Freezing, either in the initiation of or during gait, is also commonly observed and has been found to be particularly evident on turning or in narrow spaces, that is, context dependent (Giladi et al 1992). In addition to a shuffling and frozen gait, festination, that is, a progressive decrease in stride length and increase in cadence, may also be observed in some individuals.

Typically, investigations into the gait of individuals with PD have been concerned with describing the deficits in relation to able-bodied participants, the change in deficits before and after medication, and with and without visual cues. Attempts to quantify gait deficits in PD (e.g., Knutsson 1972; Blin et al 1990) have typically found slowness in gait to be associated with decreased stride length, decreased cadence and an increase in the proportion of time spent in double support (DS) phase.

In a series of studies with PD participants and age-matched controls, Morris and colleagues (1994a,b) examined the relationship between walking speed, cadence and stride length. The authors found that although PD participants could vary their gait speed similar to controls, when speed of walking was controlled, stride length was shorter and cadence higher in these participants than in control participants. An increase in stride length could be achieved in the presence of spatial visual cues, suggesting that an increase in cadence for any given speed in PD is a compensation for difficulty in regulating stride length. Morris and colleagues (1994a,b) also found that both PD participants and age-matched controls showed an increase in the time spent in DS compared with younger participants. The duration of DS when matched for speed of walking, however, was not significantly different between PD participants and their age-matched controls. Since DS is considered to be the most stable phase of the gait cycle, this finding may reflect balance deficits and reduced vigour, older participants spending a longer time in the 'safer' DS phase.

More recent studies have analysed gait under complex circumstances, such as turning, walking backwards and performing dual tasks. Huxham and colleagues (2008a,b) analysed people with PD walking straight ahead as well as turning 60° and 120° while walking. Contrary to the common clinical assumption that turning while walking is impaired due to reduced head and trunk rotation, stride length reduction was the major contributor to inefficient turning (Huxham et al 2008a). Stride length reduction was even more affected for the larger turns (Huxham et al 2008b). Similarly, decrements in speed and stride length while walking backwards are more pronounced than decrements while walking forwards (Hackney & Earhart 2008a). Further, when walking is combined with one or more additional tasks, speed and stride length are reduced to a greater degree in people with PD than controls (e.g., Bloem et al 2006). This may be due to limited central processing abilities or a failure to prioritize balance control over other tasks, increasing the risk of falls (Bloem et al 2006). Therefore, it appears that the more complex the cognitive and physical demands associated with walking, the more significant the reductions in speed and stride length and the greater the risk of falls.

Studies on gait variability have extended our understanding of the impact of PD on gait. There is evidence of variability in timing of steps early in PD (Hausdorff et al 1998; Ebersbach et al 1999; Yogev et al 2005) and this may be a precursor to the development of freezing later in the disease. Even prior to treatment with antiparkinsonian medications, 'de novo' patients show asymmetries in timing of gait (Baltadjieva et al 2006). Therefore, changes that are often described as advanced features of the disease are evident early in the disease process and are likely to reflect the direct effects of the disease, rather than adaptations or medication effects. As the disease progresses, bilateral coordination of gait is affected, especially under dual task conditions, suggesting that cognitive resources are required to maintain gait consistency (Plotnik et al 2009).

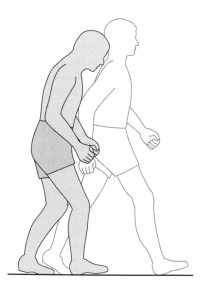

Figure 13.2 Illustration of a man with Parkinson's disease (shaded) showing relatively flexed posture compared with an able-bodied man at the point of heel contact of the right lower limb. *(From Murray et al. (1978)).*

Balance

Postural instability is considered a major contributor to the disability associated with PD (e.g., Boonstra et al 2008). Clinically, it is evident that people with PD lose their balance easily, have an increased incidence of falls (Bloem et al 2001; Wood et al 2002; Ashburn et al 2007; Latt et al 2009) and fear of falling (Adkin et al 2003) compared to able-bodied individuals. The underlying mechanism of the postural instability is not, however, clear. Studies of standing balance under different conditions have produced variable results, reflecting differences in the tasks investigated, the timing of testing in relation to ingestion of medication, disease stage, presenting impairments and each individual's adaptive behaviour.

Hypotheses regarding mechanisms underlying postural instability can be broadly categorized in two groups (Boonstra et al 2008): an 'efferent deficit', that is, reduced ability to make rapid, accurately coordinated postural responses due to bradykinesia and/or akinesia (Berardelli et al 1984, 2001); and an 'afferent deficit', that is, reduced ability to process afferent input preventing flexible adaptation in various environments (Bronstein et al 1990; Schieppati & Nardone 1991). Difficulty responding to unexpected perturbations results in instability, with a greater reliance on vision and other attentional processes as a consequence. However, changes in muscle properties and the person's own adaptive behaviour may play a part in the variations in postural adjustments seen in PD patients when they are compared with able-bodied individuals. Changes in muscle stiffness, for example in gastrocnemius muscle, have been suggested to underlie abnormalities in gait (Dietz et al 1981) and the relatively slow ankle joint displacement and speed observable in support surface perturbation studies.

What is clear, however, is that the inability to make appropriate postural adjustments (i.e., task- and context-specific muscle activations related to balancing the body mass) is deficient in any individual with a primary motor control problem. Instability is due both to abnormal coordination resulting from the brain impairment and to secondary adaptations (both behavioural and soft tissue).

Postural adjustments normally occur both in response to external perturbations (e.g., support surface movement, slips and trips) and before and during a volitional movement as an integral part of the action (see Ch. 7). Much of the early research into postural instability in PD involved studies of participants standing on a movable support surface and tests of rapid arm raising in standing. The perturbation studies provide information related to the ability of PD patients, at various clinical stages, to act in responsive ('reactive') mode. The fast arm raising studies provide information particularly related to the presence and timing of preparatory postural adjustments. Recently, the findings of studies of everyday tasks have been reported which provide information about the integration of postural adjustments with self-initiated movements during complex actions performed at their natural speeds.

The location of the centre of foot pressure (CFP) in relation to the body mass in standing affects postural muscle activation during both self-initiated and responsive movement. Given the *flexed posture* typical of individuals with PD, it is interesting that, in the group of people studied by Schieppati & Nardone (1991), the CFP was found to be shifted backward in less severe cases and forward in the more severe. The authors suggested that since maintaining the centre of body mass further back than normal is potentially destabilizing, causing the individual to overbalance backward, the movement of CFP forward (by flexing at the hips and trunk) may be an adaptive response to maintain balance.

Studies of *postural sway* during quiet standing show conflicting results, as they do in able-bodied participants, reflecting variations in stage of disease, testing protocols and variables used to quantify postural sway. Further, medication state, ON (i.e., time when medication is providing benefit with regard to mobility, slowness and stiffness) versus OFF (i.e., time when medication effects have worn off and are no longer providing benefits with regard to mobility, slowness and stiffness), is likely to affect postural sway. Most studies show an increase in postural sway, particularly in the mediolateral direction (e.g., Viitasalo et al 2002; Rocchi et al 2006a; Blaszczyk et al 2007). Further, while an increase in postural sway has been reported for eyes closed compared to eyes open conditions, the magnitude of increase in sway is greater for people with PD compared with controls (Blaszczyk et al 2007). In addition, people with more severe PD who are fallers demonstrate greater postural sway than non-fallers (Matinolli et al 2007). It is also important to note that people with PD overestimate their limits of stability (Kamata et al 2007), and as they are less able to adapt their postural adjustments to changes in the environment (De Nunzio et al 2007), this further predisposes them to falls.

One reason for poor balance in standing can be an inability to make relevant and appropriately timed *preparatory (or anticipatory) postural adjustments* (muscle activations). Preparatory postural adjustments have been studied in PD patients in relation to several different tasks. A study of rising on tiptoes (Diener et al 1990), which included individuals with PD and age-matched able-bodied participants, showed that the order of onsets for both groups of participants was tibialis anterior (to move body mass forward), quadriceps femoris (to stabilize the knee) followed by triceps surae to execute the heel-raising action. Tibialis anterior and quadriceps were active prior to the target movement as preparatory postural adjustments. Although the participants with PD showed this same basic pattern of muscle activations, the action was performed more slowly and the build-up of muscle tension appeared slower.

Some studies have reported similar preparatory muscle latencies compared to able-bodied individuals. Others have noted delays in onsets of muscle activity (e.g., Rogers et al 1987; Burleigh-Jacobs et al 1997; Rocchi et al 2006b). Still others (Frank et al 2000; Bleuse et al 2008) show decreased latencies for fast as possible movements which people with PD can prepare for in advance. One difficulty in investigating and comparing preparatory postural adjustments is the slowness of movement typical of PD. Such adjustments in able-bodied individuals are particularly evident prior to fast movement (such as arm raising) but not necessarily so when movements are slow. Hence, although preparatory muscle activations have been reported as absent or different from the able-bodied in studies of individuals with PD, this result may have been due to the relative slowness of arm movement compared with able-bodied participants (Bazalgette et al 1986; Rogers et al 1987).

More recently, postural adjustments associated with self-initiated stepping tasks in standing have been examined (Burleigh-Jacobs et al 1997; Tonolli et al 2000; Rocchi et al 2006b). In these studies, abnormally small and slow anticipatory adjustments resulted in shorter steps in people with PD compared to controls. For example, in a lateral stepping task (Tonolli et al 2000), the amplitude and speed of anticipatory weight shift onto the supporting leg, prior to stepping, was reduced.

The latency, magnitude and speed of anticipatory postural adjustments improve with dopaminergic medications, but fail to normalize completely (e.g., Burleigh-Jacobs et al 1997; Rocchi et al 2006b). Further, the response to dopaminergic medications tends to diminish as the disease progresses. In addition, a further cause of postural instability which has received little attention to date is levodopa-induced dyskinesia. Armand and colleagues (2009) showed a 125% increase in net centre of pressure displacement during quiet standing when patients were ON with dyskinesia, compared to OFF. This increased displacement occurs in both anteroposterior and mediolateral directions, with the mediolateral direction being most affected.

Several studies have investigated the response of participants with PD to *unexpected externally-induced support surface perturbations* as they stand on a movable platform. The majority of studies show latencies of muscle activations in response to the platform movement to be similar to those of able-bodied participants (e.g., Schieppati & Nardone 1991; Horak et al 1996; Carpenter et al 2004; Jacobs & Horak 2006). Responses tend, however, to be more variable than normal (Schieppati & Nardone 1991).

Some studies have employed rotational platform perturbations which project the individual into a toe-up position as a means of testing postural 'reflexes' (e.g., Scholz et al 1987; Beckley et al 1991). In one study (Beckley et al 1991), able-bodied participants used a so-called 'ankle strategy' in which tibialis anterior was active prior to vastus lateralis as a means of regaining the vertical position, whereas PD participants reversed this order and stiffened the knee. The authors pointed out that although this stiffening could contribute to postural instability, the initial posture of the participants would have affected the results by requiring a different motor response. The early activation of the more proximal muscles linking thigh and shank (and perhaps other muscles linking trunk and thigh which were not monitored) may also indicate an adaptive stiffening of the limb to counter the perturbation.

Studies have also analysed the effect of translational platform perturbations in various directions where postural responses are made between body segments without altering the base of support. A study of PD individuals (Horak et al 1992) showed normal latencies in both gastrocnemius and tibialis anterior in response to backward and forward platform translations respectively. However, excessive antagonistic activity was noted indicating poor movement control or lack of skill. Even on levodopa, individuals with PD appear to lack flexible adaptation to changing support surface conditions in standing (Horak et al 1992). It is not clear, therefore, whether difficulties with balance reflect increased intrinsic stiffness of muscle to dampen body sway (Woollacott et al 1988), or inability to activate muscles with enough force or speed to respond to a perturbation or to anticipate a forthcoming perturbation. It may also be that patients adapt to their inability to generate sufficiently fast muscle activations by self-limiting behaviours such as holding the body stiffly and by decreasing the excursion of the body mass movement and decreasing destabilization by moving very slowly (e.g., flexing the body at trunk and lower limb joints in standing or taking small shuffling steps when walking).

More recently, the role of compensatory steps to prevent falling when the centre of mass is displaced outside the base of support has been addressed (Jacobs & Horak 2006; King & Horak 2008). In one study (King & Horak 2008), participants were required to keep their balance in response to sideways platform perturbations towards the less involved side. They wore an overhead harness and an assistant stood by for safety. Able-bodied control participants stepped in the direction opposite to the perturbation with either a side step (using the leg on the opposite side to the direction of perturbation) or using the other leg to produce a cross-over step. Anticipatory lateral weight shift, which is necessary prior to stepping with either leg, was absent in half of the participants with PD and resulted in falls. Fourteen per cent of the people with PD used no stepping strategy and fell like a log. The remaining people with PD used both stepping strategies, but the cross-over step strategy resulted in a much higher rate of leg collisions and falls (75% of trials) compared to the side-step strategy (17% of trials). Even in successful trials, increased latency to step onset in response to external perturbation shows that the speed of build-up of postural responses is consistently slower, resulting in potentially ineffective postural responses. In contrast to the generally positive effect of levodopa medications on anticipatory postural adjustments, they have little effect on reactive postural adjustments (Carpenter et al 2004; Jacobs & Horak 2006; King & Horak 2008) and may have a negative impact (Horak et al 1996).

There is a suggestion in the literature that reduced spinal flexibility (measured as functional axial rotation, that is, excursion in degrees from turning and looking over one shoulder to the other) contributes to poor balance (measured as functional reach distance) in people with PD (Schenkman et al 2000). Although it remains unclear whether reduced spinal rotation is secondary to hypokinesia, rigidity, dystonia or a combination of these impairments, these results suggest that maintenance of spinal flexibility may assist in reducing balance deficits. Further, flexed posture is an independent risk factor for falling (Latt et al 2009).

The view is commonly expressed that PD individuals can generate appropriate postural muscle activation patterns and seem to be able to improve balance control by relying more than usual upon conscious effort, utilizing visual information and other external cues (Waterston et al 1993). It may be that these individuals can use cognitive strategies (e.g., by concentrating attention on preparing for a movement) to override the defective mechanisms, provided the threat to balance is not too great.

Reaching and manipulation

Numerous normative studies of the reach-to-grasp movement have shown that the movement consists of two components, the transport or reach component and the manipulation or grasp component, with both components activated in parallel. In people with PD, the effects of bradykinesia are evident in reach-to-grasp tasks which are internally timed, such as reaching at maximum possible speed to grasp a stationary ball, while speed of reaching movement is within normal limits when reaching to grasp a moving ball (Majsak et al 1998). However, reaches towards the moving ball were more frequently unsuccessful compared to control participants. Even under conditions where visual motion cues or external time constraints are present, people with PD have a slower speed of hand opening and closing, smaller maximal aperture and longer time to maximum aperture (Majsak et al 2008).

Castiello and colleagues (1993) studied the reach-to-grasp movement in both PD and control participants. The reach was either 15, 27.5 or 40 cm while the grasp was of a small (0.7 cm) or a large (8 cm) dowel. Analysis of the movement in PD participants showed a slowed MT but, similar to able-bodied controls, the PD participants had no difficulty in regulating the spatiotemporal characteristics of the movement related to changes in object distance or size. However, for the PD participants, it was the coordination of the two components that showed abnormality

in that the onset of the grasp component was delayed in relation to the onset of the transport component. In another study (Castiello et al 1994), which involved reaching to grasp a glass filled with water and take it to the lips in order to take a sip, control participants showed no transition phase between the two movements. On the other hand, PD participants showed a transition phase in 38% of trials of, on average, 337 ms or 7% of movement time. Difficulty in the transition phase has also been reported by Muller & Abbs (1990). Therefore, reach-to-grasp tasks appear to be affected by both bradykinesia and akinesia resulting in loss of dexterity as well as slowed performance of tasks.

Respiratory function

Respiratory dysfunction is a common finding in individuals with PD (e.g., Vincken et al 1984) and may be present in the absence of symptoms of pulmonary dysfunction (Pal et al 2007). This dysfunction is thought to result from the motor control deficits associated with PD. The flexed posture and immobility generally associated with PD could also contribute to respiratory impairment and cardiorespiratory deconditioning. Patients with moderate to severe PD have been found to have both decreased work capacity and exercise efficiency on a similar level of external work compared with age-matched controls performing one-legged exercise (Saltin & Landin 1975). The authors concluded that general muscle weakness secondary to the neurological disorder may have led to these results. Inactivity would also contribute.

One study (Canning et al 1997) examined the exercise capacity of participants with mild to moderate PD in order to determine whether or not respiratory dysfunction and gait disorders affect exercise capacity. The results suggest that these individuals have the potential to maintain exercise capacity within normal limits for age with regular aerobic exercise. Further, inspiratory muscle training has been shown to be an effective intervention in people with mild to moderate Parkinson's disease resulting in increased inspiratory muscle strength and endurance and decreased perception of dyspnoea (Inzelberg et al 2005).

Oromotor function

Speech disorders have been found in as many as 92% of patients (Martin et al 1973) and include abnormal voice modulation (dysphonia) with hoarseness, decreased volume and monotonous tone (Robbins et al 1986). Low speech volume (hypophonia) results in reduced speech intelligibility and consequently interferes with communication (Sadagopan & Huber 2007). Evidence supporting intensive voice treatment targeting vocal loudness (the Lee Silverman Voice Treatment) as an effective intervention for speech disorders is increasing (see Ramig et al 2008 for review).

Swallowing disorders have been reported to exist in as many as 50% of patients assessed by barium swallow (Lieberman et al 1980). Radiography (Silbiger et al 1967) and videofluoroscopy (Robbins et al 1986) have demonstrated that abnormal oropharyngeal movement patterns and timing occur in both the initial or volitional stage as well as the pharyngeal stage of swallowing. Problems include tongue tremor, slowness in initiating the swallow, difficulty forming the bolus and propelling it backward to the posterior third of the tongue for stimulating the pharyngeal stage of swallowing, and disturbances in pharyngeal motility. More recently, Gross et al (2008) reported impaired coordination of breathing and swallowing, increasing risk of aspiration. Interestingly, Robbins and colleagues (1986) found that aspiration was a problem in 33% of their participants, yet they lacked awareness of aspiration which may explain why bronchopneumonia is a major cause of death in PD (Hoehn & Yahr 1967). A recently developed swallowing disturbance questionnaire has been validated to detect early dysphagia in people with PD (Manor et al 2007).

Adaptive motor behaviour

The human system is highly adaptive and the musculoskeletal periphery, being multisegmented, has the potential to produce a variety of alternate movement patterns in order to achieve a specific goal. Normally, movement patterns appear to emerge from musculoskeletal flexibility, the goal of the task and the environmental context in which it is to be carried out (Shepherd & Carr 1991). We adapt the way we move in response to both internal and external circumstances, for example favouring the unaffected limb when shoulder movement is painful, moving more slowly than usual and seeking hand holds when balance in threatened.

In individuals with PD, moving slowly may reflect in part an adaptation to the difficulty in activating muscles fast enough. Freezing and resistance to externally-imposed movement may be options that enable the individual to avoid perturbations for which it is difficult to prepare. Less than optimal motor performance may, therefore, be adaptive in the sense that it is an attempt to avoid failure in task performance.

The view that altered motor patterns in PD may be adaptive rather than due to a primary disorder was expressed some years ago by Latash & Anson (1996). Phillips and colleagues (1993) also argued that PD bradykinesia, rather than being an inability to energize muscles (Hallett & Khoshbin 1980), may reflect a problem in specifying the appropriate rate of force production necessary for accurate movement. In investigations of targeted limb movements, it has been suggested that slowness of movement may enable greater variability and be a means of ensuring an acceptable level of accuracy (Sheridan &

Flowers 1990); that is, an adaptation. Future research may elucidate this issue. In the meantime, physiotherapy needs to focus on providing the individual with Parkinson's disease opportunities and encouragement to be physically and mentally active, preserving flexibility and agility as much as possible.

NON-MOTOR DEFICITS

When James Parkinson first described PD, he observed that the senses and intellect were unimpaired. More recent research suggests that non-motor symptoms develop during the course of the disease and some precede diagnosis. Further, it is now clear that many areas of the brain outside of the dopaminergic nigrostriatal system may be affected in PD, including the brainstem, hypothalamus, limbic system and neocortex (Poewe 2008). Common neuropsychiatric non-motor deficits include depression, anxiety, frontal executive dysfunction, dementia, psychosis, sleep disorders, restless leg syndrome and excessive daytime sleepiness. Autonomic non-motor symptoms include orthostatic hypotension, urogenital dysfunction and constipation, while sensory symptoms (pain and abnormal sensations) are also common (Chaudhuri et al 2006; Poewe 2008). Further, fatigue is common in PD and is often the most troubling of all symptoms (Friedman et al 2007). Although fatigue may be associated with depression and sleep disorders, it also occurs in non-depressed patients and in those without sleep disorders. The mechanisms underlying fatigue in PD are poorly understood and there is no known effective treatment for managing it.

Mood disturbances

Depression is common in people with PD, with approximately 40% of people with PD experiencing depression (Weintraub 2005) and/or anxiety (Menza & Dobkin 2005). Anxiety is frequently undetected and underdiagnosed and may precede diagnosis (York & Alvarez 2008). However, it may be difficult for clinicians to recognize the presence of depression in their patients if/when it occurs since many of the symptoms of depression, such as lack of variation in facial expression, slowness of movement and apparent slowness of thought and lack of variation in speech production, mimic those of PD. Because of these overlapping motor and depressive symptoms, diagnosis of depression in PD is based on subjectively experienced symptoms; that is, feelings of emptiness and hopelessness, reduced reactivity to emotional stimuli and loss of ability to enjoy and feel pleasure (anhedonia). Depression may be amenable to treatment with antidepressants as well as education to train and improve coping strategies (Lemke 2008). Further, dopamine agonists, for example pramipexole, have been shown to have antidepressive effects as well as motor benefits (Lemke et al 2005). The potential role of exercise in managing mild depressive symptoms in PD remains to be explored.

Cognitive deficits

Cognitive deficits may precede diagnosis and 25% of newly diagnosed patients present with cognitive deficits (Muslimovic et al 2005). Mild cognitive deficits in attention/executive function and memory are evident early in the disease and in the absence of dementia (Zgaljardic et al 2003) and these deficits have a significant impact on quality of life (Schrag et al 2000). Up to 40% of patients will develop clinically defined dementia, with the development of dementia associated with more rapid progression of disability (Findley et al 2003).

People with PD may have impaired performance on a wide range of neuropsychological tests including tests of psychomotor speed, language, memory, attention, executive functions and visuospatial skills, however deficits in attention/executive function and memory are most common (Muslimovic et al 2005). Specific deficits in attention/executive function include difficulty in set shifting (e.g., Lees & Smith 1983) and sequencing (e.g., Cahn et al 1998), and impaired selective attention and difficulty inhibiting attention to distracting stimuli (Deijen et al 2006). Memory deficits include impaired working memory (i.e., reduced ability to maintain and manipulate the information held in short term memory) (Muslimovic et al 2005) and impaired prospective memory, that is, reduced ability to remember to do something at a future time (Katai et al 2003). Impaired performance of visuospatial tasks is also evident reflecting both a reduction in attentional resource allocation and a specific visuospatial deficit (Kemps et al 2005).

Reduced ability to focus attention and increased reaction time variability have been shown to be associated with increased fall frequency in PD (Allcock et al 2009). These cognitive deficits may explain, in part, the deterioration in balance and gait while multitasking as well as the poor use of corrective strategies used by patients when they lose balance. Two trials have shown improvement in cognitive function with cognitive training in PD (Sinforiani et al 2004; Sammer et al 2006). Sammer and colleagues (2006) showed improvement in two executive function tests, but it is not known whether this improvement generalized to improved performance of daily activities.

It is not known whether memory deficits are amenable to training in people with PD. However, the use of devices to compensate for memory deficits such as memory notebooks, to-do lists and electronic paging systems are suggested (York & Alvarez 2008). These devices can be utilized in the context of a physiotherapy intervention programme, for example to assist patients to remember the key features of tasks to be practised or to act as a prompt to perform an exercise session.

MEDICATION AND SURGICAL INTERVENTION

In the late 1960s and early 1970s, it was reasoned that the symptoms associated with PD may be relieved if the amount of dopamine in the brain was restored to normal. Eventually oral levodopa (dopamine replacement therapy) was established as the most effective therapy for PD (Marsden & Parkes 1977; Agid et al 1987) and a significant advance in the treatment of PD was made. In particular, the most disabling symptom of the disease, bradykinesia, which had not shown any marked improvement when previously treated by anticholinergic medication and stereotaxic surgery, responded very well to levodopa (Marsden 1990). Today, levodopa or dopamine agonists are the first-line therapy in PD (see Strecker & Schwarz 2008 for review).

Motor symptoms, particularly bradykinesia, respond well to levodopa therapy, especially over the first 5–7 years. However, over time, motor fluctuations (characterized by ON and OFF periods and dyskinesia) occur and other motor symptoms which respond poorly to levodopa emerge, including gait disorders, freezing and postural instability. To enhance the availability of levodopa at this stage, catecholamine O methyltransferase (COMT) inhibitors are considered to maintain therapeutic plasma levels of levodopa over a longer time period, thereby reducing the amount of OFF time. Monoamine oxidase (MAO) inhibitors may also be used to inhibit the enzyme MAO-B which is responsible for degradation of dopamine, thereby prolonging its action. The antiviral drug, amantadine, blocks glutamate receptors and has a moderate effect on cardinal symptoms of PD (resting tremor, bradykinesia and rigidity) and reduces levodopa-induced dyskinesias. The dopamine agonist, apomorphine, given by subcutaneous injections or continuous infusions has a short half-life (approximately 10 minutes) making it an effective intervention for treating sudden unpredictable OFF periods. More recently, duodenal levodopa infusions administered via percutaneous enteral gastrostomy have also been reported to significantly reduce motor fluctuations (Strecker & Schwarz 2008).

Many of the medications used to manage PD are associated with significant side-effects including gastrointestinal complaints such as nausea and vomiting, orthostatic hypotension, confusion and delirium, behavioural changes, dyskinesia and dystonia. For a summary of the major medications used in PD and common side-effects, see Keus et al (2004), and/or the Parkinson's Disease Foundation Web site.* The pharmacological management

---

*http://www.pdf.org/en/meds_treatments

of the motor symptoms of PD is complex and in most circumstances is best managed by a neurologist with movement disorders experience. The picture is further complicated by the need to manage the non-motor symptoms from a medical point of view (see Chaudhuri et al 2006 for a review of medical management of non-motor symptoms).

With more advanced and severe disease, prolonged periods of being OFF, oscillating with ON periods characterized by severe and functionally-limiting dyskinesias, seriously compromise quality of life. At this stage, surgery or deep brain stimulation may be considered for carefully selected patients (Goetz et al 2005; Schapira 2007). Deep brain stimulation (DBS) of the subthalamic nucleus or the globus pallidus internus improves all the cardinal motor features of PD and reduces dyskinesias (Limousin et al 1998; Deuschl et al 2006) in patients with disability primarily associated with motor complications, a history of good response to levodopa and intact cognition. Long-term benefits of DBS are reported at 5-year follow-up, although progression of disability is still evident, especially for gait and postural instability (Ferraye et al 2008; Lozano & Snyder 2008).

PHYSIOTHERAPY INTERVENTION

Effective physiotherapy for people with PD relies first and foremost upon an understanding of the motor and non-motor impairments, analysis of the contribution of these impairments to activity limitations such as standing up and walking, as well as an up-to-date knowledge of the evidence base for efficacy of physiotherapy interventions. Developing interest in the ability of the movement sciences to provide the scientific basis of intervention (Carr & Shepherd 1987), developments in the medical sciences regarding the nature of the basal ganglia deficit, together with an increased understanding of the importance of physical fitness and flexibility have driven the development and testing of these new methodologies.

It is generally accepted that physiotherapy is necessary as an adjunct to medication and a theoretical framework for physiotherapy in PD has been developed (Morris 2000; Morris et al 2009) and widely adopted (Keus et al 2004, 2009) (Fig. 13.3). Over the last 10 years there has been a dramatic rise in the number of systematic reviews and randomized controlled trials (Keus et al

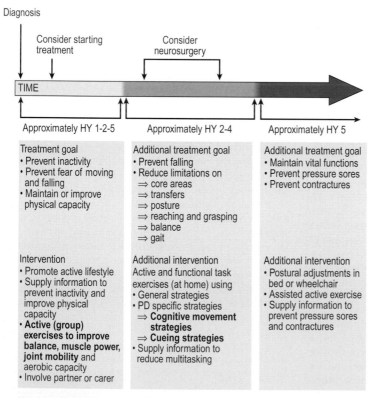

Figure 13.3 Framework for physiotherapy intervention in Parkinson's disease: goals and possible interventions according to stage of disease. *(Reprinted from Keus et al 2007, with permission).*

Diagnosis

Consider starting treatment

Consider neurosurgery

TIME

Approximately HY 1-2-5   Approximately HY 2-4   Approximately HY 5

Treatment goal
• Prevent inactivity
• Prevent fear of moving and falling
• Maintain or improve physical capacity

Additional treatment goal
• Prevent falling
• Reduce limitations on
  ⇒ core areas
  ⇒ transfers
  ⇒ posture
  ⇒ reaching and grasping
  ⇒ balance
  ⇒ gait

Additional treatment goal
• Maintain vital functions
• Prevent pressure sores
• Prevent contractures

Intervention
• Promote active lifestyle
• Supply information to prevent inactivity and improve physical capacity
• **Active (group) exercises to improve balance, muscle power, joint mobility** and aerobic capacity
• Involve partner or carer

Additional intervention
Active and functional task exercises (at home) using
• General strategies
• PD specific strategies
  ⇒ **Cognitive movement strategies**
  ⇒ **Cueing strategies**
• Supply information to reduce multitasking

Additional intervention
• Postural adjustments in bed or wheelchair
• Assisted active exercise
• Supply information to prevent pressure sores and contractures

Key recommendations are highlighted

2009) reporting the efficacy, or not, of a wide range of physiotherapy interventions. Guidelines for physical therapy in patients with PD (Plant et al 2001; Keus et al 2004) have now been established and widely distributed. The challenge for the physiotherapist is to critically evaluate this information and apply it to the individual patient, with his/her personal goals, unique set of impairments and activity limitations, in the context of the patient's environment. The emphasis in intervention should also reflect the stage of the disease. Stage of disease is characterized according to the Hoehn and Yahr staging (Hoehn & Yahr 1967) and patients are identified as being in early, middle or late stage (Keus et al 2004).

The major role for the physiotherapist in the early stage lies in promoting physical activities as a means of maintaining an active lifestyle, a flexible neuromusculoskeletal system, cardiorespiratory fitness, muscle strength and balance. In addition, in the middle stage of the disease, cueing and cognitive strategies are utilized to optimize the performance of everyday tasks. It is also necessary to consider timely and appropriate prescription of aids as the person moves from middle stage to late stage. It is likely that the physiotherapist would best assist the individual to accomplish an activity programme by working together in his/her own environment and by being available for discussion and advice by telephone and through regular visits. In the later stage of the disease, a carer may take responsibility for providing cueing and cognitive strategies during task performance and for performing strategies to minimize activity-limiting contractures and pressure sores.

The need for early physiotherapy remains controversial in the medical literature, possibly because of a lack of understanding of the potential role of physiotherapy. Nevertheless, there is the negative effect on function, wellbeing and general health caused by the decrease in activity which can occur following the diagnosis as well as due to the specific motor and non-motor impairments, and to the ageing process itself. Two obvious reasons for *early referral* of the PD individual to a physiotherapist include the need for advice in preserving musculoskeletal flexibility, including thoracic expansion, and advice in maintaining an active lifestyle and minimizing the deconditioning and mental decline which can result from reduced physical and mental activity.

To date, there are no conclusive human studies demonstrating that exercise can play a role in neuroprotection or neurorestoration. However, the evidence from animal studies suggests that this may be the case. Therefore, in addition to prevention of secondary motor and non-motor impairments, exercise may have the potential to slow the progression of the disease. Neuroprotection is suggested in the work of Faherty et al (2005) where mice have been shown to be protected against methyl-4-phenyl-1,2,3,6-tetrahydropyridine (MPTP)-induced parkinsonism following exposure to an enriched environment (a combination of exercise, social interactions and learning), where exercise appears to be the critical component. Several studies (e.g., Fisher et al 2004; Poulton & Muir 2005; Yoon et al 2007), using a variety of animal models of PD and a variety of exercise protocols, demonstrate that exercise improves motor performance. Further, the amount of exercise and the intensity of exercise appear to be important factors for mediating these effects. These results add weight to the potential role of exercise early in the disease.

Despite substantial evidence of improvement in motor behaviour in humans with PD following exercise, it is more difficult to demonstrate neurorestoration in human studies. A recent study (Fisher et al 2008) randomized people with early PD to high-intensity treadmill training (walking and running), low-intensity exercise training or an education control group. As well as measuring outcome of sit-to-stand and walking tasks, corticomotor excitability was assessed with cortical silent period (CSP) durations in response to single-pulse transcranial magnetic stimulation. The high-intensity treadmill training group (4.5 metabolic equivalents for up to 45 minutes, 24 sessions over 8 weeks) showed greater gains in walking and sit-to-stand than the other groups. The high-intensity group also showed consistent lengthening of CSP durations reflecting activity-dependent neuroplasticity coupled with improved motor performance. These findings are important for several reasons: this is the first reported study to demonstrate improvement in corticomotor excitability in people with PD, high-intensity exercise was required to demonstrate gains, and no adverse effects were reported with the high-intensity exercise.

Task- and context-related practice to improve activity levels

Intervention to improve performance of everyday actions should focus on practising tasks in the environments in which they usually take place, with emphasis on improving both motor and spatial abilities and with information and feedback provided by the physiotherapist. Motor learning (skill acquisition) is said to involve a change from controlled attention-demanding processes (Fitts' cognitive stage) to more automatic and less attention-demanding processes (Fitts' automatic stage). PD patients need to practise difficult tasks with an emphasis on 'getting the idea of' the movement (cognitive stage) in order to develop strategies for overcoming the problem. Several studies have shown recently that individuals with PD can learn to adapt their motor performance to the needs of a task or to learn a new task (e.g., Soliveri et al 1992; Wu & Hallett 2005). What seems certain is that very specific practice in an appropriate context is as necessary as it is in healthy people who want to become skilled in a particular action.

Walking and balance

The benefits of walking practice cannot be overemphasized for people with PD. There is consensus that the aim of walking practice is to increase speed by increasing stride length (rather than by increasing cadence in the absence of an increase in stride length) (Morris 2006). The challenge is to identify the most appropriate mode of walking practice, environment and level of supervision. Studies targeting overground walking over periods of 3 (Nieuwboer et al 2007) or 6 weeks (Ellis et al 2005) with or without cues (see section below on cueing strategies), in home and/or outdoor environments, combined with interventions addressing muscle strength, flexibility and balance have demonstrated positive effects on walking speed and stride length. In the early to middle stages of the disease, moderate- to high-intensity walking practice may also assist in maintaining muscle length and cardiorespiratory fitness. Given that decrements in speed and step length are compounded under more complex walking conditions, incorporation of these conditions, such as dual tasks, stepping backwards and negotiation of obstacles to demand turns of different magnitudes (e.g., Morris 2006; Nieuwboer et al 2007, 2008) is recommended.

While there is little doubt that overground walking is a necessary component of a regular exercise programme for people with PD, recent research addressing motor impairments in PD has stimulated an exploration of the value of treadmill training. Previously, treadmill training has been criticized due to concerns about safety, a perceived lack of task specificity and concern that it may trigger freezing and falling. However, treadmill walking may improve the timing of gait parameters since it forces a rhythmic movement on the lower limbs and may have the potential to delay the onset of freezing. Treadmill walking has been shown to have the immediate effect of promoting a walking consistency significantly greater than that for overground walking (Frenkel-Toledo et al 2005; Bello et al 2008). Further, a 6-week programme of treadmill walking has also been shown to improve walking consistency (Herman et al 2007). In addition, a single session of treadmill walking has shown impressive immediate effects on both walking speed and stride length in people with mild to moderate (Pohl et al 2003) and more advanced PD (Bello et al 2008).

The ability to walk faster and/or further on completion of a programme of treadmill walking has been demonstrated in several randomized controlled trials (Miyai et al 2000, 2002; Protas et al 2005; Cakit et al 2007; Canning et al 2008a) over intervention periods ranging from 4 to 12 weeks. Other demonstrated benefits include improvements in balance (Cakit et al 2007) and quality of life (Canning et al 2008a), and a reduction in fatigue (Canning et al 2008a). To date, most trials have implemented treadmill walking under fully supervised conditions with use of an overhead harness for safety (Miyai et al 2000, 2002;

Protas et al 2005, Cakit et al 2007), with some studies including initial partial body weight relief (Miyai et al 2000, 2002). However, most people with PD are not weak enough to require partial body weight support and it is likely that treadmill walking will be as effective (as demonstrated by Toole et al 2005), if not more effective, when administered without initial partial body weight support. Further, if treadmill walking is to be implemented as a feasible intervention, then protocols which can be implemented outside a rehabilitation setting and not fully supervised need to be developed and tested. Canning and colleagues (2008a) have demonstrated that a home-based treadmill walking programme can be feasibly and safely implemented in people with mild to moderate PD (Fig. 13.4).

Improvement in walking is often considered to be limited by balance impairment. Again, contrary to the traditional view, recent studies suggest that at least some individuals with PD can improve their ability to make effective postural adjustments with task-related training (Toole et al 2005; Ashburn et al 2007; Cakit et al 2007; Hackney et al 2007; Nieuwboer et al 2007; Hackney & Earhart 2008b). Essentially, training to improve balance involves methods of safely challenging the person's ability to make postural adjustments in a timely and effective manner. The challenge to balance can be achieved in a number of ways. In order to improve the ability to make anticipatory and ongoing postural adjustments, the person practises motor tasks that require movement of the body mass in relation to different bases of support. These actions require postural adjustments to be made while maintaining the base of support, or by changing the base of support. The person can be further challenged by decreasing the base of support. In more severely affected patients, reducing the amount or type of upper limb support may be sufficient to challenge balance. Randomized controlled trials which have shown improvement in balance have achieved this challenge using a variety of methods, including fully-supervised incremental treadmill walking without a harness at the highest speed for that individual without stumbling (Cakit et al 2007), home-based balance and strengthening exercises (Ashburn et al 2007), home-based cueing of functional tasks (Nieuwboer et al 2007), group Tai Chi classes (Hackney & Earhart 2008b), group tango classes (Hackney et al 2007) and supervised training of reactive postural adjustments using different directions and forces (Toole et al 2005).

It is unclear whether there is an optimal mode and dose of balance training, or whether the most critical aspect is that the person performs some type of balance training. Since impairment of reactive postural adjustments is a particular problem for people with PD and responds poorly to pharmacological intervention (Carpenter et al 2004; Jacobs & Horak 2006; King & Horak 2008), specific training of reactive postural adjustments is recommended. This type of training is difficult to implement due to safety

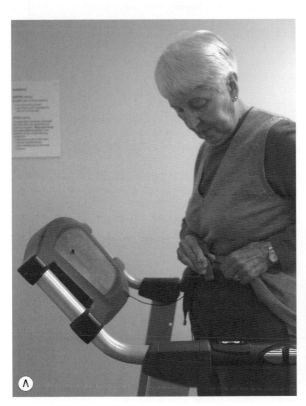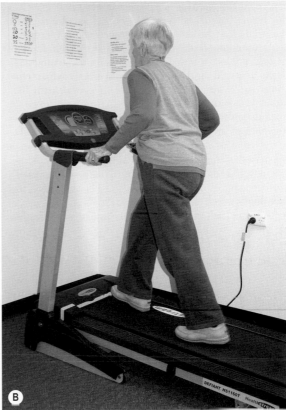

Figure 13.4 Treadmill walking. The patient practises starting/stopping the treadmill, changing speed and stopping unexpectedly with supervision from the physiotherapist, before walking on the treadmill independently. (A) The magnetic safety key on the treadmill is connected by a cord to a clip which is attached to the patient's belt. The string is kept relatively short, so that if the patient moves too far back on the treadmill while walking, the magnetic safety key will be dislodged and the treadmill will come to a stop. (B) Instructions and safety guidelines provided by the physiotherapist are attached to the wall. The patient holds lightly onto the handle bars, concentrates on taking big steps and bringing the toes forwards towards the white visual cue on each step. Notes: (i) independent treadmill walking should not be performed if the patient is OFF, and (ii) full supervision (including the use of an overhead harness) is required for patients with cognitive impairment, postural instability and/or freezing.

concerns, yet it may be a necessary component of a programme designed to reduce falls. Only two randomized controlled trials of low methodological quality have implemented training of reactive postural adjustments (Protas et al 2005; Toole et al 2005) along with anticipatory and ongoing adjustments. Toole et al (2005) conducted a combined strength and balance training programme three times a week for 10 weeks. Balance training incorporated shoulder pulls provided by the therapist in different directions with eyes open, eyes closed and on varying floor surfaces. Protas et al (2005) included walking in four different directions (forwards, backwards, sideways left and right) on a treadmill at a speed greater than overground walking speed, supported in an overhead harness for safety. The programme was conducted three times a week for 8 weeks. Simulated external perturbations were

achieved by the patient standing/walking in the same four directions and stepping to adjust to sudden and unexpected treadmill starting and stopping. The control group received no training. Although this fully-supervised training protocol, used in a small sample of patients, did not produce significant between-group differences in compensatory step length or falls, there was a positive trend in favour of the training group suggesting that this training strategy warrants further investigation.

Despite the emerging evidence that at least some elements of balance can be improved, there is no evidence of efficacy of exercise in reducing falls. To date, only three randomized controlled trials have reported falls as outcomes (Protas et al 2005; Ashburn et al 2007; Nieuwboer et al 2007) and none were adequately powered to detect an effect on falls. Nevertheless, no exercise intervention has shown an increase in falls, suggesting that exercise, both home based and fully supervised as conducted in these trials, can be safely carried out without increasing falls. Two major challenges remain for physiotherapy in this regard. First, it remains to be determined, using adequately powered randomized controlled trials, which type of exercise, if any, will reduce falls in people with PD. Further, the feasibility, viability and cost-effectiveness of interventions need to be evaluated to ensure that effective interventions are sustainable. It seems unlikely that fully-supervised exercise interventions can be sustained over a long period of time. Therefore, the second major challenge is to develop and test exercise programmes that safely target remediable risk factors, which can be tailored to the individual's needs and administered in a semi-supervised format. One such study is currently underway (Canning et al 2009).

Standing up and sitting down

People with PD are slow to stand up from sitting, probably due to reduced peak hip flexion torque and difficulty switching from the pre-extension to the extension phase of the action (Mak & Hui-Chan 2002; Mak et al 2003). By teaching the critical biomechanical features of an action, the physiotherapist helps the individual use cognitive strategies and/or cues to train a more effective motor pattern. For example, in standing up, the necessary information for the person to learn is foot placement backward, swinging the upper body forward at the hips and upward into standing. The person who cannot stand up independently may be attempting to extend the legs without doing the preparatory (pre-extension) movements which enable the sit-to-stand action to take place (see Ch. 4). Stick figure drawings may help the person develop a visual picture of the action required. A recent randomized controlled trial provides evidence of the efficacy of a 4-week programme of cueing sit-to-stand training administered three times a week for 20 minutes (Mak & Hui-Chan 2008). Visual cues of the patients' centre of mass were provided using the Equitest-Balance Master® and auditory cues were provided by the physiotherapist to 'move forward' for part-practice of sit-to-stand initiation, 'move your buttocks up' for part-practice of thighs-off and 'stand up' for practice of the whole task. Improvements in time to stand up, peak horizontal speed and peak vertical speed were significantly greater for the cued group than the general exercise group or the no-exercise control group.

Turning over in bed and getting out of bed

Difficulty turning in bed at night is frequently reported and this can be a distressing problem for people with PD. One in five people with PD are not able to turn independently and four out of five report problems in turning (Stack & Ashburn 2006). Further, difficulty turning in bed

is associated with sleep disturbance (Stack & Ashburn 2006), and those patients who use a number of different strategies in their attempts to turn (presumably because no one strategy is effective) have the poorest sleep. This suggests that specific training of this task is critical to wellbeing. In training this action, it is necessary to understand the difference between rolling over and turning in bed. The latter involves turning to the left or right side, raising the body mass sufficiently between the underneath shoulder and feet to move the hips backward. This provides a stable side-lying position. Kamsma and colleagues (1994) suggest a cognitive movement strategy be taught to patients who have difficulty turning in bed. This involves moving the arms to the sides, pulling the knees up one at a time, lifting and shifting the pelvis in the direction opposite to the intended turn, lowering the legs sideways in the turning direction and bringing the upper arm across to roll. Practice with the bedclothes in place is also necessary, so that these steps can be incorporated into the task (Kamsma et al 1995). Getting out of bed involves the steps outlined above for turning to side-lying in the first instance. Then, from side-lying, the legs are swung out of bed (serving as a counterweight), followed by pushing off with the free arm to come to sitting on the edge of the bed. Kamsma and colleagues (1995) recommend that training emphasizes practice of each step using conscious control. In a controlled trial comparing the use of these movement strategies with a non-specific group exercise programme, participants using the movement strategies demonstrated greater improvement (Kamsma et al 1995). It remains unclear whether it is possible to re-establish more normal performance of these tasks.

Performing dual tasks

There is much debate concerning the ability of people with PD to perform more than one task at a time, an ability which is critical to effective function. Undoubtedly, as the disease progresses, this ability is impaired and avoidance of dual tasks as recommended by some authors (Bloem et al 2006; Morris 2006) should be advised. Nevertheless, there is some evidence that people with mild to moderate PD can improve their ability to multitask, and therefore, dual and multitask training should be addressed. In an early study (Soliveri et al 1992), PD participants and age-matched controls were tested on the time taken to perform a skilled task, doing up buttons, a task reported to be difficult for PD individuals, and on their ability to tap their foot at the same time at two different speeds. The PD group were slower than the controls on the buttoning task but both groups improved their time (i.e., performed more quickly) over trials (i.e., as they practised). Performance of both groups on buttoning deteriorated with the addition of foot tapping, although it was more marked in the PD group. However, both the control and the PD group showed a decrease in the effect of interference over successive trials, with PD participants achieving the same performance level as the controls at the slower tapping speed. The PD group's buttoning speed and tapping speed increased. The authors suggested that by the end of practice the degree of 'learning' and the level of automaticity were similar in the two groups. Recent work utilizing functional magnetic resonance imaging indicates that compensatory neurophysiological mechanisms may underlie improvement in automaticity of finger movements after practice in people with PD (Wu & Hallett 2005).

Training more meaningful task combinations has been undertaken recently (e.g., Rochester et al 2005; Canning et al 2008b). After only four practice trials of cued dual-task walking in a single session, Rochester and colleagues (2005) reported an immediate 0.07 ms^{-1} increase in dual-task walking speed in participants with an initial single-task speed of 0.70 ms^{-1}. More recently, Canning and colleagues (2008b) used a baseline-controlled design to determine whether multiple-task training of walking is feasible and worthwhile in people with mild to moderate PD. Five participants (Hoehn and Yahr stage II–III) undertook 30 minutes of supervised walking training under dual- and triple-task conditions once a week during the 3-week training phase. Walking training was performed at fast as possible speed, and participants were challenged to maintain speed and stride length as the complexity of the additional tasks was systematically increased (see Paul et al 2005 for examples of additional tasks). Not only did multiple-task walking speed increase by 0.09 ms^{-1} between the baseline and training phase, but also this increase was maintained in the retention phase. In addition, participants reported only low levels of mental fatigue, physical fatigue, difficulty and anxiety as well as high levels of confidence associated with multiple-task training. Adverse effects were monitored and none were reported. Therefore, there is evidence that multiple-task training can be safely and effectively carried out in people with mild to moderate PD. This training strategy warrants further investigation in a large-scale randomized controlled trial.

For further information, the reader should refer to Chapters 4–7 as a guide to the critical biomechanical features of everyday actions and ways in which more effective performance can be achieved. However, given the particular motor control deficits and adaptive motor behaviours evident in individuals with PD, some ways of using external cueing to improve speed, accuracy and initiation of movement, and of developing exercise and activity programmes, are outlined below.

Cueing and attentional strategies

A large number of strategies for directing attention towards temporal and/or spatial aspects of a task with the aim of improving task performance in people with PD have been suggested and tested. It is useful to classify these strategies and it is recommended that the framework for classification used by Nieuwboer et al (2008) be adopted (Table 13.1). In essence, cueing is classified in terms of cue modality (visual, auditory, somatosensory), cue parameter (timing or spatial) and specification of the parameter (i.e., specific step length in cm or step frequency in bpm). While

Table 13.1 Framework for classifying cueing strategies, parameters and modalities

Cueing strategy	Cueing modalities	Cueing parameters	Examples of cues	Gait parameters
External generation	Visual cueing	Step amplitude	Lines on floor Patterned carpet or tiles Walking stick with laser beam	Increase step size
External generation	Auditory cueing	Step frequency	Metronome beat Musical rhythm	Modify stepping rate
External generation	Visual cueing	Step frequency	Rhythmic flash of light	Modify stepping rate
External generation	Somatosensory cueing	Step frequency	Rhythmic vibration Electrical pulse Touch Treadmill	Modify stepping rate
Associating external/ internal generation	Auditory cue and attention	Step frequency and amplitude	Metronome beat Concentrating on taking big steps in time to beat	Modify stepping rate and increase step size
Internal generation	No cue, just attention	Step amplitude	Concentrating on taking big steps	Increase step size

(Reprinted from Nieuwboer et al 2008, with permission).

cues are typically delivered from an external source, for example fixed visual cues applied to the ground or auditory cues provided by a metronome, attentional strategies (sometimes also referred to as cues), for example attending to taking big steps, are internally generated by the individual. There is evidence that both cueing and attentional strategies improve motor performance in people with PD, although the extent of carryover in the long term and into more complex activities is yet to be determined.

Systematic reviews (Rubinstein et al 2002; Lim et al 2005) confirm that cueing immediately improves walking speed, step length and cadence in PD. However, these results are largely based on single-session, laboratory experiments. It is less clear whether the benefits of cueing can be retained and maintained in the longer term, and if so, what the most effective protocol would be. The most comprehensive high-quality trial of cueing, the RESCUE trial (Nieuwboer et al 2007), implemented a home-based cueing programme for 153 people in a randomized crossover design. Participants chose one of three rhythmical cueing modalities (auditory – beeps delivered through an earpiece, somatosensory – vibrations delivered to the wrist, visual – light flashes delivered through a light-emitting diode attached to a pair of glasses), with the majority of participants choosing the auditory mode and no participants choosing the visual mode. Supervised training was performed for 30 minutes, three times a week for 3 weeks and incorporated the use of cues for walking and related activities in the home setting, both indoors and outdoors. There was evidence of improvement in stride length, walking speed, balance, freezing and walking confidence. However, there were no reported improvements in activities of daily living or participation. These results are promising and warrant further investigation of cueing, especially in terms of matching the modality (visual, auditory, somatosensory), parameter (timing or spatial) and specification of the cue to the person with impairments, both motor and non-motor (Nieuwboer et al 2008). For example, for a person with hypokinesia, an auditory cue (modality) to enhance step frequency (parameter) at 100 bpm (specification) may be used initially and adapted to the patient as required. As a general guide, when specifying a cueing frequency for non-freezers, one can begin with a frequency that is 10% higher than their baseline frequency, whereas for freezers, an initial frequency that is 10% lower than baseline is suggested (Willems et al 2006). Since two studies (Thaut et al 1996; Nieuwboer et al 2007) show that cueing strategies have no long-term effects at 6 weeks follow-up, it is necessary for further studies to develop and test protocols aimed at maintaining benefits (Nieuwboer et al 2007).

Other key issues currently being investigated, with implications for use of cueing, are the role of combined cueing (Baker et al 2007) and the effect of cues when used with individuals with cognitive impairment (Rochester et al 2009). A combined cue of walking to a metronome beat while taking big steps is effective in increasing walking speed and step length and it is suggested that this combined cue may be useful in situations where there is increased attentional demand or impaired executive function (Baker et al 2007). The same combined cue, for example 'take a big step in time with the beat', is feasible and immediately effective in increasing single- and dual-task walking speed and stride length in PD individuals with mild cognitive impairment (Rochester et al 2009).

Frequency was the parameter of interest in the RESCUE trial and this was used to reduce both bradykinesia and freezing. The trial did not examine visual spatial cueing. Visual spatial cueing has been advocated for some time, but not stringently tested for efficacy. Visual cueing with parallel lines on the walking surface was described by Martin (1967) for use by individuals with freezing episodes. He found that the optimal placement of the lines was in front (full view) of the participant so they could be 'walked over'. Lines were not effective when they were either running parallel to the walking course or off to the side of the participant. However, while visual cueing may be helpful in alleviating freezing as an incidental trick, the therapeutic potential of visual cueing to reduce freezing remains undetermined (Nieuwboer 2008).

Visual cueing to help individuals overcome episodes of freezing has also been described (Dietz et al 1990). However, one method used, which involved having individuals step over the curved portion of an inverted walking stick as a means of aborting the freezing episode (Dunne et al 1987), appears not to be as effective as was hoped. A descriptive study of eight participants compared the effect of stepping over an inverted stick, walking with a stick in the usual manner and walking over lines (Dietz et al 1990). The results (movement time and number of freezes) indicated overall that only walking over lines, as suggested originally by Martin, had a positive effect; walking with the stick, whether inverted or not, was associated with a decrease in performance. These results fit with the view that PD patients perform better when they pay attention to a visual stimulus directly related to stepping. Use of the stick in both conditions may have required a dividing of attention between the walking and the manipulation of the stick, effectively imposing a dual task, resulting in the decrement in walking performance.

Visual spatial cueing is also used to enable PD individuals to overcome the effect of bradykinesia/hypokinesia on stride length during walking, with visual cues placed on the floor at the desired step length (Bagley et al 1991; Morris et al 1994a,b). Bagley and colleagues (1991) showed that visual cues (triangular strips of coloured cardboard placed at a customized distance along a translucent walkway) improved spatial (stride length, step length) and temporal (double support time) parameters of walking and that improvement was maintained for one walk after visual cues were removed.

In another more recent study (Morris et al 1996), PD participants were found to have relatively normal stride length when they attended to their walking, during presentation of visual cues and immediately after removal of these cues. However, when they were covertly monitored immediately after testing, or asked to perform an additional task while walking, stride length deteriorated. The results suggest that PD patients are able to generate an appropriate gait at will when they attend to it. The results of these studies indicate the importance of planning training programmes that carry over beyond the training session into real life. More recent research suggests that people with PD can maintain normal stride length while performing dual tasks provided they maintain their attention on walking with big steps (Canning 2005). Therefore, specific instructions can be used to manipulate attention to enhance performance of everyday dual tasks in people with mild to moderate PD. Maintaining attention on walking may be useful as a 'safety first' strategy as suggested by Bloem et al (2001). In addition, reducing the complexity of the dual task may be considered so that both tasks can be performed without risk to safety (Canning 2005).

Cognitive strategies

It is clear that cognitive strategies, such as attending to taking big steps, have an immediate positive effect in overcoming bradykinesia/hypokinesia (Morris et al 1994b, 1996) Further, there is evidence that cognitive movement strategies, in which complex movements are broken down into separate components and conscious attention is directed toward the execution of each component, improve task performance (Kamsma et al 1995). These strategies are proposed to result in improved movement control by by-passing the defective basal ganglia and operating via alternate circuits (Morris 2000). However, it is less clear whether these effects can be maintained when the strategies are withdrawn. A recent randomized controlled trial (Morris et al 2009) compared the use of movement strategies as advocated by Morris (2006) with exercise therapy incorporating range of motion (Schenkman et al 1998) and strengthening exercises (Scandalis et al 2001; Dibble et al 2006). The movement strategies incorporated the use of visual, auditory or somatosensory cues as well as attentional strategies, including visualization and mental rehearsal, breaking long and complex sequences into components and focusing attention on performing each component. The movement strategies were performed in the context of functional tasks, including walking indoors and outdoors, turning, standing up and sitting down, and obstacle negotiation. The exercise therapy group performed exercises in supine, prone, side-lying, standing and walking. There was only one significant difference between groups; that is, the movement strategies group improved more on balance (measured using the shoulder

pull test, which evaluates the person's ability to respond to an unexpected backward perturbation to balance) than the exercise therapy group. It is important to note that gains made during the 2-week intensive inpatient programmes were not well maintained at follow-up for either group.

Two major conclusions can be drawn from this study and the current literature more broadly. First, movement strategies and exercise are both key elements of physiotherapy intervention for people with PD. Second, it is imperative that intervention models address the issue of retention of effects.

Exercise to promote physical activity

Physical activity has been shown in one structured interview study to decline more in PD individuals than in healthy elderly participants (Fertl et al 1993). It was found that, although people in both groups were similar in their physical activity profiles, once symptoms developed in the PD group there was a significant reduction in physical activity, although participation in sports such as swimming, hiking and gymnastics continued as it did in the healthy group. The assumption sometimes expressed, that sport and exercise may cause a deterioration in physical condition in PD individuals, has not been proved (Stern 1982) Further, Canning and colleagues (1997) have demonstrated that people with mild to moderate PD who performed regular aerobic exercise had better cardiorespiratory fitness than those who were sedentary, suggesting that at least in the early stages of the disease, individuals have the potential to maintain normal exercise capacity with regular exercise. Not only does physical activity improve exercise capacity (Bergen et al 2002; Bridgewater et al 1996; Burini et al 2006), it has the potential to have a number of other disease-specific benefits. Although, it is yet to be tested in the PD population, it is likely that regular, moderate- to high-intensity, weightbearing exercise may assist to minimize bone density loss, sleep disturbances, cognitive decline and depression. Furthermore, the general health benefits associated with regular exercise, such as reduced risk of cardiovascular disease and type 2 diabetes, should not be underestimated. There is also a suggestion that performing physical exercise in daily life is a factor influencing survival rate in PD by preventing decline from disuse (Kuroda et al 1992).

Three randomized trials (Bergen et al 2002; Bridgewater et al 1996; Burini et al 2006) and a recent uncontrolled trial (van Eijkeren et al 2009) have provided evidence of the positive effects of exercise on cardiorespiratory fitness. Modes of exercise which have been tested to date include overground walking and stepping exercises in a group format (Bridgewater et al 1996), fully-supervised treadmill walking and stationary cycling (Bergen et al 2002), group stationary cycling (Burini et al 2006) and group Nordic walking with poles (van Eijkeren et al 2009).

It is recommended that, within the limits of the person's motor and non-motor impairments, patients are encouraged to choose the mode of exercise which they are most likely to enjoy and to perform on a regular basis. Fully-supervised exercise is not cost-effective nor is it necessary for most individuals. However, many individuals, especially those who do not have well-established exercise habits prior to diagnosis, will need assistance and direction in identifying an appropriate environment and social support for exercise. Ongoing monitoring by a physiotherapist is recommended to ensure that risks are minimized, benefits are maximized and appropriate modifications are made as the disease progresses.

Exercise to maintain flexibility

The most effective way for an individual to preserve musculoskeletal flexibility is by maintaining an active lifestyle, involving at least three times weekly periods of walking or other aerobic activity, and general exercise. Such a regime would be expected to optimize cardiorespiratory fitness and general wellbeing as well as musculoskeletal flexibility and strength. There are particular problems associated with PD and the inactivity which commonly ensues, as well as being associated with getting older, and these are considered briefly below.

The tendency to develop an overall flexed posture (the cause of which is uncertain) is common in people with PD and this posture then predisposes to additional problems. It is likely that a flexed posture may be minimized by a simple stretching programme including lying in supine on a firm surface and stretching upper limb and upper trunk flexors by active raising and lowering of the arms, with the use of a small roll along the thoracic spine to gain further extension (Fig. 13.5). The preservation of thoracic expansion may also be aided by this type of exercise. Since the flexed posture evident in standing in some patients may be an adaptation to avoid a tendency to fall backward, activities performed in standing with the body shifted forward at the ankles and the hips extended may be effective in giving the person an alternative strategy (Fig. 13.6). Given the relationship between reduced spinal rotation and flexed posture, flexibility exercises focusing on spinal rotation should be considered (Fig. 13.7).

Exercise to maintain muscle strength and power

There is a strong rationale to include exercise to maintain muscle strength (force) and muscle power (force × velocity) in exercise programmes for people with PD. Recent research (Allen et al 2009) has confirmed that muscle weakness is evident in the leg extensors of people with mild to moderate PD, even when ON medication. In addition, reduced muscle power at low loads appears to arise due to both muscle weakness and bradykinesia (Allen et al 2009). It is evident that muscle strength (Latt et al 2009)

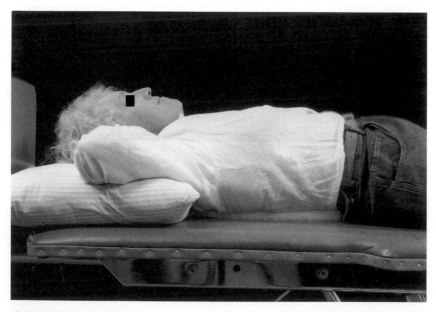

Figure 13.5 Supine lying on a firm surface with a small towel roll under the thoracic spine. Both arms are abducted and externally rotated to put a further stretch on soft tissues likely to become stiff and short. A small pillow under the knees may be necessary to prevent excessive extension of lumbar spine if spine is very stiff.

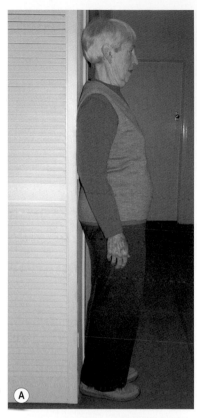

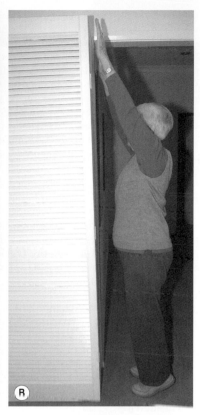

Figure 13.6 Maintaining an erect posture. (A) She concentrates on keeping her upper back against the wall while contracting the gluteal muscles and attempting to move the hips forward. Excessive cervical spine flexion is avoided by drawing the head and neck back towards the wall. (B) She raises and lowers her heels, while maintaining spinal and hip extension. Note that this exercise also challenges her balance, as she holds her hands near the wall, but only places her hands on the wall if she loses her balance.

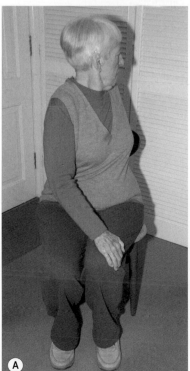

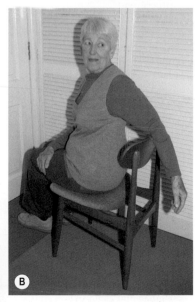

Figure 13.7 Exercise to promote maintenance of spinal rotation. The right hand is used to assist in stabilising the legs and pelvis while she rotates her trunk and neck to look over her shoulder. She concentrates on maintaining hip flexion and spinal extension while turning. Rotation to both sides is practised.

and muscle power (Allen 2010) are independent contributors to falls in people with PD. Evidence of efficacy of progressive resistance exercises for improving muscle strength has been reported (Hirsch et al 2003; Dibble et al 2006). Future investigations of training programmes designed to improve muscle power will assist to determine whether there is any advantage in using muscle power training programmes compared to muscle strength training programmes.

Evaluation and measurement

Evaluation by the physiotherapist involves seeking information from the medical notes related to general medical condition and the clinical grading used to establish the level of impairment. The most common clinical rating scale is the Unified Parkinson's Disease Rating Scale (UPDRS) (Fahn et al 1987), which has been recently updated to the Movement Disorders Society Unified Parkinson's Disease Rating Scale (MDS-UPDRS) (Goetz et al 2008).† This scale provides an excellent overview of presence and impact of impairments, both motor and non-motor as well as activity limitations experienced by the patient.

Information is also sought from the individual regarding motor performance in common everyday actions, particularly details of difficulties being experienced. This evaluation should take place in the environment in which the person is having difficulty. As a guide to the development of an exercise and training programme, the physiotherapist evaluates the individual's performance on the relevant motor actions. Pre- and post-testing needs to take into account the stability of medication and the time medication is given in relation to the time of the test. For individuals who report fluctuating motor symptoms, testing both ON and OFF should also be considered.

For the physiotherapist and patient to monitor changes occurring during motor training, exercise, fitness or stretching programmes, it is necessary to utilize methods of measurement which provide quantitative information

†http://www.movementdisorders.org/publications/rating_scales

related specifically to what is being trained or exercised. That is to say, methods of measurement need to reflect the goals of intervention which need to be relevant and meaningful. Many generic measurement methods (outlined in Ch. 3) may be utilized, for example the timed up-and-go test. For patients who have fallen or are at risk of falls, an assessment of the patient's balance confidence using the Falls Efficacy Scale-International (Yardley et al 2005) will be appropriate as well as provision of a falls diary (Keus et al 2004). Some form of self-monitoring in assessment of therapeutic effects is useful, for example the Patient-Specific Complaints Questionnaire (Keus et al 2004) which asks patients to identify activities which are difficult to perform because of their PD and to rate this difficulty on visual analogue scales. Additional PD-specific assessments/measurements may also be considered, such as the Freezing of Gait Questionnaire (FOG-Q) for assessment of FOG severity (Giladi et al 2000, 2009) and the PDQ-39 which is a PD-specific measure of quality of life (Peto et al 1995).

In conclusion, there are two principal roles of physiotherapy for the individual with PD. The first relates to the preservation of optimal musculoskeletal flexibility, physical activity and fitness. This role involves the provision of advice regarding physical activity and of a regular exercise–stretching–activity programme. The second role is more complex and relates to the provision of strategies, for example attentional cues, for dealing with motor deficits during the performance of specific everyday tasks such as sitting down and standing up in different contexts, walking on the street and in the house, with kerbs, ramps and steps, and reaching to grasp and manipulate objects. It seems evident also that physiotherapy intervention is most realistically provided by short periods of intervention by the therapist, followed by continuing, regular and monitored practice, with follow-up sessions at intervals. Overall, rehabilitation needs to focus on providing the individual with Parkinson's disease opportunities and encouragement to be physically and mentally active, preserving flexibility and agility as much as possible.

REFERENCES

Adkin AL, Frank JS, Jog MS 2003 Fear of falling and postural control in Parkinson's disease. Mov Disord 18:496–502.

Agid Y, Javoy-Agid F, Ruberg M 1987 Biochemistry of neurotransmitters in Parkinson's disease. In: Marsden CD, Fahn S (eds) Movement disorders 2. Butterworth Heinemann, Oxford:166–230.

Agid Y, Ruberg M, Raisman R et al 1990 The biochemistry of Parkinson's disease. In: Stern G (ed.) Parkinson's disease. Chapman and Hall Medical, London:99–125.

Allcock LM, Rowan EN, Steen IN et al 2009 Impaired attention predicts falling in Parkinson's disease. Parkinsonism Relat Disord 15:110–115.

Allen NE, Sherrington C, Canning CG et al 2010 Reduced muscle power is associated with slower walking velocity and falls in people with Parkinson's disease. Parkinsonism Relat Disord In press.

Allen, NE, Canning CG, Sherrington C et al 2009 Bradykinesia, muscle weakness and reduced muscle power in Parkinson's disease. Mov Disord 24:1344–1351.

Armand S, Landis T, Sztajzel R et al 2009 Dyskinesia-induced postural instability in Parkinson's disease. Parkinsomism Relat Disord 15:359–364.

Ashburn A, Fazakarley L, Ballinger C et al 2007 A randomised controlled trial of a home-based exercise program to reduce the risk of falling among people with Parkinson's disease. J Neurol Neurosurg Psychiatry 78:678–684.

Bagley S, Kelly B, Tunnicliffe N et al 1991 The effect of visual cues on the gait of independently mobile Parkinson's disease patients. Physiotherapy 77:415–420.

Baker K, Rochester L, Nieuwboer A 2007 The immediate effect of attentional, auditory and a combined cue strategy on gait during single and dual tasks in Parkinson's disease. Arch Phys Med Rehabil 88:1593–1600.

Baltadjieva R, Giladi N, Gruendlinger L et al 2006 Marked alterations in the gait timing and rhythmicity of patients with de novo Parkinson's disease. Eur J Neurosci 24:1815–1820.

Bazalgette D, Zattara M, Bathien N et al 1986 Postural adjustments associated with rapid voluntary arm movements in patients with Parkinson's disease. In: Yahr MD, Bergmann KJ (eds) Advances in neurology, 45. Raven Press, New York:371–374.

Beckley DJ, Bloem BR, van Dijk JG et al 1991 Electrophysiological correlates of postural instability in Parkinson's disease. Electroencephalogr Clin Neurophysiol 81:263–268.

Bello O, Sanchez JA, Fernandez-del-Olmo M 2008 Treadmill walking in Parkinson's disease patients: adaptation and generalization effect. Mov Disord 23:1243–1249.

Benecke R, Rothwell JC, Dick JPR et al 1986 Performance of simultaneous movements in patients with Parkinson's disease. Brain 109:739–757.

Benecke R, Rothwell JC, Dick JPR et al 1987 Disturbance of sequential movements in patients with Parkinson's disease. Brain 110:361–379.

Berardelli A, Rothwell JC, Day BL et al 1984 Movements not involved in posture are abnormal in Parkinson's disease. Neurosci Lett 47:47–50.

Berardelli A, Dick JPR, Rothwell JC et al 1986 Scaling of the size of the first agonist EMG burst during rapid wrist movements in patients with Parkinson's disease. J Neurol Neurosurg Psychiatry 49:1273–1279.

Berardelli A, Rothwell JC, Thompson PD et al 2001 Pathophysiology of bradykinesia in Parkinson's disease. Brain 124:2132–2146.

Bergen JL, Toole T, Elliott RG et al 2002 Aerobic exercise intervention improves aerobic capacity and movement initiation in Parkinson's disease patients. Neurorehab 17:161–168.

Bergman H, Deuschl G 2002 Pathophysiology of Parkinson's disease: from clinical neurology to basic neuroscience and back. Mov Disord 17:S28–S40.

Blaszczyk JW, Orawiec R, Duda-Klodowska D et al 2007 Assessment of postural instability in patients with Parkinson's disease. Exp Brain Res 183:107–114

Bleuse S, Cassim F, Blatt J-L et al 2008 Anticipatory postural adjustments associated with arm movement in Parkinson's disease: a biomechanical analysis. J Neurol Neurosurg Psychiatry 79:881–887.

Blin O, Ferrandez AM, Serratrice G 1990 Quantitive analysis of gait in Parkinson patients: increased variability of stride length. J Neurol Sci 98:91–97.

Bloem BR, Grimbergen YAM, Cramer M 2001 Prospective assessment of falls in Parkinson's disease. J Neurol 248:950–958.

Bloem BR, Hausdorff JM, Visser JE et al 2004 Falls and freezing of gait in Parkinson's disease: a review of two interconnected, episodic phenomena. Mov Disord 19:871–874.

Bloem BR, Grimbergen YA, van Dijk JG et al 2006 The 'posture second' strategy: a review of wrong priorties in Parkinson's disease. J Neurol Sci 248:196–204.

Boonstra TA, van der Kooij H, Munneke M et al 2008 Gait disorders and balance disturbances in Parkinson's disease: clinical update and pathophysiology. Curr Opin Neurol 21:461–471.

Braak H, Ghebremedhin E, Rub U et al 2004 Stages in the development of Parkinson's disease-related pathology. Cell Tissue Res 318:121–134.

Bridgewater KJ, Sharpe MH 1996 Aerobic exercise and early Parkinson's disease. J Neurol Rehabil 10:233–241.

Bronstein AM, Hood JD, Gresty MA et al 1990 Visual control of balance in cerebellar and parkinsonian syndrome. Brain 113:767–779.

Brotchie P, Iansek R, Horne MK 1991a Motor function of the globus pallidus: 1. Neuronal discharge and parameters of movement. Brain 114:1667–1683.

Brotchie P, Iansek R, Horne MK 1991b Motor function of the globus pallidus: 2. Cognitive aspects of movement and phasic neuronal activity. Brain 114:1685–1702.

Broussolle E, Drack P, Thobois S et al 2007 Contribution of Jules Froment to the study of parkinsonian rigidity. Mov Disord 22:909–914.

Burini D, Farabollini B, Iacucci S et al 2006 A randomised controlled cross-over trial of aerobic training versus Qigong in advanced Parkinson's disease. Eur Medicophys 42:231–238.

Burleigh-Jacobs A, Horak FB, Nutt JG et al 1997 Step initiation in parkinson's disease: influence of levodopa and external sensory triggers. Mov Disord 12:206–215.

Cahn DA, Sullivan EV, Shear PD et al 1998 Differential contributions of cognitive and motor component processes to physical and instrumental activities of daily living in Parkinson's disease. Arch Clin Neuropsych 13:575–583.

Cakit BD, Saracoglu M, Genc H et al 2007 The effects of incremental speed-dependent treadmill training on postural instability and fear of falling in Parkinson's disease. Clin Rehabil 21:698–705.

Canning CG 2005 The effect of directing attention during walking under dual-task conditions in Parkinson's disease. Parkinsonism Relat Disord 11:95–99.

Canning CG, Alison J, Allen N et al 1997 Parkinson's disease: an investigation of exercise, respiratory function and gait. Arch Phys Med Rehabil 78:199–206.

Canning CG, Allen NE, Fung V et al 2008a Home-based treadmill walking for individuals with Parkinson's disease: a pilot randomized controlled trial. Mov Disord 23:S210.

Canning CG, Ada L, Woodhouse E 2008b Multiple-task walking training in people with mild to moderate Parkinson's disease: a pilot study. Clin Rehabil 22:226–233.

Canning CG, Sherrington C, Lord SR et al 2009 Exercise therapy for prevention of falls in people with Parkinson's disease: a protocol for a randomized controlled trial and economic evaluation. BMC Neurol 9:4.

Carlsson A 1959 The occurrence, distribution and physiological role of catecholamines in the nervous system. Pharmacol Rev 11:490–493.

Carpenter MG, Allum JHJ, Honegger F et al 2004 Postural abnormalitites to multidirectional stance perturbations in Parkinson's disease. J Neurol Neurosurg Psychiatry 75:1245–1254.

Carr JH, Shepherd RB 1987 A motor learning model for rehabilitation. In: Carr JH, Shepherd RB (eds) Movement science. Foundations for physical therapy in rehabilitation. Aspen, Rockville, MD:31–91.

Castiello U, Stelmach GE, Lieberman AN 1993 Temporal dissociation of the prehension pattern in Parkinson's disease. Neuropsychologia 31:395–402.

Castiello U, Bennett KMB, Scarpa M 1994 The reach to grasp movement of Parkinson's disease participants. In: Bennett KMB, Castiello U (eds) Insights into the reach to grasp movement. Elsevier Science, New York:215–237.

Chaudhuri KR, Healy DG, Schapira AHV 2006 Non-motor symptoms of Parkinson's disease: diagnosis and management. Lancet Neurol 5:235–245.

Deijen JB, Stoffers D, Berendse HW et al 2006 Abnormal susceptibility to distracters hinders perception in early stage Parkinson's disease: a controlled study. BMC Neurol 6:43.

DeLong MR 2000 The basal ganglia. In: Kandel ER, Schwartz JH, Jessell TM (eds) Principles of neural science, 4th edn. McGraw-Hill, New York:854–867.

DeLong MR, Juncos JL 2008 Parkinson's disease and other extrapyramidal movement disorders. In: Fauci AS, Braunwald E, Kasper DL (eds) Harrison's principles of internal medicine, 17th edn. McGraw-Hill, New York.

Delwaide PJ, Gonce M 1988 Pathophysiology of Parkinson's signs. In: Jankovic J, Tolosa E (eds) Parkinson's disease and movement disorders. Urban and Schwarzenberg, Baltimore/Munich:59–73.

Delwaide PJ, Pepin JL, Maertens de Noordhout A 1991 Short-latency autogenic inhibition in patients with parkinsonian rigidity. Ann Neurol 30:83–89.

De Nunzio AM, Nardone A, Schieppati M 2007 The control of equilibrium in Parkinson's disease patients: delayed adaptation of balancing strategy to shifts in sensory set during a dynamic task. Brain Res Bull 74:258–270.

De Rijk MC, Launer LJ, Berger K et al 2000 Prevalence of Parkinson's disease in Europe: a collaborative study of population-based cohorts. Neurology 54:S21–S23.

Deuschl G, Schade-Brittinger C, Krack P et al 2006 German Parkinson Study Group, neurostimulation section. A randomized trial of deep-brain stimulation for Parkinson's disease. N Eng J Med 355:896–908.

Dibble LE, Hale TF, Marcus RL et al 2006 High-intensity resistance training amplifies muscle hypertrophy and functional gains in persons with Parkinson's disease. Mov Disord 21:1444–1452.

Diener H-C, Dichgans B, Guschlbauer M et al 1990 Associated postural adjustments with body movement in normal participants and patients with parkinsonism and cerebellar ataxia. Revue de Neurologie (Paris) 146:555–563.

Dietz V, Quintern J, Berger W 1981 Electrophysiological studies of gait in spasticity and rigidity: evidence that mechanical properties of muscles contribute to hypertonia. Brain 104:431–449.

Dietz V, Berger W, Horstmann GA 1988 Posture in Parkinson's disease: impairment of reflexes and programming. Ann Neurol 24:660–669.

Dietz M, Goetz CG, Stebbins GT 1990 Evaluation of a modified inverted walking stick as a treatment for Parkinsonian freezing episodes. Mov Disord 5:243–247.

Dunne JW, Hankey GJ, Edis RH 1987 Parkinsonism: upturned walking stick as an aid to locomotion. Arch Phys Med Rehabil 68:380–381.

Dural A, Atay MB, Akbostanci C et al 2003 Impairment, disability and life satisfaction in Parkinson's disease. Dis Rehab 7:318–323.

Ebersbach G, Heijmenerg M, Kindermann L et al 1999 Interference of rhythmic constraints on gait in healthy participants and patients with early Parkinson's disease: evidence for impaired locomotor pattern generation in early Parkinson's disease. Mov Disord 14:619–625.

Ellis T, de Goede CJ, Feldman RG et al 2005 Efficacy of a physical therapy program in patients with Parkinson's disease: a randomized controlled trial. Arch Phys Med Rehabil 86:626–632.

Evarts EV, Teravainen H, Calne DB 1981 Reaction time in Parkinson's disease. Brain 104:167–186.

Faherty CJ, Shepherd KR, Herasimtschuk A et al 2005 Environmental enrichment in adulthood eliminates neuronal death in experimental Parkinsonism. Mol Brain Res 134:170–179.

Fahn S, Elton RL, UPDRS Program Members 1987 Unified Parkinson's disease rating scale. In: Fahn S, Marsden CD, Goldstein M et al (eds) Recent developments in Parkinson's disease, Vol. 2, Macmillan Healthcare Information, Florham Park, NJ:153–163, 293–304.

Ferraye MU, Debu B, Fraix V et al 2008 Effects of subthalamic nucleus stimulation and levodopa on freezing of gait in Parkinson's disease. Neurology 70:1431–1437.

Fertl E, Doppelbauer A, Auff E 1993 Physical activity and sports in patients suffering from Parkinson's disease in comparison with healthy seniors. J Neural Transm 5:157–161.

Findley LJ 1988 Tremors: differential diagnosis and pharmacology. In: Jankovic J, Tolosa E (eds) Parkinson's disease and movement disorders. Urban and Schwarzenberg, Baltimore/Munich:243–261.

Findley L, Aujla M, Bain PG et al 2003 Direct economic impact of Parkinson's disease: a research survey in the United Kingdom. Mov Disord 18:1139–1145.

Fisher BE, Petzinger GM, Nixon K et al 2004 Exercise-induced behavioural recovery and neuroplasticity in the 1-methyl-4-phenyl-1,2,3,6-tetrahydropyridine-lesioned mouse basal ganglia. J Neurosci Res 77:378–390.

Fisher BE, Wu AD, Salem GJ et al 2008 The effect of exercise training in improving motor performance and corticomotor excitability in people with early Parkinson's disease. Arch Phys Med Rehabil 89:1221–1229.

Frank JS, Horak FB, Nutt JG 2000 Centrally initiated postural adjustments in Parkinsonian patients on and off levodopa. J Neurophysiol 84:2440–2448.

Frenkel-Toledo S, Giladi N, Peretz C et al 2005 Treadmill walking as an external pacemaker to improve gait rhythm and stability in Parkinson's disease. Mov Disord 20:1109–1114.

Friedman JH, Brown RG, Comella C et al 2007 Fatigue in Parkinson's disease: a review. Mov Disord 22:297–308.

Georgiou N, Iansek R, Bradshaw JL et al 1993 An evaluation of the role of internal cues in the pathogenesis of parkinsonian hypokinesia. Brain 116:1575–1587.

Giladi N, Nieuwboer A 2008 Understanding and treating freezing of gait in Parkinsonism, proposed working definition, and setting the stage. Mov Disord 23:S423–S425.

Giladi N, McMahon D, Przedborski S et al 1992 Motor blocks in Parkinson's disease. Neurology 42:333–339.

Giladi N, Shabtai H, Simon ES et al 2000 Construction of freezing of gait questionnaire for patients with parkinsonism. Parkinsonism Relat Disord 6:165–170.

Giladi N, Tal J, Azulay T et al 2009 Validation of the freezing of gait questionnaire in patients with Parkinson's disease. Mov Disord 24:655–661.

Goetz CG 2007 Textbook of clinical neurology, 3rd edn. WB Saunders, St Louis.

Goetz CG, Poewe W, Rascol O et al 2005 Evidence-based medical review update: pharmacological and surgical treatments of Parkinson's disease: 2001–2004. Mov Disord 20:533–539.

Goetz CG, Tilley BC, Shaftman SR et al 2008 Movement Disorder Society-sponsored revision of the Unified Parkinson's Disease Rating Scale (MDS-UPDRS): scale presentation and clinimetric testing results. Mov Disord 23:2129–2170.

Goldman-Rakic PS, Selemon LD 1990 New frontiers in basal ganglia

research. Trends Neurosci 13:241–244.

Gross RD, Atwood CW Jr, Ross SB et al 2008 The coordination of breathing and swallowing in Parkinson's disease. Dysphagia 23:136–145.

Hackney ME, Earhart GM 2008a Backward walking in Parkinson's disease. Mov Disord 24:218–233.

Hackney ME, Earhart GM 2008b Tai Chi improves balance and mobility in people with Parkinson's disease. Gait Posture 28:456–460.

Hackney ME, Kantorovich S, Levin R et al 2007 Effects of tango on functional mobility in Parkinson's disease: a preliminary study. J Neurol Phys Ther 31:173–179.

Hallett M, Khoshbin S 1980 A physiological mechanism of bradykinesia. Brain 103:301–314.

Halliday G, Hely M, Reid W et al 2008 The progression of pathology in longitudinally followed patients with Parkinson's disease. Acta Neuropathol 115:409–415.

Hausdorff JM, Cudkowicz ME, Firtion R et al 1998 Gait variability and basal ganglia disorders: stride-to-stride variations of gait cycle timing in Parkinson's disease and Huntington's disease. Mov Disord 13:428–437.

Havlikova E, Rosenberger J, Nagyova I et al 2008 Impact of fatigue on quality of life in patients with Parkinson's disease. Eur J Neurol 15:475–480.

Herman T, Giladi N, Gruendlinger L et al 2007 Six weeks of intensive treadmill training improves gait and quality of life in patients with Parkinson's disease: a pilot study. Arch Phys Med Rehabil 88:1154–1158.

Hirsch MA, Toole T, Maitland CG et al 2003 The effects of balance training and high-intensity resistance training on persons with idiopathic Parkinson's disease. Arch Phys Med Rehabil 84:1109–1117.

Hoehn MM, Yahr MD 1967 Parkinsonism: onset, progression and mortality. Neurology 17:427–442.

Horak FB, Nutt JG, Nashner LM 1992 Postural inflexibility in parkinsonian participants. J Neurol Sci 111:46–58.

Horak FB, Frank J, Nutt J 1996 Effects of dopamine on postural control in Parkinsonian participants: scaling, set and tone. J Neurophyiol 75:2380–2396.

Hornykiewicz O 1966 Metabolism of brain dopamine in human parkinsonism: neurochemical and clinical aspects. In: Costa E, Côté LJ, Yahr MD (eds) Biochemistry and pharmacology of the basal ganglia. Raven Press, New York:171–185.

Huxham F, Baker R, Morris ME et al 2008a Head and trunk rotation during walking turns in Parkinson's disease. Mov Disord 23:1391–1397.

Huxham F, Baker R, Morris ME et al 2008b Footsteps used to turn during walking in Parkinson's disease. Mov Disord 23:817–823.

Iansek R, Huxham F, McGinley J 2006 The sequence effect and gait festination in Parkinson's disease: contributors to freezing of gait? Mov Disord 21:1419–1424.

Inzelberg R, Peleg N, Nisipeanu P et al 2005 Inspiratory muscle training and the perception of dyspnea in Parkinson's disease. Can J Neurol Sci 32:213–217.

Jacobs JV, Horak FB 2006 Abnormal proprioceptive–motor integration contributes to hypometric postural responses of participants with Parkinson's disease. Neuroscience 141:999–1009.

Jankovic J 2008 Parkinson's disease: clinical features and diagnosis. J Neurol Neurosurg Psychiatry 79:368–376.

Kamata N, Matsuo Y, Yoneda T et al 2007 Overestimation of stability limits leads to a high frequency of falls in patients with Parkinson's disease. Clin Rehab 21:357–361.

Kamsma YPT, Brouwer WH, Lakke JPWF 1994 Prevention of early immobility in patients with Parkinson's disease: a cognitive strategy training for turning in bed and rising from a chair. In: Riddoch MJ, Humphreys GW (eds) Cognitive neuropsychology and cognitive rehabilitation. LEA, Hove, UK.

Kamsma YPT, Brouwer WH, Lakke JPWF 1995 Training of compensational strategies for impaired gross motor skills in Parkinson's disease. Physiother Theory Pract 11:209–229.

Katai S, Maruyama T, Hashimotot T et al 2003 Event based and time based prospective memory in Parkinson's disease. J Neurol Neurosurg Psychiatry 74:704–709.

Kemps E, Szmalec A, Vandierendonck A et al 2005 Visuo-spatial processing in Parkinson's disease: evidence for diminished visuo-spatial sketch pad and central executive resources. Parkinsonism Relat Disord 11:181–186.

Keus SHJ, Hendriks HJM, Bloem BR et al 2004 KNGF Guidelines for physical therapy in Parkinson's disease. Dutch Journal of Physiotherapy 114:S13. (Translated to English 2006). Available at http://www.cebp.nl.

Keus SHJ, Bloem BR, Hendriks EJM et al 2007 Evidence-based analysis of physical therapy in Parkinson's disease with recommendations for practice and research. Mov Disord 22:451–460.

Keus SHJ, Munneke M, Nijkrake MJ et al 2009 Physical therapy in Parkinson's disease: evolution and future challenges. Mov Disord 24:1–14.

King LA, Horak FB 2008 Lateral stepping for postural correction in Parkinson's disease. Arch Phys Med Rehabil 89:492–499.

Knutsson E 1972 An analysis of parkinsonian gait. Brain 95:475–486.

Korman LB, James JA 1993 Medical management of Parkinson's disease in the elderly. Top Ger Rehab 8:1–13.

Kuroda K, Tatara K, Takatorige T et al 1992 Effect of physical exercise on mortality in patients with Parkinson's disease. Acta Neurol Scand 86:55–59.

Latt M, Lord SR, Morris JGL et al 2009 Clinical and physiological assessments for elucidating falls risk in Parkinson's disease. Mov Disord 24:1280–1289.

Latash ML, Anson JG 1996 What are 'normal movements' in atypical populations? Behav Brain Sci 19:55–106.

Lees AJ, Smith E 1983 Cognitive deficits in the early stages of Parkinson's disease. Brain 106:257–270.

Lemke MR 2008 Depressive symptoms in Parkinson's disease. Eur J Neurol 15:21–25.

Lemke MR, Brecht HM, Koester J et al 2005 Anhedonia, depression and motor functioning in Parkinson's disease during treatment with paramipexole. J Neuropsychiatry Clin Neurosci 17:214–220.

Lewis SJG, Foltynie T, Blackwell AD et al 2005 Heterogeneity of Parkinson's disease in the early clinical stages using a data driven approach. J Neurol Neurosurg Psychiatry 76:343–348.

Lieberman AN, Hirowitz L, Redmond P 1980 Dysphagia in Parkinson's disease. Am J Gastroenterol 74:157–160.

Lim I, van Wegen E, de Goede C et al 2005 Effects of external rhythmical cueing on gait in patients with Parkinson's disease: a systematic review. Clin Rehabil 19:695–713.

Limousin P, Drack P, Pollak P et al 1998 Electrical stimulation of the subthalamic nucleus in advanced Parkinson's disease. N Eng J Med 339:1105–1111.

Lozano AM, Snyder BJ 2008 Deep brain stimulation for parkinsonian gait disorders. J Neurol 255:30–31.

Matinolli M, Korpelainen JT, Korpelainen R et al 2007 Postural sway and falls in Parkinson's disease: a regression approach. Mov Disord 22:1927–1935.

Majsak MJ, Kaminski T, Gentile AM et al 1998 The reaching movements of patients with Parkinson's disease under self-determined maximal speed and visually cued conditions. Brain 121:755–766.

Majsak MJ, Kaminski T, Gentile AM et al 2008 Effects of a moving target versus temporal constraint on reach and grasp in patients with Parkinson's disease. Exp Neurol 210:479–488.

Mak MKY, Hui-Chan CWY 2002 Switching of movement direction is central to parkinsonian bradykinesia in sit-to-stand. Mov Disord 17:1188–1195.

Mak MKY, Hui-Chan CWY 2008 Cued task-specific training is better than exercise in improving sit-to-stand in patients with Parkinson's disease. Mov Disord 23:501–509.

Mak MKY, Levin O, Mizrahi J et al 2003 Joint torques during sit-to-stand in healthy participants and people with Parkinson's disease. Clin Biomech 18:197–206.

Manor Y, Giladi N, Cohen A et al 2007 Validation of a swallowing disturbance questionnaire for detecting dysphagia in patients with Parkinson's disease. Mov Disord 22:1917–1921.

Marsden CD 1990 Parkinson's disease. Lancet 335:948–952.

Marsden CD 1994 Parkinson's disease. J Neurol Neurosurg Psychiatry 57:672–681.

Marsden CD, Parkes JD 1977 Success and problems of long-term levodopa therapy in Parkinson's disease. Lancet 1(1807):345–349.

Martin JP 1967 The basal ganglia and posture. Pitman, London.

Martin WE, Loewenson RB, Resch JA et al 1973 Parkinson's disease: clinical analysis of 100 patients. Neurology (Minneapolis) 23:783–790.

Menza M, Dobkin RD 2005 Anxiety and Parkinson's disease. Prim Psychiatry 12:63–68.

Miyai I, Fujimoto Y, Ueda Y et al 2000 Treadmill training with body weight support: its effect on Parkinson's disease. Arch Phys Med Rehabil 81:849–852.

Miyai I, Fujimoto Y, Ueda Y et al 2002 Long-term effect of body weight supported treadmill training in Parkinson's disease: a randomised controlled trial. Arch Phys Med Rehabil 83:1370–1373.

Morris ME 2000 Movement disorders in people with Parkinson's disease: a model for physical therapy. Phys Ther 80:578–597.

Morris M 2006 Locomotor training in people with Parkinson's disease. Phys Ther 86:1426–1435.

Morris ME, Iansek R, Matyas TA et al 1994a Ability to modulate walking cadence remains intact in Parkinson's disease. J Neurol Neurosurg Psychiatry 57:1532–1534.

Morris ME, Iansek R, Matyas TA et al 1994b The pathogenesis of gait hypokinesia in Parkinson's disease. Brain 117:1169–1181.

Morris ME, Iansek R, Summers JJ et al 1995 Motor control considerations for the rehabilitation of gait in Parkinson's disease. In: Glencross D, Piek J (eds) Motor control and sensory motor integration. Elsevier, Amsterdam:61–93.

Morris ME, Iansek R, Matyas TA et al 1996 Stride length regulation in Parkinson's disease. Normalization strategies and underlying mechanisms. Brain 119:551–568.

Morris ME, Iansek R, Kirkwood B 2009 A randomised controlled trial of movement strategies compared with exercise for people with Parkinson's disease. Mov Disord 24:64–71.

Muller F, Abbs JA 1990 Precision grip in Parkinsonian patients. In: Streifler MB, Korczyn AD, Melamed E et al (eds) Advances in neurology 53: Parkinson's disease: anatomy, pathology and therapy. Raven Press, New York.191–195.

Murray MP, Sepic SB, Gardiner GM et al 1978 Walking patterns of men with parkinsonism. Am J Phys Med 57:278–294.

Muslimovic D, Post B, Speelman JC et al 2005 Cognitive profile of patients with newly diagnosed Parkinson disease. Neurology 65:1239–1245.

Nieuwboer A 2008 Cueing for freezing of gait in patients with Parkinson's disease: a rehabilitation perspective. Mov Disord 23:S475–481.

Nieuwboer A, Kwakkel G, Rochester L et al 2007 Cueing training in the home improves gait-related mobility in Parkinson's disease: the RESCUE trial. J Neurol Neurosurg Psychiatry 78:134–140.

Nieuwboer A, Rochester L, Jones D 2008 Cueing gait and gait-related mobility in patients with Parkinson's disease. Developing a therapeutic method based on the international classification of functioning, disability and health. Top Geriatr Rehabil 24:151–165.

Pal PK, Sathyaprabha TN, Tuhina P et al 2007 Pattern of subclinical pulmonary dysfunctions in Parkinson's disease and the effect of levodopa. Mov Disord 22:420–424.

Parent A 1990 Extrinsic connections of the basal ganglia. Trends Neurosci 13:254–258.

Parkinson J 1817 An essay on the shaking palsy. Sherwood, Neely and Jones, London.

Paul SS, Ada L, Canning CG 2005 Automaticity of walking – implications for physiotherapy practice. Phys Ther Rev 10:15–23.

Peto V, Jenkinson C, Fitzpatrick R et al 1995 The development and validation of a short measure of functioning and well being for individuals with Parkinson's disease. Qual Life Res 4:241–248.

Phillips JG, Bradshaw JL, Iansek R et al 1993 Motor functions of the basal ganglia. Psychol Res 55:175–181.

Plant R, Walton G, Ashburn A et al 2001 Guidelines for physiotherapy practice in Parkinson's disease. University of Northumbria, Institute of Rehabilitation, Newcastle, UK.

Plotnik M, Giladi N, Hausdorff JM 2009 Bilateral coordination of gait and Parkinson's disease: the effects of dual tasking. J Neurol Neurosurg Psychiatry 80:347–350.

Poewe W 2008 Non-motor symptoms in Parkinson's disease. Eur J Neurol 15.14–20.

Pohl M, Rockstroh G, Rückriem S et al 2003 Immediate effects of speed-dependent treadmill training on gait parameters in early Parkinson's disease. Arch Phys Med Rehabil 84:1760–1766.

Poulton NP, Muir GC 2005 Treadmill training ameliorates dopamine loss but not behavioural deficits in hemi-Parkinsonian rats. Exp Neurol 193:181–197.

Protas EJ, Mitchell K, Williams A et al 2005 Gait and step training to reduce falls in Parkinson's disease. NeuroRehabilitation 20:183–190.

Rajput AH 1992 Frequency and cause of Parkinson's disease. Can J Neurol Sci 19:103–107.

Ramig LO, Fox C, Sapir S 2008 Speech treatment for Parkinson's disease. Expert Rev Neurother 8:297–309.

Robbins JA, Logemann JA, Kirshner HS 1986 Swallowing and speech production in Parkinson's disease. Ann Neurol 19:283–287.

Rocchi L, Chiari L, Capello A et al 2006a Identification of distinct characteristics of postural sway in Parkinson's disease: a feature selection procedure based on principal component analysis. Neurosci Lett 394:140–145.

Rocchi L, Chiari L, Mancini M et al 2006b Step initiation in Parkinson's disease: influence of initial stance conditions. Neurosci Lett 406:128–132.

Rochester L, Hetherington V, Jones D et al 2005 The effect of external rhythmic cues (auditory and visual) on walking during a functional task in homes of people with Parkinson's disease. Arch Phys Med Rehabil 86:999–1006.

Rochester L, Burn D, Woods G et al 2009 Does auditory rhythmical cueing improve gait in people with Parkinson's disease and cognitive impairment? Mov Disord 24:839–845.

Rogers MW, Kukulka CG, Soderberg GL 1987 Postural adjustments preceding rapid arm movements in parkinsonian participants. Neurosci Lett 75:246–251.

Rubinstein T, Giladi N, Hausdorff J 2002 The power of cueing to circumvent dopamine deficits: a review of physical theapy treatment

of gait disturbances in Parkinson's disease. Mov Disord 17:1148–1160.

Sadagopan N, Huber JE 2007 Effects of loudness cues on respiration in individuals with Parkinson's disease. Mov Disord 22:651–659.

Saltin B, Landin S 1975 Work capacity, muscle strength and SDH activity in both legs of hemiparetic patients and patients with Parkinson's disease. Scand J Clin Lab Invest 35:531–538.

Samii A, Nutt JG, Ransom BR 2004 Parkinson's disease. Lancet 363:1783–1793.

Sammer G, Reuter I, Hullmann K 2006 Training of executive functions in Parkinson's disease. J Neurol Sci 25:115–119.

Scandalis TA, Bosak A, Berliner JC et al 2001 Resistance training and gait function in patients with Parkinson's disease. Am J Phys Med Rehabil 80:38–43.

Schapira AHV 2007 Treatment options in the modern management of Parkinson's disease. Arch Neurol 64:1083–1088.

Schenkman M, Cutson TM, Kuchibhatla M et al 1998 Exercise to improve spinal flexibility and function for people with Parkinson's disease: a randomized, controlled trial. J Am Geriatr Soc 46:1207–1216.

Schenkman M, Morey M, Kuchibhatla M 2000 Spinal flexibility and balance control among community-dwelling adults with and without Parkinson's disease. J Gerontol A Biol Sci Med Sci 55:M441–445.

Schieppati M, Nardone A 1991 Free and supported stance in Parkinson's disease. Brain 114:1227–1244.

Scholz E, Diener HC, Noth J et al 1987 Medium and long latency EMG responses in leg muscles: Parkinson's disease. J Neurol Neurosurg Psychiatry 50:66–70.

Schrag A, Jahanshahi M, Quinn N 2000 What contributes to quality of life in patients with Parkinson's disease. J Neurol Neurosurg Psychiatry 69:308–312.

Schwab RS, Chafetz ME, Walker S 1954 Control of two simultaneous voluntary motor acts in normals and parkinsonism. Arch Neurol Psychiatry 72:591–598.

Seitz RJ, Roland PE 1992 Learning of sequential movements in man: a combined kinematic and position emission tomography (PET) study. Eur J Neurosci 4:154–165.

Sethi KD 2003 Tremor. Curr Opin Neurol 16:481–485.

Shepherd RB, Carr JH 1991 An emergent or dynamical systems view of movement dysfunction. Aust J Physiother 37:4–5.

Sheridan MR, Flowers KA 1990 Movement variability and bradykinesia in Parkinson's disease. Brain 113:1149–1161.

Silbiger MC, Pikielney R, Donner MW 1967 Neuromuscular disorders affecting the pharynx: cineradiographic analysis. Invest Radiol 2:442–448.

Sinforiani E, Banchieri L, Zucchella C et al 2004 Cognitive rehabilitation in Parkinson's disease. Arch Gerontol Geriatr Suppl 9:387–391.

Soliveri P, Brown RG, Jahanshahi M 1992 Effect of practice on performance of a skilled motor task in patients with Parkinson's disease. J Neurol Neurosurg Psychiatry 55:461–465.

Stack EL, Ashburn AM 2006 Impaired bed mobility and disordered sleep in Parkinson's disease. Mov Disord 21:1340–1342.

Stern GLA 1982 Parkinson's disease. Oxford University Press, Oxford:52–57.

Stern G, Lees A 1991 Parkinson's disease: the facts. Oxford University Press, Oxford.

Strecker K, Schwarz J 2008 Parkinson's disease: emerging pharmacotherapy. Expert Opin Emerg Drugs 13:573–591.

Talland GA, Schwab RS 1964 Performance with multiple sets in Parkinson's disease. Neuropsychologia 2:45–53.

Thaut MH, McIntosh GC, Rice RR et al 1996 Rhythmic auditory stimulation in gait training for Parkinson's disease patients. Mov Disord 11:193–200.

Tonolli I, Aurenty R, Lee RG et al 2000 Lateral leg raising in patients with Parkinson's disease: influence of equilibrium constraint. Mov Disord 15:850–861.

Toole T, Maitland CG, Warren E et al 2005 The effects of loading and unloading treadmill walking on balance, gait, fall risk and daily function in parkinsonism. Neurorehabil 20:307–322.

van Eijkeren FJ, Reijmers RS, Kleinveld MJ et al 2009 Nordic walking improves mobility in Parkinson's disease. Mov Disord 23:2239–2243.

Viitasalo MK, Kampman V, Sotaniemi KA et al 2002 Analysis of sway in Parkinson's disease using a new inclinometry-based method. Mov Disord 17:663–669.

Vincken WG, Gauthier MD, Dollfuss RE et al 1984 Involvement of upper-airway muscles in extrapyramidal disorders. A cause of airflow limitation. N Eng J Med 311:438–442.

Waterston JA, Hawken MB, Tanyeri S et al 1993 Influence of sensory manipulation on postural control in Parkinson's disease. J Neurol Neurosurg Psychiatry 56:1276–1281.

Watts RL, Wiegner AW, Young RR 1986 Elastic properties of muscles measured at the elbow in man: II. Patients with parkinsonian rigidity. J Neurol Neurosurg Psychiatry 49:1177–1181.

Weiner WJ 2008 There is no Parkinson's disease. Arch Neurol 65:705–708.

Weintraub D 2005 Depression in Parkinson's disease. Prim Psychiatry 12:45–49.

Wichmann T, DeLong MR 1993 Pathophysiology of Parkinsonian motor abnormalities. Adv Neurol 60:53–61.

Willems AM, Nieuwboer A, Chavret F et al 2006 The use of rhythmic auditory cues to influence gait in patients with Parkinson's disease, the differential effect for freezers and non-freezers, an explorative study. Disabil Rehabil 28:721–728.

Wilson SAK 1925 Disorders of motility and muscle tone, with special reference to the striatum. Lancet 2:1–53.

Wood BF, Bilclough JA, Bowron A et al 2002 Incidence and prediction of falls in Parkinson's disease: a prospective multidisciplinary study. J Neurol Neurosurg Psychiatry 72:721–725.

Woollacott MH, von Hosten C, Rosblad B 1988 Relation between muscle response onset and body segmental movements during postural perturbations in humans. Exp Brain Res 72:593–604.

Wright WG, Gurfinkel VS, Nutt J et al 2007 Axial hypertonicity in Parkinson's disease: direct measurements of trunk and hip torque. Exp Neurol 208:38–46.

Wu T, Hallett M 2005 A functional MRI study of automatic movements in patients with Parkinson's disease. Brain 128:2250–2259.

Yardley L, Beyer N, Hauer K et al 2005 Development and initial validation of the Falls Efficacy Scale-International (FES-I). Age Ageing 34:614–619.

Yogev G, Giladi N, Peretz C et al 2005 Dual tasking rhythmicity, and Parkinson's disease: which aspects of gait are attention demanding? Eur J Neurosci 22:1248–1256.

Yoon M-C, Shin M-S, Kim T-S et al 2007 Treadmill exercise suppresses nigrostriatal dopaminergic neuronal loss in 6-hydroxydopamine-induced Parkinson's rats. Neurosci Lett 423:12–17.

York MK, Alvarez JA 2008 Cognitive impairments associated with Parkinson's disease. In: Trail M, Protas ET, Lai EC (eds) Neurorehabilitation in Parkinson's disease: an evidence-based treatment model. SLACK Incorporated, Thorofare, NJ:72–100.

Zgaljardic DJ, Borod JC, Foldi N et al 2003 A review of the cognitive and behavioural sequelae of Parkinson's disease: relationship to frontostriatal circuitry. Cogn Behav Neurol 16:193–210.

Chapter | 14 |

Multiple sclerosis

Written with Phu Hoang

CHAPTER CONTENTS

Multiple sclerosis (MS) is a progressive demyelinating and neurodegenerative disease of the central nervous system (CNS) which gradually results in severe neurological deficits. MS usually presents in early adult life when it has a major impact on family, and on vocational and social life. Since lack of myelin slows down the conduction of the action potentials, MS manifests itself as impaired performance that can have a devastating effect on behaviour. MS usually involves a more or less progressive development of neurological symptoms and behavioural deficits. The exact aetiology and pathogenesis, however, are still unclear despite recent advances in understanding this mysterious disease. The disease is characterized by remissions and relapses, erratic onset and duration of symptoms that flare up acutely. There is a growing body of evidence indicating that relapses in MS are associated with stressful events. Each relapse may involve the same or quite different area of the white matter of the CNS. The remissions are rarely complete and may last for either a long or short period. Since the disease remains poorly understood, there is no effective treatment of the disease process itself. New insights into the pathophysiology, however, are suggesting new strategies for intervention. Among these are several disease-modifying pharmacological agents, which have been shown to have modest effects in slowing down the progress of the disease and to reduce the severity of relapses. Health professionals working with individuals with MS need to focus on those factors arising from the disease they can prevent or change in order to improve the quality of the individual's life.

EPIDEMIOLOGY AND AETIOLOGY

MS is thought to involve an interplay between genetic and environmental factors, which result in an immunologically mediated inflammatory response within the CNS. Although immunological abnormalities have been consistently reported, the relative role of each component of the immune response in mediating tissue damage, and the extent to which these changes are the cause or consequence of myelin injury, remain to be established

©2010 Elsevier Ltd
DOI: 10.1016/B978-0-7020-4051-1.00023-0

(Compston 1993a). There is compelling evidence for genetic susceptibility to MS (Compston 1990) while environmental influence upon MS is suggested by variation in disease incidence and prevalence according to geographical areas (Weinshenker 1996).

There is a clear pattern of latitudinal variation in the prevalence of MS. Epidemiological studies indicate that the prevalence of MS is high (>30 per 100 000) among young adults in northern Europe, North America and Australasia, medium (5–30 per 100 000) in southern Europe, southern USA and northern Australia and is less prevalent in the Orient, Africa, South America and India (Weinshenker 1996; Marrie 2004; Cristiano et al 2008). Combined data from epidemiology studies conducted in the USA, UK, Australia and New Zealand show a strong link between latitude and prevalence of MS (Richards et al 2002).

MS affects white races principally, although it has been known to affect black immigrants living in Europe and North America. In Australia and New Zealand, MS is rarely seen in the Aboriginal or Maori races but occurs in the white population. In South Africa, the disease occurs more commonly in English-speaking whites than in Afrikaaners but is not seen in native Africans. There is decreasing incidence of the disease in individuals of northern European ancestry as one approaches the tropics, suggesting that certain environments may be relatively more protective. For example, in Australians of northern European descent and in English-speaking white South Africans, the frequency of MS is only about half that of northern Europe. Age is also a factor in immigrant populations. Dean (1967) showed that the risk of MS is higher for English-speaking South African whites who migrated as adults rather than as children.

Further evidence for genetic susceptibility is provided by epidemiological studies within and between ethnic groups. The results of a survey of individuals with MS in Israel in 1973 showed that the disease was common among immigrants from Europe, and rare among immigrants from Afro-Asian countries (Leibowitz et al 1973). Similarly, immigrants from areas of low risk of MS to an area of high risk (such as the UK) retained the low risk of the area of origin (Dean et al 1976). Studies on familial aggregation showed approximately 15% of individuals with MS have an affected relative. This risk rises to 1 : 50 for offspring and 1 : 20 for siblings of affected persons (Sadovnick et al 1988). MS is 20–40 times more common in first-degree relatives, dropping off rapidly with the degree of relatedness (Kantarci & Wingerchuk 2006). Recently, large international collaborations provided strong evidence for the involvement of at least two cytokine receptor genes in the pathogenesis of MS: the interleukin 7 receptor alpha chain gene (IL7RA) on chromosome 5p13 and the interleukin 2 receptor alpha chain gene (IL2RA) (Svejgaard 2008).

Other potential environmental risk factors in MS include infection, vaccinations, stress, climate and diet.

Among these, infection is often touted as a putative causal agent, particularly childhood viral infection (Marrie 2004). Dean (1972) suggested that in countries where the disease is relatively rare, early contact with the causative agent, probably a virus, protects the population by making them immune. On the other hand, there is some evidence that exposure to viral illnesses such as measles, mumps and rubella rather late in childhood may be a factor in those who are at risk of developing the disease. In the past decade a few studies have provided preliminary data indicating that environmental stressors, which are perceived by the person as stressful (e.g., broken relationship, losing job), are associated with subsequent relapses in MS (Mohr et al 2004). The evidence of other risk factors such as climate and diet is less convincing.

It would appear, therefore, that MS does not have a single cause. New episodes of demyelination are more likely to occur following a viral infection or stressful events but no single agent or specific stressor has been implicated, suggesting that in the context of genetic susceptibility, environmental influences and immunological priming, demyelination is a physiological response to many pathogens (Compston 1993a). In summary, the epidemiological evidence implicates environmental factors, including psychosocial stressors, operating against a background of genetic susceptibility or resistance during childhood manifesting as altered immune responsiveness (Compston 1993a).

PATHOPHYSIOLOGY

Demyelination is a disintegration of the myelin sheath caused by an inflammatory and destructive process, the axon being partly or completely denuded. Destruction of the myelin sheath disrupts the normal transmission of nerve impulses resulting in neurological signs and symptoms. The axons themselves are preserved initially although some loss of axons may occur, particularly in large chronic plaques.

The hallmark features of MS lesions are perivascular inflammation followed by myelin depletion, oligodendrocyte loss and astroglial proliferation, and these processes are accompanied by limited remyelination and plaque formation. The traditional view suggests that there are four stages of evolution of focal inflammation (Compston 1993b). The initial stage is characterized by the accumulation of inflammatory cells, lymphocytes and monocytes around venules within the CNS. Inflammation is sufficient to cause a functional block in conduction through myelinated axons. Next, there is active destruction of the oligodendrocyte and its myelin sheath as a result of contact with macrophages and microglia. This is followed by depletion of oligodendrocytes in which denuded axons are seen within the lesion. Finally, the lesion heals by scar formation dependent upon astrocytic reactivity, producing hardened patches or plaques from which the disease gets its name.

This view of the mechanism underlying formations of new plaques has recently been challenged. Barnett and colleagues (Barnett & Prineas 2004; Barnett & Sutton 2006), based on recent pathological studies of initial changes in the acute MS lesion, proposed that apoptotic oligodendrocyte death precedes inflammation and demyelination in MS lesions. This means that a MS lesion starts with the death of oligodendrocytes and associated changes within the myelin sheath, which initiates local macrophage scavenger activity with subsequent amplification of inflammatory response. Over months to years the pathology of multiple sclerosis is transformed and the changes which accompany the late phase of the disease suggest that the inflammatory response becomes progressively 'compartmentalized' and therefore largely isolated from systemic influence with time (Barnett & Sutton 2006). However, the causes of oligodendrocyte death are still unknown. In summary, the relative contributions of 'immune-mediated' versus 'neurodegenerative' processes in the disease pathophysiology remain to be answered.

The most common sites of MS lesion are in the grey–white boundary in the cerebrum, the periventricular region, cerebellar white matter, optic nerves and cervical portion of the spinal cord and brainstem, but the disease can involve any part of the CNS (Fig. 14.1). Until recently MS had been widely considered as a disease of 'white matter' of the CNS. New advances in imaging techniques and post-mortem studies have shown that MS lesions are also present in cortical grey matter, with a particularly high prevalence in progressive forms of the disease (Stadelmann & Bruck 2008). At demyelinated areas, nerve conduction rates are slowed down (Reder & Antel 1983) while conduction along unaffected portions of the axon on either side of the lesion is normal (Smith & McDonald 1999). The conduction block along partially demyelinated axons is the major cause of negative symptoms such as weakness and numbness. It may also explain the fatigue complained of by many patients. These partially demyelinated axons may also discharge spontaneously, accounting for unpleasant distortions of sensation reported by a high percentage of patients (Compston 1993a). Increased temperature sensitivity experienced by many patients after exercise or immersion in hot water may also be explained by the partially demyelinated axons (Compston 1993a).

Remyelination, which involves reinvesting demyelinated axons with new myeline sheaths, does occur in MS and is an important process of 'lesion repair'. Unexpectedly, this process occurs at an early stage of lesion development in both white and grey matter lesions (Stadelmann & Bruck 2008). In contrast, remyelination does not often occur in old lesions where inflammatory activity is minimal. In these older lesions, oligodendrocytes are present but they are not engaged in active remyelination and do not seem capable of producing new myelin (Stadelmann & Bruck 2008). The extent of remyelination in MS, however, is highly variable between patients. Generally, the degree of remyelination of MS lesions is age related and correlates with both number of oligodendrocytes and macrophages in the lesions (Lucchinetti et al 1999). Animal studies (e.g., Zhao et al 2006) suggest that a critical event underlying the failure of remyelination is the impaired ability of phagocytic macrophages to clear myelin debris. This debris contains potent factors that inhibit differentiation of oligodendrocyte precursor cells, which are widely distributed throughout the adult CNS, into oligodendrocytes. Thus, the inflammation response in MS has both destructive (causing demyelination) and beneficial (facilitating remyelination) effects. Understanding of remyelination and why it fails opens up new challenges for future research and could provide development of novel therapeutic strategies (Stadelmann & Bruck 2008).

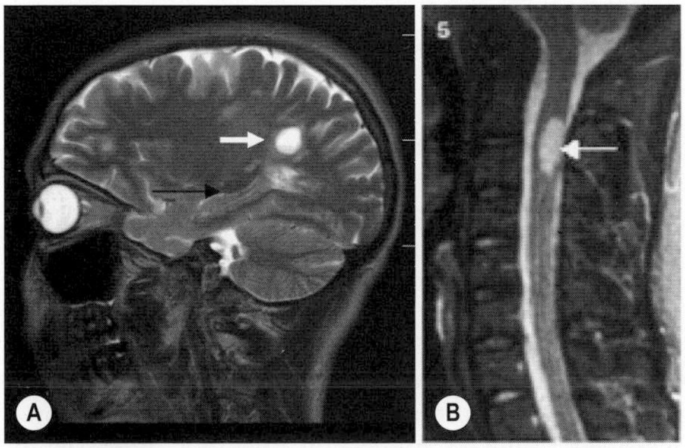

Figure 14.1 An MRI image showing MS lesions in the brain (A) and spinal cord (B).

THE DISEASE PROCESS

Reviews of large databases of MS patients have provided valuable information about its natural history. Clinical signs and symptoms in MS are variable and several patterns can be identified: benign; a relapsing–remitting (RR) course; a secondary progressive (SP) form; and a primary progressive (PP) form. Clinical onset in 80–85% of MS patients is manifested by subclinical neurological symptoms, either multifocal or anatomically discrete, which initially may recover fully. This presentation is often known as a clinically isolated syndrome (CIS). Among patients with CIS, about 20% presented with lesions involving the optic nerve, 45% with long tract signs and symptoms, 10% with a brainstem syndrome and 25% with multifocal abnormalities (Confavreux et al 2000). There is no difference in the predictive value of unifocal or multifocal presentation, but there appears a longer period to the second episode with optic neuritis presentation than with either brainstem or spinal cord presentations (Confavreux et al 2003). After the onset of CIS, 70% of patients experience further episodes during which MS symptoms worsen and then symptoms gradually diminish in severity until the next attack. Patients enter the RR phase. These RR episodes typically occur at a random frequency and for an unpredictable period involving the same or different CNS regions. Recovery after these relapses may not be complete. Over time, symptoms can increase in severity and disability becomes more pronounced. This RR phase lasts on average about 20 years, being shorter for males and those older at onset of MS (Tremlett et al 2008). The rate and severity of disease progression during RR phase may differ considerably among patients, with as many as 20–30% continuing to work 20–25 years after disease onset and with only minimal cognitive impairments (Filley et al 1990). With frequent relapses, however, a chronic progressive form of the disease may evolve. The patient is in the SP phase. The age at which individuals enter the SP phase is independent of the initial disease course (Koch et al 2007).

A small proportion of MS patients (about 10%) experience a benign course of MS after CIS; that is, further episodes are delayed for 5–10 years with minimal signs and symptoms in each episode. A benign course of MS is significantly associated with female sex, younger age of onset and absence of motor symptoms at presentations (Costelloe et al 2008). On the other hand, about 10% of patients experience a clinical course called primary progressive (PP) which is characterized by a progressive accumulation of neurological deficits from onset without relapse or remission (Dujmovic et al 2004). This group of patients has a relatively later age of onset and a lesser female preponderance compared with the general MS population.

In population studies, at the one time approximately one-third of individuals are in a quiescent phase of the disease and not significantly disabled, a further third are slowly deteriorating, and the remainder are stable but disabled having had the disease for many years (Swingler & Compston 1992). MS tends to impact on the quality of life rather than on its duration, life expectancy only decreasing slightly in individuals with MS. However, in very disabled individuals, the probability of death is more than four-fold that of the general population.

CLINICAL SYMPTOMATOLOGY

The pattern of symptoms of MS is complex, variable and unpredictable.

Sensorimotor impairments

Weakness in MS may develop gradually in one or more limbs, increasing with use and often described as a feeling of heaviness and clumsiness. Depending on the site of the lesion, signs of an upper motor neuron lesion (Ch. 8) may be present while involvement of the cerebellum and its connections produces ataxic symptoms (Ch. 9), which usually occur in combination with corticospinal damage. Spinal demyelination causes progressive weakness in both legs. In individuals where there is extensive demyelination adjacent to the dorsal root entry zones, lower motor neuron signs may be present.

People with MS who suffer from *loss of muscle activation and control* often have difficulty when participating in activities of daily living and leisure activities. This, in turn, results in a gradual decrease in physical activity. It has been shown that physical limitations are positively correlated with physiological changes in people with MS, which have been shown to be similar to those that occur in healthy people who have experienced prolonged physical inactivity.

Spasticity (along with *fatigue* and *weakness*) is one of the three most common physical signs and symptoms experienced by MS patients. Epidemiology studies show that spasticity is a significant problem for about 60–80% of people with MS (Rizzo et al 2004) and is a major contributor to disability in this population (Beard et al 2003). The most commonly used definition of spasticity is probably that of Lance (1980): 'a motor disorder characterized by a velocity-dependent increase in tonic stretch reflexes (muscle tone) with exaggerated tendon jerks resulting from hyperexcitability of the stretch reflex as one component of upper motor neuron syndrome'. Increasingly, a distinction is being made between resistance to passive movement due to reflex hyperactivity, and resistance resulting from increased mechanical stiffness. The Ashworth Scale (Ashworth 1964) is typically used to measure spasticity, although this scale cannot differentiate between intrinsic muscle stiffness and reflex hyperactivity. As discussed in Chapter 8, increased resistance to passive movement can be caused by an increase in passive stiffness of soft tissue, an increase in stiffness mediated by the stretch reflex, or an increase in intrinsic stiffness which reflects the stiffness of the contractile properties of the engaged crossbridges.

Sinkjaer and colleagues (1993) measured the passive, the intrinsic and the reflex-mediated response to stretch in the ankle extensors and flexors in subjects with MS and able-bodied subjects. The major findings suggested that spastic muscles in individuals with MS have an increased non-reflexive stiffness (passive and intrinsic) and that reflex-mediated stiffness in the ankle extensors during a sustained voluntary contraction does not differ significantly from able-bodied subjects. However, in this study the authors did not directly investigate the passive properties of muscles as the measures of stiffness were obtained from electrically stimulated muscles – the muscles were not relaxed. Moreover, the authors examined stiffness at the ankle joint. Ankle stiffness is likely to be due partly to the stiffness of muscles but also to other structures that cross the joint such as ligaments. Recently, Hoang and colleagues (2007) have developed a method that allows direct measurement of passive properties of human relaxed gastrocnemius. Using this method, they showed that the passive properties of gastrocnemius in people with MS (patients are still ambulant and have spasticity) are not different from those in healthy people (Hoang et al 2009).

Altered *sensation* occurs at some stage in almost every individual with MS. Sensory symptoms, such as paraesthesia of a limb or of the face, with numbness, tingling or burning, may be the first clinical signs. Due to the unpredictable nature of the disease, sensory deficits may affect one limb, one side of the body or all four limbs. Involvement of the posterior columns of the spinal cord results in impairments in position and movement sense, vibration sense and touch. Temperature sense may also be affected, resulting in typical heat or cold sensitivity symptoms in MS.

Pain is another common symptom in people with MS. Pain can be the direct result of demyelination and axonal loss (neurogenic pain), or a secondary consequence of another MS symptom (nociceptive pain). Several studies have reported that the incidence of pain within any one month period is between 60–80% of MS patients. Chronic pain, defined as pain of 3 months duration, is experienced by 65–70% of people with MS. Of these, 60% had chronic dysaesthetic pain and 70% experienced episodic pain. Prevalence of pain tends to increase with age and number of years since disease onset. Some studies have noted a higher pain prevalence in females with MS (Hadjimichael et al 2007) and in people who have moderate to severe mobility restriction as measured by the Expanded Disability Status Scale (EDSS) (Ehde et al 2006). However, it is important to note that pain affects people with MS at all stages of the disease, including people newly diagnosed.

Cognitive and affective symptoms

There has been considerable development in the understanding of cognitive impairments in MS over recent years. It is estimated that cognitive impairments occur in up to 65% of MS patients (Winkelmann et al 2007). Cognitive dysfunction strongly affects patients' ability to work, social relationships and quality of life. In a cross-sectional study of 250 MS patients, Lynch and colleagues (2005) found that cognitive impairment is closely associated with physical disability and this relationship appears to be stable throughout the duration of MS.

Results of recent analytical reviews suggest that the effect of MS on cognition is both general, that is all cognitive domains are affected, and specific, that is the effects are larger for the domains of mood, motor functioning, memory and learning (Prakash et al 2008). It was estimated that 40–60% of MS patients suffer deficits in memory and learning (Grafman et al 1990), even at early stages of the disease. Lezak's (1995) clinical observations suggest that slowed mental processing makes it difficult for individuals with attention deficits to grasp all aspects of a verbal message, particularly when long, complicated and delivered rapidly in a complex environment. When patients have no recollection of what has been said or what is happening around them, they and their families interpret this as a problem of memory rather than slowed processing of information. Once patients, families and health professionals understand the nature of the problem, careful attention to how, when and where information and messages are given and activities organized may greatly improve the patient's 'memory'.

Personality and psychosocial behaviour

In addition to cognitive and affective symptoms, MS may be associated with a number of behavioural changes. For example, changes in personality, preferences and attitudes tend to accompany impairments in focusing attention and distractability. Individuals with MS describe feelings of being mentally blocked, of dissatisfaction with themselves and of diminished spontaneity of action (Lezak 1995). Individuals with MS have been described as prone to 'euphoria'. Euphoria may be defined as a fixed state of wellbeing where patients may express a conviction that all is well and that they are physically fit and healthy despite the presence of considerable physical disability. The term euphoria is therefore inappropriate when applied to individuals with MS who attempt to face the future with courage (Compston 1993a). True euphoria is a relatively rare phenomenon, typically associated with advanced disease involving the frontal lobes.

Depression is said to be more commonly observed in patients with MS than in those with comparable medical disorders (Minden & Schiffer 1990). The lifetime risk for depression among MS has been estimated at 50% (Patten & Metz 1997) compared with a lifetime risk in the general population of around 10–15%. Although this is not surprising, given depression is an appropriate reaction to what can be a devastating disease, the appearance of depression does not seem to be related to the severity of the disease. Recent research suggests depression develops after disease onset and is quite stable longitudinally. Because of the stability of depression in MS and the fact that it is unlikely to remit without treatment, it can have devastating long-term consequences for the patient's day-to-day functioning (Arnett et al 2008). Recent work has suggested anxiety disorders are also common in patients with MS, but are frequently overlooked and undertreated.

Risk factors include being female, a comorbid diagnosis of depression and limited social support (Korostil & Feinstein 2007). Fortunately, anxiety disorders represent a treatable cause of disability in MS.

On the other hand, *stress* may exacerbate symptoms and precipitate onset. There is increasing evidence that stressful life events correlate with exacerbations in MS (Gold et al 2005). A systemic meta-analysis of 14 prospective studies found a consistent association between stressful life events and subsequent exacerbation in MS but there is no link of specific stressors to exacerbations (Mohr et al 2004). From several clinical studies and animal models, it was suggested that stress may be involved with the reduced sensitivity to glucocorticoid and β-adrenergic modulation, which can exacerbate overshooting inflammation in MS. The roles of the two major stress-response systems, the hypothalamic–pituitary–adrenal axis and the autonomic nervous system are topics of interest in current research on stress.

Special senses

The involvement of the visual pathways is very common. The episodic visual blurring so often described by patients early in the disease may later deteriorate further, with some patients losing sight in one eye or suffering double vision. Deafness is more often seen in individuals with established disease. Acute vestibular symptoms with severe positional vertigo (an illusion of movement in the person's relationship with the environment), vomiting, ataxia and headache are typically seen in acute brainstem demyelination. Other senses such as taste and smell may be involved.

Fatigue

Fatigue is among the most common, yet least understood, reported symptoms of MS (Krupp 2003). It may be more disabling than any of the milder symptoms, compromising the person's efficiency and sense of wellbeing (Lezak 1995). Individuals with MS report that fatigue generally occurs daily, interferes with physical and social function and worsens with heat. Individuals with MS, their families and friends can misjudge the impact of fatigue by misinterpreting it as laziness. Individuals who are working complain that they have no energy for recreational activities because of needing to rest at the weekend. Furthermore, fatigue is one of the two major reasons for unemployment among MS individuals (Edgley et al 1991). Recent data from an ongoing longitudinal study (Multiple Sclerosis Society of Australia 1990*), which involves more than 3000 patients across Australia, show that fatigue and

*http://msaustralia.org.au/msra/research/ms-life-study.php

impaired mobility are two main reasons for job loss among patients. Many patients are unable to be actively engaged for more than a few hours without fatigue and tend to limit their activity to avoid fatigue and overheating. A vicious cycle occurs, with decreased physical and social activity tending to have a further deleterious effect.

Schapiro and colleagues (1987) have described four types of fatigue: fatigue following *physical exertion*, experienced by the general population and which recovers after a period of rest; *nerve impulse* fatigue following extreme activity which, again, recovers with rest; fatigue related to *depression*, and associated with sleep disturbances, low self-esteem and mood fluctuations; and *lassitude*, or an abnormal sense of tiredness of unknown aetiology. All four types described may contribute to fatigue in MS. The sense of tiredness or lassitude is little understood and people with MS appear to be particularly vulnerable to this. However, an additional cause of fatigue is the underlying slowing of nerve impulses along partially demyelinated axons.

Krupp and colleagues (1988) devised the Fatigue Severity Scale (FSS), a nine-item questionnaire in which patients rate their agreement with statements that distinguished fatigue in MS from healthy controls. This scale has been shown to have acceptable internal consistency, stability over time and reflects the effect of fatigue on daily functioning. Interestingly, Krupp and colleagues (1989) found that the severity of fatigue did not correlate significantly with depression in individuals with MS, suggesting that fatigue and depression are separate, although overlapping, entities. Another common scale used to measure fatigue in MS is the Modified Fatigue Impact Scale or MFIS. This is a 21-item scale, developed by US National MS Society, derived from the original 40-item Fatigue Impact Scale. It has been classified as a multidimensional scale and is intended to analyse different aspects of fatigue by assessing impact on physical, cognitive and psychosocial functioning (Tellez et al 2006)

Heat in the form of hot weather, overheated rooms, immersion in hot water and increased core temperature after strenuous physical activities increases fatigue as well as other symptoms of MS, tending to weaken the individual (Lezak 1995). Increased temperature sensitivity, with a reduction in the safety factor for conduction in partially demyelinated axons, may explain the temporary increase in the severity of symptoms experienced by patients after exercise or hot baths (Honan et al 1987). MS patients may experience a temporary increase in the intensity of sensory symptoms immediately post-exercise (Smith et al 2006) but this is unlikely to have any deleterious changes in fatigue and function. On the other hand, cold may help to improve performance. Cooling nerve fibres has been shown in laboratory-based models and in some small studies of people with MS to improve the speed of messages passed along the nerves, and

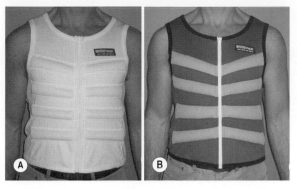

Figure 14.2 A cooling vest is useful for MS patients who suffer heat intolerance. *(With permission from Arctic Heat Pty Ltd, Burleigh Heads, Australia).*

consequently improves symptoms. There are cooling products available that may assist in decreasing or maintaining a lower body temperature to prevent worsening of symptoms (Fig. 14.2).

Autonomic involvement

Autonomic involvement occurs in most patients with MS. Bladder symptoms are more common in women than men. Impotence may be prevalent in males. Sphincter control may be lost or impaired. Disinhibition causes urgency and frequency which lead to incontinence. Bowel incontinence may also be present. Cardiovascular autonomic dysfunction is usually of minor clinical importance. However, orthostatic intolerance may be present in approximately 50% of patients (Flachenecker 2007) and can easily be detected by routine measurements of heart rate and blood pressure during rest and during standing.

Other manifestations of brainstem involvement

Compston (1993a) reports several manifestations of brainstem demyelination. Abnormalities of eye movement are common in MS. Facial palsy is reported to be present in individuals with established MS. Extensive brainstem demyelination may produce disturbances of consciousness or central respiratory failure. Paroxysmal episodes (tonic spasms), in which painful tetanic posturing of the limbs occurs for up to 1 or 2 minutes, may also be present. In a study on 483 patients, Zadro and colleagues (2008) found that isolated cranial nerve involvement was present in 10% of patients. The trigeminal nerve was most frequently involved, followed by facial, abducens, oculomotor and cochlear nerves. However, only 54% of patients had a brainstem magnetic resonance imaging (MRI) lesion that could explain the symptoms.

MEDICAL MANAGEMENT

There is at present no single accurate laboratory-supported diagnostic test for MS. Rather, diagnosis of MS requires use of both clinical and paraclinical criteria. The latter involves information obtained from MRI, motor-evoked potentials (MEPs) and cerebrospinal fluid (CSF) analysis. Investigations such as MRI, CSF analysis in individuals with MS are used to document the site and extent of lesions, to confirm the presence of intrathecal inflammation and to exclude conditions that may mimic demyelinating disease. MRI is thought to have increased the accuracy in diagnosing MS from 60% to 90% (Ebers 1994) and appears to be a more sensitive indicator of disease activity than the clinical history or neurological examination (Polman & Hartung 1995).

New diagnostic criteria for MS integrating MRI assessment with clinical and other paraclinical methods (the McDonald criteria) were introduced in 2001 (McDonald et al 2001). Since then, these criteria have been extensively assessed and used. The 2005 revisions to the McDonald diagnostic criteria for MS aim to simplify and speed diagnosis while maintaining adequate sensitivity and specificity, and are now widely accepted by the neurology community.

Medical treatments in MS can be divided into several categories. The first category is the use of medications that impact the underlying disease (disease-modifying therapies), targeting some aspect of the inflammatory process of MS with an aim of preventing inflammation which causes relapses. The second one is medications that help to decrease the severity and duration of MS relapses (steroids), which aim to suppress inflammation. The third category is medications that help ease many MS-related symptoms such as fatigue, spasticity and pain, to name a few.

A large body of experimental evidence implicating immune-mediated processes in activation and progression of MS has led to a search for immunotherapies that not only abrogate acute relapses, but also modify the progression of the disease. Consequently, many disease-modifying drugs (DMDs) or immunomodulatory treatments for MS have been developed and clinically trialed on a large scale. To date, there are enough data to support widely used DMDs that may have an effect on slowing the accumulation of disability over time. Some of these drugs are interferon beta-1a (Avonex® or Rebif®), interferon beta-1b (Betaseron®), glatiramer acetate (Copaxone®) and the latest natalizumab (Tysabri®). Each of these drugs acts to block different inflammation pathways and head-to-head studies have shown that none of them is more effective than the others. However, treatment may not be an option for every person with MS. DMDs are most effective in people with the RR type of MS while there is no treatment for people with PP MS. In addition, resistance to a drug is another concern over a long period of use of DMDs.

A short course of intravenous methylprednisolone is often used for the treatment of relapses in multiple sclerosis. But there is still no evidence to indicate that this influences the eventual outcome of the disease, although it may accelerate the onset of a remission when given during an acute relapse. In many cases, after a course of intravenous methylprednisolone, oral prednisone is prescribed and gradually tapered off. Recent observations suggest that oral prednisone following treatment with intravenous methylprednisolone for an MS relapse does not lead to improved neurologic outcome after 12 months compared with treatment with intravenous methylprednisolone only (Perumal et al 2008).

Drugs such as baclofen and diazepam may be useful in the reduction of hyperactive reflexes (spasticity). When given to individuals experiencing severe flexor and adductor spasms associated with spinal cord lesions, these agents may reduce hyperactivity sufficiently to enable the individual to sit and stand more comfortably or to be nursed more easily. However, orally administered drugs such as these, especially at high dose, can cause severe side-effects such as general muscle weakness. Studies using botulinum toxin to relieve adductor spasms have reported spasticity relief in the lower extremities and significantly increased range of passive movements in joints, making nursing care and rehabilitation easier with no significant side-effects from the toxin (e.g., Snow et al 1990; Sobolewski 2007).

Documenting the course, assessing the prognosis and validating the effects of intervention in MS require standardized measures of disability. Until recently, the most extensively used scale appears to be the Disability Status Scale (Kurtzke 1983). However, this scale is widely criticized on theoretical grounds, on its insensitivity to change, its emphasis on ambulation while neglecting other relevant functions and on its lack of objectivity and reliability (e.g., Goodkin et al 1988; Polman & Hartung 1995; Kragt et al 2008). Wade (1992) suggests that one should only consider using the Kurtzke scale in order to be able to compare results with other studies. He further suggests that it is preferable to measure change in specific impairments and motor performance using measures that are valid and reliable (see Ch. 3).

PHYSIOTHERAPY: AN OVERALL VIEW

Many of the challenges associated with progressive neurological disease are well exemplified in MS. Progressive disease presents a series of difficulties and burdens that impact on the quality of life of the individual, their families and health professionals. Coping with functional limitations, explicit uncertainty about the future and possibility

of loss of function and family role has a negative impact on quality of life, social interaction, vocational and leisure activities and are extremely stressful.

Almost any manifestation of neurological impairment can be observed in individuals with MS (see Chs 8–10). The nature of impairments and deficits in functional motor performance that arise from one individual to another, but also in the same individual at different times, are wide ranging, variable and unpredictable. Physiotherapists. as part of a team working with individuals with MS, need to be sensitive to the individual's wishes in working out strategies to enable that individual to preserve dignity and lifestyle. The physiotherapist needs to have sufficient knowledge and expertise to address wide-ranging problems, and the flexibility to cope with the unpredictable nature of the disease. If physiotherapy is to be effective, it needs to be focused and demonstrate clearly to the patient the benefits of interventions.

The overall aims of physiotherapy as part of a multidisciplinary team are to:

- optimize performance in everyday activities and skills
- maximize functional ability
- prevent unnecessary disability and handicap (Fig. 14.3C–E)
- improve the individual's quality of life.

The reader should refer to Chapters 2 and 4–7 for task-related training.

More specific aims for an individual may be to:

- preserve/improve muscle strength
- preserve/improve aerobic capacity
- preserve musculoskeletal integrity
- manage fatigue
- collaborate with the individual to ensure that interventions are relevant to the person's needs and desires
- collaborate with the individual in setting goals and defining expectations
- provide necessary aids to living.

Strengthening exercise

The need to prevent secondary adaptation to disuse is critical for the maintenance of performance of everyday actions as well as for continued participation in social and vocational activities. There has been no intervention that has proven effective in modifying long-term prognosis in multiple sclerosis but exercises are now accepted to be an important part of symptomatic treatments for people with MS (Rietberg et al 2005). Until about 20 years ago people with MS were often advised to avoid strenuous physical activities or exercises on the basis that they could worsen signs and symptoms of MS and even increase the disease activities. However, in the past 20 years a growing body of evidence has indicated that exercises are beneficial for

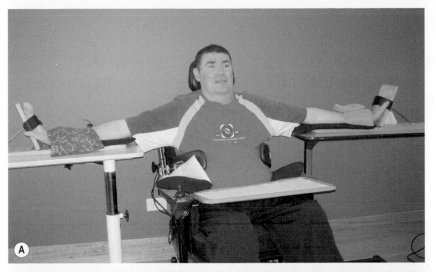

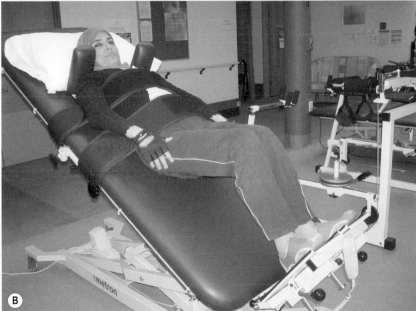

Figure 14.3 (A) Positioning can be used to prevent contracture in people with advanced MS. (B) A tilt table can be used to strengthen knee extensors if the patient is too weak to practise standing up from a seat. It can help prevent/slow down ankle contracture;

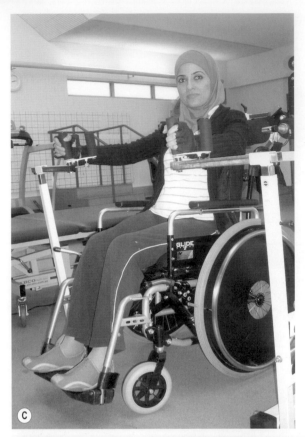

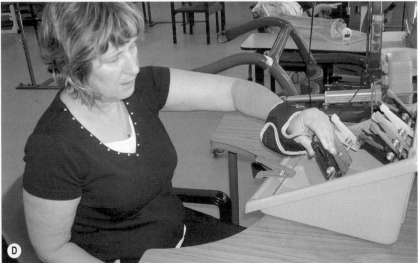

Figure 14.3 *continued* (C) Specific equipment is used for upper limb strengthening exercise for people in a wheel chair *(UpperTone, GPK Inc, El Cajon, CA, USA)*; (D) Weight is used to help reduce tremor and ataxia during functional exercise of the upper limb;

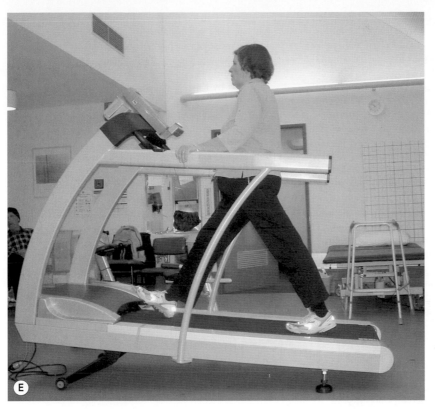

Figure 14.3 *continued* (E) Eccentric exercise by walking backward and downhill on a treadmill can help improve dorsiflexion and passively stretches the calf muscle in people with MS who are still walking. *(Scifit AC5000M Treadmill, LifeTec Inc, Wheeling, IL, USA).*

people with MS not only at impairment level but also at functional and participation levels. Strength and cardiorespiratory exercises are often prescribed to people with MS who have difficulties performing activities of daily living and/or participating in leisure activities. Results from many studies indicate that these difficulties are partly due to the primary effects of MS, such as loss of muscle activation and muscle control, fatigue and spasticity, and partly due to secondary effects, such as from prolonged disuse which results in deconditioning of the muscles and reduced fitness.

There has been considerable historical debate regarding the safety and appropriateness of prescribing strenuous physical exercise for people with MS. Concern has focused on the possibility of exacerbating MS symptoms such as fatigue or weakness which could be counterproductive to day-to-day symptom management. However, there is strong evidence indicating that exercise does not cause prolonged or permanent worsening of MS symptoms (Smith et al 2006), but rather that exercise often results in improvements in a range of MS symptoms (Gallien et al 2007). No adverse effects of strength exercise in the MS population have been documented in the literature.

There is strong evidence showing that strength training in people with MS can improve muscle force production (DeBolt & McCubbin 2004; Taylor et al 2006). Other benefits of strengthening exercise are improved walking speed and endurance (Taylor et al 2006), improved gait kinematics, reduced fatigue and physical and social disability (White et al 2004).

Some people with MS have reported that exercise preceded an MS exacerbation. However, no studies have been able to identify exercise as the cause of an exacerbation. Exercise can result in a temporary increase in existing symptoms or onset of new previously silent symptoms in people with MS (Smith et al 2006). This is probably related to a heat-induced reduction in nerve conduction velocity. Such symptoms tend to resolve within 30 minutes of rest.

Aerobic exercise

The benefits of regular exercise in the able-bodied and disabled population are well documented and include: increased wellbeing and improved mental state; increased cardiorespiratory fitness; reduction in depression and anxiety, and decreased excess body fat.

In the past two decades a large body of research has investigated the benefits of cardiorespiratory, or endurance exercise in people with MS. In a recent review by Dalgas et al (2008), at least 14 studies that have evaluated the effects of endurance training in people with MS were identified. Although there is general methodological weakness in these studies, some important clinical findings can be derived. Endurance exercise at low to moderate intensity is well tolerated and has potential physiological and psychological benefits among people with MS. However, these studies have primarily involved subjects who are minimally to moderately physically disabled with an expanded disability status scale (EDSS) score of less than 7. A single case study investigated the response to arm crank aerobic training in a wheelchair participant (EDSS 7.5) (Smith & Hale 2007). Although the subject demonstrated a trend toward improving cardiorespiratory fitness after 3 weeks of exercise, the study had to be terminated early due to the subject developing shoulder pain.

On the other hand, concerns have been voiced relating to the safe undertaking of cardiorespiratory testing and fitness training in older and long-term sedentary groups who have a number of other risk factors. In recognition of these issues, the American College of Sports Medicine (2006) recommends allocating exercise participants into one of two streams for cardiorespiratory testing and exercise prescription:

- High risk: Individuals with more than two risk factors for cardiorespiratory disease need formal testing to ascertain actual working heart rate to achieve VO_2 maximum. This eliminates the safety issues relating to blunted heart rate response, poor systolic elevation and cardiac risk factors. Exercise prescription is based on the measures obtained through this testing.
- Low to moderate risk: Individuals with two or less risk factors for cardiorespiratory disease can be prescribed exercises using heart rate and supplementary exercise intensity measures such as the Borg Rate of Perceived Exertion (RPE) (Borg 1970) scale and blood pressure monitoring.

Clinicians should adopt these guidelines when testing and prescribing exercise for people with MS who are inactive. Individuals with high risk should have a medical clearance from their treating doctors and should start at low intensity.

Many benefits from cardiorespiratory training have been identified in people with MS. A particularly interesting pioneer paper on this topic (Petajan et al 1996) demonstrated a positive impact on cardiovascular responses and facets of wellbeing in individuals with MS. The results indicated significant improvement in cardiovascular fitness, with increases in VO_{2max} comparable with those reported in studies involving healthy sedentary subjects. The improvement did not seem to be related to the degree

of neurological impairment. Although training did not involve *specific* strengthening exercises, increases in strength of most upper limb muscles and knee extensors were reported, indicating that muscle strength can be increased in a demyelinating disease. Similar results were also reported by Mostert & Kesselring (2002). Other benefits from aerobic exercise include improved lung function, improved activity levels and aerobic thresholds (Mostert & Kesselring 2002).

To date, no studies have reported adverse cardiac symptoms in response to cardiorespiratory testing or exercise participation in people with MS. This may be due to the testing of predominantly minimally to moderately physically disabled individuals (EDSS 0–6), or because most studies commenced cardiorespiratory training within the 50–60% of maximal predicted heart rate range with gradual increases in intensity over the training period.

Some particular symptoms that may prevent people with MS from undertaking aerobic exercise include fatigue, heat intolerance and spasticity. These symptoms can be managed to a certain extent for optimal patient compliance and adherence to exercise.

Preserving musculoskeletal integrity

Individuals need advice and instruction about what muscles and soft tissues are at risk of shortening and becoming stiffer, what stretches to do and how often. In the very disabled person, this may require equipment (see Fig. 14.3A, B and E). It is interesting to note that subjects participating in a baclofen drug trial reported that muscle stretching provided them with a subjective sense of control over stiffness (Brar et al 1991), although the stretches were performed for only a short period which would not be considered to be of sufficient duration to prevent contracture in inactive individuals (Williams 1990). People who are wheelchair bound should spend at least 30 minutes a day stretching hip and knee flexors and ankle plantarflexors. A tilt table is probably essential for some individuals in order to prevent severe contractures (see Fig. 14.3B).

Managing fatigue

Management of fatigue involves discussion with the individual and gathering of information about the nature, extent and precipitating factors in fatigue. Thus, managing fatigue in MS requires a multidisciplinary approach. In general, strategies to implement may include energy conservation, exercise, equipment and environmental modifications.

To conserve energy, people with MS, their families and carers should be educated about balancing rest and activity through prioritizing, delegating, pacing tasks and taking regular short rests between activities. The patient can learn how to identify aggravating lifestyle factors and apply the above strategies as their activities change and as the effects of fatigue vary over time. Practical strategies for providing exercise and treatment sessions when the person with MS is affected by fatigue include scheduling the exercise or treatment sessions early in the day, encouraging the client to work at their own pace and have regular rests, beginning with a short duration (<20 minutes) and gradually increase as tolerated. Similarly, beginning exercise with a low number of repetitions and low intensity then gradually progressing as the participant can manage more repetitions or increased intensity, mixing vigorous exercises with lighter exercises to avoid long periods of exercise at high heart rates, alternating muscle groups to rest one muscle group while exercising another and keeping body temperature down as much as possible can help. Assistive equipment for mobility, self-care and seating should be used to minimize energy consumption during activities of daily living. Changes to environmental factors, for example installing air conditioning, lifts (elevators), railings in stairwell and ergonomic office equipment, can also assist in minimizing fatigue.

There are some pharmacological agents that may help reduce fatigue in MS. However, these medications are not widely used in Australia for MS fatigue management compared with other parts of the world.

Coping with reduced activity and participation

Limitations in community participation for people with MS, including the extent of environmental modification, facilities for ongoing exercise, social, vocational and recreational availability, are to some extent dependent on national health policy. Health professionals have an important role in being familiar with and referring patients to the appropriate agency, which may include: a MS society; an independent living centre; technical aids to the disabled: accessible leisure centres; respite care provision: sporting groups for the disabled; self-help groups; carer support groups; and vocational rehabilitation services. These agencies can be valuable sources of information.

Health professionals also need to keep up to date with technological advances designed to increase environmental interaction to improve the quality of life for individuals with MS and their families. Some recent publications are helpful; for example, The Multiple Sclerosis Society of Australia has published a booklet (1990) for the newly diagnosed person or a series of handouts to help health professionals better understand specific problems in MS and provide guidelines for management of these problems.

The stress on families assisting an individual with MS can be high. A survey in the UK, for example, found that 15% of carers were depressed and 24% suffered from clinical anxiety (University of Southampton 1989). Information regarding availability of services, practical help at home and access to respite facilities appear to be some of the more important factors to address in order to relieve family stress. A hoist (Fig. 14.4) enables the person to be moved, thus diminishing some of the physical stress on family members.

A wheelchair is necessary for individuals who may be coping with walking about the house but who otherwise are confined to the house. Wheelchair training should be instituted to train the individual to negotiate a more complex environment than the home. An electric wheelchair and/or a three-wheel scooter give more freedom to a person who is unable to walk effectively and efficiently or is having difficulty operating a hand-driven chair. In some instances the energy required to walk may be better put to more beneficial activities, and the use of a wheelchair or scooter may be critical to remaining employed and maintaining social contact outside the house.

Measurement

Measures of motor performance need to be reliable and valid and be sensitive to changes important for the individual (Ch. 3). Paltamaa and colleagues (2008) found that

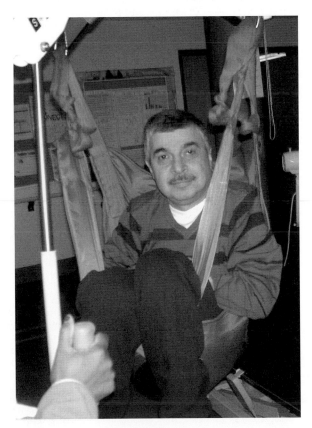

Figure 14.4 A hoist decreases the physical burden for carers and ensures greater comfort for the individual when being moved from one place to another.

the measures most responsive to deterioration in MS were self-reported scores in self-care, mobility and domestic life; distance walked and change in heart rate during a 6-minute walk test; 10-m walk test speeds, stride length and cadence; repetitive squatting; and box-and-block test scores. MS-specific measures have been developed in recent years. One is the Multiple Sclerosis Spasticity Scale (MSSS-88) that is used to measure spasticity from a patient's perspective (Hobart et al 2006). The Modified Fatigue Impact Scale (MFIS) is a modified form of the Fatigue Impact Scale (Fisk et al 1994) based on items derived from interviews with MS patients concerning how fatigue impacts their lives. This instrument provides an assessment of the effects of fatigue in terms of physical, cognitive and psychosocial functioning. The full-length MFIS consists of 21 items while the abbreviated version has five items. The abbreviated version can be used if time is limited but the full-length version has the advantage of generating subscales. Although these measures have been shown to be valid and clinically relevant, further research is needed to establish their reliability.

Coping with chronic illness and uncertainty can be very stressful. Schwartz and colleagues (1996) have developed and tested a *self-efficacy scale* specifically for MS. Self-efficacy is a term used to describe the degree of confidence an individual has in his/her ability to cope with a specific situation or condition. The test was found to have high internal consistency and test–retest reliability. This scale should be valuable in measuring the outcome of intervention in terms of enhancing the patient's wellbeing and confidence. High self-efficacy in individuals with MS has previously been found to be associated with better adjustment and less psychological dysfunction (e.g., Schnek et al 1995).

The use of *integrated care pathways* (ICPs) appears to be useful in identifying key factors influencing outcome of intervention. An ICP is a document that details the interventions expected to occur during a specific period of clinical intervention (Rossiter & Thompson 1995). Several audits have shown that the introduction of ICPs in an inpatient setting resulted in decreased length of stay, a framework for identifying not just how many goals were achieved but also for identifying why goals were not met, and improved record keeping (Rossiter & Thompson 1996).

In summary, as Compston (1990) has pointed out, a clearer understanding of the epidemiological and biological factors that determine the geographical and anatomical dissemination of MS may provide a solution to this disease. The most exciting development in neurological rehabilitation for persons with MS is the impact of strengthening and aerobic training, with adequate temperature control, on strength and fitness, together with factors related to quality of life. Therapists are encouraged to become familiar with the literature on strengthening and aerobic training in order to prescribe effective exercise programmes. Other critical interventions include prevention of unnecessary limitations in activity and participation and advice on reducing unnecessary fatigue in everyday, social and vocational activities.

REFERENCES

American College of Sports Medicine 2006 ACSM's guidelines for exercise testing and prescription, 7th edn. Lippincott Williams & Wilkins, New York.

Arnett PA, Barwick FH, Beeney JE 2008 Depression in multiple sclerosis: review and theoretical proposal. J Int Neuropsychol Soc 14:691–724.

Ashworth B 1964 Preliminary trial of carisoprodol in multiple sclerosis. Practitioner 192:540–542.

Barnett MH, Prineas JW 2004 Relapsing and remitting multiple sclerosis: pathology of the newly forming lesion. Ann Neurol 55:458–468.

Barnett MH, Sutton I 2006 The pathology of multiple sclerosis: a paradigm shift. Curr Opin Neurol 19:242–247.

Beard S, Hunn A, Wight J 2003 Treatments for spasticity and pain in multiple sclerosis: a systematic review. Health Technol Assess 7:ix–x, 1–111.

Borg G 1970 Perceived exertion as an indicator of somatic stress. Scand J Rehabil Med 2–3:92–98.

Brar P, Smith MB, Nelson LM et al 1991 Evaluation of treatment protocols on minimal to moderate spasticity in multiple sclerosis. Arch Phys Med Rehabil 72:186–189.

Compston DAS 1990 The dissemination of multiple sclerosis. The Lanfdon-Brown Lecture (1989). J R Coll Physicians Lond 24:207–218.

Compston A 1993a Multiple sclerosis. In: Walton J (ed.) Brain's diseases of the nervous system. Oxford University Press, Oxford:366–382.

Compston A 1993b Limiting and repairing the damage in multiple sclerosis. Schweiz Med Wochenschr 123:1145–1152.

Confavreux C, Vukusic S, Moreau T et al 2000 Relapses and progression of disability in multiple sclerosis. N Engl J Med 343:1430–1438.

Confavreux C, Vukusic S, Adeleine P 2003 Early clinical predictors and progression of irreversible disability in multiple sclerosis: an amnesic process. Brain 126:770–782.

Costelloe L, Thompson A, Walsh C et al 2008 Long-term clinical relevance of criteria for designating multiple sclerosis as benign after 10 years of disease. J Neurol Neurosurg Psychiatry 79:1245–1248.

Cristiano E, Patrucco L, Rojas JI 2008 A systematic review of the epidemiology of multiple sclerosis in South America. Eur J Neurol 15:1273–1278.

Dalgas U, Stenager E, Ingemann-Hansen T 2008 Multiple sclerosis and physical exercise: recommendations for the application of resistance-, endurance- and combined training. Mult Scler 14:35–53.

Dean G 1967 Anual incidence, prevalence and mortality of multiple sclerosis in white South-African-born and in white immigrants to South Africa. Br Med J 2:724.

Dean G 1972 On the risk of multiple sclerosis according to age at immigration. In: Field EJ, Bell TM, Carnegie PR (eds) Multiple sclerosis progress in research. North-Holland, Amsterdam and London:197–207.

Dean G, McLoughlin H, Brady R et al 1976 Multiple sclerosis among immigrants in Greater London. Br Med J 1:861–864.

DeBolt LS, McCubbin JA 2004 The effects of home-based resistance exercise on balance, power, and mobility in adults with multiple sclerosis. Arch Phys Med Rehabil 85:290–297.

Dujmovic I, Mesaros S, Pekmezovic T et al 2004 Primary progressive multiple sclerosis: clinical and paraclinical characteristics with application of the new diagnostic criteria. Eur J Neurol 11:439–444.

Ebers GC 1994 Treatment of multiple sclerosis. Lancet 343:275–279.

Edgley K, Sullivan M, Dehoux E 1991 A survey of multiple sclerosis: 11. Determinants of employment status. Can J Rehabil 4:127–132.

Elide DM, Osborne TL, Hanley MA et al 2006 The scope and nature of pain in persons with multiple sclerosis. Mult Scler 12:629–638.

Filley CM, Heaton RK, Thompson LL et al 1990 Effects of disease course on neuropsychological functioning. In: Rao SM (ed.) Neurohehavioural aspects of multiple sclerosis. Oxford University Press, New York:136–148.

Fisk JD, Pontefract A, Ritvo PG et al 1994 The impact of fatigue on patients with multiple sclerosis. Can J Neurol Sci 21:9–14.

Flachenecker P 2007 Autonomic dysfunction in Guillain–Barré syndrome and multiple sclerosis. J Neurol 254(Suppl 2):II96–101.

Gallien P, Nicolas B, Robineau S et al 2007 Physical training and multiple sclerosis. Ann Readapt Med Phys 50:373–376, 369–372.

Gold SM, Mohr DC, Huitinga I et al 2005 The role of stress–response systems for the pathogenesis and progression of MS. Trends Immunol 26:644–652.

Goodkin DE, Hertsgaard D, Seminary J 1988 Upper extremity function in multiple sclerosis: improving assessment sensitivity with box-and-block and nine-hole peg tests. Arch Phys Med Rehabil 69:850–854.

Grafman J, Rao S, Litvan I 1990 Disorders of memory. In: Rao SM (ed.) Neurobehavioural aspects of multiple sclerosis. Oxford University Press, New York:102–117.

Hadjimichael O, Kerns RD, Rizzo MA et al 2007 Persistent pain and uncomfortable sensations in persons with multiple sclerosis. Pain 127:35–41.

Hoang PD, Herbert RD, Todd G et al 2007 Passive mechanical properties of human gastrocnemius muscle tendon units, muscle fascicles and tendons in vivo. J Exp Biol 210:4159–4168.

Hoang P, Saboisky JP, Gandevia SC et al 2009 Passive mechanical properties of gastrocnemius in people with multiple sclerosis. Clin Biomech 24:291–298.

Hobart JC, Riazi A, Thompson AJ et al 2006 Getting the measure of spasticity in multiple sclerosis: the Multiple Sclerosis Spasticity Scale (MSSS-88). Brain 129:224–234.

Honan WP, Heron JR, Foster DH et al 1987 Paradoxical effects of temperature in multiple sclerosis. J Neurol Neurosurg Psychiatry 50:1160–1164.

Kantarci O, Wingerchuk D 2006 Epidemiology and natural history of multiple sclerosis: new insights. Curr Opin Neurol 19:248–254.

Koch M, Mostert J, Heersema D et al 2007 Progression in multiple sclerosis: further evidence of an age-dependent process. J Neurol Sci 255:35–41.

Korostil M, Feinstein A 2007 Anxiety disorders and their clinical correlates in multiple sclerosis patients. Mult Scler 13:67–72.

Kragt JJ, Thompson AJ, Montalban X et al 2008 Responsiveness and predictive value of EDSS and MSFC in primary progressive MS. Neurology 70:1084–1091.

Krupp LB 2003 Fatigue in multiple sclerosis: definition, pathophysiology and treatment. CNS Drugs 17:225–234.

Krupp LB, Alvarez LA, LaRocca NG et al 1988 Fatigue in multiple sclerosis. Arch Neurol 45:435–437.

Krupp LB, LaRocca NG, Muir-Nash J et al 1989 The fatigue severity scale. Application to patients with multiple sclerosis and systemic lupus erythematosus. Arch Neurol 46:1121–1123.

Kurtzke JF 1983 Rating neurologic impairment in multiple sclerosis: an expanded disability status scale (EDSS). Neurology 33:1444–1452.

Lance JW 1980 The control of muscle tone, reflexes, and movement: Robert Wartenberg Lecture. Neurology 30:1303–1313.

Lezak MD 1995 Neuropsychological assessment, 3rd edn. Oxford University Press, New York:241–248.

Leibowitz S, Kahana E, Alter M 1973 The changing frequency of multiple sclerosis in Israel. Arch Neurol 29:107.

Lucchinetti C, Bruck W, Parisi J et al 1999 A quantitative analysis of oligodendrocytes in multiple sclerosis lesions. A study of 113 cases. Brain 122:2279–2295.

Lynch SG, Parmenter BA, Denney DR 2005 The association between cognitive impairment and physical disability in multiple sclerosis. Mult Scler 11:469–476.

McDonald WI, Compston A, Edan G et al 2001 Recommended diagnostic criteria for multiple sclerosis: guidelines from the International Panel on the Diagnosis of Multiple Sclerosis. Ann Neurol 50:121–127.

Marrie RA 2004 Environmental risk factors in multiple sclerosis aetiology. Lancet Neurol 3:709–718.

Minden SL, Schiffer RB 1990 Affective disorders in multiple sclerosis. Arch Neurol 47:98–104.

Mohr DC, Hart SL, Julian L et al 2004 Association between stressful life events and exacerbation in multiple sclerosis: a meta-analysis. Br Med J 328:731.

Mostert S, Kesselring J 2002 Effects of a short-term exercise training program on aerobic fitness, fatigue, health perception and activity level of subjects with multiple sclerosis. Mult Scler 8:161–168.

Multiple Sclerosis Society of Australia 1990 Living with multiple sclerosis – a book for the newly diagnosed. Multiple Sclerosis Society of Australia, Sydney, Australia.

Paltamaa J, Sarasoja T, Leskinen E et al 2008 Measuring deterioration in international classification of functioning domains of people with multiple sclerosis who are ambulatory. Phys Ther 88:176–190.

Patten SB, Metz M 1997 Depression in multiple sclerosis. Psychother Psychosom 66:286–292.

Perumal JS, Caon C, Hreha S et al 2008 Oral prednisone taper following intravenous steroids fails to improve disability or recovery from relapses in multiple sclerosis. Eur J Neurol 15:677–680.

Petajan JH, Gappmaier E, White AT et al 1996 Impact of aerobic training on fitness and quality of life in multiple sclerosis. Ann Neurol 39:432–441.

Polman CH, Hartung H 1995 The treatment of multiple sclerosis: current and future. Curr Opin Neurol 8:200–209.

Prakash RS, Snook EM, Lewis JM et al 2008 Cognitive impairments in relapsing–remitting multiple sclerosis: a meta-analysis. Mult Scler 14:1250–1261.

Reder AT, Antel JP 1983 Clinical spectrum of multiple sclerosis. In: Antel JP (ed.) Neurologic clinics: symposium on multiple sclerosis. WB Saunders, Philadelphia.

Richards RG, Sampson FC, Beard SM et al 2002 A review of the natural history and epidemiology of multiple sclerosis: implications for resource allocation and health economic models. Health Technol Assess 6:1–73.

Rietberg MB, Brooks D, Uitdehaag BM et al 2005 Exercise therapy for multiple sclerosis. Cochrane Database Syst Rev Issue 3. Art. No.: CD003980. DOI: 10.1002/14651858. CD003980.pub2.

Rizzo MA, Hadjimichael OC, Preiningerova J et al 2004 Prevalence and treatment of spasticity reported by multiple sclerosis patients. Mult Scler 10:589–595.

Rossiter D, Thompson AJ 1995 Introduction of integrated care pathways for patients with multiple sclerosis in an inpatient neurorehabilitation setting. Disabil Rehabil 17:443–448.

Rossiter D, Thompson AJ 1996 Integrated care pathways (ICPs) in multiple sclerosis management: a three series audit review. Eur J Neurol 3:49.

Sadovnick AD, Baird PA, Ward RH 1988 Multiple sclerosis: updated risks for relatives. Am J Med Genet 29:533–541.

Schapiro RT, Harris L, Lenling M et al 1987 Fatigue. In: Schapiro RT (ed.) Symptom management in multiple sclerosis. Demos, New York:23–28.

Schnek ZM, Foley FW, LaRocca NG et al 1995 Psychological predictors of depression in multiple sclerosis. J Neurol Rehabil 9:15–23.

Schwartz C, Coulthard-Morris L, Zeng Q 1996 Psychosocial correlates of fatigue in multiple sclerosis. Arch Phys Med Rehabil 77:165–170.

Sinkjaer T, Toft E, Larsen K et al 1993 Non-reflex and reflex mediated ankle joint stiffness in multiple sclerosis patients with spasticity. Muscle Nerve 16:69–76.

Smith C, Hale L 2007 Arm cranking: an exercise intervention for a severely disabled adult with multiple sclerosis. N Z J Physiother 34:172–178.

Smith KJ, McDonald WI 1999 The pathophysiology of multiple sclerosis: the mechanisms underlying the production of symptoms and the natural history of the disease. Philos Trans R Soc Lond B Biol Sci 354:1649–1673.

Smith RM, Adeney-Steel M, Fulcher G et al 2006 Symptom change with exercise is a temporary phenomenon for people with multiple sclerosis. Arch Phys Med Rehabil 87:723–727.

Snow BJ, Tsui JKC, Bhatt MH et al 1990 Treatment of spasticity with botulinum toxin: a double blind study. Ann Neurol 28:512–515.

Sobolewski P 2007 The application of botulinum toxin type A in the treatment of spastic paraparesis. Przegl Lek 64(Suppl 2):3–7.

Stadelmann C, Bruck W 2008 Interplay between mechanisms of damage and repair in multiple sclerosis. J Neurol 255(Suppl 1):12–18.

Svejgaard A 2008 The immunogenetics of multiple sclerosis. Immunogenetics 60:275–286.

Swingler RJ, Compston DAS 1992 The morbidity of multiple sclerosis in south east Wales. Q J Med 83:325–337.

Taylor NF, Dodd KJ, Prasad D et al 2006 Progressive resistance exercise for people with multiple sclerosis. Disabil Rehabil 28:1119–1126.

Tellez N, Rio J, Tintore M et al 2006 Fatigue in multiple sclerosis persists over time: a longitudinal study. J Neurol 253:1466–1470.

Tremlett H, Yinshan Z, Devonshire V 2008 Natural history of secondary-progressive multiple sclerosis. Mult Scler 14:314–324.

University of Southampton 1989 Multiple sclerosis in the Southampton district. Rehabilitation Unit and Department of Sociology and Social Policy, University of Southampton, UK.

Wade DT 1992 Measurement in neurological rehabilitation, Oxford University Press, New York.

Weinshenker BG 1996 Epidemiology of multiple sclerosis. Neurol Clin 14:291–308.

White LJ, McCoy SC, Castellano V et al 2004 Resistance training improves strength and functional capacity in persons with multiple sclerosis. Mult Scler 10:668–674.

Williams PE 1990 Use of intermittent stretch in the prevention of serial sarcomere loss in immobilised muscles. Ann Rheum Dis 47:316–317.

Winkelmann A, Engel C, Apel A et al 2007 Cognitive impairment in multiple sclerosis. J Neurol 254(Suppl 2):II35–42.

Zadro I, Barun B, Habek M et al 2008 Isolated cranial nerve palsies in multiple sclerosis. Clin Neurol Neurosurg 110:886–888.

Zhao C, Li WW, Franklin RJ 2006 Differences in the early inflammatory responses to toxin-induced demyelination are associated with the age-related decline in CNS remyelination. Neurobiol Aging 27:1298–1307.

Index

Note: Page references in *italics* refer to Figures, Tables or Boxes.

A

Abductor digiti minimi 130
Abstract goals 38–39
Action research arm test (ARAT) 64
Active exercises, early post-stroke 253
Active stretching 28–32, *30f*
   gait training 115
   stroke rehabilitation 258
Activities-Specific Balance Confidence (ABC) Scale 64
Adaptability 35
Adaptations
   cerebellar function 220
   post-stroke 205–210
   upper motor neuron lesions 193–194, *194f*, 205–208, *207b*
   weakness or paralysis 35–37, *36f*
Adaptive motor behaviour 9, 207–208
   cerebellar lesions 224, *224f–225f*
   Parkinson's disease 316
   post-stroke 208, 256–257
Adaptive system 3–14
Adhesive capsulitis, shoulder 273–274
Aerobic capacity
   age-related changes 102
   peak (VO$_{2peak}$) 66–67
Aerobic testing, peak 66
Aerobic training 32–33
   multiple sclerosis 345–346
   specificity 18
   stroke 260
   traumatic brain injury 298
   see also Fitness training
Ageing
   brain plasticity and 6
   training issues 16
   see also Older people

Aggressive behaviour 294
Agility, improving 25
Agnosia 240–241
Akinesia 309–310
Alcohol use 253, 282
Amantadine 317
Amnesia
   anterograde 291
   post-traumatic *see* Post-traumatic amnesia
Amputation, cortical reorganization after 4
Angle-specific training effects 19
Ankle dorsiflexion
   decreased *105f–106f*, 173
   stair walking 101
   standing up 78, *79f*
Ankle extensors, strength training 111–113, *112f*
Ankle–foot orthoses (AFO) 118, 261
Ankle joint mobility, reduced 102, 173
Ankle movements
   standing up 78–79
   walking 98
Ankle plantarflexors
   paretic leg, activating 89, *89f*
   reduced strength 173
   strength training 89–91, 112
   walking 99–101
Ankle strategy, balance during standing 171
Anosognosia 241
Anticoagulation 252–253
Anxiety
   multiple sclerosis 339–340
   Parkinson's disease 316–317
Aphasia 240, 261–264

Broca's 261
   expressive 261
   global 261
   nominal 261
   receptive 261
   Wernicke's 261
Apomorphine 317
Apraxia 240
   ideational 240
   ideomotor 240
Arm cycling *145f–146f*
Arm function 123
   see also Upper limb function
Aspirin, acute stroke 252
Associated movements 204
Astereognosis 237–238
Ataxia 217, 221–224
Ataxic gait 224–227
Atrial fibrillation 253
Attention 37–42
   balance training 182
   internal and external focus 38–39
   maintenance of balance 164
   role of feedback 40–41
   unilateral 241, 244
Attentional deficits
   Parkinson's disease 317
   training 243–244
   traumatic brain injury 293
   see also Neglect, unilateral
Attentional strategies 37, 47
   Parkinson's disease 323–325
Auditory feedback 41
Auditory perception
   impaired 240
   test 242

DOI: 10.1016/B978-0-7020-4051-1.00024-2